Handbook of
Psychological Approaches with Violent Offenders

Contemporary Strategies and Issues

THE PLENUM SERIES IN CRIME AND JUSTICE

Series Editors:
James Alan Fox, *Northeastern University, Boston, Massachusetts*
Joseph Weis, *University of Washington, Seattle, Washington*

A Continuation Order Plan is available for this series. A continuation order will bring delivery of each new volume immediately upon publication. Volumes are billed only upon actual shipment. For further information please contact the publisher.

Handbook of
Psychological Approaches
with Violent Offenders

Contemporary Strategies and Issues

Edited by

Vincent B. Van Hasselt

Nova Southeastern University
Fort Lauderdale, Florida

and

Michel Hersen

Pacific University
Forest Grove, Oregon

KLUWER ACADEMIC / PLENUM PUBLISHERS
NEW YORK, BOSTON, DORDRECHT, LONDON, MOSCOW

Library of Congress Cataloging-in-Publication Data

```
Handbook of psychological approaches with violent offenders :
contemporary strategies and issues / edited by Vincent B. Van
Hasselt and Michel Hersen.
      p. cm. -- (The Plenum series in crime and justice)
    Includes bibliographical references and index.
    ISBN 0-306-45845-4
    1. Violence--Psychological aspects. 2. Violent
crimes--Psychological aspects. I. Van Hasselt, Vincent B. II.
Hersen, Michel. III. Series.
    RC569.V55 H36 1998
    616.85'82--ddc21
```

98-40748
CIP

ISBN 0-306-45845-4

© 1999 Kluwer Academic / Plenum Publishers, New York
233 Spring Street, New York, N.Y. 10013

10 9 8 7 6 5 4 3 2 1

A C.I.P. record for this book is available from the Library of Congress.

Printed in the United States of America

Contributors

PAUL F. BRAIN, School of Biological Sciences, University of Wales, Swansea SA2 8PP, United Kingdom

ALISA BRICKLIN, Center for Psychological Studies, Nova Southeastern University, Fort Lauderdale, Florida 33314

ALLEN G. BURGESS, School of Business, Northeastern University, Boston, Massachusetts 02115-5096

ANN W. BURGESS, School of Nursing, University of Pennsylvania, Philadelphia, Pennsylvania 19104-6096

DEWEY G. CORNELL, Curry Programs in Clinical and School Psychology, School of Education, University of Virginia, Charlottesville, Virginia 22903-2495

FRANCA CORTONI, Department of Psychology, Queen's University, Kingston, Ontario, K7L 3N6, Canada

JOHN E. DOUGLAS, Midhunters, Inc., Box 1957, Vienna, Virginia 22183

FRANK A. ELLIOTT, Neurology Department, Pennsylvania Hospital, Philadelphia, Pennsylvania 19107

YOLANDA M. FERNANDEZ, Department of Psychology, Queen's University, Kingston, Ontario, K7L 3N6, Canada

JAMES ALAN FOX, College of Criminal Justice, Northeastern University, Boston, Massachusetts 02115

GORDON P. GARY, Bureau of Alcohol, Tobacco, and Firearms, Arson and Bombing Investigative Services Subunit, National Center for the Analysis of Violent Crime, FBI Academy, Quantico, Virginia 22135

PAUL J. GEARAN, Department of Psychiatry, University of Massachusetts Memorial Health Care System, Worcester, Massachusetts 01655

DAVID J. HANSEN, Department of Psychology, University of Nebraska–Lincoln, Lincoln, Nebraska 68588-0308

DAWN M. HASEMANN, Department of Psychology, University of Kentucky, Lexington, Kentucky 40506-0044

DEBRA B. HECHT, Department of Psychology, University of Nebraska–Lincoln, Lincoln, Nebraska 68588-0308

MICHEL HERSEN, School of Professional Psychology, Pacific University, Forest Grove, Oregon 97116

TIMOTHY G. HUFF, Federal Bureau of Investigation, Arson and Bombing Investigative Services Subunit, National Center for the Analysis of Violent Crime, FBI Academy, Quantico, Virginia 22135

JOHN A. HUNTER, JR., University of Virginia Department of Health Evaluation Sciences, Health Sciences Center, Charlottesville, Virginia 22908

DAVID J. ICOVE, Tennessee Valley Authority, TVA Police, Knoxville, Tennessee 37902-1499

OTTO KAUSCH, Department of Psychiatry, Case Western Reserve University, Cleveland, Ohio 44106

DAVID J. KOLKO, Director, Special Services Unit, Western Psychiatric Institute and Clinic; Associate Professor of Child Psychiatry and Psychology, University of Pittsburgh Medical Center, Pittsburgh, Pennsylvania 15213

JEFF KOVNICK, Department of Psychiatry, Neuropsychiatry Institute, University of Utah School of Medicine, Salt Lake City, Utah 84103

KENNETH E. LEONARD, Research Institute on Addictions, and Department of Psychiatry at the State University of New York at Buffalo Medical School, Buffalo, New York 14203-1016

HOWARD D. LERNER, Michigan Psychoanalytic Institute and Department of Psychiatry, University of Michigan, Ann Arbor, Michigan 48104-2427

JACK LEVIN, Department of Sociology and Anthropology, College of Arts and Sciences, Northeastern University, Boston, Massachusetts 02115

DONALD R. LYNAM, Department of Psychology, University of Kentucky, Lexington, Kentucky 40506-0044

WILLIAM L. MARSHALL, Department of Psychology, Queen's University, Kingston, Ontario, K7L 3N6, Canada

NATHANIEL MCCONAGHY, Psychiatric Unit, The Prince of Wales Hospital, Randwick, New South Wales, Australia 2031

WILEY MITTENBERG, Center for Psychological Studies, Nova Southeastern University, Fort Lauderdale, Florida 33314

WADE C. MYERS, Department of Psychiatry, Health Sciences Center, University of Florida, Gainesville, Florida 32610

MICHAEL T. NIETZEL, Department of Psychology and Graduate School, University of Kentucky, Lexington, Kentucky 40506-0044

NORMAN G. POYTHRESS, JR., Department of Mental Health, Law & Policy, F.M.H.I.— University of South Florida, Tampa, Florida 33612-3899

ROBERT A. PRENTKY, Justice Resource Institute at the Massachusetts Treatment Center, Bridgewater, Massachusetts 02324

KATRINA R. RAYLS, Department of Psychiatry, Medical University of South Carolina, Charleston, South Carolina 29401

PHILLIP J. RESNICK, Department of Psychiatry, Case Western Reserve University, Cleveland, Ohio 44106

CATON F. ROBERTS, Department of Psychology, University of Wisconsin, Madison, and Mendota Mental Health Center, Madison, Wisconsin 53706

LINDA J. ROBERTS, Department of Child and Family Studies, University of Wisconsin, Madison, Madison, Wisconsin 53706

ALAN ROSENBAUM, Department of Psychiatry, University of Massachusetts Medical Center, Worcester, Massachusetts 01655

ALLEN D. SAPP, Department of Criminal Justice, Central Missouri State University, Warrensburg, Missouri 64093

SUZANNE K. STEINMETZ, Department of Sociology, University of Indiana, Indianapolis, Indiana 46202

VINCENT B. VAN HASSELT, Family Violence Program, Center for Psychological Studies, Nova Southeastern University, Fort Lauderdale, Florida 33314

JODY E. WARNER-ROGERS, MRC Child Psychiatry Unit, de Crespigny Park, Denmark Hill, London SE5 8AF United Kingdom

JANET I. WARREN, Clinical Psychiatric Medicine, University of Virginia, and Institute of Law, Psychiatry, and Public Policy, Charlottesville, Virginia 22908

ROSALIE S. WOLF, Institute on Aging, UMass Memorial Health Care, Worcester, Massachusetts 01605-2982

Preface

The past quarter-century has witnessed a dramatic upsurge of violent crime in the United States and abroad. In this country, the rise in violent criminal activity has been consistently documented in such published accounts as the *Uniform Crime Reports* and the *Statistical Handbook on Violence in America*, published by the FBI and the Violence Research Group, respectively. Further, social scientists—particularly those working in the fields of sociology and psychology—have provided a convergence of findings attesting to the magnitude of one of today's most significant social problems: domestic violence (e.g., spouse, child, and elder abuse). Such efforts have served as the impetus for heightened clinical and investigative activity in the area of violent behavior. Indeed, a wide range of mental health experts (such as psychologists, psychiatrists, social workers, counselors, and rehabilitation specialists) have endeavored to focus on strategies and issues in research and treatment for violent individuals and their victims.

The purpose of this book is to provide a comprehensive and timely examination of current psychological approaches with violent criminal offenders. Despite the fact that we continue to have much to learn about perpetrators of violent acts, in recent years an increasingly large body of empirical data have been adduced about this issue. However, these data generally have appeared in disparate journals and books. That being the case, it is our belief that such a handbook now is warranted.

Handbook of Psychological Approaches with Violent Criminal Offenders: Contemporary Strategies and Issues is divided into six parts and includes 24 chapters. Part I (Overview and Theoretical Perspectives) consists of an overview of the field followed by four chapters representing the sociological, behavioral, psychodynamic, and biological perspectives. In Part II, we include three chapters (firesetting, adolescent sex offenders, and child and adolescent homicide) related to the largest growing violent offender population in our nation: children and youth. Part III (Homicide) contains contributions on topics that have perhaps received some of the most recent attention from the public and media: serial murder and sexual homicide, mass and spree murder, and women who kill.

In Part IV (Sexual Deviance and Assault), we include chapters on paraphilias, rape, and child molestation, all of which have received considerable attention from mental health professionals for several years now. Part V provides in-depth presentations on the major forms of family violence: child sexual abuse, physical abuse, and neglect, as well as spouse and elder abuse. We end with a Special Topics section (Part VI) which consists of six chapters on a variety of issues ranging from neurological factors to neuropsychological assessment, and the prediction of dangerousness in violent offenders.

Many people have contributed their time and effort to bring this volume to fruition. First, we thank our gracious contributors for sharing their expertise with us. Second, we thank our technical assistants for their contributions: Virginia Basil, Burt Bolton, Melissa Brymer, Eleanor Gill, Carole Londerée, Claudia Lopez, Sue Warshal, and Erika Qualls. And finally, once again we thank our friend and Editor at Plenum Press, Eliot Werner, for agreeing about the timeliness of this project and for his support and guidance throughout.

Vincent B. Van Hasselt
Fort Lauderdale, Florida

Michel Hersen
Forest Grove, Oregon

Contents

IV. SEXUAL DEVIANCE AND ASSAULT

V. FAMILY VIOLENCE

VI. SPECIAL TOPICS

I

OVERVIEW AND THEORETICAL PERSPECTIVES

Overview

Alisa Bricklin, Michel Hersen, and Vincent B. Van Hasselt

Introduction

As Americans watch television, read newspapers, or listen to the radio, they are continuously faced with stories of the violent offenses that occur relentlessly in our society on a daily basis. Whether the offense is random, premeditated, or accidental, it is almost impossible to escape this dismal and frightening reality of violence. Despite the fact that the United States is no stranger to violence, the nature of it appears to be changing. The offenses themselves seem to be increasing in intensity and becoming progressively more shocking to the public. In addition, throughout the years, careful examination of violent crime has shown the perpetrators to be younger and with much greater access to dangerous weapons than in earlier years.

According to Shreve and Mango (1994), the increase in violent crime has significantly affected the activities of individuals, including the method in which they protect themselves. Previously, Americans were concerned about how to protect themselves from burglary and theft of property. With the surge of more violent crime, citizens are now securing their homes with metal and steel bars and purchasing weapons to protect themselves and their residences from intrusion. One result of America's increasing focus on violent crime is that one group constructed a "Death Clock," displayed at 47th Street and Broadway in New York City. This clock, situated at the top of the building, keeps a continual count of Americans killed by guns each year. The purpose of such visual demonstration is to attract the attention of the public to the prevalence of violence that occurs as a function of the proliferation of guns in our society (Shreve & Mango, 1994).

A survey that appeared in the *Wall Street Journal* (NBC News Poll, 1994) documented the public's response to increasing fear of violent crime. Ninety-three percent of the individuals questioned emphasized that addressing the crime problem in this country should be "an absolute priority" for the federal government; 57% stated that

Alisa Bricklin • Center for Psychological Studies, Nova Southeastern University, Fort Lauderdale, Florida 33314. *Michel Hersen* • School of Professional Psychology, Pacific University, Forest Grove, Oregon 97116. *Vincent B. Van Hasselt* • Family Violence Program, Center for Psychological Studies, Nova Southeastern University, Fort Lauderdale, Florida 33314.

Handbook of Psychological Approaches with Violent Offenders: Contemporary Strategies and Issues, edited by Van Hasselt and Hersen. Kluwer Academic/Plenum Publishers, New York, 1999.

crime was a "critical" or "major" problem in their communities. On the basis of this poll, there appears to be increasing intolerance toward perpetrators who commit violent offenses. Seventy-six percent of respondents supported mandatory life sentences for three-time violent offenders, and a majority of Americans indicated that "making more crimes subject to the death penalty and toughening punishment for juvenile offenders would make a big difference" (p. 1A).

Scope of the Problem

"Violent crime has reached record levels" (Shreve & Mango, 1994, p. 128). "From 1973 to 1992, the number of violent crimes (murder, rape, robbery, and aggravated assault) rose 121%." According to the Federal Bureau of Investigation's Uniform Crime Reports (1993), with the exception of an 8.4% decrease from 1980 to 1983, rape has increased every year since 1973, with a 75% increase overall from 1973 to 1992. Aggravated assault has followed the same trend, with an initial 6.4% decrease from 1980 to 1983, and then a substantial increase of 120% from 1973 to 1992. Robbery increased by 44% from 1973 to 1992. However, although the crime rate had an overall increase, homicide fluctuated the least during this time period, with its highest level in 1980 (10.2%), and lowest level of in 1984 (7.9%). In 1991, the homicide level had reached 9.8%.

According to the Federal Bureau of Investigation (FBI) (1995) in 1994, a violent crime occurred every 17 seconds: one murder every 23 seconds, one forcible rape every 5 minutes, and one aggravated assault every 28 seconds. A violent crime rate of 716 per 100,000 inhabitants was registered nationally in 1994. This is 29% above the 1985 figure. Total arrests for violent crimes rose 1% from 1993 to 1994; juvenile arrests (under age 18) increased 7%. As noted in the report, overall violent crime arrests rose 1% in the nation's cities and 2% in suburban counties (FBI, 1995).

The following statistics further illustrate frequency with which humans inflict harm on one another. Physical violence between spouses occurs in almost one third of marriages in the United States (Straus, Gelles, & Steinmetz, 1980). A woman is beaten every 12 seconds (Waits, 1985) and murdered by her boyfriend or husband every 6 hours. Three to five thousand children die each year in the United States from parental abuse (Pagelow, 1984) and homicide deaths of infants are three times greater than for toddlers. Each year 4% of elderly Americans are abused by family members (Pagelow, 1984). Sixteen percent of children report "beating up" their siblings (Straus *et al.*, 1980). More than one million violent crimes occur in the United States each year, of which 20,000 are murders, (U.S. Bureau of Census, 1988). Homicide is the 11th leading cause of death in the United States (Baker, 1986) and the leading killer of 15- to 34-year-old Black males (Butterfield, 1992). In a separate survey of 25 countries, infanticide tended to be as high as, or higher than, the rate for adult homicide, which has remained relatively consistent through the years.

Fifty percent of the people arrested in 1994 were under the age of 25 (Freeh, 1995). Greenwood (1995) reported that 3–4 out of every 10 boys growing up today in urban America will be arrested before their 18th birthdays. A brief look at previous juvenile statistics on homicide shows that 10% of homicides were committed by juveniles in 1980 and 13.6% in 1990. The number of juveniles under the age of 15 arrested for homicide increased by 50% from 1984 to 1992. Stories found in local newspapers document the tragic results of violent offenses committed by juveniles. Consider the case of a 13-year-old boy who shot his friend to death during the course of an argument because the victim allegedly was interested in the boy's "woman." Next, consider the 6-year-old child who, along with 8-year-old twins, beat and kicked a 4-week-old infant almost to death because of that infant's crying. Another case involves three preadolescents who dropped a 5-year-old boy 14 stories to his death because he would not steal candies for them. Finally, consider the 10-year-old boy who shot his 5-year- old sister to death because she would not go to her room, and a group of youngsters, ages 10–15 years, who gang-raped a 13-year-old girl (Coudroglou, 1996).

Next to assault and homicide, sexual assault is one of the most frequently committed offenses. According to Uniform Crime Reports (FBI, 1995), an estimated 77 of every 100,000 females in the country were victims of rape in 1994. Results from the National Crime Survey showed that incidents involving sexual assault fell from 607,000 in 1992 to 485,000 in 1993 (Englander, 1994). Despite these encouraging figures, however, sexual assaults are still of major concern to the American public.

Where Does Violent Crime Occur?

Acts of violence can occur anywhere, including, but not limited to, home, streets, bars, cars, stores, the workplace, and schools. Nevertheless, despite the public's awareness of the increasing frequency of violence, it appears that the vast majority of people are still under the impression that violent acts are most likely to occur are on the streets. Women, in particular, are usually taught to defend themselves against street crime (Englander, 1994). The rationale for this is that a majority of women are led to believe that city streets hold the greatest threat when it comes to being attacked, raped, or beaten. The reality is that the average American woman is much more likely to encounter violent behavior in her own home than on the streets, and the leading cause of injury to U.S. women is domestic, not street, violence (Jones, 1990).

The Home

When considering different locations of violent behavior, Romero (1985) found the home to be the most frequent setting for sexual assault. His study included children, adolescents, young adults, and older adults, ranging in age from 40 to 76. Gelles (1972) conducted an interesting study that examined exact locations in the home where assaults occur for different types of offenders. The only room in the house in which there appeared to be no violence was the bathroom. On the basis of the homicide data gathered by Gelles (1972), Pokorny (1965), and Wolfgang (1958), the bedroom is considered the deadliest room in the house. Results from the aforementioned studies also revealed that the second most frequented room in the house for violence is the kitchen, with the living room a close third. Findings suggest that a male is the most likely perpetrator in the bedroom and a female the most likely offender in the kitchen (Gelles, 1972; Pokorny, 1965; Wolfgang, 1958).

The Streets

"The street is many places, a site for much of the best and much of the worst in human interaction" (Goldstein, 1994, p. 20). The media constantly reminds us of the level of danger in American streets. Brown, Flanagan, and McLeod (1984) report that 53% of assaults occur in the streets or another outside location. Although incidence of street violence is high, Campbell (1986) points out that it is also the most public place for aggressive and violent behavior, thus making it more observable and measurable. Areas such as vacant lots and spaces between buildings (Angel, 1968), poorly lit areas, areas with difficult access (Brill, 1977), sites that are concealed, have low pedestrian traffic, or have a poor opportunity for surveillance (Harries, 1976), are all reported as likely locations for violent crime. Stoks (1982) examined 590 rape sites in the city of Seattle in 1981. One of the objectives of the study was to identify where such rapes took place. Results indicated the most frequent outdoor locations as follows: a vehicle (38%), on or next to a sidewalk (19%), in an alley (9%), a wooded area (7%), a park (6%), a parking lot (5%), and a school (4%).

Alcohol

Ingestion of alcoholic beverages has been found to facilitate aggressive behavior (Goldstein, 1994). A meta-analytic review by Bushman and Cooper (1990) of 30 experimental studies showed that a causal relationship between aggression and alcohol can safely be inferred, suggesting that alcohol, in fact, does serve as an antecedent to aggressive behavior. MacDonald (1961), on the basis of a review of numerous studies, found that perpetrators had consumed alcohol prior to committing murder in 50% of the cases. Holcomb and Anderson (1982) and Sorrells (1977) reported similar findings in their analyses of adult and juvenile murderers. Alcohol intoxication also has been found to be an antecedent in cases of assault, wife abuse, and rape (Gayford, 1975; S. D. Johnson, Gibson, & Linden, 1978; Myers, 1982).

Driving

More recently, the roadways of America have become a dangerous outlet for many frustrated and distressed motorists. Violence frequently is the consequence of such displaced aggression and has resulted in a surprising number of fatalities. A study conducted in Texas (McAlhany, 1984) showed that the most frequent expressions of aggression included tailgating, rude gestures or shaking fists, deliberate blinding by high headlight beams, deliberate preventing of passing or changing lanes, swearing at another motorist, blocking a motorist from leaving a stop sign or traffic light, throwing an object, and threatening with a weapon. Novaco (1991) has specifically studied the increased violence seen on U.S. roadways and has developed a typology of such aggressive actions. Included are roadway shootings, throwing of objects, assault with a vehicle, sniper or robber attacks, drive-by shootings, suicide or murder crashes, and roadside confrontations.

Convenience Stores

Duffalo (1976) reported that convenience stores are a vulnerable crime target, particularly those located near major transportation routes, on streets with little traffic, next to vacant lots, or in areas with minimal commercial activity. Other important factors relating to convenience stores were parking-lot size, hours of operation, gas service, and degree of disorganization (D'Alessio & Stolzenberg, 1990).

Workplace

"Prior to 1980, violence in the workplace was a virtually unheard of phenomenon" (P. W. Johnson, Myer, & Feldmann, 1995, p. 262). However, according to the 1993 U.S. Bureau of Labor Statistics, approximately 17% of all occupational deaths were the result of homicide. In fact, it has been reported that homicide is the third leading cause of death in the workplace nationally, except for five states, where it is the leading cause of death (D. L. Johnson, 1994). Indeed, the fastest growing category of homicide is employee-on employee (D. L. Johnson, 1994).

Schools

"For decades, it seemed, school was neutral turf. Aggression in the community and in near proximity to the school generally remained there, and school problem behaviors were largely of the throwing-spitballs or talking-out-of-turn variety" (Goldstein, 1994, p. 34). The following statistics confirm the dramatic rise of aggression and violence that has taken place in the schools in more recent years. Siegel and Senna (1991) have stated that "although teenagers spend only 25 percent of their time in school, 40 percent of the robberies and 36 percent of the physical attacks involving this age group occur in school" (p. 43). When considering the role of firearms in school violence, *Caught in the Crossfire* (Center to Prevent Handgun Violence, 1990) reported that from 1986 to 1990, 71 people (65 students and 6 employees) were killed by guns in American schools. An additional 201 were wounded seriously, and 242 were held hostage at gunpoint. Eighteen percent of school gun violence was the result of gang or drug disputes, 15% stemmed from longstanding arguments, 12% were over romantic disagreements, 10% were fights over possession, and 13% were the result of accidents. Apparently an estimated 270,000 students carry handguns to school one or more times each year, and a survey conducted by the American School Health Association (1989) found that 7% of boys and 2% of girls carry a knife to school every day.

Violence in the United States

"The United States was born in the crucible of individual and collective violence, a relationship which has persisted with but infrequent interruption for over two centuries" (Goldstein, 1994, p. 72). Throughout history, the United States has been no stranger to violence, dating back as early as the American Revolution, where acts of violence (including guerrilla tactics) were used to gain independence from British rule. Subsequent examples of our apparently violent culture include riots, demonstrations, and a large variety of violent crimes. Moreover, the Civil War (1861–1865) is the most dramatic example of violence in America, with more combatants killed than the total for all wars since that time. Reiss and Roth (1993) reported, based on the National Research Council report: "Homicide rates in the United States far exceed those in any other industrialized nation. For other violent crimes, rates in the United States are among the world's highest. . . . Among 16 industrialized countries surveyed in 1988, the United States had the highest prevalence rates for serious sexual assaults and for other assaults including threats of physical harm" (p. 3).

Relationships Between Offenders and Victims

Previous statistics on relationships of victims to offenders demonstrated that the majority of murder victims knew their killers (FBI, 1995). However, according to Uniform Crime Reports (FBI, 1995), 1991 through 1994 saw the relationship percentages change. In 1994, only 12% of murder victims were related to their assailants were 35%, acquaintances and 13% of the victims were murdered by strangers. Fortunately, overall homicide rates in the United States seem to be declining. The Federal Bureau of Investigation reported a 12% decrease in the number of homicides in the first half of 1995 (Ostrow, 1995). Homicide rates declined in cities of more than 1 million citizens. However, despite this finding, Americans remain concerned about the occurrence of stranger homicide for a few reasons: First, the number of juveniles responsible for killings is continuously increasing (Freeh, 1995); second, the nature of homicides is becoming more grotesque, shocking, and unnecessarily violent; and third, violent crime is occurring more frequently in response to minimal provocation.

Preview of the Book

In light of the increased intensity of crime in our society, this handbook takes an investigative journey into the world of violent offenders. The purpose of this effort is threefold: (1) to provide a compelling and thorough examination of salient strategies and issues in research and treatment of a wide variety of violent offenders; (2) to discuss relevant clinical implications of working with the disparate groups that are covered; (3) to offer coverage of a range of special topics and factors that are common to populations of violent individuals.

In Part I, chapters 2 through 5 provide an overview of sociological, behavioral, psychodynamic, and biological theories and perspectives on violence.

Part II examines violent crimes committed by children and adolescents. Chapter 6 takes a look at firesetting in these groups with consideration of such areas as assessment and evaluation, clinical characteristics and correlates, and intervention. Chapter 7 covers adolescent sex offenders, a population that has received increased clinical and investigative attention in recent years. Chapter 8 focuses on child and adolescent homicide and discusses characteristics of offenders, family patterns, assessment and diagnosis, course and prognosis-recidivism, clinical management, and treatment.

Part III explores the most extreme end of the violent behavior continuum: homicide. Specifically, Chapter 9 examines the burgeoning problems of serial murder and sexual homicide, providing definitions, classification efforts, case examples, FBI research, epidemiology, and family patterns. Offender characteristics that are covered include organized versus disorganized offenders (and their crime scenes), mobility classification, social background, etiology, and the role of fantasy in their acts of homicide. The assessment and diagnosis, course, prognosis-recidivism, psychological profiling, and clinical management and treatment of these offenders also are discussed. Chapter 10 targets mass and spree murder and addresses patterns, typology, and factors contributing to this growing trend. Chapter 11 investigates the phenomenon of women who kill, and includes such topics as maternal filicide, spousal homicide, and the psychopathic female murderer.

Part IV offers comprehensive coverage of sexual deviance and assault. In chapters 12, 13 and 14, paraphilia, rape, and child sexual molestation, respectively, are covered. Each of these chapters provides a description and historical background and an overview of epidemiology, offender characteristics, family patterns, assessment and diagnosis, course and prognosis-recidivism, clinical management, and treatment.

Part V examines disparate forms of family violence. In chapters 15 and 16, adolescent victims, intergenerational issues in sexual abuse, and child physical abuse and neglect. Chapter 17 explores relationship aggression between partners and provides individual and couple characteristics. Relevant strategies and issues in research and treatment are outlined (e.g., effects of arrest, current findings on treatment outcome). The chapter on elder abuse, Chapter 18, provides information on this more recently acknowledged form of family violence. Crimes against older adults, epidemiology, theoretical explanations, risk factors, case profiles, and assessment and intervention strategies are provided in this chapter.

Part VI is dedicated to special topics concerning violent offenders. Chapter 19 discusses arson and fire-related crimes and offers a statement of the problem, relevant definitions, and a classification of motivations for this act. Chapter 20 provides a neurological perspective of violent offenders and includes coverage of affective aggression, epilepsy and violence, anatomical and chemical substrates of violent aggression, neurophysiological correlates and neuropathological correlates of criminal violence, and the clinical evolution of violence with age. This chapter also examines the neuropathology in a sample of 161 murderers. In Chapter 21, the authors guide the reader through the psychiatric assessment of violent offenders, including an assessment of risk factors. Civil commitment, release of insanity acquittees, probation, parole, and stalking are discussed. The neuropsychology of aggression is the focus of Chapter 22, where the functional neuroanatomy of the central nervous system is examined. The problems of head trauma, epilepsy, Alzheimer's disease, metabolic conditions, developmental disorders, and their role in violent behavior, are discussed. Of considerable social concern and controversy is the prediction of dangerousness in violent offenders and release decision making. These areas are explored in Chapter 23, which covers criminal justice psychiatric release decisions, policy development involving administration and substantive issues, documentation, and implementation of release decisions. Finally, Chapter 24 looks at the relationship between alcohol, drugs, and interpersonal violence. This chapter offers an extensive overview of current etiological models and epidemiological research on alcohol and drug use and violence; experimental studies of the effects of alcohol and other drugs on aggressive behavior are reviewed. The complexity of the alcohol–violence relationship is explored, and relevant clinical implications including risk assessment and treatment are discussed.

References

American School Health Association (1989). *National adolescent student health survey*. Denver, CO: Author.
Angel, S. (1968). *Discouraging crime through city planning*. Berkeley: University of California Press.
Baker, S. (1986). A plague called violence. *Omni, 8*(11), 43–47, 88.
Brill, W. (1977). *Controlling access in highrise buildings: Approaches and guidelines*. Washington, DC: U.S. Government Printing Office.

Brown, E., Flanagan, T., & McLeod, M. (Eds.). (1984). *Sourcebook of criminal justice statistics—1983.* Washington, DC: U.S. Government Printing Office.

Bushman, B. J., & Cooper, H. M. (1990). Effects of alcohol on human aggression: An integrative research review. *Psychological Bulletin, 107,* 341–354.

Butterfield, F. (1992, October 23). Dispute threatens U.S. plan on violence. *New York Times,* p. A8.

Campbell, A. (1986). The streets and violence. In A. Campbell & J. J. Gibbs (Eds.), *Violent transactions: The limits of personality* (pp. 115–132). Oxford, England: Blackwell.

Center to Prevent Handgun Violence. (1990). *Caught in the crossfire: A report on gun violence in our nation's schools.* Washington, DC: Author.

Coudroglou, A. (1996). Violence as a social mutation. *American Journal of Orthopsychiatry, 66,* 323–328.

D'Alessio, S., & Stolzenberg, L. (1990). A crime of convenience. *Environment and Behavior, 22,* 255–271.

Duffalo, D. C. (1976). Convenience stores, armed robbery and physical environment features. *American Behavioral Scientist, 20,* 227–246.

Englander, E. K. (1994). *Understanding violence.* Hillsdale, NJ: Erlbaum.

Federal Bureau of Investigation. (1993). *Uniform Crime Report, 1992.* Washington, DC: U.S. Government Printing Office.

Federal Bureau of Investigation. (1995). *Uniform Crime Report, 1994.* Washington, DC: U.S. Government Printing Office.

Freeh, L. J. (1995). *Uniform crime report press release.* Washington, DC: U.S. Department of Justice.

Gayford, J. J. (1975). Ten types of battered wives. *Welfare Officer, 25,* 5–9.

Gelles, R. J. (1972). "It takes two": The roles of victim and offender. In R. J. Gelles (Ed.), *The violent home: A study of physical aggression between husband and wives.* Newbury Park, CA: Sage.

Goldstein, A. P. (1994). *The ecology of aggression.* New York: Plenum.

Greenwood, P. (1995). Juvenile crime and juvenile justice. In J. Q. Wilson & J. Petersilia (Eds.), *Crime* (pp. 91–117). San Francisco: ICS.

Harries, K. D. (1976). Cities and crime: A geographic model. *Criminology, 14,* 369–386.

Holcomb, W. R., & Anderson, W. P. (1982). Alcohol and drug abuse in accused murderers. *Psychological Reports, 52,* 159–164.

Johnson, D. L. (1994, August). *Violence in the workplace.* Violence in America: Selected readings. Major City Chiefs Administrators National Executive Institute, FBI Academy 1994.

Johnson, P. W., Myer, R. G., & Feldman, T. B. (1995). Violence in the workplace: New empirical data. Paper presented at the sixth annual national symposium, *Mental health and the law, aggression and abuse: Clinical and legal issues,* April 13, 1996, Ft. Lauderdale, Florida.

Johnson, S. D., Gibson, L., & Linden, R. (1978). Alcohol and rape in Winnipeg, 1966–1975. *Journal of Studies on Alcohol, 39,* 1887–1894.

Jones, J. (1990, October). Violent statistics. *American Psychological Association Monitor,* 4.

MacDonald, J. M. (1961). *The murderer and his victim.* Springfield, IL: Thomas.

McAlhany, D. A. (1984). *Highway abuse and violence: Motorists' experiences as victims.* Unpublished master's thesis, North Texas State University, Denton, TX.

Myers, T. (1982). Alcohol and violent crime re-examined: Self-reports from two subgroups of Scottish male prisoners. *British Journal of Addiction, 77,* 399–413.

NBC News poll. (1994) *Wall Street Journal,* p. 1A.

Novaco, R. W. (1991). Aggression on roadways. In R. Baenniger (Ed.), *Targets of violence and aggression.* Amsterdam: Elsevier Science.

Ostrow, R. J. (1995, December 18). Homicides in US drop sharply, FBI reports. *The Boston Globe,* p. 3.

Pagelow, M. D. (1984). *Family violence.* New York: Praeger.

Pokorny, A. D. (1965). Human violence: A comparison of homicide, aggravated assault, suicide and attempted suicide. *Journal of Criminal Law, Criminology and Police Science, 56,* 488–497.

Reiss, A. J., & Roth, J. A. (Eds.). (1993). Panel on the Understanding and Control of Violent Behavior, Committee on Law and Justice, Commission on Behavioral and Social Sciences and Education, National Research Council, Patterns of Violence in American Society. *Understanding and preventing violence.* Washington, DC: National Academy Press.

Romero, J. J. (1985). *A situational analysis of sexual assault among age-groups of female victims.* Unpublished doctoral dissertation, Temple University, Philadelphia.

Shreve, D., & Mango, N. F. (1994, August). *Violence in America: Changes and trends.* Violence in America: Selected readings. Major City Chiefs Administrators National Executive Institute, FBI Academy.

Siegel, L. M., & Senna, J. J. (1991). *Juvenile delinquency: Theory, practice and law.* St. Paul, MN: West.

Sorrells, J. M. (1977). Kids who kill. *Crime and Delinquency, 23,* 312–320.

Stoks, F. G. (1982). *Assessing urban public space environments for danger of violent crime—Especially rape.* Unpublished doctoral dissertation, University of Washington, Seattle.

Straus, M. A., Gelles, R. J., & Steinmetz, S. K. (1980). *Behind closed doors: Violence in the American family.* New York: Doubleday.

U. S. Bureau of the Census. (1988). *Statistical abstracts of the United States* (108th ed.). Washington, DC: U.S. Department of Commerce.

Wolfgang, M. E. (1958). *Patterns in criminal homicide.* Philadelphia: University of Pennsylvania Press.

Sociological Theories of Violence

Suzanne K. Steinmetz

Introduction

Violence is pervasive in the United States. The U.S. Department of Justice reported that during 1995, there were 7,947 hate crime incidents involving 9,895 separate offenses, 10,469 victims, and 8,433 known offenders reported to the FBI during 1995. And these data cover only 45 states and the District of Columbia—about 75% of the United States.

On a global level, during 1995 acts of terrorism that threatened society and caused major political, psychological, and economic damage occurred in 51 countries and this does not even consider the politically and religiously motivated violence that occurs daily in numerous countries. U.S. citizens are increasingly becoming targets of acts of terrorism abroad as well as in their own country.

Interpersonal violence appears to be an inter- and intra-generational phenomenon, and persons who experience one form of violence (e.g., violence in the school, family, or streets) are much more likely to experience subsequent violence in a variety of forms (Steinmetz, 1990, 1996). Studies of adolescents demonstrate the extent to which they experience family violence, rape, and street crime, which continues intergenerationally (Steinmetz, 1996; Steinmetz, 1999). Experience with violence begins early in children's lives in their own home when they experience child abuse and sibling violence and witness violence between their parents (Steinmetz 1987; Straus, Gelles, & Steinmetz, 1980). Such violence continues in the early school years where 10% of the boys and 6% of girls reported being bullied, often over a period of 6 months or more (Slee & Rigby, 1993), and throughout their years in school, which is a violent setting for both teachers and students (Steinmetz, 1990).

Homicides were the second leading cause of death for individuals 15–24 years of age (accounting for over 18% of all deaths) and the third leading cause of death among youth ages 5–14 during 1996 (Ventura, Peters, Martin, & Mauer, 1977). Three out of every 10 homicides are committed by juveniles who have killed other children. Furthermore, 4173 teenagers ages 15–19 are killed each year in incidents involving firearms, which is not surprising since 200 million firearms are owned by Americans

Suzanne K. Steinmetz • Department of Sociology, University of Indiana, Indianapolis, Indiana 46202.

Handbook of Psychological Approaches with Violent Offenders: Contemporary Strategies and Issues, edited by Van Hasselt and Hersen. Kluwer Academic/Plenum Publishers, New York, 1999.

in the United States (Sells & Blum, 1996). Although homicides are decreasing in major cities, other forms of violence have been increasing with three disturbing trends observed. First, violence is occurring at consistently younger ages. Second, it appears that sex-related acts of violence tend to be increasing. And, third, girls and women are increasingly being identified as perpetrators of violence.

The 1995 National Youth Gang Study provided estimated that there were over 650,000 youth who were members of over 25,000 gangs (Curry, 1996; Curry, Ball, & Decker, 1996). Furthermore, the percentage of students reporting street gangs in their school increased from 15% to 28% between 1989 and 1995 (Chandler, Chapman, Rand, & Taylor, 1998). Since the mid-1980s two trends have been observed. Gangs have been increasing in upscale communities and female membership in gangs has increased with estimates from 5%–10% in suburban gangs to 25% in urban gangs. This trend towards gangs in the more affluent communities is seen as youth searching for a replacement for family (Korem, 1995).

Television has perhaps become the principal cultural and social force in the United States with children watching more than 50 hour per week (Donner, 1990). Television violence has been linked to violence in society (Davis, 1980; Gerbner, 1972; Huston, Donnerstein, Fairchild, Feshbach, Katz, Murray, Rubinstein, Wilcox & Zuckerman, 1992; Paik & Comstock, 1994; Phillips, 1983; Radecki, 1981). There also have been a number of studies that documented a strong relationship between viewing sexually violent material and rape (Allison & Wrightsman, 1993; Linz, Donnerstein, & Penrod, 1987; Malamuth & Donnerstein, 1982; Russell, 1988). A National Institute of Mental Health report that reviewed 2,500 research studies found a strong relationship between violence portrayed on television and violence in our society (Pearl, 1982). According to the National Television Study (1996), programming continues to have a heavy violent content: 57% of TV programming had violence and 25% of violent interaction involved handguns.

Can one theory explain all forms of violence? It appears that violence at all levels of society is very much a part of our landscape. We need to ask, therefore, whether one theory can be applied to all forms of violence or whether it is necessary to have specific theories to explain different types of violence such as family violence, street crime, or large-scale national or international violence. Gelles and Straus (1979) argued that, although violence itself is not unique, the special relationship of family members, the intimacy, privacy, amount of time spent together, and the interdependency of the members makes family violence a somewhat special case.

Taking a different stance, Glaser (1986) suggested that all type of physical assaults among humans, whether between individuals, family members, large groups, or nations share similar characteristics: The ideas are verbally expressed to justify the use of violence, the violence tends to evoke counter violence, and violence in one setting tends to spread to other settings.

The commonality that makes it possible to discuss theories that are applicable to all forms of violence is the emphasis on group or social phenomena for explaining violence rather than intra-individual processes. Factors, such as inequality in the distribution of resources, power, status, money, and the differential ability to access knowledge, that are based on age, gender, race, ethnicity, and the social class of one's parents appear to underlie all forms of violence. It is the relative importance of these and whether the outcome of violence is considered to be justified that takes on a different appearance based on the specific theory being used to explain violence.

This chapter will examine factors contributing to violence in the more general form, drawing more from classical and more general theories, with a focus on sociological theories of violence that are useful in understanding why a group of individuals or a society engages in violence. It is not the function of these theories to provide explanations or understanding regarding the intra-individual factors that might influence any one individual to engage in violence. To make this task more manageable, we will examine theories that offer insights into a variety of forms of violence, but will limit our examples, for the most part, to violence which occurs on the street and in the home.

One of the major difficulties facing the social scientist is the untangling of the effect of one variable from another—a difficulty intensified because individuals' day-to-day interactions cannot be studied in a controlled experimental setting. For example, the abused wife is often a member of a family that exhibits numerous characteristics (e.g., alcohol abuse, economic instability, unplanned or unwanted pregnancy, lack of resources) that produce a high level of stress and have been shown to contribute to violence; therefore the researcher, without the ability to manipulate family members, finds it difficult to discover which of these variables is the major contributor or which variables interact to intensify the violence. Similarly, the rapist or murderer often has background characteristics, such as being raised in a disorganized family, poverty, educational deficiencies, minority status, and experience as a victim of violence, which all contribute to the tendency to rape or murder. The choice of a theoretical perspective is important not only for attempting to understand the process by which violence is initiated and maintained but, more important, for developing mechanisms to help reduce or eliminate violence and, one hopes, preventing it from occurring.

Definition of Terms

To begin, it is important to make clear the disciplinary boundaries that encompass sociology. The general definition of sociology is the study of patterned human interaction. The focus is on groups—family, peer, work, and so on. Sociology examines the patterned micro and macro influences on group behavior.

Violence has been defined in a variety of ways, all with a similarity in theme. Graham and Gurr (1969) defined violence as behavior designed to inflict personal injury on people or damage to property; Skolnick (1969) defines violence as the intentional use of force to injure, kill, or to destroy property. MacFarlane (1974) differentiated between force and violence. When one imposes his or her will on another and the position held is legitimate, this is considered force; when the position held is considered illegitimate then it is defined as violence. From this position, using a gun to protect oneself would be labeled as "force." Using a gun during the commission of a crime would be considered an example of "violence."

In this chapter, violence is defined as an act carried out with the intention of physically hurting another person (Steinmetz & Straus, 1974). Such "physical hurt" can range from a slap to murder. Although this is the basic definition of violence, Steinmetz (1977, 1987) suggested that there are four dimensions to violence. The first dimension is intent. Was the violence accidental or intentional? In the definition provided that the act must be intentional to be considered violence. The second dimension is purpose. Was the act instrumental to some other purpose, such as disciplining a child for a specific wrongdoing or self-defense in a street crime, or was it expressive, an end in itself (which appeared to be the situation in the Rodney King beating and similar incidents)?

The third dimension is legitimacy. Is the violent act a culturally permitted or required act, such as spanking a disobedient child or self-defense—a legitimate act, as opposed to one that runs counter to cultural norms such as murder which is considered to be illegitimate violence? Thus, the basis for the "intent to hurt" may range from concern for a child's safety (as when a child is spanked for going into the street) to hostility so intense that the death of the other is desired. The former would be an example of "legitimate instrumental violence" and the latter of "illegitimate expressive violence."

The last dimension is the outcome: the perceived success or failure of the use of violence to resolve the problem or express one's will. In earlier articles (Steinmetz, 1977, 1987), it was hypothesized that the conflict resolution methods most likely to be repeated are those deliberate acts that are considered legitimate behavior by society (or at least are perceived as such by the respondents), that are aimed at changing another's behavior (instrumental), and that area perceived to be successful by the individuals participating.

These relationships are illustrated by the following quotation that reflects family violence but certainly has counterparts in other forms of violence:

> I've heard that you shouldn't spank when you're angry, but I can't agree with that, because I think that the time you should spank; before you have to completely cool off, too. I think that the that the spanking helps the mother or dad as well as impresses the child that they did something wrong and when they do something bad, they are going to be physically punished for it. You don't hit them with a stick or a belt, or a hairbrush, but a good back of the hand . . . they remember it. (Steinmetz, 1977, p. 27)

The four dimensions just discussed are illustrated in this quotation. First, the respondent suggests an expressive dimension ("spanking helps the mother or dad" get rid of frustration). Second, the instrumental dimension ("impresses the child that he did something wrong") is mentioned. A third point is the respondent's differentiation between what she considers legitimate ("a good back of the hand") and illegitimate ("you don't hit them with a stick or belt or a hairbrush"). Furthermore, her action is deliberate ("I think that's the time you should spank; before you have a chance to completely cool off, too") and perceived to be successful ("they remember it").

In the following section we examine some major sociological theories that are useful in explaining violence. We discuss functional theories, structural theories, cultural theories, exchange and resource theory, conflict theory, symbolic interaction theory, feminist theory, and postpositivistic theory, which has also been called postmodernism or deconstruction theory. Within each of these theories, variants or subtheories are also examined.

Theories of Violence

Historical Influences

Early sociological theorists were educated in the natural sciences, philosophy, and theology, and their theories reflect their religious, cultural, and educational background. As Vargus (1999) noted, Francis Bacon and Isaac Newton had established science as an important means to understand the nonhuman world, but it required modern social philosophy to lay the foundation for the development of social theory.

Classical philosophy, which forms the foundation of most early sociological theories, tends to have two distinct views of human behavior. John Locke (1632–1704) saw humans as capable of reason, but needing a government to uphold the natural laws. Jean-Jacques Rousseau (1712–1778) had a similar view of society noting that the growth of society resulted in unbridled individualism, greed, violence, lack of responsibility, and general corruption—society's downfall. Rousseau believed that humans were born moral, but society and the corruption and evil that develops in society resulted in a breakdown of the social order.

An opposing view was presented by Thomas Hobbes, who viewed humans as evil and violent and requiring society's control mechanisms to establish social order and civility. The social order as a product of civilization is a social control mechanism requiring individuals to act in ways that benefit others. Social-conservative paradigms see individuals as morally deficient, irrational, and requiring a strong authority to control impulses and maintain order.

In an attempt to reconcile these two opposing views, Etzioni (1988) rephrased the same issues: "Assuming human beings see themselves both as members of a community and as self-seeking individuals, how are the lines drawn between the commitments to the commons and to one's self?" (p. 1x). Etzioni asked if we are single-minded individuals, each out to maximize our own well-being, and if society is a marketplace where individuals compete with each other, do we try to do what is both correct and individually pleasurable? He noted that the utilitarian, rationalistic-individualistic, neoclassical paradigm is applied not only to economic relations, but also to other social relations such as crime and family. Etzioni proposed a new paradigm which sees individuals able to act rationally and advance the position of each (the "I") but doing so within a strong moral commitment to the community's well-being (the "we").

Functionalism

Auguste Comte, who coined the term *sociology,* advocated a science of society and is credited with influencing social thought known as functionalism. Comte and other functionalists were greatly influenced by the scientific discoveries being made in the natural and physical sciences. Comte was also reacting to the chaos of the French Revolution, especially the individualistic, utilitarian philosophies in vogue at that time, Comte wanted to discover a way to create a society that exhibited order and harmony. He believed that human evolution in the 19th century had reached a "positive" stage with sufficient empirical knowledge to be able to study and understand society and use this scientific knowledge to create a better society.

Comte and other functionalists considered societies to be analogous to organisms and the various components of the society to be analogous to the parts of the organism. The social control mechanism of a society, such as power, authority, rewards, and punishment served a function similar to the mechanisms that enabled an organism to survive. If the organism flourished, this was seen as an example of Herbert Spencer's (1860) use of the phrase "survival of the fittest," a concept that had been adopted by Darwin and used in his *On the Origin of Species* (1859), and credited to Spencer in the introduction. However, unlike Comte, Spencer believed that change in the structure of an organism or a social organization cannot occur without changes occurring in the functions of the organism.

From a Darwinian perspective, societies that were flourishing, for example, western European societies, were considered to be examples of better, more fit, superior societies. It was this basic type of thought, transformed into social Darwinism, that laid the foundation for the theories propagated by Hitler in the 1930s to 1940s and by current white supremist groups.

Durkheim was also influenced by Comte in both the emphasis on empiricism and the importance of the group as an explanation. Durkheim developed the most comprehensive systematic formulation of the analogy between social and organic life. His theories were grounded in the belief that the ultimate social reality was the group rather than the individual; social facts rather than individual facts define human behavior. Durkheim's book *Suicide* (1966), originally published in 1897, is a distinguished example of using social data to formulate a sociological theory to explain individual acts of violence. Using census data, Durkheim was able to define three types of suicide based on the social structural characteristic of the society under study: egoistic, altruistic, anomic. A fourth type, fatalistic, is identified in a footnote (p. 276), according to Vargus (1999).

Functionalism, the progenitor of American structural-functionalism emerged in the early 1930s with heavy moralistic tones (Kingsbury & Scanzoni, 1993). There are four defining properties of a social system: differentiated or specialized roles, shared values, and norms that define rights and obligations; mechanism to maintain boundaries because members of the system are more closely bounded to each other than those outside the system; and a tendency toward homeostasis or a dynamic equilibrium (McIntyre, 1966; Kingsbury & Scanzoni, 1993).

Individuals have the ability to make choices and do so because of normative standards. Parsons (1937), a major American social theorist, believed that solidarity, the idea that social systems function because the members conform to a set of standards that promotes the goals of society, was a critical component of functionalism. Gouldner (1970), in discussing Parsons's concept of shared values and norms as a mechanism to maintain the social order, suggested that Parsons believed that individuals conform to normative expectations regarding behavior because of an internalized moral code rather than fear of consequences. If, as Parsons posits, shared values and norms are critical in keeping the social order, then shared values and norms might be equally functional for groups that are outside of mainstream society, for example, cults, gangs, and militia as for mainstream society.

Merton's (1938) concept of functional equivalent, that is, nontraditional ways to meet societal goals, was operationalized in his typology of deviant behavior. His essay "Social Structure and Anomie" one of the most widely read and influential of his works, builds on Durkheim's concept of anomie. Merton proposed, as an explanation of deviance, five modes of adaptation that are available to an individual who is unable to fulfill cultural goals through socially acceptable institutional means.

Using functional analysis, Merton notes that, on the whole, deviance is dysfunctional for the majority group although deviance might provide an adaptation with positive consequences for one segment of society. According to Merton, a social system is based on culturally defined goals and the structural paths for achieving these goals. However, some individuals and groups will not be able to achieve these culturally defined goals through the socially acceptable means. To be in equilibrium, a social system must integrate the cultural goals with the structural means for achieving these goals.

His topology, presented below, suggests ways in which individuals for whom normal control mechanisms (e.g., rewards and punishments) do not result in conforming behavior, might adapt. Merton (1957) noted that those individuals who use rebellion are seeking "to bring into being a new . . . greatly modified social structure," (p. 155), which suggests similarities to assumptions found in conflict theory.

Adaptation to anomie	Cultural goals	Institutionalized means
Conformity	+	+
Innovation	+	−
Ritualism	+	
Retreatism	−	+
Rebellion	±	±

Sutherland and Cressey (1974) explain criminal behavior using an approach that is similar to that used by Merton. Likewise Reiss (1951), Hirschi (1969), and G. Marx (1981) suggested that absence of social control explains deviance and violence. Functional theory asserts that conflict is important in maintaining the adaptability of the family. Coser (1956) noted that violence can serve three positive functions.

First, it provides an area of achievement for an individual, such as violence or compulsive masculinity as illustrated in Brown (1965) and Toby (1966). Second, violence can also act as a danger signal for the community. The numerous videos documenting police brutality have stirred public outrage and resulted in law enforcement agencies reevaluating their selection and training procedures as well as developing mechanisms for review and removal from the force. Third, violence can act as a catalyst for change. For example, horrifying, extremely sadistic accounts of child abuse stirred the public consciousness to support state laws for dealing with child abuse, as well as the federal Child Abuse Prevention and Treatment Act. Publicizing ordeals faced by beaten wives, especially celebrity wives such as Charlotte Fedders or, more recently, Nicole Simpson, has been instrumental in instituting legislation to provide protection from abuse, as well as services for victims and their children.

Social Frustration Theory

Social frustration theory is a variant of functional theory that posits that individuals become frustrated when they are no longer able to fulfill their goal according to the socially expected means, which is similar to Merton's ideas. One of the first studies to document the relationship between violence and the business cycle was a British study done in 1925 that compared government statistics on unemployment, production, and prices with crime statistics (D. S. Thomas, 1925, as cited in Gunn, 1973). This study found that years characterized by a poorer financial outlook had higher numbers of suicides. Henry and Short (1954) found that burglary, robbery, suicide, and lynching of Blacks seemed to go up during years characterized by a depressed economic status, while homicides increased during periods of prosperity. More recent studies have confirmed the relationship between economic conditions and violence—both in the street and in the home (Steinmetz, 1987; Steinmetz & Straus, 1974).

Poverty and the inability to fulfill one's goal through socially acceptable means have been presented as explanations for child abuse. In summarizing the research on poverty, the Children Defense Fund publication *Wasting America's Future* (1994), notes that child abuse increased with growing economic hardships and declined as economic prospect improved; infant mortality rates increased during period of high joblessness and fell as employment improved across the nation; and children were better nourished, performed better in school, and completed more education when families were financial secure (p. xxiv). Similarly, abuse is five times more likely and neglect nine times more likely when families with income less than $15,000 were compared with those making $15,000 or more.

Sociobiology

Another variant of functional theory, sociobiology, traces its roots to the work of ethnologists. A sociobiological perspective would explain the higher rates of child neglect or abuse among handicapped, foster, or adopted children as a lack of parental bonding between parent and child resulting from the inability of these offspring to continue the genetic line of the parents.

Gunn (1973), in reviewing early writers' theories about the evolutionary behavior, noted that Carveth Read in 1917 believed that man's violence was a direct outgrowth of his being an omnivore and a hunter who deliberately catches and kills. This led to hunting behavior that resulted in more aggressiveness as well as more cooperation. This group bonding and cooperation among males is posited by Tiger (1969) as an explanation for gender differences. Although, as Gunn noted, herbivorous animals can also be quite violent, he further noted that other theories suggest that man learns to be dominant over other species by defining them as less worthy; this is similar to the stance taken by the contemporary military regarding the enemy (e.g., our definition of Vietnamese as less-than-human "gooks").

Sociobiology has also been used to explain how child abuse, especially infanticide, serves as a population control mechanism (Bakan, 1971). Although it is doubtful that the estimated 1,215 children who died from abuse and neglect in 1995 (Lung & Daro, 1996) could be considered a population control measure in most contemporary societies, infanticide was a very effective population control mechanism in the past (Radbill, 1968). Infanticide is also a solution chosen by families in China who desire a son but have given birth to a daughter and under the one-child certificate are not permitted to have another child (Johansson & Nygren, 1991). Another option has been to batter the wife so she will divorce her husband, or murder the wife, both of which enable the husband to remarry and have another child.

Rape also has been explained using sociobiology theory (Gibson, Linden, & Johnson, 1980; Hagen, 1979). The rapist commits rape in an attempt to spread his sperm so that there is a greater chance that his offspring will populate the earth (thus reflecting the rules of natural selection by a dominant, aggressive male).

Catharsis Theory

A final variant of structural-functionalist theory, catharsis theory, postulates the necessity of "moderate violence" in order to release pent-up frustration and hostility, thus reducing the likelihood of severe violence. Although this position has not been supported by research in child rearing (Bandura & Walters, 1963) or husband–wife interaction (Straus, 1974), it continues to form the basis of treatment offered by some family therapists (Bach & Wyden, 1968), in which freely expressing controlled, lower-level violence is seen as a mechanism for preventing explosive, violent interaction as a result of "stored-up" anger.

Structural Theory of Violence

Structural theories of violence identify the source of violence as the differential distribution of violence-producing factors such as stress, frustration, and deprivation. Therefore, one would expect a greater prevalence of violence among certain groups, such as those who live in poverty, with large numbers of children, and in crowded living quarters.

Status Inconsistency Theory

Social structural characteristics that can produce status inconsistency have also been linked to violence (Kelly & Chambliss, 1966; Lenski, 1954). This might occur when there is an unstable transition of power, which often occurs in third-world countries; the former leader may hold status and some residual accouterments of power, but no longer has the authority to demand actions or the power to enforce his or her will.

Differences between an individual's ascribed status (what one has accomplished) may also account for violence. O'Brian (1971) found that when the husband felt threatened in his traditional status by a wife who was more educated or had more resources or skills, he resorted to violence to maintain his dominance. This may be useful in understanding why seemingly successful, powerful individuals resort to violence. For example, in a study of political violence that examined the backgrounds of men who assassinated or attempted to assassinate presidents of the United States, it was found that many of these men had come from prominent families, but the assassins considered themselves failures and were viewed similarly by their families and associates (Steinmetz, 1974).

In addition to the husband's and the wife's occupational, educational, and financial achievement and their social status, the compatibility of their statuses is important. Status inconsistency (inconsistent educational and occupational attainment) and status incompatibility (husband and wife with unequal status) were found to predict marital violence (Hornung, McCullough, & Sugimoto, 1981). Although both status inconsistency and incompatibility in general increase psychological abuse, physical aggression, and life-threatening violence, certain types of status inconsistency (e.g., husband's occupational underachievement) and status incompatibility (e.g., a woman's high-status occupation relative to her husband's) are particularly likely to result in severe marital violence.

Gender-Based Inequality

Because gender-based inequality has been considered a major force behind the abuse of wives, reducing sexual inequality is considered to be necessary in order to reduce wife abuse (Dobash & Dobash, 1979; Martin, 1976). However, some researchers (Marsden, 1978; Steinmetz & Straus, 1974; Straus, 1976; Whitehurst, 1974) suggest that violence may actually increase as women strive to obtain greater income, power, and status, while men attempt to maintain their dominant position in these areas.

Fortunately, the data from the two national surveys found a 28% decrease in spouse abuse between the 1975 survey (Straus *et al.*, 1980) and the 1985 survey (Gelles & Straus, 1988). Using American states as a unit of analysis, Yllö (1983), obtained measures for the economic status of women, their educational accomplishments, their role in politics, and the laws protecting women's rights. The relationship between the overall status of women and the levels of violence, as measured by the Conflict Tactic Scales (CTS) (Straus *et al.*, 1980), was curvilinear; violence is highest in those states where the status of women is lowest; violence decreases as a status improves, but violence increases among states in which the status of women is the highest. This relationship was not affected by measures of urbanization, statewide levels of education, or the state level of violent crime, and was only slightly affected by state levels of income.

Structural–Functional Theories

The structural–functional theories just discussed tend to be conservative. The goal is to preserve the system and maintain the status quo. Thus a theory of wife abuse from this perspective might locate the factors leading up to the abuse as role conflict resulting from women's occupying roles and status traditionally assigned to men. These might include employment, having a car registered in the wife's name only, holding positions of power and authority at work or in the community, or having an independent income and individual credit rating. If women had adhered to fulfilling the expressive (caregiving, nurturing) roles and men to instrumental (employment, car maintenance) roles, role conflict and concomitant domestic violence would not occur. Likewise, if youth and their families performed their roles as prescribed, they would have legitimate means for accomplishing goals and would not have to resort to criminal activity.

Cultural Theory of Violence

The culture of violence theory suggests that the differential distribution of violence is a function of cultural norms and values concerning violence (Wolfgang & Ferracuti, 1967). This theory predicts that a greater degree of violence would occur in those families belonging to a culture or a subculture in which socialization practices are deeply embedded in violence, rather than resulting from an excess of deprivation and stress, or from the lack of alternative resources for resolving a conflict. Thus Merton's (1938) paradigm of alternative pathways to fulfilling cultural goals fits nicely.

Throughout the history of the United States some segment of the population, ethnic, social class, or geographic, has experienced severe conflict and violence (Steinmetz & Straus, 1973). Use of physical force to suppress conflict and the general societal sanctioning of these acts can be seen in more recent events such as the Kent State University shooting, the 1968 Chicago Democratic National Convention, the school-desegregation busing programs, the bombing of abortion clinics, the Olympic games in Atlanta, Georgia, and the federal building in Oklahoma, numerous other acts of violence including those in Waco, Texas, and less publicized acts of violence perpetrated by various groups for political and religious reasons. It is not surprising that the United States ranks among the highest of all Western countries in violent crime (Feierbend, Feierbend, & Nesvold, 1969; Gurr, 1969; Gurr & Bishop, 1976).

The image of machismo among Latino males has often been used as an example of a cultural attitude supporting the appropriateness of violence. Wolfgang and Ferracuti (1967) found that groups with high rates of homicide were also characterized by extremely high rates of rape and aggravated assault, which constituted evidence of a subculture of violence.

Cultural values have also been found to determine differences in the rates of violence among societies in studies conducted by anthropologists. In Ruth Benedict's (1934) *Patterns of Culture* she contrasted the peaceful Zuni Indians of New Mexico with the hostility and violence among natives residing in the Island of Dobu in Melanesia; Margaret Mead's (1935) *Sex and Temperament in Three Primitive Societies* demonstrated that aggression was defined by society, not by biology. More recently scholars have examined street violence and political violence cross-culturally (Archer & Gartner, 1984; Gurr, 1969; Gurr & Bishop, 1976; Hibbs, 1973), marital and sibling violence cross-culturally (Steinmetz, 1981, 1982, 1987), and national and regional differences in wife abuse, (Yllö, 1983), homicide (Phillips, 1983), and rape (Baron & Straus, 1989).

Glaser (1986) has suggested that our frontier mentality during early colonial days with emphasis on gun ownership to protect the early settlers from Native Americans, slaves, and convicts "sentenced" to deportation to America, made gun ownership necessary. In contrast, only the upper class had guns in Europe, and the formalized concept of dueling was the gentleman's way of resolving serious conflicts. This, according to Glaser, was translated into the gunfights of the western frontier that are emulated in gang-related turf and drive-by shootings in contemporary American society. Other scholars have suggested that beginning in the 1870s, as a result of rapid immigration and the development of slums, violence was a fact of daily life (Taff & Ross, 1969). This trend of violence as commonplace in America is present today.

Cultural values are also a prominent part of the explanation of child abuse and sibling violence (Steinmetz, 1977), courtship violence (Goodchild & Zellman, 1984; Lundberg-Love & Geffner, 1986), partner abuse (Davies, 1994; Hanmer, Radford, & Stanko, 1989; Lazarus-Black & Hirsch, 1994), and elder abuse (Block & Sennott, 1980; Steinmetz, 1988). Finkelhor (1979) argued that the sexual abuse of children is legitimated in our society by prevalence of child pornography, relatively weak criminal sanctions against sexual abuse of children, and toleration of a sexual interest in children as portrayed in advertisement. Most recently the sensationalist killing of Jonbenet Ramsey, a 6-year-old, whose videos of her performances during beauty contests portrayed her more like a sultry 20-year-old exotic dancer than a wholesome 6-year-old child, provided further evidence of the tendency in our society to eroticize the actions of even the youngest girls.

Sociocultural theories of violence focus on the macro-level conditions that lead to violence such as sexism, racism, ageism, poverty, inadequate housing, unemployment or underemployment, and unequal opportunity. Although caution must be used when linking societal levels of aggression to interpersonal and familial levels of aggression, Steinmetz (1977, 1987, 1988) found both theoretical and empirical support for this position. Langman (1973) linked child-rearing methods that parents used and the amount of interpersonal aggression considered tolerable. Bellak and Antell (1974) found that the aggressive treatment of a child by his or her parents was correlated as well as measures of suicide and homicide with the aggressiveness displayed by the child on the playground in Germany, Italy, and Denmark.

Studies based on the data in the Human Relations Area Files reveal that incidence of wife beating in 71 primitive societies was positively correlated with invidious displays of wealth, pursuit of military glory, bellicosity, institutionalized boasting, exhibitionistic dancing, and sensitivity to insults (Slater & Slater, 1965). Lester (1980) and Masumura (1979), in studies of less modernized cultures, found that wife beating was more common in societies characterized by marital instability, societies with higher levels of homicide, suicide, feuding, warfare, personal crime, and aggression, and societies in which women were devalued. Matrilocal societies were found to be characterized by intrasocietal "peacefulness" (Divale, 1974; Van Valzen & Wetering, 1960) and exhibited less feuding (Otterbein & Otterbein, 1965).

Whiting (1965) reported less wife beating in societies that lived in extended-family forms. Steinmetz (1981, 1982, 1987) compared the societal violence profiles from a number of studies with marital violence scores for Finland, Puerto Rico, Canada, Israel, Belize (British Honduras), and the United States. In general, political and civil profiles of violence and marital violence scores were similar within each society. One exception was the high levels of violence among kibbutz families in Israel, where norms of sexual equality and the availability of numerous kin would have predicted lower levels of spousal violence. One explanation for these findings can be extrapolated from the Demos (1970) study of the early American colonists, who lived in cramped quarters and went to great lengths to avoid family conflict, but had high rates of conflict with their neighbors. It is possible that the reverse was occurring on the kibbutz, where preserving the community peace is of extreme importance so the kibbutz family keeps the conflicts within the family in order to preserve the more important communal tranquillity.

Steinmetz (1981, 1987) also examined sibling violence cross-culturally. Finland and Puerto Rico, societies shown to be consistently low on all societal measures of violence, had relatively low scores on sibling violence. However, Canada and the United States, societies that scored fairly high on all measures of societal violence, had somewhat higher sibling scores.

Subcultural Theories

Subcultural theories are based on the notion that violent traditions, norms, and skills are present among certain groups within society (Gunn, 1973). Wolfgang and Ferracuti (1967) postulate that violence is primarily confined to a relatively homogeneous subcultural group in which members learn that power, money, respect, and success are achieved through the use of violence. These subcultures exist among underprivileged, lower class males, especially in minority ghettos.

Wolfgang and Ferracuti's (1967) concept of a subculture of violence is based on the premise that rates of violence among certain segments of the population are higher or lower due to differential acceptance and approval of the use of violence. They suggested that individuals in the lower class have a greater emphasis on force and violence because they are powerless to achieve their goals through other means. These researchers suggested that the documented high rates of homicide and aggravated assault in the South are indications of acceptability of using violence to resolve conflicts.

Gastil (1971) developed an index of "southernness," which was based on the percentage of population that was of southern origin. This accounted for more variance in state homicide rate than other demographic indices such as income, urbanization, or median age. Amir (1971) found that 77% of the rapes reported during the study year were committed by offenders who were identified as low status and poor. The southern culture of violence has been challenged by other researchers (Doerner, 1978; Erlanger, 1975). However, Lundsgaarde (1977) reported that Houston police did not classify a crime as murder, and sometimes the crime was not prosecuted at all when the police regarded it as a legitimate provocation, such as adultery.

Poverty (Lewis, 1966; Liebow, 1967) and relative poverty (Blau & Blau, 1982; Merton, 1957; Williams, 1984) have been offered as subcultural explanations for violence. Loftin and Hill (1974) found that extreme poverty accounted for the variation in state homicide rates. J. R. Blau and Blau (1982) used the Gini Coefficient, which is a measure of inequality in income, and differences in income between races to account for variation in homicide rates in the 125 largest metropolitan areas.

Other subcultural explanations for violence include masculinity or machismo (Glaser, 1986; Steinmetz & Straus, 1974); ethnic difference in child abuse (Garbarino & Ebata, 1983); social class and ethnic variation in marital, child, and sibling violence (Gelles & Straus, 1988; Straus *et al.*, 1980); race and ethnicity, in sexual abuse (Pierce & Pierce, 1984); rural environment (Russell, 1984); and lower-class status (Finkelhor, 1979; Steinmetz, 1987).

Rather than seeing violence as pathological, functional theory focuses on the purpose that violence serves in society such as defining group boundaries for "acceptable" violence and punishing those who cross the boundaries, thus strengthening the group norms regarding acceptable behavior. As an example, we can examine the murder of Nichole Simpson and the trial of her ex-husband which held the national interest for nearly 2 years. In part this was because of O. J. Simpson's status as a former football star and recent movie star, but in part it was also because of the difficulty of reconciling the public view of this hero with the atrocity of the act he was charged with committing. This event served a positive function. Simpson's acquittal of the criminal charge by a predominant African American jury and conviction on the civil charge by a white jury gave the appearance that law enforcement and the judicial system are not color blind, stimulating considerable discussion over needed reforms.

Symbolic Interaction Theory

Symbolic interaction theory is concerned with the processes involved in defining action such as an act of violence. Symbolic Interaction has two schools of thought (Meltzer & Petras, 1972). The first was the Chicago school, led by Blumer with an emphasis on the interpretive process in the social construction of meaning, and the use of life histories, autobiographies, and case studies so richly demonstrated in *The Polish Peasant* (W. I. Thomas & Znaniecki, 1918–1920). The second school of thought, the Iowa School, was led by Manfred Kuhn (1964) and was concerned with efforts to construct and test hypotheses based on symbolic interaction propositions.

Symbolic interaction theory considers the interpretation that is placed on social phenomena, not the phenomena in a pure sense, to provide an understanding of human behavior. W. I. Thomas's definition of the situation "If men define situations as real, they are real in their consequences" (W. I. Thomas & Thomas, 1928, p. 572) is the key to this theory. As LaRossa and Reitz (1993) note, if a parent believes that a crying infant is doing so to be malicious, then that reality will have implications for how the parents will interact with that child.

Street crime frequently caught on videotape likewise will be interpreted differently based on the social class, ethnicity, and residential proximity to the incident. Outsiders may interpret the violence as an indication of crime, poverty, disrespect for laws, and predilection of people in the community toward violence. Insiders, on the other hand, might see the incident as an isolated event that was given media attention to reinforce negative impressions of minorities.

A symbolic interaction perspective also focuses on roles, shared norms, and systems of meaning that are attached to social positions (Heiss, 1981). These roles have several purposes: They encompass knowledge, ability, and motivation (Brim, 1966); they consist of the emotional content attached to the roles (Hochschild, 1979); and they are complementary to other roles, vary based on social position, and have "careers" that change over time (Goffman, 1959).

In spouse abuse the degree to which a spouse does not fill the role expectations of the partner predicts the likelihood of abuse in a violent family. Numerous accounts of battering incidents lay the blame on the wife for not having dinner on the table on time, not having the house cleaned as expected, and not obeying the rules set out by the husband. Likewise the child who does not fill the parents' expectations for some real reason (disability or chronic illness) or perceived reason (refusal to stop crying or soiling his or her diapers) is at risk of abuse.

Gelles (1974) and Steinmetz (1977) suggest that the perception of the individual is an important component of this process. The individual's perception of the family relationship has been a critical factor in child abuse (Friedrich & Borisking, 1976), family interaction (Niemi, 1974), suicide (Lester, 1968), family violence (Steinmetz, 1977, 1987), and elder abuse (Steinmetz, 1988). From a symbolic interaction perspective, it is not just the interaction itself that is important, but also the symbolic interpretation placed on the act that must be considered. Thus, a slap may be labeled as unacceptable violence by one wife who seeks help from a crisis center whereas a 2-minute beating is viewed by another wife as a loss of temper not worthy of mentioning.

Initiation rites into membership of various groups and organizations such as gangs, fraternities, and special groups in the military, have used violence to test a member's willingness to obey unquestioningly. The gratuitous violence often associated with initiation rites is embedded in a context that for members fills the role expectations of loyalty, character, and obedience.

Identity Theory

Identities are the meanings that individuals give to the roles they fulfill; the greater the salience of an identity, the more motivated an individual will be to perform the role according to cultural expectations. Stets (1990), using a symbolic interaction perspective, found that an aggressive identity encourages violence. Identities, used in this way, serve a function similar to the mechanism in a subculture of violence theory. The major difference is that the identity is personal, whereas the subcultural meaning is a shared group belief and behavior.

Labeling Theory

Developed by Howard Becker (1963), labeling theory is based on the premise that it is not solely the act that is defined as deviant or criminal but also the rules and sanctions that others in positions of power and dominance place on the act. This is often the case with rape, in which the character, appearance, location of the crime, and time of day appear to be important considerations in a jury's or the public's view of whether the act was consensual or forced (LaFree, 1989). A similar case existed for wife abuse which was, until recently, labeled as a private matter between spouses and the right of a husband to discipline his wife, not a criminal act of assault and battery.

The label placed on the behavior by others frequently takes precedence in the definition of the behavior to a greater degree than either the actual behavior or the individual's definition of the behavior. The definition of child abuse by a welfare caseworker carries the power to define the parents' behavior as abuse or neglect even when the parents, child, or other family members do not define the behavior as abusive.

Escalation as a result of social controllers (police) labeling an incident as potentially violent can lead to further violence (G. Marx, 1981; McNamara, 1967). McNamara (1967) conducted a 3-year study of police–citizen incidents and found that police frequently escalated relatively minor situations such as traffic violations and husband–wife disputes into more serious situations. G. Marx provides the example of the high-speed chase in which a 15-year-old was being chased by two police cars at 95 miles an hour. When the young driver killed a patrolman on the street, he was charged not only with speeding, but with manslaughter.

On a larger scale, this was demonstrated by the fire bombing of the Move cult in Philadelphia and the more recent bombing of the cult in Waco, Texas. These acts and similar ones were undertaken by the government because of a fear that these groups might commit acts of violence.

Social-Learning–Role-Modeling Theories

General

Social-learning theory, which views violence as a learned phenomenon, has received support in studies utilizing a laboratory setting (Bandura, 1973; Bandura & Walters, 1963; Bandura, Ross, & Ross, 1961; Singer, 1971) as well as clinical studies (Walker, 1977–1978) and survey research (see Steinmetz, 1987, for a review of these studies).

The social-learning and role modeling theories assume that individuals learn violent behavior first as children when they see their parents or significant others resolving problems with violence. They model this role of violent interpersonal interactions when they become parents. Social-learning theory, specifically as it explains learned helplessness, has been used to describe the processes of battering (Walker, 1977–1978). Social learning has also been used to explain rape as an aggressive behavior that was learned from observing violent acts against women usually through the mass media (Ellis, 1989).

Although we have attempted to group the theories into specific categories, it appears that most theories have been influenced and modified by other theories. For example, Glaser (1986), drawing from the symbolic interaction approach (Blumer, 1969; Mead, 1935), and social learning theory (Baldwin & Baldwin, 1978; Bandura, 1973) noted that violence among humans tends to evoke counterviolence and violence in one setting or relationship tends to spread to their settings. Unless interrupted, violence tends to escalate and to become more widespread.

Sex-Role Theory

This theory proposes that gender-based childhood socialization serves as a foundation for violence (McCall & Shields, 1986). For example, traditional sex-role socialization has the effect of "training" young girls to be submissive and boys to be dominant. This socialization results in women's accepting their victimization as abused wives and their male partners' belief that their use of violence against their partners is their right (Steinmetz, 1979; Walker, 1977–1978).

In a similar manner, Watkins (1982, as cited in McCall & Shields, 1986) has suggested that sexual socialization during childhood wherein boys are taught to be sexual aggressors and girls are taught to be physically and sexually attractive to men sets the stage for sexual abuse of women. Finkelhor (1979) and Russell (1984) have linked sexual abuse of children to role confusion in which the incestuous father or father figure treats the child as a wife rather than a daughter. Similar role confusion has been labeled as role reversal when children are physically abused because they do not fulfill the parents' needs by behaving as an adult (Steele & Pollock, 1974); role reversal also occurs as elder abuse in generationally inversed families (Steinmetz, 1988).

It appears that over the past few decades girls are being socialized to be more similar to males in their use of violence. This position is supported by the substantial increase in violent crimes committed by adolescent girls and women, as well as the increase in exclusively female gangs and female membership in male gangs (Steinmetz, 1999).

Exchange and Resource Theory

Exchange theory has some basis in Etzioni's concept that one will attempt to maximize individual benefit. Exchange theorists (P. M. Blau, 1964; Homans, 1961, 1974) posit that individuals will engage in behavior either to avoid punishment or earn rewards. The rule of distributive justice is key in Homans's view of exchange interactions. This rule, according to Homans (1961), states: "A man in an exchange relation will expect that the rewards of each man be proportional to his costs—the greater the rewards, the greater the costs—and that the new rewards, or profits, of each man be proportional to his investments" (p. 75).

Exchange theory asserts that marital interaction is governed by an attempt to maximize rewards and minimize costs. Therefore, violence would be used as a method for attempting to restore distributive justice when the costs are perceived by one individual to be exceeding the rewards.

In some ways, this theory is similar to resource theory, in which violence is used as a resource to gain one's wishes in a manner similar to money, status, and the individual's personal attributes. Goode (1971) hypothesized that the greater the nonviolent resources available to an individual, the more force that individual has the ability to use, but the less he or she will actually deploy this force overtly. Thus, violence is used as a resource when all else fails or is perceived to have failed. Gelles (1976) reported that the fewer the resources a woman has, the more likely she is to remain with a severely abusive husband.

Other research has demonstrated the impact of power differential as relative resources in explanation of spousal violence (Gelles, 1976; Gelles & Straus, 1979, 1988;

Straus *et al.*, 1980), parental violence against children as a last resort (Gelles & Straus, 1979, 1988; Steinmetz, 1987), and elder abuse (Steinmetz, 1988).

Conflict Theory

Farrington and Chertok (1993), in their historical overview of conflict theories, trace the early beginnings of conflict theory to Niccolo Machiavelli (1469–1527) and Thomas Hobbes (1588–1679). Both of these social philosophers viewed human nature as resulting in conflict among individuals because of pure self-interests; this conflict needed to be controlled by the state. Competition over scarce resources was viewed by Thomas Malthus (1766–1834) and later Karl Marx (1867/1967) as inevitable sources of conflict. Malthus and Darwin believed that when these self-interests (or species needs) were not fulfilled, the individuals or species became extinct. Thus some individuals were able to meet their needs and survived; other were not as fortunate, or as fit, and they perished. Violence, in order to meet the group's needs when other means fail, is the end product.

Other early conceptions of conflict theory are presented by Hegel, who was concerned with dialectics, a process of change that results when the "thesis" is challenged and resulting in "antithesis." Over time, alterations or modification occur, which Hegel called "synthesis." Marx's (1867/1967) theory, based on class conflict between the bourgeois owners of the means of production and the proletariat who are the instruments of production, provided the foundation for modern conflict theory which examines power differentials based on social class, race, gender, age, and so on.

The connection between Hegel's dialectic theory and Marxian conflict theory are evident; change brought about by reactions to circumstances considered to be unfair or against one's best interest results in changes in social structure or social relations.

A conflict theory of violence assumes that conflict is an inevitable part of all dyads or groups characterized by positions of dominance and submission (which may be reversed with each new interaction) and competing goals. One can examine society's treatment of domestic violence from this perspective. Prior to the 1970s, battering men were frequently given a slap on the wrist or at most a stern lecture by the courts for battering their partner. With the changing attitudes and laws with regard to domestic violence, batterers now faced stiffer penalties, often with prison terms. However, women, fearing retribution, frequently withdrew charges or failed to appear in court. The synthesis, an altering of the laws so that battering was a crime against the state, not the woman, removed the victim from the burden of bringing charges of battering.

Because the family can be viewed as an arena of confrontation and conflicting interests (Sprey, 1969), violence is a likely outcome and a powerful mode of advancing one's interests when all others fail. Important to an understanding of a conflict theory of violence is Weber's (1947) clarification and differentiation of the terms authority and power as used by Dahrendorf (1958) in his discussion of a theory of social conflict. Authority is defined as the probability that a command content will be obeyed by a given group of persons, whereas power is the probability that one actor within a social relationship will be in a position to carry out his own will despite resistance.

Confrontations within the family often occur when an individual has the authority but not the power to demand certain behavior. Numerous reports exist of parents severely battering an infant who would not stop crying, or a toddler who would not stop wetting the bed. These parents felt that their authority was being questioned by the child, and that they lacked the power to control the child's undesirable behavior.

A widespread example of incongruity between authority and power occurs when parents of teenagers realize that, although they still have the legal authority to "control" their child, they may not have the "power" to carry out their desires if the child rebels (Steinmetz, 1977). When this happens, parents resort to physical violence (Bachman, 1967; Steinmetz, 1974, 1987; Straus *et al.*, 1980). This authority, sans power, has also been offered as an explanation of marital conflict and wife beating (Allen & Straus, 1979; Kolb & Straus, 1974; O'Brian, 1971).

Conflict theory has also been useful in explaining civil disruption when leaders of a faction are unable to obtain their goals, or perceive that they are unable to obtain their goals, through other means.

Marxist Theory

The Marxist approach sees the source of violence as an economic and political phenomenon. Women and minorities are an oppressed economic class deprived of economic control, political power, and status. They are victimized by the Euro-American, patriarchal, capitalistic system, which fosters control of the oppressed (female, minority) class by their oppressors. Violence, as a male's mechanism of controlling females or as the Euro-Americans' control over minorities is a logical extension of this theory.

Interest-Group Theory

Thorsten Sellin was one of the earliest scholars using the perspective of interest-group theory to explain criminal behavior in his monograph *Culture, Conflict and Crime* (1938). Sellin claims that during periods of rapid social change, often resulting from immigration to the United States (or mass migration from one part of the country to another such as the patterns of migration of rural Blacks to the northern manufacturing states), groups with different values and norms border each other. The behavior of one group may appear deviant to the other groups, producing cultural conflict.

Turk's (1969) theory of criminalization explains how the more powerful group defines the behaviors of the less powerful group as criminal. This theoretical approach has been utilized by Quinney (1970) and Chambliss and Seidman (1971) to illustrate how laws and social policy reflect the views of the more dominant and powerful sectors of society. From this perspective, which shares many similarities with Merton's topology discussed under functionalism, it is predicted that as women continue to gain more power in the political, economic, and policy-making realms, rape will more consistently be defined as a violent crime with severe penalties, rather than a sexual behavior incited by women. Likewise, the derogatory treatment of minorities, including police brutality, will no longer be tolerated, in part because of the increased power of minorities in decision-making and political positions.

Feminist Theories

Although feminist theory is closely identified with Marxist theory, Osmond and Thorne (1993) suggested that there is a wide range of feminist-oriented theories and not all are Marxist in philosophy. They note, however, that a common theme in feminine thought is the "Centrality, normality, and value of women's (and girls') experiences" (p.

592). Feminist theory is an action-oriented theory with a goal of not only understanding phenomena from a women's perspective, but trying to change the phenomena.

Radical feminist theory emerged from the women's movement in the late 1960s; this perspective is based on the patriarch with male power and dominance who oppresses women. Radical feminist theory has been used to explain wife beating as an example of the victimization of a gender-oppressed class that is a socially produced, male-dominated, sanctioned pattern of interaction. From this perspective, the abusive husband is simply an expected product of his society. Only by eliminating socially instituted sexism can women reduce their victimization. A feminist theory of rape is seen as resulting from the powerlessness of women, which produces dependency and subservience to men and gives them the right to dominate and control women by any means (Dworkin, 1981; Ellis, 1989; Brownmiller, 1975).

Socialist feminist theory, which is most closely tied to classical Marxist theory, sees wife beating as a political act resulting from the patriarchal capitalistic society's domination over women. The radical feminist and social feminist theories have limited utility in explaining violence that is perpetrated by women against men or violence in gay relationships because men are assumed power holders. Explaining lesbian violence, from these perspectives, because both partners are members of the oppressed gender, is also problematic. Unfortunately, abuse exists in both gay and lesbian relationships (Coleman, 1994; Island & Letellier, 1991; Letellier, 1994; Renzetti, 1992), and males are abused by their female partners (see Steinmetz, 1987; Miller, Knudsen, and Coperhaver, 1999, for reviews of this research).

A liberal feminist theory assumes that men and women are endowed with equal capabilities and they reject competitive individualism and a strict division between public and private spheres. Liberal feminists are committed to changing social policy and legal barriers to equality. Liberal feminist theory is essentially a resource theory in which the goal is to equalize the resources between males and females in order to produce equal status. It is the unequal distribution of resources, a resource theory perspective, that produces violence. Unlike radical and socialist feminist theory, liberal feminist theory is useful in explaining both women and men as victims of domestic violence and supports research on violence in gay and lesbian relationships.

Feminist theories can also be considered an example of a social structural theory. The basic assumption in many of these theories is that the patriarchal, capitalistic nature of society reinforces the ideal of male dominance and power over women (Dobash & Dobash, 1979; Russell, 1984, 1988). Thus the male's use of violence against his partner is an extension of his right to control all his property. Although we no longer uphold the old English law that permitted men to whip their wives with a stick no bigger than their thumb; or a later Missouri law that told citizens to look away if there was no permanent damage (Steinmetz, 1977), punishment for men who beat their partners is likely to be less harsh than punishment for men who use similar violence against a stranger.

Postpositivistic, Postmodernism, Deconstructionism

Doherty, Boss, LaRossa, Schumm, & Steinmetz (1993) suggested that postpositivism, which has also been called postmodernism or deconstructionism, demands a recognition that theory is socially constructed and precedes observation and that without theory there are no facts. Theory is the lens through which social phenomena are viewed and without the lens one is blind. Jeffrey Alexander (1988) has noted that social scientists evaluate human behavior as well as describe it—the discourse as well as traditional scientific verification and explanation.

Postmodernism, like feminist theory, questions the basic Enlightenment assumptions that truth can be discovered through the scientific method of logic and reason in a value-free, unbiased way. Rather than universal truths, most positivistic theories are based on the Eurocentric views derived from the experiences of privileged males.

Postmodern theory would deconstruct our view of violence and attempt to explore the motivations from the actors' perspectives. For example, the positivist view of assault would be based on observation and recording of data based on the facts, for example, an individual is arrested for stealing another's wallet. When we deconstruct this act, we may see a poor person who steals another's wallet by force in order to get money to survive—violence as an act of self-defense. Deconstructed, violence may be the result of hunger or lack of adequate clothing and medicine. Those viewed as committing violence might be the restaurant owner who throws away great quantities of food and the health department administrators who developed codes that require restaurants to discard unserved food; the clothing manufacturer who exploits women and children's labor but prices the clothing out of the reach of the poor; and the pharmaceutical companies and the FDA because of costly requirements to test and produce life-saving medicine.

Summary

The definition of an act as violent, the punishment administered, the rehabilitation (if any), are all shaped by the particular lens through which the act has been viewed. No longer are the lenses those of Eurocentric, privileged males. The lenses now have many voices: female, African American, Hispanic American, Asian American, Native American, middle class, working class, underclass, the poor, and the disenfranchised. Thus we must examine more critically the assumptions behind the explanation we select to explain violence.

Durkheim in *The Rules of Sociological Method* (1964: 68) noted that "for murder to disappear, the horror of bloodshed must become greater in those social strata from which murderers are recruited; but, first, it must become greater throughout the entire society" (pp. 78–79). More recently, the *Journal of the American Medical Association* (Fingerhut and Kleinmen, 1990) suggested that any plan to reduce homicides must also address strategies to promote nonviolent resolution of interpersonal conflict as well as strategies to prevent crime.

The violence in our society and in the world is so prevalent that regardless of the theoretical lens through which we view it, we can no longer ignore it. Unfortunately, as the mechanisms to find socially defined success within the socially accepted means diminish, violence can be expected to be a way that individuals and groups select when there are no other means for fulfilling their needs.

ACKNOWLEDGMENT

I wish to thank my husband, Thomas E. Pickett, for research and editorial assistance, and William Stuckey for his dedication in getting my incorrigible computer running without the use of violence.

References

Alexander, J. C. (1988). The new theoretical movement. In N. J. Smelser (Ed.), *Handbook of Sociology* (pp. 77–101). Newbury Park, CA: Sage.

Allen, C. M. & Straus, M. A. (1979). Resources, power, and husband–wife violence. In M. A. Straus & G. T. Hotaling (Eds.), *The social causes of husband–wife violence* (pp. 188–208). Minneapolis: University of Minnesota Press.

Allison, J. A., & Wrightsman, L. S. (1993). *Rape: The misunderstood crime.* Newbury Park, CA: Sage.

Amir, M. (1971). *Patterns in forcible rape.* Chicago: University of Chicago Press.

Archer, D., & Gartner, M. R. (1984) *Violence and crime in cross-national perspective.* New Haven, CT: Yale University Press.

Bach, G. R., & Wyden, P. (1968). *The intimate enemy: How to fight fair in love and marriage.* New York: Morrow.

Bachman, J. G. (1967). *Youth in transition.* Ann Arbor: University of Michigan Institute for Social Research.

Bakan, D. (1971). *Slaughter of the innocents: A study of the battered child phenomenon.* Boston: Beacon.

Baldwin, J. D., & Baldwin, J. I. (1978). Behaviorism on Versteen and Erklaren. *American Sociological Review, 43,* 335–347.

Bandura, A. (1973). *Aggression: A social learning analysis.* Englewood Cliffs, NJ, Prentice-Hall.

Bandura, A., & Walters, R. H. (1963). *Social learning and personality development.* New York: Holt, Rinehart, & Winston.

Bandura, A., Ross, D., & Ross, A. (1961). Transmission of aggression through imitation of aggressive models. *Journal of Abnormal Social Psychology, 63,* 575–582.

Baron, L., & Straus, M. A. (1989). *Four theories of rape in American society: A state level analysis.* New Haven, CT: Yale University Press.

Becker, H. (1963). *Outsiders: Studies in the sociology of deviance.* Glencoe, IL: Free Press.

Bellak, L., & Antell, M. (1974). An intellectual study of aggressive behavior on children's playgrounds. *American Journal of Orthopsychiatry, 44*(4), 503–511.

Benedict, R. (1934). *Patterns of culture.* Boston: Houghton Mifflin.

Blau, J. R., & Blau, P. M. (1982). The cost of inequality: Metropolitan structure and violent crime. *American Sociological Review, 47,* 114–128.

Blau, P. M. (1964). *Exchange and power in social life.* New York: Wiley.

Block, M., & Sennott, J. P. (1980). Elder abuse: The hidden problem. Prepared statement briefing by the Select Committee on Aging, U.S. House of Representatives (96) June 23, 1979, pp. 10–12, Boston, MA. Washington DC: Government Printing Office.

Blumer, H. (1969). *Symbolic interactionism: Perspective and methods.* Englewood Cliffs, NJ: Prentice-Hall.

Brim, O. G. (1966). Socialization through the life cycle. In O. G. Brim & S. Wheeler (Eds.), *Socialization after childhood* (pp. 1–49). New York: Wiley.

Brown, C. (1965). *Manchild in the promised land.* New York: New American Library.

Brownmiller, S. (1975). *Against our will: Men, women and rape.* New York: Simon & Schuster.

Chambliss, W. J., & Seidman, R. (1971). *Law, order and power.* Reading MA: Addison-Wesley.

Children's Defense Fund. (1994). *Wasting America's future: The Children's Defense Fund report on the costs of child poverty.* Washington, DC: Author.

Chandler, K. A., Chapman, C. D., Rand, M. R., & Taylor, D. M. (1998). *Students' reports of school crime: 1989 and 1995.* U.S. Departments of Education and Justice. NCES 98–241/NCJ-169607. Washington, DC.

Coleman, V. E. (1994). Lesbian battering: The relationship between personality and the perpetration of violence. *Violence and Victims, 9,* 139–152.

Coser, L. (1956). *The functions of social conflict.* New York: Free Press.

Curry, G. D. (1996). *National youth gang surveys: A review of methods and findings.* Office of Juvenile Justice and Delinquency Prevention. Washington, DC: U.S. Department of Justice.

Curry, G. D., Ball, R. A., & Decker, S. H. (1996). Estimating the national scope of gang crime from law enforcement data. In C. R. Huff (ed.), *Gangs in America,* 2nd ed. (pp. 21–36). Thousand Oaks, CA: Sage.

Dahrendorf, R. (1958). Towards a theory of social conflict. *Journal of Conflict Resolution, 2,* 170–183.

Darwin, C. R. (1859). *On the origin of species.* London: John Murray.

Davies, M. (Ed.). (1994). *Women and violence: Realities and responses worldwide.* London: Zed Books.

Davis, R. H. (1980). *Television and the aging audience.* Los Angeles: University of Southern California Press.

Demos, J. (1970). *A little commonwealth.* New York: Oxford University Press.

Divale, W. T. (1974). Migration extended warfare and matrilocal residence. *Behavior Science Research, 9,* 75–133.

Dobash, R. E., & Dobash, R. (1979). *Violence against wives*. New York: Free Press.

Doherty, W. J., Boss, P. G., LaRossa, R., Schumm, W. R., & Steinmetz, S. K. (1993). Family theories and methods: A contextual approach. In P. G. Boss, W. J. Doherty, R. LaRossa, W. R. Schumm, & S. K. Steinmetz (Eds.), *Sourcebook of family theories and methods: A contextual approach* (pp. 3–30). New York: Plenum.

Doerner, W. G. (1978). The index of Southernness revisited: The influence of where from upon whodunit (with comments by Loftin & Hill, and by Gastil). *Criminology, 16,* 47–88.

Donner, L. (1990). Television and violence. In L J. Hertzberg, G. F. Ostrum, & J. R. Field (Eds.), *Violent behavior: Vol 1. Assessment and intervention* (pp. 151–166). Great Neck, NY: PMA.

Durkheim, E. (1964). *The Rules of sociological method*. Glencoe, IL: Free Press.

Durkheim, E. (1966). *Suicide*. New York: Free Press. (Originally published in 1897)

Dworkin, A. (1981). *Pornography: Men possessing women*. New York: Perigee.

Ellis, L. (1989). *Theories of rape: Inquiries into the causes of sexual aggression*. New York: Hemisphere.

Erlanger, H. (1975). Is there a "Subculture of Violence" in the South? *Journal of Criminal Law and Criminology, 66,* 483–490.

Etzioni, A. (1988). *The moral dimension: Toward a new economics*. New York: Free Press.

Farrington, K., & Chertok, E. (1933). Social conflict theories of the family. In P. C. Boss, W. J. Doherty, R. LaRossa, W. R. Schumm, & S. K. Steinmetz (Eds.), *Sourcebook of family theories and methods: A contextual approach* (pp. 357–381). New York: Plenum.

Feierbend, I. K., Feierbend, R. L. (1966). Aggressive behaviors within politics, 1948–1962: A cross-national study. *Journal of Conflict Resolution, 10,* pp. 249–271

Feierbend, I. K., Feierbend, R. L., & Nesvold, B. A. (1969). Social change and political violence: Cross national pattern. In H. D. Graham & T. R. Gurr (Eds.), *Violence in America: Historical and comparative perspective* (pp. 632–687). Washington, DC: U.S. Government Printing Office.

Finkelhor, D. (1979). *Sexually victimized children*. New York: Free Press.

Friedrich, W. N., & Borisking, J. A. (1976). The role of the child in abuse: A review of the literature. *American Journal of Orthopsychiatry, 46,* 580–590.

Garbarino, J., &d Ebata, A. (1983). The significance of ethnic and cultural differences in child maltreatment. *Journal of Marriage and the Family, 45,* 773–783.

Gastil, R. D. (1971). Homicide and a regional culture of violence. *American Sociological Review, 36,* 412–427.

Gelles, R. J. (1974). Abused wives: Why do they stay? *Journal of Marriage and the Family, 38,* 659–668.

Gelles, R. J., & Straus, M. A. 91979). Determinants of violence in the family: Toward a theoretical integration. In W. R. Burr, R. Hill, F. I. Nye, & I. L. Reiss (Eds.), *Contemporary theories about the family* (Vol. 1, pp. 549–581). New York: Free Press.

Gelles, R. J., & Straus, M. A. (1988). *Intimate violence*. New York: Simon and Schuster.

Gerbner, G. (1972). Violence in television drama: Trends and symbolic functions. In G. A. Comstock & E. A. Rubinstein (Eds.), *Television and social behavior: Vol. 1. Media content and control* (pp. 28–188). Washington, DC: U.S. Government Printing Office.

Gibson, L., Linden, R., & Johnson, S. (1980). A situational theory of rape. *Canadian Journal of Criminology, 22,* 51–63.

Glaser, D. (1986). Violence in the society. In M. Lystad (Ed.), *Violence in the home: interdisciplinary perspectives* (pp. 5–31). New York: Brunner/Mazel.

Goffman, E. (1959). The moral career of the mental patient. *Psychiatry: Journal for the Study of Interpersonal Process, 22,* 123–142.

Goodchild, J. D., & Zellman, G. L. (1984). Sexual signaling and sexual aggression in adolescent relationships. In N. Malamuth & E. Donnerstein (Eds.), *Pornography and sexual aggression* (pp. 233–243). New York: Academic Press.

Goode, W. J. (1971). Force and violence in the family. *Journal of Marriage and the Family, 33* (November), 624–636.

Gouldner, A. (1970). *The coming crisis of Western sociology*. New York: Basic Books.

Graham, H. D., & Gurr, T. R. (1969). *The history of violence in America: A report to the National Commission on the Causes and Prevention of Violence*. New York: Bantam.

Gunn, J. (1973). *Violence*. New York: Praeger.

Gurr, T. R. 91969). A comparative study of civil strife. In H. D. Graham & T. R. Gurr (Eds.), *Violence in America: Historical and comparative perspectives* (pp. 572–626). Washington, DC: U.S. Government Printing Office.

Gurr, T. R., & Bishop, V. F. (1976). Violent nation and others. *Journal of Conflict Resolution, 20,* 79–110.

Hagen, R. (1979). *The bio-sexual factor*. Garden City, NY: Doubleday.

Hanmer, J., Radford, J., & Stanko, E. A. (Eds.). (1989). *Women, policing, and male violence: International perspectives.* New York: Routledge.

Heiss, J. (1981). Social Roles. In M. Rosenberg & R. H. Turner (Eds.), *Social psychology: Sociological perspectives* (pp. 94–132). New York: Basic Books.

Henry, A. F., & Short, J. F., Jr. (1954). *Suicide and homicide.* New York: Free Press.

Hibbs, D. A., Jr. (1973). *Mass political violence: A cross-national causal analysis.* New York: Wiley.

Hirschi, T. (1969). *The causes of delinquency.* Berkeley: University of California Press.

Hochschild, A. R. (1979). Emotional work, feeling rules, and social structure. *American Journal of Sociology, 85,* 551–575.

Homans, G. C. (1961). *Social behavior: Its elemental forms.* New York: Harcourt, Brace and World.

Homans, G. C. (1974). *Social behavior: Its Elementary forms* (Rev. ed.). New York: Harcourt, Brace and Jovanovich.

Hornung, C. A., McCullough, B. C., & Sugimoto, T. (1981). Status relationships in marriage: Risk factors in spouse abuse. *Journal of Marriage and the Family, 43,* 675–692.

Huston, A. C., Donnerstein, F., Fairchild, II., Feshback, N. D., Katz, P. A., Murray, J. P., Rubinstein, E. A., Wilcox, B., & Zuckerman, D. (1992). *Big world, small screen: The role of television in American society.* Lincoln: NE: University of Nebraska Press.

Island, D., & Letellier, P. (1991). *Men who beat the men who love them: Battered gay men and domestic violence.* New York: Haworth.

Johansson, S., & Nygren, O. (1991). The missing girls of China: A new demographic account. *Population and Development Review, 17* (March), 35–51.

Kelly, K. D., & Chambliss, W. J. (1966). Status consistency and political attitudes. *American Sociological Review, 31,* 375–382.

Kingsbury, N., & Scanzoni, J. (1993). Structural-functionalism. In P. C. Boss, W. J. Doherty, R. LaRossa, W. R. Schumm, & S. K. Steinmetz (Eds.), *Sourcebook of family theories and methods: A contextual approach* (pp. 195–217). New York: Plenum.

Kolb, T. M., & Straus, M. A. (1974). Marital power and marital happiness in relation to problem solving ability. *Journal of Marriage and the Family, 36,* 756–766.

Korem, D. (1995). *Suburban gangs—The affluent rebels.* Richardson, TX: International Focus Press.

Kuhn, M. (1964). Major trends in symbolic interaction theory in the past twenty-five years. *Sociological Quarterly, 5,* 61–84.

LaFree, G. D. (1989). *Rape and criminal justice: The social construction of sexual assault.* Belmont, CA: Wadsworth.

Langman, L. (1973, August). *Economic practices and socialization in three societies.* Paper presented at the annual meeting of the American Sociological Association, New York.

LaRossa, R., & Reitz, D. C. (1993). Symbolic interactionism and family studies. In P. C. Boss, W. J. Doherty, R. LaRossa, W. R. Schumm, & S. K. Steinmetz (Eds.), *Sourcebook of family theories and methods: A contextual approach* (pp. 135–162). New York: Plenum.

Lazarus-Black, M., & Hirsch, S. F. (Eds.). (1994). *Contested states: Law, hegemony and resistance.* New York: Routledge.

Lenski, G. E. (1954). Status crystallization: As a non-vertical dimension of social status. *American Sociological Review, 19,* 405–413.

Lester, D. (1968). Punishment experiences and suicidal preoccupation. *Journal of Genetic Psychology, 113,* 89–94.

Letellier, P. (1994). Gay and bisexual male domestic violence victimization: Challenges to feminist theory and responses to violence. *Violence and Victims, 9,* 95–106.

Lewis, O. (1966). *La vida: A Puerto Rican family in the culture of poverty.* New York: Random House.

Liebow, E. (1967). *Talley's corner.* Boston: Little, Brown.

Linz, D., Donnerstein, E., & Penrod, S. (1987). The findings and recommendations of the Attorney General's Commission on Pornography: Do the psychological facts fit the political fury? *American Psychologist, 42,* 946–953.

Loftin, C., & Hill, R. H. (1974). Regional subculture and homicide: An examination of Gastil–Hackney thesis. *American Sociological Review, 39,* 714–724.

Lundberg-Love, P., & Geffner, R. (1986). Date rape: Prevalence, risk factors, and a proposed model. In M. A. Pirog-Good & J. E. Stets (Eds.), *Violence in Dating Relationships* (pp. 168–184). New York: Praeger.

Lung, C. T., & Daro, D. (1996). *Current trends in child abuse reporting and fatalities: The results of the 1995 Annual Fifty State Survey.* Chicago, IL: National Committee for the Prevention of Child Abuse.

Lundsgaarde, P. (1977). *Murder in Space City*. New York: Oxford University Press.

MacFarlane, L. S. (1974). *Violence and the state*. London England: Nelson.

Malamuth, N. M., & Donnerstein, E. (1982). The effects of aggressive pornographic mass media stimuli. In L. Berkowitz (Ed.), *Advances in Experimental Social Psychology* (Vol. 15, pp. 103–136). New York: Academic Press.

Malamuth, N. M., & Donnerstein, E. (1984). (Eds.). *Pornography and sexual aggression*. Orlando, FL: Academic Press.

Marsden, D. (1978). Sociological perspectives on family violence. In J. P. Martin (Ed., *Violence and the family* (pp. 103–133). New York: Wiley.

Martin, D. (1976). *Battered wives* (Rev. ed.). San Francisco: Volcano Press.

Marx, G. (1981). Ironies of social control: Authorities as contributors to deviance through escalation, non-enforcement, and covert facilitation. *Social Problems, 18*(3), 221–233.

Marx, K. (1967). *Capital: A critique of political economy: Vol. 1. The process of capitalist production* (S. Moore & E. Aveline, Trans., & F. Engels, Ed.). New York: International Universities Press. (Original work published 1867).

Masumura, W. R. (1979). Wife abuse and other forms of aggression. *Victimology: An International Journal, 4*(1), 46–59.

McCall, G., & Shields, N. M. (1986). Social and structural factors in family violence. In M. Lystad (Ed.), *Violence in the Home* (pp. 98–123). New York: Brunner/Mazel.

McIntyre, D., Jr. (1967). *Law enforcement in the metropolis*. Chicago: American Bar Foundation.

McNamara, J. H. (1967). Uncertainties in police work: The relevance of police recruit's backgrounds and training. In D. J. Bordua (Ed.), *The police: Six sociological essays*, (pp. 163–252). New York: John Wiley.

Mead, M. (1935). *Sex and temperament in three primitive societies*. New York: Morrow.

Meltzer, B. N., & Petras, J. (1972). The Chicago and Iowa schools of symbolic interactionism. In J. G. Manis & B. N. Meltzer (Eds.), *Symbolic interaction: A reader in social psychology* (2nd ed., pp. 43–57). Boston: Allen & Bacon.

Merton, R. K. (1938). Social structure and anomie. *American Sociological Review, 3,*672–682.

Merton, R. K. (1957). *Social theory and social structure*. Glencoe, IL: Free Press.

Miller, J. L., Knudsen, D. D., & Copenhaver, S. (1999). Family violence. In M. B. Sussman, S. K. Steinmetz, & G. P. Peterson (Eds.), *Handbook of marriage and the family* (pp. 705–742). New York: Plenum.

Murray, J. P. (1994). The impact of televised violence. Hofstra Law Review, 22 (4), 809–825.

National Institute of Mental Health (1982). Television and behavior: Ten years of scientific progress and implications for the eighties (vol. 1). Summary report. Washington, D.C.: United States Government Printing Office.

National Television Violence Study: Part One, 1994–5. (1996). Studio City, CA: Mediascope, Inc.

Niemi, R. G. (1974). *How family members perceive each other*. New Haven, CT: Yale University Press.

O'Brian, J. E. (1971). Violence in divorce prone families. *Journal of Marriage and the Family, 30,* 692–698.

Osmond, M. W., & Thorne, B. (1993). Feminist theories: The social construction of gender in families and society. In P. G. Boss, W. J. Doherty, R. LaRossa, W. R. Schumm, & S. K. Steinmetz (Eds.), *Sourcebook of family theories and methods: A contextual approach* (pp. 591–625). New York: Plenum.

Otterbein, K. F., & Otterbein, C. S. (1965). An eye for an eye, a tooth for a tooth: A cross-cultural study of feuding. *American Anthropologist, 67,* 1470–1482.

Paik, H. & Comstock, G. (1994). The effects of television violence on antisocial behavior: A meta-analysis. *Communication Research. 21*(4), 516–546.

Parsons, T. (1937). *The structure of social action*. New York: McGraw-Hill.

Pearl, D. (1982, June 4). Another look at TV and behavior. *ADAMHA News*, p. 4.

Phillips, D. P. (1983). The impact of mass media violence on U.S. homicides. *American Sociological Review, 48,* 560–568.

Pierce, L. H., & Pierce, R. L. (1984). Race as a factor in the sexual abuse of children. *Social Work Research and Abstracts, 20,* 9–14.

Quinney, R. (1970). *The social reality of crime*. Boston: Little, Brown.

Radbill, S. X. (1968). A history of child abuse and infanticide. In R. E. Helper & C. H. Kempe (Eds.), *The Battered Child* (pp. 3–24). Chicago: University of Chicago Press.

Radecki, T. (1981). National Coalition on Television Violence. *(NCTV) News, 2*(3).

Reiss, A., Jr. (1951). Delinquency as the failure of personal and social control. *American Sociological Reviews, 16,* 196–207.

Renzetti, C. M. (1992). *Violent betrayal: Partner abuse in lesbian relationships*. Newbury Park, CA: Sage.

Russell, D. E. H. (1984). *Sexual exploitation: Rape, child sexual abuse and workplace harassment*. Beverly Hills, CA: Sage.

Russell, D. E. H. (1988). Pornography and rape: A causal model. *Political Psychology, 9*, 4173.

Sellin, T. (1938). *Culture, conflict and crime*. Bulletin #41, Social Science Research Council.

Sells, C. W., & Blum, R. W. (1996). Morbidity and mortality among U.S. adolescents: An overview of data and trends. *American Journal of Public Health, 86*(4), 513–519.

Singer, J. L. (1971). The influence of violence portrayed in television or motion pictures upon overt aggressive behavior. In J. L. Singer (Ed.), *The control of aggression and violence: Cognitive and physiological factors* (pp. 19–60). New York: Academic Press.

Skolnick, J. H. (1969). *The politics of protest*. New York: Clarion.

Slater, P., & Slater, D. (1965). Maternal ambivalence and narcissism. *Merrill Palmer Quarterly, 11*, 241–259.

Slee, P. T., & Rigby, K. (1933). Australian school children's self appraisal of interpersonal relations: The bullying experience. *Child Psychiatry and Human Development, 23*(4), 273–282.

Spencer, H. (1888). *Social statics. On the conditions essential to human happiness specified, and first of them developed*. New York: Appleton. (Work originally published in 1852).

Sprey, J. (1969). The family as a system in conflict. *Journal of Marriage and the Family, 33*, 722–31.

Steele, B. F., & Pollock, C. B. (1974). A psychiatric study of parents who abuse infants. In R. E. Helfer & C. H. Kempe (Eds.), *The battered child* (2nd ed., pp. 103–148). Chicago: University of Chicago Press.

Steinmetz, S. K. (1974). *Family backgrounds of political assassins*. Paper presented at the meeting of the American Orthopsychiatric Association, 1973 (Reviewed in *Human Behavior*, 1974).

Steinmetz, S. K. (1977). *The cycle of violence: Assertive, aggressive and abusive family interaction*. New York: Praeger.

Steinmetz, S. K. (1979). Wife beating: A critique and reformulation of existing theory. *Bulletin of the American Academy of Psychiatry and the Law, 6*(3), 322–334.

Steinmetz, S. K. (1981). Marital abuse: A cross-cultural comparison. *Sociology and Social Welfare, 8*(2), 404–414.

Steinmetz, S. K. (1982). A cross-cultural comparison of sibling violence. *International Journal of Family Psychiatry, 2*(3–4), 337–351.

Steinmetz, S. K. (1987). Family violence: Past, present, and future. In M. B. Sussman & S. K. Steinmetz (Eds.), *Handbook of marriage and the family* (pp. 725–765). New York: Plenum.

Steinmetz, S. K. (1988). *Duty bound: Elder abuse and family care*. Beverly Hills, CA: Sage.

Steinmetz, S. K. (1990). Confronting violence in the 1980s: In the streets, schools and home. In L. J. Hertzberg, G. F. Ostrum, & J. R. Field (Eds.), *Violent Behavior: Vol. 1. Assessment and Intervention* (pp. 167–180). Great Neck, NY: PMA.

Steinmetz, S. K. (1996). *Marion County residents of Boys' School: A demographic analysis*. Final report to the Marion County Community Corrections, Indiana Department of Corrections, Indianapolis.

Steinmetz, S. K. (1999). Adolescence. In M. B. Sussman, S. K. Steinmetz, & G. W. Peterson (Eds.), *Handbook of marriage and the family* (2nd. ed.) pp. 371–423. New York: Plenum.

Steinmetz, S. K., & Straus, M. A. (1973). The family as cradle of violence. *Society, 10*(6), 50–56.

Steinmetz, S. K., & Straus, M. A. (Eds.). 1974. Editor's introduction. In *Violence in the Family* (pp. 3–24). New York: Harper & Row.

Stets, J. E. (1990). Verbal and physical aggression in marriage. *Journal of Marriage and the Family, 52*, 501–514.

Straus, M. A. (1974). Leveling, civility, and violence in the family. *Journal of Marriage and the Family, 36*, 13–29.

Straus, M. A. (1976). Sexual inequality, cultural norms and wife-beating. *Victimology, 1*, 54–76.

Straus, M. A., Gelles, R. J., & Steinmetz, S. K. (1980). *Behind closed doors: Violence in the American family*. New York: Doubleday.

Sutherland, E. H., & Cressey, D. (1974). *Criminology*. Philadelphia: Lippincott.

Taff, P., & Ross, P. (1969). American labor violence: Its causes, character and outcome. In H. G. Graham & T. R. Gurr (Eds.). *The history of violence in America* (pp. 221–301). Washington, DC: U.S. Government Printing Press.

Thomas, D. S. (1925). *Social aspects of the business cycle*. In J. Gunn, *Violence*. New York: Praeger.

Thomas, W. I., & Thomas D. S. (1928). *The child in America: Behavior, problems and programs*. New York: Knopf.

Thomas, W. I., & Znaniecki, F. (1918–1920). *The Polish Peasant in Europe and America* (5 vols.). Boston: Badger.

Tiger, L. (1969). *Men in groups*. New York: Random House.

Toby, J. (1966). Violence and the masculine ideal: Some quantitative data. *Annals of the American Academy of Political and Social Science, 364*, 20–27.

Turk, A. T. (1969). *Criminology and legal order*. Chicago: Rand McNally.

Van Valzen, H. U. E., & Wetering, W. (1960). Residence, power groups, and intra-societal aggression. *International Archives of Ethnography, 49,* 169–200.

Vargus, B. S. (1999). Classical social theory and family studies: The triumph of reactionary thought in contemporary family studies. In M. B. Sussman, S. K. Steinmetz, & G. W. Peterson (Eds.), *Handbook of marriage and the family* (2nd. ed., pp. 179–204). New York: Plenum.

Walker, L. E., (1977–1978). Battered women and learned helplessness. *Victimology, 2,* 525–534.

Watkins, C. R. (1982). *Victims, aggressors and the family secret: An exploration into family violence.* Minneapolis: Minnesota Department of Public Welfare.

Weber, M. (1947). *The Theory of social and economic organization* (A. M. Henderson & T. Parsons, Trans., & T. Parsons, Ed.) New York: Oxford University Press.

Whitehurst, R. (1974). Violence in husband–wife interaction. In S. K. Steinmetz & M. A. Straus (Eds.), *Violence in the family* (pp. 75–82). New York: Harper & Row.

Whiting, B. (1965). Sex identity conflict and physical violence: A comparative study. *American Anthropologist, 67,* 123–140.

Williams, K. R. (1984). Economic sources of homicide: Reestimating the effects of poverty and inequality. *American Sociological Review, 49,* 283–289.

Wolfgang, M. E., & Ferracuti, F. (1967). *The subculture of violence: Towards an integrated theory of criminology.* London: Tavistock.

Yllö, K. (1983). Sexual equality and violence against wives in American states. *Journal of Comparative Family Studies, 14*(1), 67–86.

Behavioral Perspectives on Violent Behavior

Michael T. Nietzel, Dawn M. Hasemann, and Donald R. Lynam

Introduction

In 1994, the most recent year for which we had official police statistics, 23,310 Americans were murdered, 102,100 were raped, 618, 820 were robbed, and 1,119,950 were assaulted by someone using a weapon (Federal Bureau of Investigation [FBI], 1995). These figures underestimate the extent of violent crime in America because many crimes are never reported to the police, particularly those involving intrafamily violence. Although the rate of violent crime in the United States has flattened or, for some crimes, even declined in the 1990s, most Americans continue to list the fear of violent crime as one of their most important concerns.

What are the causes of violent behavior? How can we best explain the development of violent offenders? Several behaviorally oriented answers to these questions have been proposed. In fact, the range of criminological theories laying claim to being "behavioral" is extensive. Various labels have been applied to these theories; social-psychological, control, operant learning, classical conditioning, social learning, and cognitive-behavioral are all now a standard part of the criminological lexicon.

What unifies and what distinguishes behavioral perspectives on violent crime? They are unified by an attempt to explain criminal violence as the result of one or more learning processes. These processes are usually embedded in social interactions; hence, behavioral theories are sometimes categorized under the rubric of social-psychological explanations of criminality. Behavioral formulations focus their attention on those historical and contemporary experiences by which an individual learns to become violent or criminal. In some theories, learning involves acquisition of antiso-

Michael T. Nietzel • Department of Psychology and Graduate School, University of Kentucky, Lexington, Kentucky 40506-0044. *Dawn M. Hasemann and Donald R. Lynam* • Department of Psychology, University of Kentucky, Lexington, Kentucky 40506-0044.

Handbook of Psychological Approaches with Violent Offenders: Contemporary Strategies and Issues, edited by Van Hasselt and Hersen. Kluwer Academic/Plenum Publishers, New York, 1999.

cial behaviors; in others it involves failure to learn prosocial behaviors. In either case, most behavioral theories occupy a theoretical middle ground, situated between the narrow individualism of biological positivism and the abstract environmentalism of purely sociological theories.

The major distinctions among "behaviorists" involve the relative emphasis they place on different processes of learning and different crucial responses to be learned. Most behavioral theories of violent behavior are crafted broadly as theories of crime rather than violence specifically. Some (e.g., Bandura, 1973) focus on aggressive behavior; others are more concerned with explaining deviance in general (e.g., Akers, 1977).

This diversity of focus creates problems for reviewers. Although deviance, crime, aggression, and violence are overlapping concepts, they describe behaviors that differ in severity, topography, intensity, and intentionality. We define violent behavior as actions that involve use of physical force or threatened physical force to injure another person. Aggression is behavior that is intended to injure or irritate another person. Researchers often use these two terms interchangeably, although one usually associates violence with a narrower, more physically dangerous level of behavior than aggression, which can include physical or verbal behavior. Further, some researchers (e.g., L. Eron, 1987) do not include intentionality in their definition of aggression because of difficulties in measuring intent, especially in children. However, intention is an important quality of the behavior we discuss in this chapter.

Violent behavior is often criminal behavior, behavior that is legally prohibited and subject to state-inflicted punishment. It includes offenses such as assault, aggravated assault, murder, rape, and sexual assaults against children. We are aware that some scholars construe other offenses, such as business crime, environmental plunder, and price fixing to be violent because of the harm they cause. We also acknowledge that slugging an opponent in a boxing match or shooting an enemy in war are violent behaviors. However, we do not concern ourselves with these classes of behavior in this chapter. We limit our discussion to violent offending as people conventionally understand it: legally proscribed behavior in which one or more persons deliberately attack and often inflict physical injury on others.

We had to decide whether to limit our review only to theories that focus on aggression and violent behavior or to include theories of criminality that cover more versatile antisocial conduct. In an attempt to be comprehensive in our review and because many behavioral theories do not distinguish between types of criminal behavior, we review behavioral theories of aggression, violence, and crime in general. This inclusion is justifiable, as most violent offenders are very similar to nonviolent frequent offenders in childhood, adolescent, and adult features (Farrington, 1995). In fact, most violent offenses occur in the course of long, active criminal careers dominated by property offenses.

We devote the remainder of the chapter to two topics. First, we review briefly what we believe are the major behavioral theories of criminal offending. Second, in the concluding section, we attempt to integrate behaviorally based explanations of violent offending with empirically supported biological and sociological findings on violence in order to arrive at a comprehensive, multifactor theory of violent offending.

Behavioral Theories of Crime, Violence, and Aggression

Control Theories

Control theories claim that people behave antisocially unless they are encouraged or trained to avoid doing so (Conger, 1980). Some people never form bonds with significant others so they do not internalize necessary controls over antisocial behavior. The most influential example of this perspective is Travis Hirschi's (1969, 1978) *social-control* model, which stresses four control variables, each of which represents a major social bond. Young people can be bonded to conventional society at several levels, and they can differ in the degree to which they are affected by the opinions and expectations of others, the payoffs they receive for conventional behavior, and the extent to which they subscribe to prevailing norms. This theory predicts that the odds of violent offending are lowered when youths

- are *attached* emotionally to other people
- are *committed* to conventional social goals
- are *involved* in traditional school and family activities
- *believe* that laws are morally justified and must be obeyed

Another example of a control theory is Walter Reckless's (1967) *containment theory.* Reckless proposed that it is largely external containment; that is, social pressure, that controls crime. When a society is well integrated, enforces well-defined social roles, places clear limits on behavior, encourages effective family discipline and supervision, and reliably reinforces positive accomplishments, crime will be contained. However, if social disorganization or adversities undermine these external controls, control of crime increasingly depends on internal restraints, or what psychologists usually call the conscience or superego. Thus, a positive self-concept serves as an important insulator against offending. Strong inner containment is inferred from the following indicators:

- the ability to tolerate frustration
- to be directed toward goals
- to resist distractions
- to find substitute satisfactions (Reckless, 1967)

The British psychologist Hans Eysenck (1964) elaborated a different version of containment theory in which "heredity plays an important, and possibly a vital part, in predisposing a given individual to crime" (p. 55). Socialization practices then translate these innate tendencies into criminal acts. According to Eysenck, effective socialization depends on two kinds of learning. First, *operant learning* explains how behavior is acquired and maintained by its consequences: responses followed by rewards are strengthened, responses followed by aversive events are weakened. A mainstay principle of operant conditioning is that immediate consequences influence behavior more than delayed consequences. However, according to Eysenck (1964) in the real world the effects of punishment are usually "long delayed and uncertain (while) the acquisition of the desired object is immediate; therefore, although the acquisition and the pleasure derived from it may, on the whole, be less than the pain derived from the in-carceration which ultimately follows, the time element very much favors the acquisi-tion as compared with the deterrent effects of the incarceration" (p. 101).

Because of punishment's ineffectiveness, restraint of antisocial behavior must de-pend on a second process: the conscience, which develops through *classical condition-ing*. Eysenck believed that the conscience is conditioned through multiple, temporally close pairings of a child's undesirable behaviors with prompt punishment of these be-haviors. Taboo acts are *conditioned stimuli* which, when associated frequently enough with the *unconditioned stimulus* of punishment, produce unpleasant physiological and emotional responses. Conscience becomes a private voice of inhibition that deters wrongdoing through the emotions of anxiety and guilt.

Whether conditioning builds a strong conscience depends to a large extent on the strength of the autonomic nervous system. According to Eysenck, conditioned re-sponses develop slowly and extinguish quickly in some individuals. In others, condi-tioning progresses rapidly and produces strong resistance to extinction.

Underlying these differences are the three major dimensions of Eysenck's per-sonality theory: *extraversion, neuroticism,* and *psychoticism* (Eysenck & Gudjonson, 1989). Extraverted people are active, aggressive, and impulsive. Persons high in neu-roticism are restless, emotionally volatile, and hypersensitive. Persons high in psy-choticism are troublesome, lacking in empathy, and insensitive to the point of cruelty.

Extraversion, neuroticism, and psychoticism are also associated with important physiological differences, many of which describe traditional notions of psychopathy. High extraverts have low levels of arousal which slow their ability to be conditioned and also render any responses that are conditioned likely to be extinguished easily. Conditioning is also impaired because physiological arousal dissipates more slowly in extraverted people and psychopaths. As a result, avoiding a previously punished act is less reinforcing for such people because they experience less reduction in fear following avoidance of taboo behavior (Mednick, Gabrielli, & Hutchings, 1984).

Because persons high in neuroticism have a reactive autonomic nervous system they overreact to stimuli. Therefore, high neuroticism interferes with efficient learn-ing because of the irrelevant arousal that is evoked. In addition, high neuroticism leads to greater drive to carry out behavior of all sorts, including crimes.

Eysenck believed that high extraversion and neuroticism would result in poor conditioning, and consequently, inadequate socialization. Poor conditioning leads to a faulty conscience which in turn produces a higher risk for criminality. Finally, if the person is high on psychoticism, she or he will tend to be a primary "tough-minded" psychopath.

One problem with the theory is that Eysenck did not separate the predisposition to be conditioned from the different conditioning opportunities that children experi-ence. Genetic differences are accompanied by different conditioning histories. A fam-ily of extraverts transmits a potential for crime not only through inherited personality qualities but also through laissez-faire discipline where conditioning is too scarce or inconsistent to be effective.

Differential Association–Reinforcement Theory

Several behavioral theories focus on the way specific criminal behaviors are learned. Historically, the best-known version of this approach was Edwin H. Sutherland's (1947) theory of differential association. According to Sutherland, criminal behavior requires socialization into a system of values that is conducive to offending; thus, the potential criminal learns "definitions" that are favorable to deviant behavior. If definitions of criminal acts as acceptable are stronger and more frequent than definitions unfavorable to deviant behavior, the person is more likely to commit criminal acts.

Definitions favorable to crime need group support; crime will not persist in the absence of a "subculture of violence." It is not necessary to associate with criminals directly. Children might learn pro-violence definitions from watching their father behave abusively toward their mother or by watching repeated examples of violence on TV.

In 1965, C. R. Jeffery proposed a straightforward translation of Sutherland's formulation into behavioral terminology: "A criminal act occurs in an environment in which in the past the actor has been reinforced for behaving in this manner, and the aversive consequences attached to the behavior have been of such a nature that they do not control or prevent the response" (p. 295). About a decade after Jeffery's translation, Robert Burgess and Ronald Akers (Akers, 1977; Akers, Krohn, Lanz-Kaduce, & Radosevich, 1996; Burgess & Akers, 1966) authored a more systematic operant elaboration of differential association theory. As described in *differential association–reinforcement theory*, criminal behavior is acquired through operant conditioning and modeling. A person behaves criminally when such behavior is favored by greater reinforcement than punishment contingencies. The principal contingencies are those that involve "groups which control individuals' major sources of reinforcement and punishment and expose them to behavioral models and normative definitions" (Akers *et al.*, 1996, p. 12). These groups include one's family, peers, and schools.

Differential association attempts to explain crime in places where it would not ordinarily be expected—for example, among lawbreakers who grew up in affluent environments. But it has difficulty explaining crimes of impulsive violence, and it does not explain why certain individuals, even within the same family, have the different associations they do. Why are some people more likely than others to form criminal associations?

Social-Learning Theory

Although social-learning theory acknowledges the importance of differential reinforcement for developing new behaviors, it gives more importance to cognitive factors and to observational or *vicarious learning*. Its chief architect is Albert Bandura (1986), who claims that "most human behavior is learned by observation through modeling" (p. 47). Learning through modeling is more efficient than learning through differential reinforcement. Sophisticated behaviors such as speech and complex chains of behavior (e.g., driving a car) require models. In all likelihood, so does violent crime.

Observational learning depends on

- *attention* to the important features of modeled behavior
- *retention* of these features in memory to guide later performance
- *reproduction* of the observed behaviors
- *reinforcement* of attempted behaviors which determines not whether they are learned but influences whether they will be performed again

The most prominent attempt to apply social learning theory to criminal behavior is Bandura's (1973) book, *Aggression: A Social Learning Analysis* (see also Platt & Prout, 1987; Ribes-Inesta & Bandura, 1976). The theory emphasizes modeling of aggression in three social contexts.

1. *Familial influences.* Familial aggression assumes many forms, from child abuse at one extreme to aggressive parental attitudes and language at the other. It is the arena of discipline, however, where children are exposed most frequently to vivid examples of coercion and aggression as a preferred style for resolving conflicts and asserting desires.
2. *Subcultural influences.* Some subcultures provide a rich diet of aggression and a full schedule of rewards for their most combative members. "The highest rates of aggressive behavior are found in environments where aggressive models abound and where aggressiveness is regarded as a highly valued attribute" (Bandura, 1976, p. 207).
3. *Symbolic models.* The major influence of symbolic models on aggression has been attributed to the mass media, particularly television. Numerous studies have investigated the effects that televised violence has on viewers, especially in children. Interpretations of this literature vary as to whether viewing televised violence causes later aggression in viewers. The consensus is that TV violence does increase aggression for children and adolescents, that this influence is of small, but meaningful, magnitude, that short-term effects have been demonstrated more clearly than long-term effects, and that TV violence might have a larger impact on children who are initially more aggressive (Friedrich-Cofer & Huston, 1986; Pearl, Bouthilet, & Lazar, 1982; Surgeon General's Scientific Advisory Committee on Television and Social Behavior, 1972; for a dissenting view, see Freedman, 1984, 1986).

Several types of environmental cues increase antisocial behavior. These "instigators" (Bandura, 1976) signal when it will be rewarding to behave antisocially versus when it is risky to do so. Six instigators deserve special mention: (1) aggressive *models* can prompt others to behave aggressively; (2) *prior aversive treatment* can increase the perceived awards for aggression; (3) *incentives* can induce individuals to behave aggressively especially if they cause the individuals to underestimate the chances of apprehension; (4) certain individuals might behave aggressively if they are simply *instructed* to do so; (5) *delusions. hallucinations, or paranoid jealousies* may stimulate aggression in a few individuals; and (6) *alcohol and drug abuse* lowers people's responsiveness to other cues that might inhibit aggression.

According to social learning theorists, people also regulate their behavior through self-reinforcement. Individuals who derive pleasure, pride, revenge, or self-worth from their ability to harm others will persist in these activities, enjoying an almost sensual pleasure in the tactics and "feel" of criminal behavior (Katz, 1988). Conversely, people will discontinue conduct that results in self-criticism and self-contempt. Bandura discusses several cognitive maneuvers by which people exempt themselves from their own conscience after behaving antisocially. These tactics of "self-exoneration" assume many forms: minimizing the seriousness of one's acts by pointing to more serious offenses by others, justifying aggression by appealing to higher values, displacing the responsibility for misbehavior onto a higher authority, blaming victims for their misfortune, diffusing responsibility for wrongdoing, dehumanizing victims so they are stripped of sympathetic qualities, and underestimating the damage of one's actions.

The social-learning approach can explain how specific patterns of criminality might have developed in individual offenders and it applies to a wide range of offending behavior. Its major limitation is that there is little empirical evidence that "real life" criminal behaviors are learned according to behavioral principles. Most data come from laboratory research where the experimental setting nullifies all the legal and social sanctions that actual offenders must risk.

A second problem is that social-learning theory does not explain why some people fall prey to "bad" learning experiences while others resist them. Learning is probably a necessary ingredient in developing criminality, but it is unlikely to be a sufficient one. Individual differences in the way people respond to reinforcement need to be considered.

Multiple-Factor Learning Theories

Some theorists have integrated multiple learning processes into a comprehensive, learning-based formulation of criminality. For example, Philip Feldman (1977) assimilated modern learning theory, individual predispositions, and social labeling theory into a comprehensive sociopsychological explanation of crime. James Wilson and Richard Herrnstein (1985) accomplished a similar integration that paid extra attention to biologically influenced individual differences.

Feldman (1977)

According to Feldman, learning affects acquisition, performance, and maintenance of criminal behavior. Individual predispositions influence the ease with which criminal behaviors are acquired, and labeling variables affect the maintenance of aggressive behavior. The learning component is the most pervasive influence across different types of offenders. Individual predispositions play a more important role for persons who suffer psychological problems or are at the extremes of the major dimensions of personality.

People learn not to offend due to early socialization practices, the restraining power of which is maintained by positive consequences for rule keeping and negative consequences for rule breaking. Faulty training in socially acceptable behavior leads to a behavioral repertoire dominated by legally forbidden activities.

People also learn to offend through the direct effects of differential reinforcement, social modeling, and situational inducements to harmful behavior. Criminal behavior is maintained by certain cognitive processes accompanying overt performance. One such mechanism is cognitive dissonance, which, like the techniques of neutralization or Bandura's techniques of self-exoneration, self-servingly underestimate the aversiveness of one's offenses. Another is self-reinforcement for successful criminal acts which helps maintain such behaviors.

The effects of learning variables are often moderated by social situations. In Feldman's (1977) words, "membership of a particular class or culture, or living in a particular geographical area might affect the probabilities of acquiring and performing criminal behaviors, and of such behaviors being maintained or reduced" (p. 284).

Just as social settings might lead to more criminal behavior among certain groups, so might personality differences. Successful socialization depends on an optimal match between training techniques and the personality of the learner. Feldman uses Eysenck's personality theory to explain the differential acquisition of conditioned responses unfavorable to law breaking. Extroverted neurotics have the poorest potential for effective socialization, and people high on psychoticism are relatively insensitive to the plight of their victims. The role of personality predispositions remains secondary to the effects of learning. Small, initial differences in personality may grow into major ones through differential social shaping. "The Eysenckian personality dimensions are likely to make a useful contribution to the explanation of criminal behavior, but more to acquisition than its performance or maintenance, and much more in the case of extreme, than in the case of medium, scorers. Even in acquisition, by extreme scorers, personality will be only part of the story; situational variables will play a significant role" (Feldman, 1977, p. 161).

The final component of Feldman's (1977) framework is labeling theory, which "points to the important role of the social reactions of those in positions of power within the law enforcement and penal systems in maintaining, perhaps even enhancing, the criminal behavior of over-represented groups" (p. 285). The person whose predispositions, in concert with a specific learning history, produce a high susceptibility to offending is often pushed into more permanent deviance by criminalizing contacts with the legal system.

Wilson and Herrnstein (1985)

The most controversial multiple-component learning theory is found in James Wilson and the late Richard Herrnstein's (1985) *Crime and Human Nature*. Wilson and Herrnstein argue that both criminal and noncriminal behavior have gains and losses. Gains from crime include revenge and peer approval. Gains associated from "noncrime" include avoiding punishment and having a clear conscience. Whether a crime is committed depends, in part, on the net ratio of these gains and losses for criminal and noncriminal behavior. When the ratio for committing a crime exceeds that for not committing it, the likelihood of the crime being committed increases, a proposition that nonbehaviorists (Cornish & Clark, 1986) call *rational choice* theory.

Wilson and Herrnstein argue that individual differences determine these ratios and help explain whether a given individual is likely to commit a crime. Like Eysenck, they propose that people differ in the ease with which they learn to associate, through classical conditioning, negative emotions with misbehaviors and positive emotions with proper behaviors. These conditioned responses are the building blocks of a strong conscience which increases the gains associated with noncrime and increases the losses associated with crime.

Another personality factor is impulsivity or what Wilson and Herrnstein call "time discounting." All reinforcers lose strength the more remote they are from a behavior, but persons differ in their ability to delay gratification and obtain reinforcement from long-term gains. More impulsive persons have greater difficulty deriving benefits from distant reinforcers. Time discounting is important to understanding crime because the gains associated with crime (e.g., revenge, money) occur immediately, whereas the losses from such behavior (e.g., punishment) occur much later in time, if at all. Thus, for impulsive persons, the ratio of gains to losses shifts in a direction that favors criminal behavior.

Equity is another important influence on criminality. Equity theory states that people compare what they feel they deserve with what they observe other people receiving. Inequitable transactions are perceived when one's own ratio of gains to losses is less than that of others. Judgments of inequity change the reinforcing value of crime. If one perceives oneself as having been treated unfairly by society, this sense of inequity increases the perceived gains associated with robbery because such behavior helps restore one's sense of equity.

Another major component is what Wilson and Herrnstein call "constitutional factors" that are present at birth or soon after. These factors include gender, intelligence, variations in physiological arousal, and impulsivity, all of which conspire to make some persons more attracted to wrongdoing and less deterred by the potential aversive consequences of crime.

Of several social factors linked to criminal behavior, Wilson and Herrnstein believe that family influences and early school experiences are most important. Families that foster (l) *attachment* of children to their parents, (2) *longer time horizons* where children consider the distant consequences of their behavior, and (3) strong *consciences* about misbehavior can successfully counteract criminal predispositions. The work of Gerald Patterson and his colleagues is pertinent to this aspect of Wilson and Herrnstein's theory. Based on elaborate observation of families with and without aggressive and conduct-disordered children, G. R. Patterson (1982, 1986), identified four family interaction patterns associated with later delinquency: (1) poor disciplinary techniques involving either overinvolved nagging or indifferent laxness; (2) lack of positive parenting and affection toward children; (3) ineffective parental monitoring of a child's behavior, and (4) failure to employ adequate problem-solving strategies thereby increasing stress and irritability within a family.

The remedies for these harmful patterns involve warm supportiveness combined with consistent enforcement of clear rules for proper behavior. Of course, these methods are least likely to be practiced by parents whose own traits reflect the predispositions they have passed to their children. Therefore, many at-risk children face the double difficulty of problematic predispositions coupled with inadequate parental control.

Biological factors interact with early school experiences. Impulsive, poorly socialized children of lower intelligence not only are more directly at risk for criminality, their interactions with cold, indifferent schools that do not improve educational achievements is an additional liability that pushes them away from traditional social conformity.

Because they took hereditary and biological factors seriously, Wilson and Herrnstein came under heavy fire from critics who portrayed their ideas as a purely genetic theory. It is not. However, it does restore psychological factors (some heritable, some not) and family interaction variables to a place of importance in criminology.

Integration: A Multifactor Behavioral Model of Violent Offending

Where do all these theories lead us? Do any of them offer a sufficient explanation of crime? While we still await a completely convincing theory of crime, we believe an increasing fund of knowledge about the causes of serious crime points to an integrated set of valid explanations for how some violent criminality develops.

Historically, theories of crime and violent behavior have been very territorial. Each discipline or subdiscipline has defended its favorite explanatory turf with a con-

fidence usually reserved for religious zealots. Integration of theories or even accom-
modations of one theory to the obviously insightful ideas of another have been only
grudgingly achieved (see Andrews & Bonta, 1994; Pearson & Weiner, 1985 for exceptions along with the aforementioned theories of Feldman and Wilson and Herrnstein).
Some theories—genetic and sociological examples come quickly to mind—are usually
contrasted as arch rivals. More often, most theories of crime, violence, and aggression
stand alone; independent and aloof from competitors, isolated even from complementary perspectives. Economists, ecologists, sociologists, behavior geneticists, Marxists,
psychologists, and theologians have had much to say on the causes of violence, but
they appear to have seldom said it to one another or listened while the others spoke.

Serious criminality is extraordinarily versatile, involving careers that include violent crime, property crime, vandalism, and substance abuse. One implication of this
diversity is that several causal pathways or tributaries may lead to specific criminal careers. No single variable causes all crime, just as no one agent causes all fever or upset
stomachs.[1] However, several etiological factors are associated reliably with criminality.
Any one of these factors is sometimes a sufficient explanation for criminal conduct;
more often, however, we believe they act in concert to cause violent criminality.

Our attempt to integrate behavioral theories with other criminological perspectives is summarized in Figure 3.1. We emphasize four main contributions to violent
offending, occurring in a developmental sequence. This model emphasizes the following four etiological principles, which we believe are among the best-supported
empirical findings in the criminological literature:

- The chances of repeated violent offending are increased by three types of *distal antecedents:* biological, psychological, and environmental factors that make
it easier for some individuals to learn violent offending and easier for such
learning to occur in certain settings.
- Repetitive violent offending is relatively stable over time. Aggressive children
often grow up to be aggressive adults, and precedents for adult violence are
often seen in *early indicators* of aggressiveness in preschool and elementary
school–aged children. Of course, not all violent offenders were violent children, but a large percentage of repetitively aggressive adults began early.
- Whether these early indicators of violent offending harden into patterns of recidivistic antisocial behavior or soften into reasonably prosocial, nonviolent conduct depends on a variety of *developmental processes.* These processes occur in
families, schools, peer groups, the media, and in the cognitions of the individual.
- Once violent behavior has been learned and performed, several *maintenance
variables* are encountered which lead either to a further entrenching or even
escalation of antisocial conduct or to a decline in aggression that may also be
accompanied by an increase in prosocial behavior.

Distal Antecedents

Environments

Certain environments are rich in opportunities and temptations for crime. They
achieve this quality because of social impoverishment and disorganization, fundamental economic inequalities, a tradition of tolerating if not encouraging crime, social

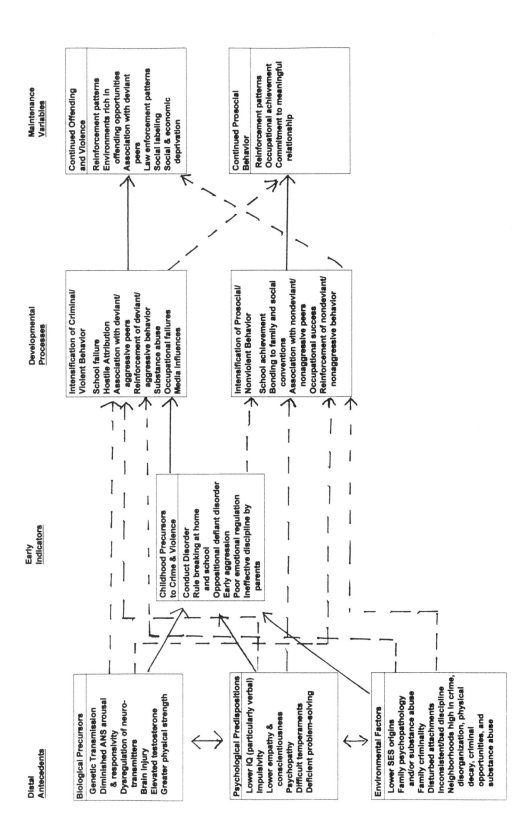

NOTE: Solid lines indicate probable paths; dotted lines indicate possible, but less likely, paths.

FIGURE 3.1. The development of violent offenders.

dissension, pathology, and strife, and an abundance of inviting targets and easy victims (E. B. Patterson, 1996). Criminogenic environments make it easier for some individuals to behave violently because they are full of discriminative stimuli for violence; antagonists provoke violence, at the same time that high density increases the targets for violence, and high rates of alcohol and substance abuse lower inhibitions against it.

Within family environments, high levels of psychopathology, criminality, and substance abuse are also linked with higher rates of aggression among children. These links may be forged through genetic influences, modeling, the development of hostility as a result of living in harsh or frustrating family environments, disturbed attachments with parents, or through lax or punitive discipline that does not teach children how to control their behavior (Loeber & Dishion, 1983; Loeber & Stouthamer-Loeber, 1986).

Likewise, certain *persons* are particularly vulnerable to behaving criminally: a predisposition that becomes stronger when such persons find themselves in risky environments. Some predispositions to criminality are biologically rooted, some are psychological in nature, and still others involve a complex interaction of both biological and psychological factors.

Biological Precursors

An abundant literature has now implicated genetic transmission, neurochemical abnormalities, brain dysfunction, hormonal dysregulation, and autonomic nervous system irregularities in aggressive and violent behavior (for reviews see DiLalla & Gottesman, 1991; Garza-Treviño, 1994).

Twin and adoption studies consistently lead to the conclusion that aggression and antisocial behavior are heritable to an appreciable degree, although environmental factors are also related to these behaviors (DiLalla & Gottesman, 1989; 1991; Mednick & Kandel, 1988; Widom, 1989). Adoption studies have yielded evidence of a small genetic link to crime (Walters, 1992); they more strongly support the conclusion that the children at highest risk for criminal behavior are born to parents who were criminal and are then adopted into criminal environments (Cloninger, Sigvardsson, Bohman, & von Knorring, 1982). Heritability for crimes against property tends to be higher than for crimes against persons (Cloninger & Gottesman, 1987; Mednick, Gabrielli, & Hutchings, 1987).

The question remains as to what exactly is inherited as part of this genetic risk. One possibility is abnormal activity of one of the major neurotransmitters such as dopamine, serotonin, or GABA (Ellis, 1991a; Garza-Treviño, 1994). For example, evidence points strongly to depletions or insufficient activity of serotonin as one factor underlying impulsive aggression (Brown, Botsis, & Van Praag, 1994; Coccaro, Kavoussi, & Lesser, 1992). Another contributor may be elevated testosterone levels, which have been associated with increased aggression in adolescent boys (Olweus, 1987), although whether these elevations precede or follow aggression is still not clear (Archer, 1991). Olweus's (1995) research on youths' aggression toward peers has also consistently found that bullies are simply physically stronger than either their victims or boys in general.

Differences in autonomic nervous system reactivity are often proposed as a biological risk factor for aggressive offending. Several researchers have suggested that repetitively antisocial persons suffer chronically low levels of autonomic arousal, causing them to have a high need for stimulation that they gratify through aggressive thrill seeking.

Brain injury is also related to aggression in humans; several aggressive syndromes subsequent to head injury have been documented (Miller, 1994). Aggressive behavior occurs spontaneously in individuals who suffer seizure disorders. Frontal lobe damage can result in disinhibited behavior and dysregulated emotional responses, or it can exacerbate premorbid antisociality. Finally, temporal lobe damage has been linked to specific types of sexual violence (Mills & Raine, 1994).

Psychological Predispositions

With respect to psychological predispositions, individuals with lower verbal ability, poor impulse control, and personalities and temperaments marked by undercontrol, irritability, and low empathy are at great risk for antisocial conduct. Consequently, they are well stocked in psychological qualities that encourage violent offending, discourage prosocial behavior, and render these individuals relatively immune to negative consequences for misconduct.

Verbal Ability

There is a robust relation between low verbal ability and serious antisocial behavior across the life course. The evidence is present in studies using standard IQ tests and investigations using more specific neuropsychological measures of verbal ability.

There is overwhelming evidence that low Verbal IQ (VIQ) scores are associated with the most serious offending across the life course (Lynam, Moffitt, & Stouthamer-Loeber, 1993; Moffitt & Lynam, 1994). Ever since Wechsler (1974) remarked on the utility of a Performance IQ (PIQ) greater than VIQ score to identify delinquents, a plethora of studies have examined the relation between VIQ and antisocial behavior. Children with severe conduct problems (CP) have lower VIQ scores than their non-CP peers (Lahey *et al.*, 1995; Schonfeld, Shaffer, O'Connor, & Portnoy, 1988). Severely delinquent adolescent have lower VIQs than their nondelinquent counterparts (Haynes & Bensch, 1981; Lynam *et al.*, 1993; Prentice & Kelly, 1963; Walsh, Petee, & Beyer, 1987; West & Farrington, 1973). Serious adult offenders have lower VIQ scores than less serious offenders and nonoffending adults (Valliant, Asu, Cooper, & Mammola, 1984; Yeudall, Fedora, Fedora, & Wardell, 1981). In addition, there is evidence that the deficit is even greater in violent than in nonviolent offenders (DeWolfe & Ryan, 1984; Heilbrun & Heilbrun, 1985; Holland & Holt, 1975; Holland, Beckett, & Levi, 1981).

The impressive replicability of the relation between low VIQ and severe antisocial behavior has been interpreted as strongly supporting a specific deficit in language manipulation for antisocials. This position is strengthened by neuropsychological studies employing more specific measures of verbal and language functioning. As for VIQ, robust relations between severe antisocial behavior (including violence) and impaired performance on standard neuropsychological tests of verbal and language functioning have been observed. This finding is true across child, adolescent, and adult populations (see Moffitt, 1990b; Moffitt & Henry, 1991; Moffitt & Lynam, 1994).

The causal relation seems to run from low VIQ to antisocial behavior and not vice versa. The deficit is present before onset of offending (Denno, 1990), suggesting that it does not result from consequences of antisocial behavior. For example, in his longitudinal study of 411 London boys, Farrington (1995) found that low VIQ at ages 8–10 was linked to persistent criminality and a high number of convictions for violent offenses up to age 32. The deficit is present whether one assesses offending with official or self-reports, indicating that the results are not due to the differential detection of less intellectually competent antisocials (for a direct test of this hypothesis, see Moffitt & Silva, 1988). Finally, the relation does not disappear when one controls for social class, race, or test motivation (Lynam *et al.*, 1993).

Impulsivity

Another area in which severely antisocial and violent offenders can be distinguished from nonoffenders is impulsivity, which, broadly defined, involves a tendency to act without thinking and an inability to delay gratification. Impulsivity goes by many names: ego-undercontrol, self-control, response modulation, and executive function to name a few. By whatever name, though, impulsivity is implicated in many theories of severe antisocial behavior. Gorenstein and Newman (1980) proposed a "disinhibitory" personality style that may result in severe and chronic antisocial behavior. In her developmental taxonomy, Moffitt (1993) placed impulsivity at the core of what she termed Life-course Persistent antisocial behavior. Impulsivity is a hallmark of the psychopath; theorists and observers have all underscored the psychopath's inability to constrain his impulses (Buss, 1966; Cleckley, 1976; Hare, 1970; McCord & McCord, 1964; Millon, 1981; D. Shapiro, 1965).

There are also strong empirical links between impulsivity and antisocial behavior. In one of the best studies, White and colleagues (1994) gathered data on "self-control and impulsivity" from 430 12-year-old boys. Twelve measures of impulsivity were taken from multiple sources (mother, teacher, self, observer) via multiple methods (rating scales, neuropsychological tests, computer games, Q-sorts, and videotaped observations). A linear composite of the impulsivity measures strongly predicted the 3-year longevity of antisocial behavior, even after controlling for IQ and social class. Boys who had severe conduct problems from ages 10 to 13 scored 1.75 standard deviations higher on impulsivity than their age-mates without conduct problems. Deficient executive functioning has been specifically related to stable aggression; boys who were aggressive at three of four ages scored more poorly than nonaggressive and unstable aggressive boys on a battery of tests assessing executive functioning (Seguin, Pihl, Harden, Tremblay, & Boulerice, 1995). Many studies that have applied batteries of formal tests of executive functions to adolescent samples have found that these batteries can discriminate antisocial adolescents from their nonantisocial counterparts (see Moffitt, 1990b, Moffitt & Henry, 1991; Moffitt & Lynam, 1994, for reviews). Newman and his colleagues (Newman, 1987; Newman & Kosson, 1986; Newman, Patterson, & Kosson, 1987; Newman, Patterson, Howland, & Nichols, 1990), working at the adult level, have demonstrated that the psychopath is characterized by a specific type of impulsive responding that they refer to as a deficit in response modulation.

Somewhat related to impulsivity, Hyperactive-Impulsive-Attention problems (HIA) in childhood are associated with severe antisocial behavior, although the nature of the relation is not clear (Lynam, 1996). Children with HIA in childhood are more likely to be serious offenders in adolescence and adulthood (Farrington, Loeber, & Van Kammen, 1990; Loeber, Brinthaupt, & Green, 1990; Magnusson, 1988; Moffitt, 1990a). At any given time, HIA offenders are among the most frequent, severe, and varied (Loeber *et al.*, 1990; McGee, Silva, & Williams, 1984; Moffitt, 1990a; Offord, Sullivan, Allen, & Abrams, 1979; S. K. Shapiro & Garfinkel, 1986; Szatmari, Boyle, & Offord, 1989), and are the most likely to offend across situations (Walker, Lahey, Hynd, & Frame, 1987); all portend later chronic offending (Loeber, 1982; Loeber & Dishion, 1983).

Personality

Given the stability of personality across the life course (Caspi & Bem, 1990), personality traits represent an especially important class of individual factors. Across a 10-year period, two personality dimensions, Negative Emotionality and Constraint (discussed later), yielded cross-age correlations of .60 and .58 (McGue, Bacon, & Lykken, 1993). Robust relations between crime and several dimensions of personality have been demonstrated.[2]

Using the Five Factor Model as an organizing framework,[3] two dimensions of personality are robustly related to serious antisocial behavior: low Agreeableness and low Conscientiousness. Persons high in Agreeableness are described as trusting, helpful, unselfish, compliant, and soft-hearted, whereas persons scoring low are described as unfriendly, unkind, quarrelsome, and hard-hearted. Those scoring high in Conscientiousness are described as planful, reliable, deliberate, and cautious, whereas low scorers are described as careless, irresponsible, and impulsive. Moffitt and her colleagues have found that Negative Emotionality (a composite of Agreeableness and Neuroticism) and Constraint (Conscientiousness), are robustly related to serious conduct problems in childhood and delinquency in adolescence and young adulthood (Krueger *et al.*, 1994; Moffitt, Caspi, Silva, & Stouthamer-Loeber 1995). Delinquents and conduct-problem children are impulsive, danger-seeking, and rejecting of conventional values (low in Constraint); they are also prone to respond to frustration with negative emotions, to feel stressed or harassed, and to approach interpersonal relationships with adversarial attitudes (high in Negative Emotionality). These relations hold across gender, race, nations (New Zealand and Pittsburgh), neighborhoods (good vs. disadvantaged), gender, and methods of delinquency assessment (self-, informant-, and official reports) (Moffitt *et al.*, 1995). Similarly, Farrington found that children who were impulsive, risk-taking, unable to delay gratification (low in Conscientiousness), and lacking in empathy (low in Agreeableness) were the most likely to be violent offenders in adulthood (Farrington, 1989). Finally, numerous investigators have found relations between scores on Eysenck's Psychoticism scale (a combination of low Agreeableness and low Conscientiousness) and conduct disorder in childhood (Lane, 1978, 1987; Lane & Hymans, 1982) and serious violent offending in adulthood (Af Klintberg, Humble, & Schalling, 1992; Allsop & Feldman, 1974; Eysenck & Eysenck, 1976; Lane, 1987).

Finally, a specific configuration of personality traits—psychopathy—is strongly related to antisocial behavior in adulthood. Interpersonally, the psychopath has been described as grandiose, egocentric, manipulative, forceful, and cold-hearted; affectively, he displays shallow emotions, is unable to maintain close relationships, and lacks empathy, anxiety, and remorse. Behaviorally, he commits more types of crime, more crimes of any type and more violent crimes, in or out of prison than his nonpsychopathic counterpart (Hare, 1981; Hare & McPherson, 1984; Hare, McPherson, & Forth, 1988; Kosson, Smith, & Newman, 1990). Importantly, psychopathy also appears to have a childhood manifestation (Frick, O'Brien, Wootton, & McBurnett, 1994; Lynam, 1996). Lynam (1996) has demonstrated that psychopathy can be reliably assessed in 12–13-year-old boys and that "psychopathic" boys are the most serious, violent, and stable offenders across a 3-year span.

Two additional dimensions, Neuroticism and Extraversion, have been theorized to be related to antisocial behavior (Eysenck, 1970, 1977). The support for Neuroticism (N) and Extraversion (E), however, is equivocal at best. Several studies have reported the predicted positive relations between N and antisocial behavior (Eysenck & Eysenck, 1974; Shuck, Dubeck, Cymbalisty, & Green, 1972), whereas other studies have reported negative relations (Lane, 1987; Pierson, 1969; Rushton & Chrisjohn, 1981). Similarly, evidence indicates that Extraversion bears little consistent relation to antisocial behavior (Af Klintberg *et al.*, 1992; Cochrane, 1974; Feldman, 1977; Lane, 1987; Pasingham, 1972; Putnins, 1982). Although Eysenck and Gudjonsson (1989) have suggested that lack of consistency in these relations may be due to age effects, this possibility awaits demonstration.

Temperament

A "difficult temperament" in infancy has been shown to predict behavioral problems in late childhood and adolescence. In an attempt to specify the dimensions of "difficulty," Caspi and his colleagues (Caspi & Silva, 1995; Caspi, Henry, McGee, Moffitt, & Silva, 1995) examined the relations between factor-analytically derived temperament dimensions and late adolescent outcomes in a sample of more than 800 children. The factor most strongly associated with negative outcomes in late adolescence was Lack of Control which combined elements of emotional liability, restlessness, short attention span, and irritability. Researchers found that 3-year-olds who scored high on Lack of Control were much more likely to be rated as aggressive and interpersonally alienated by their parents at ages 13 and 15. In addition, as young adults (18 years of age), these undercontrolled children scored high on personality measures of impulsivity, danger seeking, aggression, and interpersonal alienation; as noted earlier, each of these dimensions has been linked with serious antisocial behavior in early adulthood (Krueger *et al.*, 1994). Most recently, Henry, Caspi, Moffitt, and Silva (1996) found that Lack of Control in childhood was related to convictions by age 18 and uniquely related to convictions for a violent offense.

Early Indicators

As a result of these predisposing antecedents acting in isolation or interacting with one another, certain early indicators of aggression or antisocial conduct will be observed in children. Such early indicators include Conduct Problems (CP), oppositional and defiant behaviors, Hyperactive-Impulsive-Attention problems (HIA), and early aggressiveness, each of which is discussed in the following.

A frequently stated truism in psychology is that "the best predictor of future behavior is past behavior." Nowhere is this truer than in the area of antisocial behavior.

Rarely, if ever, does antisocial behavior spring *de novo* in adults (L. Robins, 1978); rather, severe antisocial behavior in adolescence and adulthood is almost always preceded by antisocial behavior in childhood. In what follows, several, often overlapping, early indicators of future antisocial behavior are discussed.

The Topography of Childhood Conduct Problems

The most frequently examined early manifestations of antisocial behavior are conduct problems in childhood which include hurting animals, fighting, stealing, damaging property, setting fires, lying, conning, breaking curfew, truancy, and running away from home. Whereas no single act is particularly predictive of later antisocial outcomes, the topography of conduct problems is an excellent predictor. Several reviews (Loeber, 1982; Loeber & Dishion, 1983) have concluded that the main predictors of antisocial outcome for children are the age at onset of conduct problems, the frequency, severity, and variety of conduct problems, and the manifestation of these conduct problems across situations (i.e., school and home). Children who manifest these problems earlier rather than later (before 10 years of age) and who manifest several of the more serious problems across settings are at the highest risk for later severe criminal offending. The Fourth Edition of the *Diagnostic and Statistical Manual of Mental Disorders* (*DSM-IV*; American Psychiatric Association, 1994) has incorporated these findings in its Conduct Disorder diagnosis, which requires presence of multiple problems, makes a distinction between early and late onset, and allows specification of seriousness. Important to our purposes here, youth with childhood onset Conduct Disorder are markedly more aggressive than youth with adolescent Conduct Disorder (McGee, Feehan, Williams, & Anderson, 1992).

Oppositional and Defiant Behavior

Oppositional and defiant behaviors in early childhood (Oppositional Defiant Disorder in *DSM-III-R* and *DSM-IV*) are even earlier manifestations of antisocial tendencies than are conduct problems. Oppositional and defiant behaviors include temper tantrums, arguing with adults, active defiance of adult requests, deliberately annoying others, blaming others for one's mistakes, irritability, angry resentment, and vindictiveness. Some of these behaviors can be seen as early as 3 years of age, and most are present before 7 years. Although little evidence is available on the relation between oppositional and defiant behaviors in childhood and later adolescent and adult outcomes, it is clear that oppositional and defiant behaviors are precursors to more serious conduct problems. Boys with childhood-onset CD almost always meet criteria for a diagnosis of Oppositional Defiant Disorder (ODD) as well. In addition, although ODD does not always predict the development of CD, ODD almost always precedes the development of CD (Hinshaw, Lahey, & Hart, 1993).

Hyperactive-Impulsive-Attention Problems and Conduct Problems

One of the earliest and most predictive manifestations of antisocial behavior is the co-occurrence of HIA and CP in the same child (HIA+CP). Lynam (1996) has argued that this combination represents the earliest presentation of the future psychopath. Longitudinal studies demonstrate that children with both types of symptoms (HIA+CP children) are more likely than their counterparts (CP-only, HIA-only, and controls) to have high rates of delinquency in adolescence and to continue their offending into adulthood (Farrington *et al.,* 1990; Loeber *et al.,* 1990; Magnusson, 1988; Moffitt, 1990a). Cross-sectional studies demonstrate that HIA+CP children are the most likely to manifest the high-risk topography of conduct problems discussed earlier (see Lynam, 1996). Family and genetic studies demonstrate that HIA-CP in the proband is related to more severe antisocial behavior in the relatives of these proband than in the relatives of CP-only proband (Lahey *et al.,* 1987). Finally, children with HIA and CP symptoms show patterns of performance on laboratory tasks and psychophysiological profiles that are similar to those of adult psychopaths (see Lynam, 1996, 1997).

Aggression

Perhaps most relevant to the present discussion, aggression and violence in childhood predict aggression and violence in adulthood. Huesmann, Eron, Lefkowitz, and Walder (1984) have tracked, across 22 years, a group of men and women who had been rated as aggressive by their peers in late childhood. They found that aggressive children became aggressive adults; aggressive men were more likely to commit serious criminal acts, abuse their spouses, and drive while intoxicated, whereas the women were likely to punish their children severely. These investigators have also shown that aggression is stable across generations; they tracked its transmission across three generations. In fact, the stability coefficients of aggressive behavior rival, in magnitude, those of IQ (Olweus, 1979). Thus, the child who is aggressive (e.g., tries to hurt others) at an early age can be expected to grow into an aggressive adult; in fact, L. D. Eron (1990) has suggested that aggressive antisocial behavior crystallizes at about 8 years of age.

Developmental Processes

Whether early forms of aggressive behavior intensify into more serious violent offending depends on several developmental processes, beginning in the middle-school years and stretching across adolescence into young adulthood.

Delinquency has often been linked to poor school achievement. In their review of predictors of male delinquency, Loeber and Dishion (1983) listed poor academic achievement as one of five variables with the best predictive validity for official offending. However, grade-point average does not emerge as a strong predictor of delinquency until around age 15 (Loeber & Dishion, 1983), suggesting that poor academic achievement is one of the consequences of early dyscontrol problems. Its relevance to delinquency increases during middle school and adolescence primarily because as youths fall farther and farther behind in school, they have fewer and fewer opportunities or motives to stay bonded to school and committed to the conventional norms of educational achievement (Cernkovich & Giordano, 1996). School failure appears to be one more factor that narrows the options for prosocial behavior; its long-term consequences include impaired employability and job success. In fact, the association between unemployment and arrests becomes strongest for men in their 20s and 30s (Seidman & Rapkin, 1983). As young people perceive their options for prosocial behavior and success to be dwindling, their commitments to antisocial norms increase.

A vast array of modeling and peer influences can intensify investment in antisocial norms and overt criminality. Criminal behavior increases when peers support it. The more delinquent friends a juvenile has, the more likely he or she is to behave criminally (Elliott, Huizinga, & Menard, 1989). Repeated associations with deviant, aggressive peers help youths learn to tolerate deviance, to rationalize antisocial behavior, to imitate new forms of aggressive behavior, and to vicariously enjoy the immediate positive reinforcers that aggression can provide (Warr & Stafford, 1996).

These same modeling influences can be mediated through media displays of violent behavior, particularly via television. In Leonard Eron's large-scale longitudinal study of aggression, children who watched aggression on TV were more likely to behave aggressively themselves, particularly when they were frustrated, than children who had not watched such models (L. Eron, 1987). Of greater interest to our thesis that models help escalate or maintain violence, children's viewing of TV violence at age 8 correlated .41 with a variety of aggressive behaviors at age 30, even after controlling for initial aggressiveness, IQ, and socioeconomic status (L. Eron, 1987; see Wiegman, Kuttschreuter, & Baarda, 1992, for a contrasting view of the effects of TV violence on a sample in the Netherlands).

Why does televised violence have such effects? One possibility is that it provides opportunities for adolescents to rehearse various aggressive strategies that, as a result of many repetitions, ascend their behavioral hierarchies until they are a dominant response to many kinds of difficult situations. Another possibility is that a steady diet of televised violence teaches youngsters to construe their interpersonal world as hostile and competitive. TV might provide the scripts that adolescents work into their personal crime stories. The work of Ken Dodge (1986) indicates that aggression is linked to tendencies to make hostile attributions about the behavior of others. Aggressive youngsters are more likely to interpret ambiguous behavior as hostile; they display what Dodge calls a hostile attributional bias. By assuming hostile intent by others, youngsters feel more justified in retaliating aggressively. Of course this behavior initiates a vicious cycle in which the aggressive youngster is more often avoided, condemned, or attacked, further confirming their "dog eat dog" view of the world.

An additional intensifier of aggression among adolescents is alcohol or substance abuse. A large body of evidence confirms a positive correlation between amount of alcohol consumed and aggressive behavior (Murdoch, Pilh, & Ross, 1990). The mechanisms by which substance abuse can lead to increased aggression are numerous. Alcohol's depressant effects may selectively suppress certain inhibitory centers in the brain, leading to disinhibited behavior. Drug abuse is associated with fewer positive achievements; the more time a youth spends drinking and drugging, the less time he or she has available for prosocial, proacademic activities. Substance abuse during adolescence is usually a peer activity so these habits typically involve differential association with deviant peers, thereby increasing the opportunities for antisocial behavior to be reinforced. In general, repeated substance abuse during adolescence functions as one more "trap" that gradually limits adolescents' options for prosocial activities and achievements. These limits, in turn, increase the reinforcing properties of antisocial conduct.

It should be noted that such intensifiers are not randomly distributed. Rather, youth already at risk are more likely to experience each of them. The impulsive, low-IQ child is more likely to fail at school. The process of homophyly ensures that the antisocial child will associate with antisocial peers (Cairns, Cairns, Neckerman, Gest, & Gariepy, 1988). Parents who fail to monitor and sanction their children when they misbehave are unlikely to show much concern about what their children are watching on television. Finally, early conduct problems are strongly related to later substance use and abuse (L. N. Robins & McEvoy, 1990). In the world of antisocial behavior, the at-risk youth stay at risk.

Maintenance Processes

Violent offending can become an adult way of life when individuals

- continue to live in environments that are rich in opportunities for offending and low in apprehension rates;
- are reinforced, as they will intermittently always be in such environments, for behaving violently;
- persist in associating with aggressive peers, who are abundant in these environments;
- begin, following their inevitable arrests and incarcerations, to associate increasingly with more serious offenders and to be more frequently labeled as dangerous or unrehabilitable;
- feel, as the ultimate consequence of a long list of earlier disengagements from conventional norms, resentment or contempt toward social rules thereby increasing the perceived value of violent behavior.

Empirical support for these maintenance variables is less direct than for other components of the model. However, research sheds some light on one of the processes: the effects of social labeling. The basic assumption of labeling theory is that deviance is created by the labels that society assigns to certain acts. Deviance is not simply based on the quality of the act; rather, it stems also from official reactions to the act. The stigma of being labeled a deviant can create a self-fulfilling prophecy. Even former offenders who seek an honest life in a law-abiding society are sometimes spurned by prospective employers and by their families and are labeled "ex-cons." Frustrated in their efforts to make good, they may adopt this label and engage in further lawbreaking. Consistent with the perspective that the criminal justice system produces some of the deviance it is intended to correct are meta-analytic data (Andrews, Bonta, & Hodge, 1990) indicating that the severity of criminal sanctions is *negatively* correlated (–.07) with decreased recidivism. This relationship suggests that more official processing within the criminal justice system is associated with increased repetition of criminal activity.

On the prosocial side of this equation is recent evidence that "entering into a satisfying occupation and enriching personal relationships during early adulthood" can break patterns of antisocial offending for some individuals (Basic Behavioral Science Task Force of the National Advisory Mental Health Council, 1996). Likewise, evidence that some adults can "turn around" a life of violent offending is provided by meta-analyses showing that treatment programs that strengthen social and cognitive skills, that model and reward prosocial behavior, and that are targeted to the specific contingencies and needs of individual offenders do reduce criminal recidivism (see Andrews & Bonta, 1994, for a review of these studies).

Despite occasional success stories, however, much evidence suggests that interventions with lifelong offenders are frequently unsuccessful (Lipton, Martinson, & Wilks, 1975; Palmer, 1984; Sechrest, White, & Brown, 1975). For example, adult psychopaths are a group known to be recalcitrant to efforts at rehabilitation; the psychopath is more likely than other offenders to recidivate upon release from prison (Hart, Kropp, & Hare, 1988; Serin, Peters, & Barbaree, 1990), and he benefits less from attempts at treatment (Ogloff, Wong, & Greenwood, 1990). This should not be surprising. After a protracted history of learning antisocial behavior, failing to learn prosocial behavior, and closing the doors of legitimate opportunity, attempts to suppress antisocial behavior will not easily bring prosocial behavior to the surface. Thus, we close with a call for increased efforts at primary and secondary prevention of violent offending. If at-risk youth can be reliably identified, we have the opportunity to intervene in multiple areas (e.g., school, family, peers, and individually) before youths are "ensnared" into an antisocial lifestyle by hostile environments and their own previous decisions and actions (e.g., addiction to drugs or alcohol, school dropout, injuries, patchy work histories, and multiple incarcerations).

Summary

Behavioral theories of violent crime have traditionally focused on a variety of learning processes embedded in social interactions that lead to the acquisition of antisocial behaviors and the failure to learn prosocial behaviors. Most prominent among the behavioral explanations are processes involved in (1) the formation of bonds with antisocial role models and lack of commitments to conventional rules, (2) lack of close parental supervision of children that is coupled with emotionally warm but consistent discipline, (3) individual personality differences that either enhance or deter socialization and the formation of internal controls over behavior, and (4) direct and vicarious reinforcement experiences that encourage antisocial behavior.

Other behaviorally oriented theories of violent behavior have integrated multiple learning processes into a comprehensive formulation of criminality. Included in this group are the multiple-component theory of Philip Feldman and the biopsychosocial theory of James Wilson and the late Richard Herrnstein. Based on our attempt to synthesize what is known about the empirical relationships between violent crime and various criminogenic factors, we propose that violent crime results from the influence of four categories of variables, unfolding in a developmental sequence. Specifically, we suggest that the probability of violent crime is increased by (1) distal antecedents involving biological, psychological, and environmental factors that make it easy for certain individuals to learn violent offending, (2) early indicators of dyscontrol and externalizing behavior problems that begin to surface in preschool and elementary school–aged children, (3) any of a set of family, peer, school, social, and individual factors that harden the early indicators of behavior problems into chronic antisocial conduct, and (4) several maintenance variables that lead to a further entrenchment or escalation of violent behavior in adulthood, often culminating in recidivistic violence. A major implication of this model is the need for preventive interventions that target multiple risk factors for violence in developmentally appropriate ways.

Notes

1. Excluded from our model are behavioral accounts of violence that are usually limited to specific contexts or are committed by special types of offenders. For example, we do not review social-learning explanations of spouse abuse or domestic violence even though some excellent multifactor theories (e.g., Dutton, 1995) have been proposed. Likewise, we do not survey learning-based accounts of violence committed by the mentally ill (Monahan, 1992) or crimes involving sexual aggression (Ellis, 1991b; Hall & Hirschman, 1991). Some of these theories would be particularly useful in explaining violent offending that has not been preceded by the early behavioral indicators we discuss in our model.
2. Several scales from commonly used personality instruments are not discussed; these scales include the Psychopathic Deviate scale from the Minnesota Multiphasic Personality Inventory and the Socialization scale from the California Psychological Inventory. Although these scales differentiate very well between criminal and noncriminal samples (Arbuthnot, Gordon, & Jurkovic, 1987), they were designed to do so and it is therefore unclear how relevant they are to understanding the relation between individual factors and crime. For example, the MMPI Pd scale was standardized on a group of incarcerated offenders (Dahlstrom, Welsh, & Dahlstrom, 1972). Both the MMPI and the CPI include items such as "I have never been in trouble with the law" and "Sometimes when I was young I stole things."
3. The Five Factor Model consists of Extraversion (E), Neuroticism (N), Openness to Experience (O), Conscientiousness (C), and Agreeableness (A) (John, 1990). Because combinations and subsets of these five dimensions can be found in other personality systems; these five dimensions can be used as a common language with which to organize findings.

References

Af Klintberg, B., Humble, K., & Schalling, D. (1992). Personality and psychopathy of males with a history of early criminal behavior. *European Journal of Personality, 6,* 245–266.

Akers, R. L. (1977). *Deviant behavior: A social learning approach* (2nd ed.). Belmont, CA: Wadsworth.

Akers, R. L., Krohn, M. D., Lanz-Kaduce, L., & Radosevich, M. (1996). Social learning and deviant behavior: A specific test of a general theory. In D. G. Rojek & G. F. Jensen (Eds.), *Exploring delinquency: Causes and control* (pp. 109–119). Los Angeles: Roxbury.

Allsop, J. F., & Feldman, M. P. (1974). Extraversion, neuroticism, psychoticism, and antisocial behaviour in school girls. *Social Behavior and Personality, 2,* 184–190.

American Psychiatric Association (1994). *Diagnostic and statistical manual of mental disorders* (4th ed.). Washington, DC: Author.

Andrews, D. A., & Bonta, J. (1994). *The psychology of criminal conduct.* Cincinnati, OH: Anderson.

Andrews, D. A., Bonta, J., & Hodge, R. D. (1990). Classification for effective rehabilitation: Rediscovering psychology. *Criminal Justice and Behavior, 17,* 19–52.

Arbuthnot, J., Gordon, D. A., & Jurkovic, G. J. (1987). Personality. In H. C. Quay (Ed.), *Handbook of juvenile delinquency* (pp. 139–183). New York: Wiley.

Archer, J. (1991). The influence of testosterone on human aggression. *British Journal of Psychology, 82,* 1–28.

Bandura, A. (1973). *Aggression: A social learning analysis.* Englewood Cliffs, NJ: Prentice-Hall.

Bandura, A. (1976). Social learning analysis of aggression. In E. Ribes-Inesta & A. Bandura (Eds.), *Analysis of delinquency and aggression* (pp. 203–232). Hillsdale, NJ: Erlbaum.

Bandura, A. (1986). *Social foundations of thought and action: A social cognitive theory.* Englewood Cliffs, NJ: Prentice-Hall.

Basic Behavioral Science Task Force of the National Advisory Mental Health Council. (1996). Basic behavioral science research for mental health: Vulnerability and resilience. *American Psychologist, 51,* 22–28.

Brown, S., Botsis, A., & Van Praag, H. (1994). Serotonin and aggression. *Journal of Offender Rehabilitation, 21,* 27–39.

Burgess, R. L., & Akers, R. L. (1966). A differential association–reinforcement theory of criminal behavior. *Social Problems, 14,* 128–147.

Buss, A. H. (1966). *Psychopathology.* New York: Wiley.

Cairns, R. B., Cairns, B. D., Neckerman, H. J., Gest, S. D., & Gariepy, J. L. (1988). Social networks and aggressive behavior: Peer support or peer rejection? *Developmental Psychology, 24,* 815–823.

Caspi, A., & Bem, D. (1990). Personality continuity and change across the life course. In L. Pervin (Ed.), *Handbook of personality: Theory and research* (pp. 549–575). New York: Guilford.

Caspi, A., & Silva, P. A. (1995). Temperamental qualities at age 3 predict personality traits in young adulthood: Longitudinal evidence from a birth cohort. *Child Development, 66,* 486–498.

Caspi, A., Henry, B., McGee, R. O., Moffitt, T. E., & Silva, P. A. (1995). Temperamental origins of child and adolescent behavior problems: From age 3 to age 15. *Child Development, 66,* 55–68.

Cernkovich, S. A., & Giordano, P. C. (1996). School bonding, race, and delinquency. In D. G. Rojek & G. F. Jensen (Eds.), *Exploring delinquency: Causes and control* (pp. 210–218). Los Angeles: Roxbury.

Cleckley, H. (1976). *The mask of sanity.* St. Louis, MO: Mosby.

Cloninger, C., & Gottesman, I. (1987). Genetic and environmental factors in antisocial behavior disorders. In S. A. Mednick, T. Moffitt, & S. Stack (Eds.)., *The causes of crime: New biological approaches* (pp. 92–109). Cambridge, England: Cambridge University Press.

Cloninger, C., Sigvardsson, S., Bohman, M., & von Knorring, A. (1982). Predisposition to petty criminality in Swedish Adoptees: II. Cross-fostering analysis of gene–environment interaction. *Archives of General Psychiatry, 39,* 1242–1249.

Coccaro, E., Kavoussi, R., & Lesser, J. (1992). Self- and other-directed human aggression: The role of the central serotonergic system. *International Clinical Psychopharmacology, 6,* 70–83.

Cochrane, R. (1974). Crime and personality: Theory and evidence. *Bulletin of the British Psychological Society, 27,* 19–22.

Conger, R. (1980). Juvenile delinquency: Behavior restraint or behavior facilitation? In T. Hirschi & M. Gottfredson (Eds.), *Understanding crime: Current theory and research* (pp. 131–142). Newbury Park, CA: Sage.

Cornish, D. B., & Clark, R. V. (1986). *The reasoning criminal: Rational choice perspectives on offending.* New York: Springer.

Dahlstrom, W. G., Welsh, G. S., & Dahlstrom, L. E. (1972). *An MMPI handbook* (Vol. 1). Minneapolis: University of Minnesota Press.

Denno, D. J. (1990). *Biology, crime and violence: New evidence: From birth to adulthood.* Cambridge, England: Cambridge University Press.

DeWolfe, A. S., & Ryan, J. J. (1984). Wechsler Performance IQ > Verbal IQ index in a forensic sample: A reconsideration. *Journal of Clinical Psychology, 40,* 291–294.

DiLalla, L. F., & Gottesman, I. (1989). Heterogeneity of causes for delinquency and criminality: Lifespan perspectives. *Development and Psychopathology, 1,* 339–349.

DiLalla, L. F., & Gottesman, I. (1991). Biological and genetic contributors to violence—Widom's untold tale. *Psychological Bulletin, 109,* 125–129.

Dodge, K. (1986). A social information processing model of social competence in children. In M. Perlmutter (Ed.), *Minnesota symposium on child psychology* (pp. 77–125). Hillsdale, NJ: Erlbaum.

Dutton, D. (1995). Male abusiveness in intimate relationships. *Clinical Psychology Review, 15,* 567–582.

Elliott, D., Huizinga, D., & Menard, S. M. (1985). *Multiple problem youth: Delinquency, substance use, and mental health problems.* New York: Springer-Verlag.

Ellis, L. (1991a). Monoamine oxidase and criminality: Identifying an apparent biological marker for antisocial behavior. *Journal of Research in Crime and Delinquency, 28,* 227–251.

Ellis, L. (1991b). A synthesized (biosocial) theory of rape. *Journal of Consulting and Clinical Psychology, 59,* 631–642.

Eron, L. (1987). The development of aggressive behavior from the perspective of a developing behaviorism. *American Psychologist, 42,* 435–442.

Eron, L. D. (1990). Understanding aggression. *Bulletin of the International Society for Research on Aggression, 12,* 5–9.

Eysenck, H. J. (1964). *Crime and personality.* Boston: Houghton Mifflin.

Eysenck, H. J. (1970). *The structure of human personality.* London: Methuen.

Eysenck, H. J. (1977). *Crime and personality.* London: Routledge & Kegan Paul.

Eysenck, H. J., & Eysenck, S. B. G. (1974). Personality and recidivism in Borstal Boys. *British Journal of Criminology, 14,* 385–387.

Eysenck, H. J., & Eysenck, S. B. G. (1976). *Psychoticism as a dimension of personality.* London: Hodder and Stoughton.

Eysenck, H. J., & Gudjonson, G. H. (1989). *The causes and cures of criminality.* New York: Plenum.

Farrington, D. P. (1989). Early predictors of adolescent aggression and adult violence. *Violence and Victims, 4,* 79–100.

Farrington, D. P. (1995). The twelfth Jack Tizard Memorial Lecture. The development of offending and antisocial behavior from childhood: Key findings from the Cambridge Study in Delinquent Development. *Journal of Child Psychology and Psychiatry, 360,* 929–964.

Farrington, D. P., Loeber, R., & Van Kammen, W. (1990). Long-term criminal outcomes of hyperactivity-impulsivity-attention deficit and conduct problems in childhood. In L. N. Robins & M. Rutter (Eds.), *Straight and devious pathways from childhood to adulthood* (pp. 62–81). Cambridge, England: Cambridge University Press.

Federal Bureau of Investigation. (1995). *Uniform Crime Reports for the United States: 1994.* Washington, DC: U.S. Department of Justice.

Feldman, M. P. (1977). *Criminal behavior: A psychological analysis.* New York: Wiley.

Freedman, J. L. (1984). Effect of television violence on aggressiveness. *Psychological Bulletin, 96,* 227–246.

Freedman, J. L. (1986). Television violence and aggression: A rejoinder. *Psychological Bulletin, 100,* 372–378.

Frick, P. J., O'Brien, B. S., Wootton, J. M., & McBurnett, K. (1994). Psychopathy and conduct problems in children. *Journal of Abnormal Psychology, 103,* 700–707.

Friedrich-Cofer, L., & Huston, A. C. (1986). Television violence and aggression: A rejoinder. *Psychological Bulletin, 100,* 364–371.

Garza-Treviño, E. (1994). Neurobiological factors in aggressive behavior. *Hospital and Community Psychiatry, 45,* 690–699.

Gorenstein, E. E., & Newman, J. P. (1980). Disinhibitory psychopathology: A new perspective and a model for research. *Psychological Review, 87,* 301–315.

Hall, G., & Hirschman, R. (1991). Toward a theory of sexual aggression: A quadripartite model. *Journal of Consulting and Clinical Psychology, 59,* 662–669.

Hare, R. D. (1970). *Psychopathy: Theory and practice.* New York: Wiley.

Hare, R. D. (1981). Psychopathy and violence. In J. R. Hayes, T. K. Roberts, & K. S. Solway (Eds.), *Violence and the violent individual* (pp. 53–74). Jamaica, NY: Spectrum.

Hare, R. D., & McPherson, L. M. (1984). Violent and aggressive behavior by criminal psychopaths. *International Journal of Law and Psychiatry, 7,* 329–337.

Hare, R. D., McPherson, L. M., & Forth, A. E. (1988). Male psychopaths and their criminal careers. *Journal of Consulting and Clinical Psychology, 56,* 710–714.

Harris, G. T., Rice, M. E., & Cormier, C. A. (1989). Violent recidivism among psychopaths and nonpsychopaths treated in a therapeutic community. *Penetanguishene Mental Health Center Research Report, 6,* 181.

Hart, S. D., & Hare, R. D. (1989). Discriminant validity of the Psychopathy Checklist in a forensic psychiatric population. *Psychological Assessment: A Journal of Consulting and Clinical Psychology, 1,* 211–218.

Hart, S. D., Kropp, P. R., & Hare, R. D. (1988). Performance of male psychopaths following conditional release from prison. *Journal of Consulting and Clinical Psychology, 56,* 227–232.

Haynes, J. P., & Bensch, M. (1981). The P > V sign of the WISC-R and recidivism in delinquents. *Journal of Consulting and Clinical Psychology, 49,* 480–481.

Heilbrun, A. B., & Heilbrun, M. R. (1985). Psychopathy and dangerousness: Comparison, integration and extension of two psychopathic typologies. *British Journal of Clinical Psychology, 24,* 181–195.

Henry, B., Caspi, A., Moffitt, T. E., & Silva, P. A. (1996). Temperamental and familial predictors of violent and nonviolent criminal convictions: From age 3 to age 18. *Developmental Psychology, 32,* 614–623.

Hinshaw, S. P., Lahey, B. B., & Hart, E. L. (1993). Issues of taxonomy and comorbidity in the development of conduct disorder. *Development and Psychopathology 5,* 31–49.

Hirschi, T. (1969). *Causes of delinquency.* Berkeley: University of California Press.

Hirschi, T. (1978). Causes and prevention of juvenile delinquency. In H. M. Johnson (Ed.), *Social systems and legal process.* San Francisco: Jossey-Bass.

Holland, T. R., & Holt, N. (1975). Prisoner intellectual and personality correlates of offense severity and recidivism probability. *Journal of Clinical Psychology, 31,* 667–672.

Holland, T. R., Beckett, G. E., & Levi, M. (1981). Intelligence, personality, and criminal violence: A multivariage analysis. *Journal of Consulting and Clinical Psychology, 49,* 106–111.

Huesmann, L. R., Eron, L. D., Lefkowitz, M. M., & Walder, L. O. (1984). Stability of aggression over time and generations. *Developmental Psychology, 20,* 1120–1134.

Jeffery, C. R. (1965). Criminal behavior and learning theory. *Journal of Criminal Law, Criminology, and Police Science, 56,* 294–300.

John, O. P. (1990). The "Big Five" factor taxonomy: Dimensions of personality in the natural language and questionnaires. In L. A. Pervin (Ed.), *Handbook of personality: Theory and research* (pp. 66–100). New York: Guilford.

Katz, J. (1988). *Seductions of crime.* New York: Basic Books.

Kosson, D. S., Smith, S. S., & Newman, J. P. (1990). Evaluating the construct validity of psychopathy on Black and White male inmates: Three preliminary studies. *Journal of Abnormal Psychology, 99,* 250–259.

Krueger, R. F., Schmutte, P. S., Caspi, A., Moffitt, T. E., Campbell, K., & Silva, P. A. (1994). Personality traits are linked to crime among men and women: Evidence from a birth cohort. *Journal of Abnormal Psychology, 103,* 328–338.

Lahey, B. B., Piacentini, J. C., McBurnett, K., Stone, P., Hartdagen, S., & Hynd, G. (1987). Psychopathology in the parents of children with conduct disorder and hyperactivity. *Journal of the American Academy of Child and Adolescent Psychiatry, 27,* 163–170.

Lahey, B. B., Loeber, R., Hart, E. L., Frick, P. J., Applegate, B., Zhang, Q., Green, S. M., & Russo, M. F. (1995). Four-year longitudinal study of conduct disorder in boys: Patterns and predictors of persistence. *Journal of Abnormal Psychology, 104,* 83–93.

Lane, D. A. (1978). *The impossible child* (Vols. 1–2). London: ILEA.

Lane, D. A. (1987). Personality and antisocial behaviour: A long-term study. *Personality and Individual Differences, 8,* 799–806.

Lane, D. A., & Hymans, M. H. (1982). The prediction of delinquency. *Personality and Individual Differences, 3,* 87–88.

Lipton, D., Martinson, R., & Wilks, J. (1975). *The effectiveness of correctional treatment: A survey of treatment evaluation studies.* New York: Praeger.

Loeber, R. (1982). The stability of antisocial behavior and delinquent child behavior: A review. *Child Development, 53,* 1431–1446.

Loeber, R., & Dishion, T. J. (1983). Early predictors of male adolescent delinquency: A review. *Psychological Bulletin, 94,* 68–99.

Loeber, R., & Stouthamer-Loeber, M. (1986). Family factors as correlates and predictors of juvenile conduct problems and delinquency. In M. Tonry & N. Morris (Eds.), *Crime and justice: An annual review of research* (Vol. 7, pp. 29–149). Chicago: University of Chicago Press.

Loeber, R., Brinthaupt, V. P., & Green, S. (1990). Attention deficits, impulsivity, and hyperactivity with or without conduct problems: Relationships to delinquency and unique contextual factors. In R. J. McMahon & R. DeV. Peters (Eds.), *Behavior disorders of adolescence: Research, intervention, and policy in clinical and school settings* (pp. 39–61). New York: Plenum.

Lynam, D. R. (1996). The early identification of chronic offenders: Who is the fledgling psychopath? *Psychological Bulletin, 120,* 209–234.

Lynam, D. (1997). Pursuing the Psychapath: Capturing the fledgling psychopath in the nomological net. *Journal of Abnormal Psychology, 106,* 425–438.

Lynam, D., Moffitt, T., & Stouthamer-Loeber, M. (1993). Explaining the relation between IQ and delinquency: Class, race, test motivation, school failure, or self-control? *Journal of Abnormal Psychology, 102,* 187–196.

Magnusson, D. (1988). *Individual development from an interactional perspective: A longitudinal study.* Hillsdale, NJ: Erlbaum.

McCord, W., & McCord, J. (1964). *The psychopath: An essay on the criminal mind.* Princeton, NJ: Van Nostrand.

McGee, R., Silva, P. A., & Williams, S. (1984). Behavior problems in a population of seven-year-old children: Prevalence, stability, and types of disorder—A research note. *Journal of Child Psychology and Psychiatry, 25,* 251–259.

McGee, R., Feehan, M., Williams, S., & Anderson, J. (1992). DSM-III disorders from age 11 to age 15 years. *Journal of the American Academy of Child and Adolescent Psychiatry, 31,* 50–59.

McGue, M., Bacon, S., & Lykken, D. T. (1993). Personality stability and change in early adulthood: A behavioral genetic analysis. *Developmental Psychology, 29,* 96–109.

Mednick, S., & Kandel, E. (1988). Congenital determinants of violence. *Bulletin of the American Academy of Psychiatry and the Law, 16,* 101–109.

Mednick, S. A., Gabrielli, W. F., Jr., & Hutchings, B. (1984). Genetic factors in the etiology of criminal behavior. In S. A. Mednick, T. E. Moffitt, & S. A. Stack (Eds.), *The causes of crime: New biological approaches* (pp. 74–91). Cambridge, England: Cambridge University Press.

Mednick, S., Gabrielli, W., & Hutchings, B. (1987). Genetic influences in the etiology of criminal behavior. In S. A. Mednick, T. Moffitt, & S. Stack (Eds.), *The causes of crime: New biological approaches* (pp. 74–91). Cambridge, England: Cambridge University Press.

Merton, R. K. (1968). *Social theory and social structure.* Revised edition. New York: The Free Press.

Miller, L. (1994). Traumatic brain injury and aggression. *Journal of Offender Rehabilitation, 21,* 91–103.

Millon, T. D. (1981). *Disorders of personality: DSM-III Axis II.* New York: Wiley.

Mills, S., & Raine, A. (1994). Neuroimaging and aggression. *Journal of Offender Rehabilitation, 21,* 145–158.

Moffitt, T. E. (1990a). Juvenile delinquency and attention deficit disorder: Boys' developmental trajectories from age 3 to age 15. *Child Development, 61,* 893–910.

Moffitt, T. E. (1990b). The neuropsychology of delinquency: A critical review of theory and research. In N. Morris & M. Tonry (Eds.), *Crime and justice: An annual review of research* (Vol. 12, pp. 99–169). Chicago: University of Chicago Press.

Moffitt, T. E. (1993). Adolescence-limited and life-course persistent antisocial behavior: A developmental taxonomy. *Psychological Review, 100,* 674–701.

Moffitt, T. E., & Henry, B. (1991). Neuropsychological studies of juvenile delinquency and violence: A review. In J. Milner (Ed.), *The neuropsychology of aggression* (pp. 67–91). Norwell, MA: Kluwer Academic Publishers.

Moffitt, T. E., & Lynam, D. R. (1994). The neuropsychology of Conduct Disorder and delinquency: Implications for understanding antisocial behavior. In D. Fowles, P. Sutker, & S. Goodman (Eds.), *Psychopathy and Antisocial Personality: A developmental perspective* (pp. 233–262). Vol. 18 in the series, Progress in Experimental Personality and Psychopathology Research. New York: Springer.

Moffitt, T. E., & Silva, P. A. (1988). IQ and delinquency: A direct test of the differential detection hypothesis. *Journal of Abnormal Psychology, 97,* 330–333.

Moffitt, T. E., Caspi, A., Silva, P., & Stouthamer-Loeber, M. (1995). Individual differences in personality and intelligence are linked to crime: Cross-context evidence from nations, neighborhoods, genders, and age-cohort. In J. Hagan (Ed.), *Current perspectives on aging and the life-cycle: Vol. 4. Delinquency and disrepute in the life-course: Contextual and dynamic analyses* (pp. 1–34) Greenwich, CT: JAI.

Monahan, J. (1992). Mental disorder and violent behavior: Perceptions and evidence. *American Psychologist, 47,* 511–521.

Murdoch, D., Pihl, R., & Ross, D. (1990). Alcohol and crimes of violence: Present issues. *International Journal on Addiction, 25,* 1065–1081.

Newman, J. P. (1987). Reaction to punishment in extraverts and psychopaths: Implications for the impulsive behavior of disinhibited individuals. *Journal of Research in Personality, 21,* 464–480.

Newman, J. P., & Kosson, D. S. (1986). Passive avoidance learning in psychopathic and nonpsychopathic offenders. *Journal of Abnormal Psychology, 95,* 257–263.

Newman, J. P., Patterson, C. M., & Kosson, D. S. (1987). Response preservation in psychopaths. *Journal of Abnormal Psychology, 96,* 145–148.

Newman, J. P., Patterson, C. M., Howland, E. W., & Nichols, S. L. (1990). Passive avoidance in psychopaths: The effects of reward. *Personality and Individual Differences, 11,* 1101–1114.

Offord, D. R., Sullivan, K., Allen, N., & Abrams, N. (1979). Delinquency and hyperactivity. *Journal of Nervous and Mental Disease, 167,* 734–741.

Ogloff, J., Wong, S., & Greenwood, A. (1990). Treating criminal psychopaths in a therapeutic community program. *Behavioral Sciences and the Law, 8,* 181–189.

Olweus, D. (1979). Stability of aggressive reaction patterns in males: A review. *Psychological Bulletin, 86,* 852–875.

Olweus, D. (1987). Testosterone and adrenaline: Aggressive antisocial behavior in normal adolescent males. In S. A. Mednick, T. E. Moffitt, & S. A. Stack (Eds.), *The causes of crime: New biological approaches* (pp. 263–282). Cambridge, England: Cambridge University Press.

Olweus, D. (1995). Bullying or peer abuse at school: Facts and intervention. *Current Directions in Psychological Science, 4,* 196–200.

Palmer, T. (1984). Treatment and the role of classification: A review of basic issues. *Crime and Delinquency, 30,* 245–267.

Pasingham, R. E. (1972). Crime and personality: A review of Eysenck's theory. In V. D. Nebylitsyn & J. A. Gray (Eds.), *Biological bases of individual behavior* (pp. 342–371). New York: Academic Press.

Patterson, E. B. (1996). Poverty, income inequality, and community crime rates. In D. G. Rojet & G. F. Jensen (Eds.), *Exploring delinquency: Causes and control* (pp. 142–149). Los Angeles: Roxbury.

Patterson, G. R. (1982). *Coercive family process.* Eugene, OR: Castalia.

Patterson, G. R. (1986). Performance models for antisocial boys. *American Psychologist, 41,* 432–444.

Pearl, D., Bouthilet, L., & Lazar, J. (Eds.). (1982). *Television and behavior: Ten years of scientific progress and implications for the eighties* (Vols. 1–2). Washington, DC: U.S. Government Printing Office.

Pearson, F., & Weiner, N. (1985). Criminology: Toward an integration of criminological theories. *Journal of Criminal Law and Criminology, 76,* 116–150.

Pierson, G. R. (1969). The role of the HSPQ in the Greenhill Programme. In R. B. Cattell & M. D. Cattell (Eds.), *Handbook for the H.S.P.O.* Champaign, IL: IPAT.:

Platt, J. J., & Prout, M. F. (1987). Cognitive-behavioral theory and interventions for crime and delinquency. In E. K. Morris & C. J. Braukmann (Eds.), *Behavioral approaches to crime and delinquency: A handbook of application, research, and concepts* (pp. 477–497). New York; Plenum.

Prentice, N. M., & Kelly, F. J. (1963). Intelligence and delinquency: A reconsideration. *Journal of Social Psychology, 60,* 327–337.

Putnins, A. C. (1982). The Eysenck Personality Questionnaires and delinquency prediction. *Personality and Individual Differences, 3,* 339–340.

Reckless, W. (1967). *The crime problem* (4th ed.). New York: Meredith.

Ribes-Inesta, E., & Bandura, A. (Eds.). (1976). *Analysis of delinquency and aggression.* Hillsdale, NJ: Erlbaum.

Robins, L. (1978). Sturdy childhood predictors of adult antisocial behavior: Replications from longitudinal studies. *Psychological Medicine, 8,* 611–622.

Robins, L. N., & McEvoy, L. (1990). Conduct problems as predictors of substance abuse. In L. Robins & M. Rutter (Eds.), *Straight and devious pathways from childhood to adulthood* (pp. 182–204). Cambridge, England: Cambridge University Press.

Rushton, J. P., & Chrisjohn, R. D. (1981). Extraversion, neuroticism, psychoticism, and self-reported delinquency: Evidence from eight separate samples. *Personality and Individual Differences, 2,* 11–20.

Schonfeld, I. S., Shaffer, D., O'Connor, P., & Portnoy, S. (1988). Conduct disorder and cognitive functioning: Testing three causal hypotheses. *Child Development, 39,* 993–1007.

Sechrest, L., White, S. O., & Brown, E. D. (Eds.). (1975). *The rehabilitation of criminal offenders: Problems and prospects.* Washington, DC: National Academy of Sciences.

Seguin, J. R., Pihl, R. O., Harden, P. W., Tremblay, R. E., & Boulerice, B. (1995). Cognitive and neuropsychological characteristics of physically aggressive boys. *Journal of Abnormal Psychology, 104,* 614-624.

Seidman, E., & Rapkin, B. (1983). Economics and psychosocial dysfunction: Toward a conceptual framework and prevention strategies. In R. D. Felner, L. A. Jason, J. N. Moritsugu, & S. S. Farber (Eds.), *Preventive psychology* (pp. 175–198). New York: Pergamon.

Serin, R. C., Peters, R. D., & Barbaree, H. E. (1990). Predictors of psychopathy and release outcome in a criminal population. *Psychological Assessment, 2,* 419–422.

Shapiro, D. (1965). *Neurotic styles.* New York: Basic Books.

Shapiro, S. K., & Garfinkel, H. D. (1986). The occurrence of behavior disorders in children. *Journal of the American Academy of Child and Adolescent Psychiatry, 25,* 809–819.

Shuck, S., Dubeck, J. A., Cymbalisty, B. Y., & Green, C. (1972). Delinquency, personality tests, and relationships to measures of guilt and adjustment. *Psychological Reports, 31,* 219–226.

Surgeon General's Scientific Advisory Committee on Television and Social Behavior. (1972). *Television and growing up: The impact of televised violence.* Washington, DC: U.S. Government Printing Office.

Sutherland, E. H. (1947). *Principles of criminology* (4th ed.). Philadelphia: Lippincott.

Szatmari, P., Boyle, M., & Offord, D. R. (1989). ADDH and conduct disorder: Degree of diagnostic overlap and differences among correlates. *Journal of the American Academy of Child and Adolescent Psychiatry, 28,* 865–872.

Valliant, P. M., Asu, M. E., Cooper, D., & Mammola, D. (1984). Profile of dangerous and nondangerous offenders referred for pretrial psychiatric assessment. *Psychological Reports, 54,* 411–418.

Walker, J. L., Lahey, B. B., Hynd, G. W., & Frame, C. L. (1987). Comparison of specific patterns of antisocial behavior in children with conduct disorder with or without coexisting hyperactivity. *Journal of Consulting and Clinical Psychology, 55,* 910–913.

Walsh, A., Petee, T. A., & Beyer, J. A. (1987). Intellectual imbalance and delinquency: Comparing high verbal and high performance IQ delinquents. *Criminal Justice and Behavior, 14*(3), 370–379.

Walters, G. D. (1992). A meta-analysis of the gene–crime relationship. *Criminology, 30,* 595–613.

Warr, E. M., & Stafford, M. (1996). The influence of delinquent peers: What they think or what they do? In D. G. Rojet & G. F. Jensen (Eds.), *Exploring delinquency: Causes and control* (pp. 219–227). Los Angeles: Roxbury.

Wechsler, D. (1974). *Manual for the Wechsler Intelligence Scale for Children–Revised.* San Antonio, TX: Psychological Corporation.

West, D. J., & Farrington, D. P. (1973). *Who becomes delinquent?* London; Heineman Educational Books.

White, J., Moffitt, T. E., Caspi, A., Bartusch, D. J., Needles, D., & Stouthamer-Loeber, M. (1994). Measuring impulsivity and examining its relation to delinquency. *Journal of Abnormal Psychology, 103,* 192–205.

Widom, C. (1989). Does violence beget violence? A critical examination of the literature. *Psychological Bulletin, 106,* 3–28.

Wiegman, O., Kuttschreuter, M., & Baarda, B. (1992). A longitudinal study of the effects of television view-
    ing on aggressive and prosocial behaviours. *British Journal of Social Psychology, 31*, 147–164.

Wilson, J. Q., & Herrnstein, R. (1985). *Crime and human nature*. New York: Simon & Schuster.

Yeudall, L. T., Fedora, O., Fedora, S., & Wardell, D. (1981). Neurosocial perspective on the assessment and
    etiology of persistent criminality. *Australian Journal of Forensic Science, 13*, 131–159; *14,* 20–44.

4

Psychodynamic Theories

Howard D. Lerner

Introduction

In approaching the topic of the violent criminal offender from a psychoanalytic point of view, it is important to realize that contemporary psychoanalysis is not a unified theory. The original Freudian theory has been modified and expanded into several overlapping but coherent and distinct approaches to human development, psychopathology, and treatment. Most prominent among these are modern structural theory (most closely associated with Freud's drive theory), self psychology (associated with the theories of Heinz Kohut), and object relations theory (stressing the formative developmental impact of interpersonal relationships).

In regard to violence and aggression, a fundamental disagreement exists, for example, between structural theorists who tend to see aggression as an innate drive, and self psychologists, who view aggression as secondary to narcissistic injury. Despite such differences, psychoanalysts share certain basic views: aggression plays a crucial role in the infant–parent and child–parent dyads, the successful modulation of aggression is crucial to healthy development, and managing aggression successfully is critical to the therapeutic endeavor. Psychoanalysts also concur in understanding that difficulties in modulating or integrating aggression, on a continuum from its milder to its more severe forms, is core to psychopathology.

In this chapter, a brief review of Freud's approach to aggression is outlined and some of its recent modifications presented. Violence and aggression are then explored, using Kernberg's (1975) notion of personality organization. A prominent contemporary theorist who has addressed severe psychopathology at length, Kernberg used a conceptual framework that broadly integrates both drive theory and object relations theory. Seven structural variables that determine levels of personality organization are defined. Most violent criminal offenders fall in the borderline level of personality organization. This level of personality organization will be explored in depth in terms of pathological narcissism and what is referred to as the antisocial personality. The role of dehumanization in violent crime is discussed in terms of the dynamics of externaliza-

Howard D. Lerner • Michigan Psychoanalytic Institute, and Department of Psychiatry, University of Michigan, Ann Arbor, Michigan 48104-2427.

Handbook of Psychological Approaches with Violent Offenders: Contemporary Strategies and Issues, edited by Van Hasselt and Hersen. Kluwer Academic/Plenum Publishers, New York, 1999.

tion and omnipotence. The chapter concludes with a brief overview of psychoanalytic approaches to the treatment of the violent criminal offender.

The Concept of Aggression in Freud's Work

As H. Lerner and Ehrlich (1994) outlined, at a time when prevailing cultural and scientific opinion held that childhood was free of any evidence of sexuality, Freud proclaimed the opposite. He advanced the libido theory which stressed the influence of sexuality on mental life. His vast clinical experience, including his self-analysis and the analysis of his patients' fantasies, associations, and memories from childhood, led him to conclude that sexual urges provided the prime motivation for psychological functioning. He postulated that a force or psychic energy propelled sexual behavior, and he termed this energy *libido*.

As more clinical data accumulated, Freud (1920) expanded his instinctual drive or libido theory to include an aggressive or destructive component. His clinical observations and experience led him to the compelling conclusion that feelings of anger and hostility result in conflict and unconscious guilt in the same manner that sexual wishes do, and that these affects initiate defensive activity. He observed that many impulses contain both sexual and aggressive components, and that many clinical manifestations, including sadism and masochism, can be explained in terms of varying degrees of conflict between these drives or their fusion. Freud also believed that nondestructive dimensions of aggression provide motivation for activity and mastery. In essence, he postulated that the libidinal and aggressive drives are fundamental aspects of human nature.

In his first model of the mind, Freud (1905) viewed aggression as a component of the sexual drive: "The history of civilization shows beyond any doubt that there is an innate connection between cruelty and the sexual instinct" (p. 159). The observation that aggressive impulses often appear to be a reaction to external stimuli led Freud (1915) to describe aggression as an attitude in the service of self-preservation. In a more philosophical context, Freud (1920) hypothesized existence of a fundamental and lifelong conflict between the death instinct (Thanatos) and a life instinct (Eros). He viewed the aggressive drive as originating from an organically based death instinct. The principle by which the death instinct operated was that of an organism striving to discharge excitation and reach an ultimate state of nirvana, or the total absence of excitation. This revision in theory provided fuel for theoretical controversy for many years.

According to Schengold (1989), "Freud believed that destructiveness and the abuse of power are part of our inherited biological nature, flowing from our bodies to our minds in the form of instinctual drives. He viewed our attempts at civilization as transcending our murderous, polymorphous perverse and incestuous human nature, as heroic and tragic—capable at best of achieving a partial success, a compromise that leaves us inherently neurotic, with a discontent that can easily regress to hatred and misery (Freud, 1930, p. 15)."

Contemporary psychoanalytic theories of aggression revolve around the nature–nurture debate. Following directly from Freud, some theorists consider aggression to be an innate part of the person's constitution, an instinct for destruction. Core to these formulations is a view of aggression as an annihilating presence in the infant.

It is an anti-life, anti-self force; an impediment to development. Kernberg offers the most sophisticated statement of the "innate destructiveness" model. In his view of aggression as a drive that is integrated from a variety of inborn feeling states, these negative feeling states and associated proprioceptive and perceptual experiences are the innate components of complex affects such as hatred and rage. They are, in turn, integrated into the drive structure of aggression.

Other theorists, particularly self psychologists, regard aggression as a reactive and protective phenomenon, provoked in the individual by external circumstances that ultimately lead to frustration. From this vantage point, aggression has been seen as a reaction to the conflicts inherent in the process of adaptation, a reaction to unpleasure, a striving to overcome obstacles, and as a part of a healthy struggle to oppose pathological interactions. This point of view roots aggression in a "failure of fit" between the child's needs and the response of the mother. For self psychologists, aggression is a reaction to narcissistic threat, a signal of potential injury to the self.

Structural Variables

Almost a century of cumulative psychoanalytic knowledge has contributed to an appreciation that each individual processes external events to give them unique internal meaning and mental representation. In a major theoretical and clinical contribution, Kernberg (1975) formulated a classification of personality organizations, which provides a useful framework for examining the spectrum of meanings and expressions of aggression in violent criminal offenders. Kernberg describes three levels of personality structures: normal–neurotic, borderline (including narcissistic and antisocial personalities), and psychotic personality organizations. These hierarchical levels of personality organization are determined by constitutional, developmental, psychosocial, genetic, and intrafamilial factors. Kernberg's classification of personality organizations involves a systematic appraisal of levels of instinctual development, manifestations of ego strength, level of defensive organization, quality of internalized object relations or representations, level of superego or moral development, and attainment of ego identity. The degree of differentiation, articulation, and integration of these, both individually and as a gestalt, determines the overall level of personality organization and, in turn, determines the intensity and personal meanings as well as the expression of violent criminal behavior. According to Kernberg, the personality organization, once formed, functions as the underlying matrix or structure out of which behavioral symptoms develop, and it serves to stabilize psychological functioning. Kernberg's schema suggests that the quality, intensity, and meaning of aggression for an individual with a psychotic personality organization will differ significantly from the aggression of the borderline individual, which, in turn, will differ from the quality of aggression in an individual with a neurotic personality organization.

A consideration of aggression in the context of levels of personality organization has important treatment implications and prognostic value. Personality organization serves as a key prognostic indicator of specific treatment needs and helps determine treatment response. Kernberg's classification schema has received wide currency in the literature related to psychopathology, and the structural variables he has identified and described have proven especially useful in empirical investigations of more severe psychopathology (Giacono & Meloy, 1994; Kwawer, Lerner, Lerner, & Sugarman, 1980; H. Lerner & Lerner, 1988; P. Lerner, 1991).

In what follows, the three levels of personality organization—normal–neurotic, borderline, and psychotic—are examined to illustrate specific characteristics of each and how these determine the experience and expression of violent crime. Each is explored in terms of seven structural variables of personality function that have been demonstrated to distinguish them and to contribute to differences in aggression, ego identity defensive organization, reality testing, ego strength, superego formation, and genetic-dynamic considerations. First, the structural variables are defined.

Object Representation

In psychoanalytic theory, the term "object" can refer to interpersonal relationships, but it generally refers to an individual's underlying *internal* relationships with others. According to Greenberg and Mitchell (1983), individuals carry "internal images" of self and others that determine the individual's experience of the world. According to these authors, "What is generally agreed upon about the internal images is that they constitute a residue within the mind of relationships with significant others. In some way crucial exchanges with others leave their mark; they are 'internalized' and so come to shape subsequent attitudes, reactions, and perceptions" (p. 11). From a psychoanalytic perspective, insight into and assessment of an individual's internalized object relations or representations is crucial to an understanding of that individual's developmental experience, level of personality organization, and experience of the world. Psychoanalysts have increasingly focused on the complex interactions among early formative interpersonal relationships and how these transactions result in the formation of intrapsychic structures that can be best understood in terms of self and object representations. Representations of self and other in turn shape and direct subsequent interpersonal relationships.

Broadly defined, object representation refers to the conscious and unconscious mental schemata, including cognitive, affective, and experiential dimensions, of significant interpersonal transactions. Beginning as vague, diffuse, variable sensory motor experience of pleasure and unpleasure, schemata gradually develop into differentiated, consistent, relatively realistic representations of the self and others. Earlier forms of representation are thought to be based on action sequences associated with need gratification, intermediate forms are based on specific perceptual and functional features, and higher forms of representation are more symbolic and conceptual. There is a constant and reciprocal interaction between past and current interpersonal relations and the development of representations. Schemata evolve from the internalization of object relations and new levels of object and self representation provide a revised organization for subsequent interpersonal relationships (Blatt & Lerner, 1991).

Ego Identity

According to Kernberg (1976), ego identity "is the highest level of organization of the world of object relations in the broader sense" (p. 32). Ego identity is developed, according to Kernberg, through the gradual internalization of object relations at progressively higher, more differentiated levels. In its more integrated form, ego identity provides a sense of continuity within the self, a sense of consistency in one's interpersonal interactions, and a sense of sameness across different situations and along a time dimension.

Defensive Organization

According to Brenner (1982), defenses constitute an aspect of mental functioning that reduces anxiety or depressive affect. Psychoanalysts have identified a wide spectrum of defenses that Kernberg arranges hierarchically—from "upper level" defenses such as repression and sublimation, found in individuals with a neurotic personality organization, to what are termed more "primitive" defenses such as splitting and devaluation, found in individuals with borderline and psychotic organizations. According to Kernberg (1976), different levels of personality organization reflect different constellations of defenses, which in turn reflect the individual's overall level of ego functioning and are employed to contend with particular conflicts and dilemmas associated with each level of personality organization.

Reality Testing

Frosch (1964) has identified three types of involvement with reality: the relation to reality (adaptive social behavior), the feeling of reality (absence of depersonalization and derealization), and the capacity to test reality. Reality testing can be conceptualized on a continuum, including (1) the ability to distinguish self from others; (2) the ability to distinguish between internal ideas, images, and affects (internal stimuli) and perceptions (external stimuli); and (3) the ability to assess accurately one's own actions, impulses, and thoughts in the context of the culture in which one lives (social judgment).

Ego Strength

Ego strength refers to the capacity to tolerate anxiety (to regulate increased levels of stress without developing symptoms or regressing), the capacity for impulse control (to experience intense affects, fantasies, and experiences without acting on them against one's best interest), and the capacity for sublimation (to develop creative outlets for gratification and self-interest). Ego weakness refers to a difficulty in these three domains. Ego strength permits individuals to sublimate both aggressive and sexual impulses in adaptive activities rather than through non-self-reflective action in the pursuit of instant gratification or pleasure.

Superego Integration

Superego integration refers to the degree to which an individual is able to regulate behavior according to ethical principles; that is, to refrain from exploitation, manipulation, or mistreatment of others and to maintain honesty and moral integrity in the absence of external control. Brenner (1982) identifies five superego functions: the internal approval or disapproval of actions and wishes on the grounds of moral considerations, a critical self-observation capacity, self-punishment, the demand for reparation or repentance of wrongdoing, and self-praise or self-love as a reward for virtuous behavior and thoughts. Extremes of any of these functions are thought to be pathological. The internalization of object relations is thought to constitute the major organizing factor for superego development.

Genetic–Dynamic Considerations

Within psychoanalytic theory, "genetic" refers to how conflicts develop from multiple origins in childhood. The term "dynamic" refers to competing, conflicting forces that prevent an idea or feeling from becoming conscious or allow it to enter consciousness only in disguised form. While genetic–dynamic issues vary from individual to individual, certain themes predominate at different levels of personality organization.

Aggression and Levels of Personality Organization

Normal–Neurotic Personality Organization

The normal–neurotic level of personality organization is characterized by a cohesive ego identity, including a relatively stable self-concept and a stable representational world. Values tend to be consistent, goals tend to be realistic, and the sense of reality provides an organizing function for guiding and directing behavior. In terms of superego functioning and moral considerations, neurotic individuals tend to be guided by ethical principles in their daily lives and respond to difficult choices with modulated, goal-directed behavior. Relatively direct or fantasized expressions of aggression are likely to be accompanied by guilt, which, among other things, provides a modulating force and self-regulating function. Neurotic individuals are prone to experience excessive guilt or depression around specific internal, conflictual areas, aggression being prominent among them. Many neurotics suffer from severe inhibitions around aggression.

Individuals with a normal–neurotic level of personality organization utilize higher level, more adaptive defenses than individuals with either borderline or psychotic personality organization. These defenses function largely to restrict anxiety-provoking thoughts and feelings from reaching consciousness. Such defense mechanisms as repression, intellectualization, reaction formation, and rationalization are typical. These defenses often lead to inhibitions of sexuality, aggression, or both. Generally, however, these defenses do not compromise reality testing or contribute to chaotic interpersonal relationships, as do defenses found in the borderline or psychotic personality organization. Individuals with neurotic personality organization exhibit intact reality testing, although they may experience difficulty in assessing their own actions, emotions, and thoughts, secondary to internal conflict and in circumscribed areas of their lives. In contrast to the often chaotic and destructive aggression in individuals with borderline and psychotic personality organizations, the neurotic's greater ego strength and more mature defenses, bolstered by mature superego functioning, contribute to an ability to integrate, modulate, and use aggression in more adaptive, law-abiding ways.

The neurotic tends to maintain a high degree of adaptation to reality, interpersonal stability, and a compliance with societal expectations. The excessive bottling up of aggression in the form of rigid defenses and inhibitions often contributes to the neurotic's experience of unsatisfying interpersonal relationships, frequently experienced as fear of success in the workplace and other domains. Often, this is what leads neurotic individuals to seek treatment. In psychotherapy, in stark contrast to the chaotic presentation of more disturbed individuals, neurotics are well able to explain their problems and conflicts in an integrated fashion, they can empathize with others with whom they are in conflict, and frequently experience excessive guilt. Their internal world is well integrated but in conflict.

The neurotic individual is not immune from antisocial behavior. In fact, Freud (1916) referred to some neurotics who commit crimes out of an unconscious sense of guilt. Nevertheless, their sometimes dramatic antisocial behavior occurs in the context of a neurotic personality organization which has an excellent prognosis for psychotherapy. Kernberg (1992) described a patient with an obsessive-compulsive neurosis who stole minor objects from public places where he worked, exposing himself to the humiliating possibility of being caught and fired. The individual had the good sense to seek psychotherapy and responded very well.

Borderline Personality Organization

Psychoanalysts generally agree that most violent criminal offenders present an underlying borderline personality organization. The lack of an integrated self-concept (identity diffusion) is a core conflict for those individuals with a borderline level of personality organization. Lack of a stable self-concept involves two dimensions: (1) split self-images resulting in contradictory attitudes, feelings, and behavior directed toward the self and personal choices, and (2) splits in the image of significant others, with subsequent chaos and turmoil in interpersonal relationships. These individuals tend to rely on others, even penal institutions, for what is missing in the self—the ability to evaluate oneself and others realistically over time and across situations. Consequently, borderline individuals' perceptions and relationships become increasingly chaotic and distorted over time because of their inability to evaluate themselves and others realistically. Despite what often initially appears to be a stable veneer, these individuals are often "stable in their instability" (Schmideberg, 1959, p. 398), because over time and with increased personal closeness they regress and rely on primitive cognitive-affective states to relate to others in increasingly manipulative and infantile ways. It is extremely difficult for these individuals to maintain empathy and understanding in a relationship once conflict arises; yet, paradoxically, they are unable to separate or take perspective. This is one reason that relationships of borderline individuals are often chaotic and embellished with aggression. Manipulation often replaces empathy as a way of relating. Deficits in reality testing also contribute to this presentation. Borderline individuals experience difficulty in distinguishing between external perceptions and their own intense affective reaction to those perceptions. This contributes to the borderline's propensity to overreact to external stimuli, often aggressively.

According to Kernberg (1976, 1992), individuals with borderline personality structure rely on more primitive defenses, such as splitting, idealization, devaluation, denial, projective identification, and omnipotence. These defenses are thought to "protect the ego from conflicts by means of dissociating or actively keeping apart contradictory experiences of the self and significant others" (Kernberg, 1977, p. 107). Reliance on such defenses is thought to weaken the individual's overall level of functioning and capacity for adaptation.

Kernberg's formulation of primitive defenses encompasses several areas. Core to these defensive operations are contradictory ego states which are actively kept separate from one another. These states are activated alternatively as a way of either reducing or eliminating painful feelings such as anxiety or depression. On the borderline level, individuals can cognitively acknowledge different ego states but either emotionally deny or are emotionally indifferent to this contradictory state of affairs. This state of indifference can protect the borderline individual from potential psychotic experience.

Splitting is the central defense that supports and maintains other primitive defense mechanisms. Splitting is the division of self and others into "all good" or "all bad" representations. These splits are often accompanied by rapid shifts from an all-good to an all-bad array of affective reactions. Clinical implications of splitting frequently involve an inability to experience ambivalence, leading to a rapid devaluation and idealization of others, a rapid shift in allegiances and chaotic relationships; impaired decision-making capacity; rapid oscillation of self-esteem; nonconflicted impulsive behavior such as shoplifting, promiscuity, substance abuse, or wanton violence with little guilt; and an intensification of affect such that positive feelings are often experienced euphorically, while negative feelings are overwhelming, frequently rageful and murderous or suicidal in their intensity.

Primitive idealization, a common defense mechanism in borderline individuals, refers to the tendency to experience some people as all good in order to feel protected from others who are experienced as all bad. Envy and aggression are thought to underlie idealization. Devaluation, another borderline defense, refers to the tendency to deprecate, tarnish, and lessen the importance of others. The devaluation of others is often accompanied by an omnipotent and grandiose self-presentation.

Projective identification, a typical borderline defense, has important interpersonal implications. Kernberg (1975) defined projective identification as a "group of fantasies and accompanying object relations having to do with the ridding of the self of unwanted aspects of the self, the depositing of these unwanted 'parts' into another person; and finally, with the 'recovery' of a modified version of what was extruded" (p. 357). Borderline individuals are thought to be exquisitely sensitive and often have their antennae out, looking for others who accept their projections; that is, people who unconsciously resonate with them and can be manipulated. For example, most people have conflicts in the area of self-esteem as well as a desire to help others. Therefore, when borderline individuals project their rage with the fantasy of being entitled, the projection will resonate with the internal conflicts of others who will be willing to accept them.

Presentation of a contradictory, misleading, and vexing clinical picture has become the *sine qua non* of the borderline individual. Many serial killers, such as Ted Bundy, show this confusing picture. There is compelling clinical and research evidence indicating that more disturbed borderline individuals, unlike many floridly psychotic individuals, are unable to escape from the experience of interpersonal distortions, malevolence, and destruction into an idyllic fantasy world of benevolence, stability, and order (H. Lerner & St. Peter, 1984). Interpersonal distortions, angry affect storms, and the turbulent enactment of subjective experience swiftly become available in interpersonal relationships and often lead to impulsive behavior.

Kernberg (1976) posited heightened constitutional aggression or temperament as the major underlying etiological factor for borderline conditions. Excessive aggression results in splitting, which prevents integration in terms of the capacity to synthesize loving and hating feelings toward the same individual. Lack of integration leaves the individual vulnerable to impulsive action because of inability to regulate aggression. In fact, it is the relative degree to which aggression embellishes superego or moral development in interpersonal relationships that serves as the major prognostic indicator for these individuals. In discussing clinical aspects of superego psychopathology, Kernberg (1984, 1992) offers several examples of the antisocial or psychopathic personality, a variant of borderline personality organization. One patient entered treatment under pressure from his parents and to avoid going to prison because of his involvement in several break-ins. He talked openly about planning a robbery. He made it clear through "subtle but unmistakable threats, that he would know how to protect himself in case the therapist reported him to legal authorities. Kernberg described this patient as conveying an "overpowering sense of superiority and security." His relaxed smile conveyed a deprecation of the therapist, and in turn the therapist experienced difficulty thinking constructively in intervening. Treatment was interrupted after the therapist reached the conclusion that the combination of legal problems and treatment issues was beyond his capacity. The antisocial personality is examined in greater detail later in the chapter.

Psychotic Personality Organization

As with individuals exhibiting a borderline personality organization, an individual with a psychotic personality organization is unable to maintain a stable integration of the concept of self or others. Such inability interferes with the capacity to realistically assess oneself and others over time and across situations. Like the borderline, patients with a psychotic-level personality organization employ a range of primitive defenses which further weakens their ego functioning. The reasons, however, for the employment of such defensive operations are different in borderline and psychotic individuals. In the borderline, as noted, splitting and other defenses protect the individual from intolerable feelings of ambivalence and the overwhelming rage that interferes with all significant relationships. In contrast, the psychotic employs these defenses in an effort to avoid the subjective experience of disintegration or merger. Merger refers to the intrapsychic fusion of self and object representations. The experience of merger manifests in a total and frightening loss of reality testing: in delusions, hallucinations, and confusion between self and others.

Not unlike the borderline, primitive defenses in the psychotic often lead to chaotic, contradictory, and impulsive forms of behavior. For example, a patient who had just attacked a staff member on an inpatient unit might insist that he or she was feeling absolutely calm and content at the time of the attack. In contrast to borderline individuals, who often are able to acknowledge such contradictions, psychotics usually decompensate when these contradictions are pointed out; they become overwhelmed by disorganizing affects and chaotic fantasies, which often prompt further behavioral regressions. Often, especially under stress, psychotic individuals experience a frightening blurring of interpersonal boundaries, which they attempt to deal with through aggressive, destructive behavior.

T., a 19-year-old, single white male, had progressively decompensated, beginning at age 15, shortly after his first lengthy separation from his mother in order to attend prep school. T., a tall, slender, gangly adolescent, was bodily and inter-personally awkward, stiff, constricted, mechanical, vague, and indefinite. He pre-sented a startlingly painful sense of reality and history of thought disorder, auditory hallucinations, poor school performance, and seriously impaired social skills. He had few friends.

T. was raised in an extended family in which there were two divorces. He had an overly enmeshed symbiotic-like relationship with his infantilizing mother. The mother was strikingly attractive, overly seductive, overstimulating, and intrusive. She used her close relationship with T. to gain some relief from her own intense de-pression and loneliness. Her intrusiveness often left T. feeling passive, withdrawn, and unable to differentiate or express his own independent strivings. He seemed paralyzed by intense feelings of anxiety, rage, helplessness, and despair. His room at school was described as a "virtual altar" to his mother, with her pictures and let-ters arranged throughout the room in almost religious fashion. He felt "lost," iso-lated, listless, distant from others, and unable to concentrate. As his disjointed speech, hallucinations, and withdrawal gradually increased in school, he began to behave in an increasingly bizarre fashion, which culminated with him attacking his mother with a knife.

Antisocial Personality

Gabbard (1990) noted that antisocial personality disorders are the most exten-sively studied of all those in the borderline range of personality organization. These are also those individuals whom clinicians most tend to avoid. Most psychoanalysts agree that the label "antisocial personality" is applied to a broad spectrum of patients ranging from the totally untreatable to those who can be treated under certain condi-tions. Meloy (1988) utilized the term "psychopath" to describe individuals with a complete absence of empathy and a marked sadomasochistic interactional style based on power rather than emotional attachment. There is a consensus that the antisocial personality is best understood as a more psychopathological variant of the narcissis-tic personality disorder (Kernberg, 1984), with the same underlying borderline per-sonality organization that utilizes primitive defenses and highly pathological internal object relations (Gabbard, 1990; Kernberg, 1975; Meloy, 1988; Reid, 1985). One can conceptualize a narcissistic continuum of antisocial pathology within the borderline realm, ranging from the most severe psychopath in its purest form, to the narcissistic personality disorder with ego-syntonic antisocial features, to those narcissistic pa-tients who tend to be dishonest in their day-to-day interactions. In the remainder of this chapter I refer to the antisocial personality as those at the lower end of Kernberg's (1984) continuum.

Kernberg viewed most narcissistic individuals as organized on a borderline level of personality organization and describes such individuals as exhibiting a heightened degree of self-absorption, an inordinate need to be loved and admired, an overin-flated sense of themselves, and a desperate desire for adoration. He suggested further that their emotional life is shallow, that they show little empathy for others, and that they feel restless and bored unless their self-regard is being nourished. In relation-ships, potential providers of self-esteem are idealized, while those from whom little is expected are deprecated and treated with contempt. Beneath their veneer of charm, Kernberg argued, such individuals are cold, arrogant, ruthless, and exploitative. According to Gabbard (1990), a complete understanding of the antisocial personality must begin with the realization that biological factors contribute to the etiology and pathogenesis of the disorder. There is a high concordance for criminality in twins (Wilson & Herrnstein, 1985); many are thought to be neuropsychologically impaired (Yeudall, 1977); and studies have linked hormonal and neurochemical factors (Meloy, 1988). These findings certainly do not rule out the role of trauma and other environmental factors, and in turn, biological factors may contribute to early problems in the infant–mother relationship. Many individuals with antisocial personality disorders have histories of childhood neglect, deprivation, and abuse by parental figures. Regardless of etiology, however, it is clear that those with antisocial personalities have not attained the developmental level of object constancy, meaning that their sense of others and of themselves is not consistent over time and across situations. As a result, they lack a capacity to soothe themselves and show little capacity to draw on and internalize relationships with others. To compensate, they form a pathological "grandiose self," described by Kernberg as a fusion of the real self, the ideal self, and the ideal internal other. In the antisocial personality, however, the "ideal object" is often an aggressive introject (Meloy, 1988). This internal object representation may be derived from real experience of parental cruelty and deprivation.

Absence of basic trust, coupled with loss of loving experiences with maternal figures, have significant implications for the antisocial personality's development. The mother is often experienced as not only a stranger but a malignant presence. Meloy (1988) outlines two separate developmental processes that coexist in such individuals. The first is characterized by a profound detachment from all relationships and from all emotional experience; the second is characterized by sadistic attempts to relate to others through the exercise of power, destructiveness, and control. In early childhood, the antisocial personality never becomes aware of others as separate individuals with feelings of their own, and as a result, does not develop a capacity for depression or guilt stemming from concerns that his own actions can hurt others.

Impairment in internalization leads to a massive failure of superego or moral development. It is this quality, more than any other, that makes the antisocial personality seem to lack fundamental humanness. His value system appears to revolve around the exercise of aggressive power. Another quality of what is termed "superego pathology" that distinguishes these individuals from those with higher-level narcissistic personality disorders is a lack of effort to morally justify or ethically rationalize their antisocial behavior.

Formation of a sadistic, grandiose self structure, a defensive response to recurrent experiences of helplessness and rage in relationship to early caretaking objects, aborts later internalizations necessary for moral development. Kernberg (1984) described a number of internal scenarios that are common to antisocial personalities: (1) the experience of others as omnipotent and cruel; (2) the conviction that any good, loving relationship with another is fragile, easily destroyed, and, even worse, contains the threat for attack by an overpowering and cruel other; (3) a sense that complete submission to the other is the only condition for survival and, as a result, all ties to a good object have to be severed; (4) once identification with the omnipotent other is achieved, an intoxicating sense of power and freedom from fear and pain, as well as the feeling that gratification of aggression is the only important way of relating to others; and (5) the need for an escape route from any genuine relationship and the negation of the importance of any other person. A major consequence of this internal condition is a defensive dehumanization of all interpersonal relationships so that there is no longer a threat of love being destroyed by hate.

Dehumanization and Violent Crime

Violent criminal behavior, including murder, is viewed by most analysts as an interpersonal interaction that reflects a distorted perception of human relationships on the part of the offender. The way the offender perceives the victim and his or her relationship with the victim is thought to have paramount importance to the act. The murderer–victim relationship is not reciprocal; that is, it is an attempt on the murderer's part to express a wish or satisfy a need through the relationship but against the wishes of the other (Kennedy, 1994). Murder is conceptualized by Kennedy as an object relationship and the act of murder is seen as a manifestation of distorted, internal self and object representations.

Kennedy (1994), in a comprehensive study of the psychological structure of violent criminal offenders, hypothesized an empathy–dehumanization continuum. While empathy for others inhibits violence and aggression, when disturbances in the empathic capacity occur, there is a greater likelihood for harm. The diminished capacity for empathic understanding and modes of relating to others permits one to be exploitative and ruthless (Kernberg, 1984; Meloy, 1988). Dehumanization was viewed by Kennedy as a construct that provides a deeper understanding of how empathic inhibition and interpersonal detachment occurs. Dehumanization helps an individual avoid or lessen the emotional significance of others. Kennedy conceptualized dehumanization as a component of intrapsychic structure which creates a powerful "psychological wedge" that separates the internal and socialized inhibition to kill from the actual physical act. According to Bernard, Ottenberg, and Redl (1965), dehumanization can be defined as "a composite psychological defense which results in a diminished perception of and feeling for humanness in oneself and others" (p. 64). Kennedy formulated the extent to which one dehumanizes as ranging from temporary or recurrent episodes, which are situation- or person-dependent, to partial or permanent conditions, which are more characterologically embedded. She defines three gradients of dehumanization: temporary, partial, and permanent.

Temporary dehumanization in murder is associated with dissociation, intellectualization, rationalization, and splitting (Armstrong & Loewenstein, 1990). Temporary dehumanization requires psychological support for murder to occur, and murder is often justified for ideological reasons. Gault (1971), in a study of Vietnam veterans, made the significant observation that relatively ordinary people have the psychological capacity to temporarily dehumanize and murder when the emotional significance for others is circumvented. In this context, perpetrators unrealistically view their victim as the "enemy" who is not individualized and regarded as human. Gault noted: (l) the pressure to act aggressively is increased by the sight of wounded or dead peers; (2) realistic self-appraisal and responsibility for action is disowned; and (3) any identification with the humanness of the victim is absent. The ability to empathize with the other is unavailable. Kennedy (1994) cited the dramatic example of members of the Third Reich who implemented the so-called Final Solution of the Jews during World War II. Their ability to isolate affect, disown responsibility, rationalize behavior, idealize Hitler, and devalue their victims as nonhuman "vermin" enabled them to mute their conscience while conducting genocide, yet retain access to empathic feelings for their families (Kelman, 1993).

Partial dehumanization is associated with predatory murderers (Meloy, 1998), who murder as part of their job or as the successful completion of a duty. Motivation for murder can be material gain or protection of territory, such as in organized crime or gangs. Stark (1990) suggested that a pervasive form of socially sanctioned partial dehumanization is spouse battering. Victims of these murders become the repository of split-off, bad, frustrating, depriving, pain-inducing objects who induce rage sufficient to distort accurate perceptions of the real person.

According to Kennedy (1994), permanent or complete object-directed dehumanization "results in the perception of others as non-human; as objects to be used, discarded or destroyed" (p. 25). Permanent dehumanizers murder without conflict; that is, it is ego-syntonic. They lack any conscious feeling of empathy for others.

Meloy (1988) termed permanent dehumanizers "severe psychopaths," whom he describes as seeking interpersonal contact to use others and to reinforce their own grandiose self. He further characterized these individuals as extremely distant, as inflicting pain on others for pleasure, and lacking in empathic capacity. Often these individuals have a paradoxical yet exquisite capacity to establish "pseudo-identifications" (Meloy, 1988), which Krohn (1974) described as "borderline empathy." Kennedy (1994) discussed the infamous serial sexual murderer, Theodore Bundy, as an example of a permanent dehumanizer whom some considered sensitive, empathic, and caring. While Bundy appeared to have some empathic qualities, Kennedy cited forensic evidence that unquestionably illustrated this killer's capacity to place a "psychological wedge" between those pseudo-qualities and the desire to kill.

In summary, an empathic identification with others can be regarded as the developmental component of intrapsychic structure that matures in direct proportion to the stability and depth of interpersonal relationships. Failure in empathic identification is the hallmark of a psychopathic or antisocial personality. Kennedy's (1994) review identified dehumanization in individuals who murder as reflecting cognitive limitations, attachment disturbances, inadequate internalizations, and extreme environmental stress. Further, dehumanization is temporarily, partially, or permanently ego-syntonic and serves as an important barometer of prognosis.

Treatment

Psychoanalysts uniformly agree that individuals with serious antisocial violent behavior are unlikely to benefit from a treatment approach based exclusively on outpatient psychotherapy (Gabbard, 1990; Gabbard & Coyne, 1987). An institutional setting is necessary for even slight improvement. It is generally believed among psychoanalysts that only long-term hospital-like treatment can produce any meaningful change in these individuals. Because individuals with antisocial personalities are so prone to act on impulses and translate their feelings into actions, treatment must revolve around a tightly controlled structure. From the onset, treaters must anticipate and deal with acting out. The general strategy is to establish control over the lives of the patients and block their usual channels for discharging unpleasant feelings into actions. When impulsivity and acting-out is blocked, the emergence of depression, anxiety, and aggression can be expected. A staff's predictable and consistent response to all breaches in structure attempts to frustrate usual efforts to get around "the system" (Gabbard, 1990) and help transform actions into feelings and thoughts which can then be worked with, using language.

Meloy (1988) has identified five clinical features of psychopathic individuals that absolutely contraindicate psychotherapy: sadistic cruelty toward others, complete absence of remorse, and a lack of emotional attachment distinguishes psychopathic patients from more treatable narcissistic individuals. Meloy also identified the paradox of both high and low intelligence and the intense countertransference or counterreactions that these individuals evoke in clinicians.

Several analysts have attempted to treat antisocial personalities in individual psychotherapy. Gabbard (1990) has distilled six basic principles of technique based upon his review of the literature. First, the therapist must be stable, persistent, and completely incorruptible. Second, the therapist must repeatedly confront the antisocial patient's denial and minimization of antisocial behavior. Third, the therapist must attempt to help the patient connect actions with internal states. Fourth, confrontation of here-and-now behaviors are more effective than interpretations of unconscious material from the past. In this regard, the patient's deprecation of the therapist and devaluation of the therapeutic process must consistently be challenged. Fifth, counterreactions on the therapist's part must be rigorously monitored to avoid acting out by the therapist. Finally, the therapist must avoid having excessive expectations for improvement. It must be understood that progress with these individuals is slow because they experience therapy as a threat to their grandiose self which protects them from profound feelings of helplessness and hopelessness. As Gabbard notes: "Despite these pitfalls, however, many experienced clinicians believe that psychotherapeutic efforts with these patients pay off frequently enough to warrant such heroic treatment" (p. 420).

Summary

In approaching the topic of the violent criminal offender, most psychoanalysts share certain basic views: Aggression plays a crucial role in the infant–parent and child–parent dyads, the successful modulation of aggression is crucial to healthy development, and managing aggression successfully is critical to the therapeutic endeavor. Psychoanalysts also agree that understanding difficulties in modulating, regulating, and integrating aggression is core to viewing psychopathology on a continuum from its milder to its more severe forms. Violence and aggression is explored using Kernberg's notion of personality organization, based on a continuum model ranging from normal–neurotic, to borderline (including antisocial personality) and psychotic organizations. Most violent criminal offenders fall within the borderline level of personality organization. This level is explored in depth in terms of a psychoanalytic understanding of pathological narcissism and the antisocial personality.

The capacity to indulge in violent criminal behavior is understood in terms of Kennedy's (1994) hypothesis of an empathy–dehumanization continuum. Core to dehumanization is an empathic inhibition and interpersonal detachment. Dehumanization helps an individual avoid or lessen the emotional significance of others and creates a powerful "psychological wedge" that separates the internal and socialized inhibition to kill from the actual physical act. Three gradients of dehumanization are posited: temporary, partial, and permanent. Severe dehumanization reflects cognitive limitations, attachment disturbances, inadequate internalizations, and extreme environmental stress. Psychoanalysts uniformly agree that individuals with serious antisocial violent behavior require extensive structure, preferably in institutional settings, to benefit even slightly from psychotherapy. Treatment progress with these individuals is slow because they experience therapy as a threat to their grandiose self, which protects them from profound feelings of helplessness and hopelessness.

References

Armstrong, J., & Loewenstein, R. (1990). Characteristics of patients with multiple personality and dissociative disorders on psychological testing. *Journal of Nervous and Mental Diseases, 178*(7), 448–454.

Bernard, V., Ottenberg, P., & Redl, F. (1965). Dehumanization: A composite psychological defense in relation to modern war. In M. Schwebel (Ed.) *Behavioral science and human survival* (pp. 64–82). Palo Alto, CA: Science and Behavior Books.

Blatt, S., & Lerner, H. (1991). Psychodynamic perspectives on personality theory. In M. Herson, A. Kazdin, & A. Bellack (Eds.), *The clinical psychology handbook* (2nd ed., pp. 87–106). New York: Pergamon.

Brenner, C. (1982). *The mind in conflict.* New York: International Universities Press.

Freud S. (1905). Three essays on the theory of sexuality In J. Strachey (Ed. and trans.), *The standard edition of the complete psychological works of Sigmund Freud* (Vol. II, 11, pp. 31–122). London Hogarth. (Original work published 1905)

Freud, S. (1915). Instincts and their vicissitudes *(Standard edition,* (Vol. 14). London: Hogarth. (Original work published 1915)

Freud, S. (1916). Some character-types met with in psychoanalytic work. *Standard edition,* (Vol. 14, pp. 309–333). London: Hogarth. (Original work published 1916)

Freud, S. (1920). Beyond the pleasure principle. *Standard edition* (Vol. 16, pp. 7–64) London: Hogarth. (Original work published 1920)

Freud S. (1930). Civilization and its discontent. *Standard edition* (Vol. 21, pp. 59–145). London: Hogarth. (Original work published 1930)

Frosch, J. (1964). The psychotic character: Clinical psychiatric considerations. *Psychiatric Quarterly, 38,* 81–96.

Gabbard, G. (1990). *Psychodynamic psychiatry in clinical practice.* Washington, DC.: American Psychiatric Press.

Gabbard, G., & Coyne, L. (1987). Predictors of response of antisocial patients to hospital treatment. *Hospital and Community Psychiatry, 38,* 118–185.

Gault, W. (1971). Some remarks on slaughter. *American Journal of Psychiatry, 4,* 450–454.

Giacono, C., & Meloy, J. (1994). *The Rorschach Assessment of Aggressive and Psychopathic Personalities.* Hillsdale, NJ: Erlbaum.

Greenberg, J., & Mitchell, S. (1983) . *Object relations in psychoanalytic theory.* Cambridge, MA: Harvard University Press.

Kelman, H. (1973). Violence without moral restraint: Reflections on the dehumanization of victims and victimizers. *Journal of Social Issues, 4,* 25–61.

Kennedy, R. (1994). *A study of intrapsychic structure and dehumanization in subgroups of men who murder.* Unpublished, doctoral dissertation, Boston University, Boston, MA.

Kernberg, O. (1975). *Borderline conditions in pathological narcissism.* New York: Aronson.

Kernberg, O. (1976). *Object relations theory in clinical psychoanalysis.* New York: Aronson.

Kernberg, O. (1977). Normal psychology of the aging process revisited—II. *Journal of Geriatric Psychiatry, 10,* 27–45.

Kernberg, O. (1984). *Severe personality disorders.* New Haven, CT: Yale University Press.

Kernberg, O. (1992). *Aggression in personality disorders and perversions.* New Haven, CT: Yale University Press.

Krohn, A. (1974). Borderline "empathy" and differentiation of object relationship: A contribution to the psychology of object relations. *International Journal of Psychoanalytic Psychotherapy, 3,* 142–165.

Kwawer, J. Lerner, H., Lerner, P., & Sugarman, A. (1980). *Borderline phenomena in the Rorschach test.* New York: International Universities Press.

Lerner, H., & Ehrlich, J. (1994). Psychoanalytic perspectives. In M. Hersen, R. Ammerman, & L. Sisson (Eds.), *Handbook of aggressive and destructive behavior in psychiatric patients* (pp. 65–86). New York: Plenum.

Lerner, H., & Lerner, P. (1988). *Primitive mental states and the Rorschach*. Madison, CT: International Universities Press.

Lerner, H., & St. Peter, S. (1984). Patterns of object relations in neurotic, borderline, and schizophrenic patients. *Psychiatry, 47,* 77–92.

Lerner, P. (1991). *Psychoanalytic theory and the Rorschach*. Hillsdale, NJ: Analytic Press.

Meloy, J. (1988). *The psychopathic mind: Origins, dynamics and treatment*. Northvale, NJ: Aronson.

Reid, W. (1985). The antisocial personality: A review. *Hospital and Community Psychiatry, 36,* 831–837.

Schengold, L. (1989). *Soul murder: The effects of childhood abuse and deprivation*. New Haven, CT: Yale University Press.

Schmideberg, M. (1959). The borderline patient. In S. Arieti (Ed.), *American handbook of psychiatry* (Vol. 1, pp. 398–416). New York; Basic Books.

Stark, E. (1990). Rethinking homicide: Violence, race, and the police of gender. *International Journal of Health Services, 20,* 3–26.

Wilson, J., & Hernstein, R. (1985). *Crime in human nature*. New York: Simon & Schuster.

Yeudall, L. (1977). Neuropsychological assessment of forensic disorders. *Canada Mental Health, 25,* 8–15.

The Role of Biological Factors

Paul F. Brain

Introduction

Although aggression and violent behavior are clearly heterogenous concepts with etiologies in which biology, environmental factors and social learning play complex roles, the debate about their causes frequently disintegrates into argument about whether biological factors should be considered at all. The arguments for not doing so include the fact that biology is generally outside social control, a view that such approaches are reductionist, and the problem of unfairly labeling particular groups. In spite of these reservations, there have been consistent attempts to assess the potential effects of genes, drugs, neural systems, hormones and diet on violence. The suggested reasons for doing so include the argument that, if violence is a complex phenomenon, one must consider the roles of *all* potential factors: the view that biological factors may have a predictive role (with all the ethical problems that would be associated with such properties) and the view that an individual with a greatly disordered biology could not be regarded as wholly responsible for his/her actions.

This brief review provides an overview of some of the more recent writings on the role or roles of biological factors in aggression and violent behavior, with a view to illustrating the current prevailing views and concerns.

Problems With Terminology

Brain (1990, 1994a) has considered some of the difficulties raised by the use of the terms "aggression" and "violence." I have pointed out (Brain, 1994a) that they "are used with enormous flexibility, making it difficult to tie down firm associations with biologic factors (such as hormones)" (p. 174). If one considers the various attributes that have been used to characterize aggression and violence (potential for harm or damage, intentionality of the act, arousal, aversiveness to the victim), one can see that none of them, individually or in combination, will consistently label an act as "aggressive" or "violent." One can find perfectly "legitimate" acts with such characteristics

Paul F. Brain • School of Biological Sciences, University of Wales, Swansea SA2 8PP, United Kingdom.
Handbook of Psychological Approaches with Violent Offenders: Contemporary Strategies and Issues, edited by Van Hasselt and Hersen. Kluwer Academic/Plenum Publishers, New York, 1999.

and acts characterized as violent by most people that lack one or more of these features. The obvious conclusion is that aggression and violence are concepts or, essentially, somewhat ambiguous categories of items created to enable the human mind to make some sense of a complex world. As concepts are not capable of precise definition (a concept is judged by its utility and not by its scientific rigor), the items judged to constitute aggression and violence are much influenced by individual and collective value judgments. Indeed, the same act can be viewed by a variety of individuals (the "aggressor," the victim, and an outside observer) as being clearly violent or a legitimate response to real or perceived threats. Obviously, this makes correlating biologic variables with such activities extremely difficult.

A further problem with terminology is that the wide array of tests for animal aggression clearly tap a wide range of motivations including offense, defense and even predation. Broadly similar acts may be used with apparently different aims (Brain, 1984). There is clear evidence that certain biologic factors (e.g., levels of male sex hormone, a particular modification of fine neural architecture) are only important in *some* of these events. This means that even in "simple" animals, such as rats and mice, there is no such thing as *a* physiology of aggression. This is not the same as maintaining that physiological variables are not important in studies on aggression (see Brain, 1984; 1990, 1994a, 1994b, Brain & Haug, 1992; Brain & Susman, 1997).

As mentioned earlier, "aggression" is influenced by at least three sets of variables that are difficult to separate clearly, as follows:

1. Biologic factors (such as genes, neural systems, neurochemicals, and hormones)
2. Situational factors (or the context in which the behavior is expressed)
3. Individual learning experiences

Brain (1994b) has maintained that, because the labeling of behavior as aggression actually involves profound value judgments, it is highly unlikely that one will find simple relationships between any biologic factor and this class of behavior. Although Brain (1984) argued that the roles of particular biologic factors in aggressive and destructive behaviors do not form mutually exclusive categories, using the traditional specialties to look at real and potential relationships has some merit. One must emphasize, however, that the actual contribution of individual biologic factors to examples of aggression will vary on a case-by-case basis (i.e., genes, brain circuits, and particular hormones are not exclusively linked to all expressions of such behaviors).

Genes and Aggression

Brain (1984, 1994b) essentially reviewed the claims made in this area of behavior-genetics. He maintained that animal studies now suggest that genes do not directly cause behavior, but provide (as a result of gene–environment interactions) modifications of anatomy and physiology that can alter predispositions for behaving in particular ways (i.e., they alter behavioral traits and "mood"). Brain (1994b) also reviewed some of the older human data, such as Christiansen's (1978) Danish twin studies and the Jacobs, Brunton, and Melville (1965) claims concerning the 47 XYY karyotype. The conclusion, at the time, was that "[i]t is obviously true that genetic endowment can influence an individual's predisposition to show particular mood changes and alter the efficiency of the processing mechanism facilitating social interactions, but there is *no* evidence (in humans or animals) of specific genes for aggressive and destructive behavior" (p. 6; emphasis added).

Carey (1994) comprehensively reviewed the area of genetics and violence. So far as human data are concerned, he suggested that most studies support the view that there is a genetic effect on adult and possibly adolescent antisocial behavior. The genetics of antisocial behavior do not, however, fit a simple model and there is evidence of imitation, collusion, and reciprocal interactions between twins (especially identical twins) in many studies. Adoption studies have consistently reported correlations between antisocial behavior in the adopted child and some variable intervening between birth and final placement in the adoptive home. Indeed, selection of adoptive families makes it difficult to generalize about the impact of family environment on criminal behavior. There is a strong tendency, especially in juvenile antisocial behavior, for some correlate of the home environment (e.g., urban vs. rural) to influence antisocial behavior. Carey (1994) also noted that the evidence for genetic effects on offenses involving physical aggression is weak and the available data does not suggest that human antisocial behavior can be linked with a major polymorphism of the Y chromosome. There *is* support for a genetic link between antisocial behavior and alcohol (and possibly other substance) abuse.

The recent Ciba Foundation Conference on "Genetics of Criminal and Antisocial Behaviour" with a resulting volume edited by Bock and Goode (1996) also reexamined the issues in some detail. In that volume, Rutter (1996) concluded, that despite the problems of methodological hazards (which must be avoided), inconsistencies across studies (which require explanation) and the marked limitations of the inferences that can be drawn from findings to date, "it is evident that genetic factors do play a significant role in antisocial behavior and that their investigation is likely to be useful, with respect to both theory and practice" (p. 265). He also said, however, that the media view that researchers are involved in a search for the "gene for crime" is greatly mistaken and that current genetic research takes full account of the technological problems and does not assume there is a single homogeneous entity we can refer to as antisocial behavior (see the "Problems with Terminology" section). He maintained that twin studies strongly suggest that genetic factors are especially important in varieties of antisocial behavior associated with "early-onset, pervasive hyperactivity" rather than "adolescent-onset delinquency" (p. 65). There is consequently evidence from twin studies of a stronger genetic effect on adult rather than juvenile crime. Of direct relevance to this review is the finding from adoption studies that the genetic component in violent crime is less than that in property crime. Such studies also indicate that criminality associated with alcohol abuse should be differentiated from that which is not linked to alcohol problems. There are data suggesting links between an inherited predisposition to schizophrenia and violent crime as well as evidence that genes can be implicated in the serotonin (5HT) neurotransmitter system correlated with certain expressions of violent behavior (probably by altering risk-taking behavior including suicidal as well as antisocial activities).

Glover (1996), although of the opinion that genetic determinism is unlikely to be true of most human behavior, did suggest that "when genetic causes are combined with others, including environmental ones, the resulting picture may be a more determinist one than we are used to" (p. 237). This would, he thought, not necessarily undermine responsibility: an important feature of Western legal systems. Denno (1996) also looked at the legal implications of genetics and crime research and concluded that "no doubt, genetic evidence and comparable kinds of biological evidence will have a major impact on juries when such evidence is more fully accepted by the legal and scientific communities" (p. 248).

Neurobiology and Human Violence

Brain (1990) has pointed out that there has long been considerable interest in the potential involvement of parts of the brain in aggression. This interest was stimulated by animal experiments (notably cats) apparently demonstrating that one could modify "sham rage" by hypothalamically positioned stimulatory electrodes or discrete lesions. The initial view that the brain has "on" and "off" centers in the central nervous systems of higher vertebrates regulating aggression has been complicated by recognition that there are different kinds of aggression and that results of neural manipulations can be influenced by the social context in which the animals are placed.

The initial enthusiasm for treating human violence with psychosurgery (e.g., Mark & Ervin, 1970), as well as equating all aggression with neurological disorders, has been tempered by recently revealed complications. Mirsky and Siegel (1994) critically reviewed the involvement of the central nervous system in human aggression and violence. Looking at studies involving patients with neuropsychiatric disorders, they concluded that there is tentative evidence of a connection between violence and alcohol abuse mediated via alcohol-induced damage to the brain. Brain (1986, 1994c) suggested that associations between alcohol ingestion and violence are complex in some cases, as they are related to alcohol-induced impairments in cognitive ability and social skills.

Mirsky and Siegel (1994) focused on the studies involving associations between violence and epilepsy. Ictal (concomitant with the seizure) violence is reportedly very rare (around 0.25% of epileptics show this), only occasionally associated with angry feelings (fear is much more common), and can scarcely be described as directed attack on another person. The picture concerning interictal (the period between the seizures) violence is much more obscure. Claims range from maintaining that the violence represents an occult (hidden) seizure to the view that such events are traits associated with the primary cerebral disorder (i.e., that the emotional mechanisms of the brain are damaged so that violent outbursts are much more common than in "normal" individuals). A particular question, not yet resolved, is whether interictal violence can be abolished by the equivalent of removal of a seizure focus (as has been used to treat intractable seizures per se).

In studies where violence is the independent variable (rather than alcoholism or epilepsy), the available data suggest that there are no conclusive links between violence and brain dysfunction in individuals involved in non-sex and sex crimes. There are some provocative but inconclusive findings concerning subtle brain abnormalities in sexual offenders (e.g., Langevin, Wortzman, Wright, & Handy, 1989) but these may be different in different types of offenders (pedophiles and sadists).

Mirsky and Siegel (1994) concluded that "the issue of whether or not human aggression and violence can be linked unequivocally to disordered brain mechanisms remains very much in doubt" (p. 96). They thought that available literature suggested some relationship between "pathophysiologic processes in the limbic system and the tendency to engage in assaultive and violent behavior" (p. 96), but pointed out the difficulty of controlling for effects of lifestyle (brain injuries may be more common in some groups).

Miczek, Mirsky, Carey, DeBold, and Raine (1994) reviewed the neurochemistry and (related) pharmacotherapeutic management of violence. They suggested that although norepinephrine and dopamine can be implicated in aggressive responses, there is particular evidence that 5HT metabolism is involved in certain expressions of human aggression. Virkkunen, Goldman, and Linnoila (1996) claimed that there are many polymorphisms of 5HT metabolism and function-related genes in impulsive violent offenders and healthy volunteers, but their significance remains to be determined. Brunner (1996) suggested that there is evidence of monoamine oxidase A deficiency in human males with increased impulsive aggression and other types of abnormal behavior, but a number of problems must be resolved in these data. Miczek and colleagues (1994) concluded that "an important objective of future research is to delineate unique characteristics of the GABA$_A$-benzodiazepine receptor complex or 5HT receptors that predict propensity to engage in violent behavior" (p. 280).

Hormones and Human Aggression

Brain (1994a) reviewed the enormous body of diverse information associating the varied secretions of the endocrine system to various manifestations of human aggressive and destructive behaviors. A major conclusion was that, while " 'raging hormones' do not cause violence" (p. 228), these factors do have diverse and subtle influences on the developing and developed individuals that can change the predispositions for showing particular behavioral responses. The data relating to hormones can be effectively subdivided into the following categories:

a. Investigations on the effects of perinatal "programming" of adult aggressiveness
b. Direct motivational effects (mediated by the central nervous system?) on fighting and threat
c. Indirect effects (seemingly mediated by altered social signaling) on fighting and threat
d. The effects of fighting and threat on hormonal production

Brain and Susman (1997) recently reviewed this area. The major components of the endocrine system that are generally linked to human aggression are the hypothalamus–pituitary–gonadal (HPG) and the hypothalamus–pituitary–adrenal (HPA) axes, although other endocrine factors (notably the thyroid and the adrenal medulla) also have been correlated with some direct and indirect actions.

In terms of their early programming effects, there has been a repeated suggestion that early exposure to androgens modifies temperament, increasing it in the direction of "impetuous and active." In humans, gonadal steroids during prenatal life produce structural, organizational changes that masculinize and defeminize the brain (Meyer-Bahlberg *et al.*, 1995) resulting in sexual dimorphisms in behavior. Many reproductive and nonreproductive behaviors are seemingly influenced by gonadal steroid-induced sexual dimorphisms in behavior. Nonreproductive behaviors apparently mediated by prenatal organizational influences include spatial cognition, sex-typed behavior (e.g., activity level), and sexual orientation. The research approach adopted for detecting such organizational influences on behavior consists of showing the degree of masculine or feminine responses in cognitive or behavioral measures. Populations considered generally consist of individuals in whom the levels of early hormone are altered endogenously (e.g., by congenital adrenal hyperphasia in the mother) or exogenously (via treatment with sex steroids to prevent miscarriage). In studies attempting to link prenatal hormonal effects and behavior, it is now recognized that there are multiple sociocultural influences in addition to those directly attributable to hormones. Socialization processes can augment or override hormonal influences on behavior at many points in development. Such processes may have progressive effects on cognition and behavior with each succeeding year of life.

There have been numerous speculative attempts to relate hormones of the HPG axis to "rebellious attitude" in adolescents. Indeed, the "storm and stress theory" of adolescence (Hall, 1904) was directly rooted in the presumed activational influence of hormones at puberty. Modern notions view antisocial behavior, emotions and cognition as being linked. The past decade of hormone–behavior research with adolescents has simultaneously assessed hormonal profiles and behavior, facilitating deriving definitive conclusions about the reciprocal nature of hormone–behavior interactions. There is evidence that testosterone and adrenal androgens can influence antisocial behavior in adolescents. These effects may be complicated by the variety of ways in which behavior is assessed, other hormonal factors (e.g., cortisol, estrogen), and the impact of hormones and emotions.

In adult humans, hormones have been suggested to partially account for the often recorded sexual dimorphisms in this behavior. Maccoby and Jacklin (1974) famously suggested that males are "biologically disposed" toward violent behavior, but Kruttschnitt (1994) argued that "the most challenging issues appear in the area of understanding how social, situational or cultural factors ameliorate or aggravate aggressive or violent patterns in males and females" (p. 325). It has been suggested that males and females view aggression differently, generally have different experiences of giving and receiving aggressive behavior, and vary in "anger proneness," which make accounting for the apparent sexual dimorphism in violent behavior difficult.

Although manipulations of the HPG axis via castration or treatment with estrogens or anti-hormones have, at various times, been used to control hostile behavior in humans, there is currently a reduced enthusiasm for "treating" human violence by such means. This seems to be partially due to a growing recognition of the interpretational difficulties of existing studies and the recognition of side effects, but also due to an appreciation of the ethical problems associated with such approaches.

In attempts to correlate levels of androgen with human aggression, there has been a growing appreciation that single plasma testosterone determinations are not easy to relate to behavior. There is a weak positive relationship between testosterone level and some measures (e.g., the Buss–Durkee Hostility Inventory) of aggression in males. Self-perceptions of aggressive offenders, however, rarely accord with other people's views of their behavior. The hormonal profiles in different kinds of offenders may be subtly different (adrenal androgens may be important here) and "winning" in a variety of situations (athletic, examination, and laboratory task) elevates testosterone levels apparently as a consequence of altered mood and perceived status.

The basic conclusion (Brain, 1994a) is that "it seems unlikely that androgens have a simple causal effect on human aggression and violence, but the patterns of production of sex steroids do appear to alter several factors (e.g., 'aggressive feelings,' self-image, and social signalling) that predispose individuals toward carrying out actions that can receive this label" (p. 221).

Brain (1994a) concluded that "genuine progress in this area (which has lagged in sophistication behind developments in the study of sexual behavior) is likely if the quality of the behavioral analysis (which should be as direct and as detailed as possible) is matched to the sophistication of the endocrine manipulations and measures" (pp. 226–227). He suggested that the technique of measuring multiple steroids in saliva samples by enzyme immunoassays and the eventual development of techniques to noninvasively estimate the impact of hormones on the central nervous system hold the keys to a better appreciation of this area. Brain and Susman (1997) briefly reviewed evidence that hormones may produce subtle structural changes in the brains of adults (changing cognition, affective expression, and aggressive behavior) as well as in fetuses.

Nutrition and Human Aggression

Kanarek (1994) and Benton (1996) independently reviewed the literature looking at the impact of diet on aggressive behavior. Kanarek looked, for example, at the claims concerning sugar (sucrose) and behavior (violent behavior and Attention-Deficit/Hyperactivity Disorder—ADHD). Kanarek concluded that evidence in neither case is clear. So far as violent behavior is concerned, the evidence is often confounded by extraneous variables (e.g., overcrowding, drug use), a failure to measure food intake, and inadequately specified antisocial behaviors. Benton (1996), reviewing this area, looking at items as diverse as low blood sugar levels in the Quolla Indians of Peru, violent criminals, and populations of 6–7-year-old children subjected to a deliberately frustrating computer game, concluded that "moderate falls in blood glucose may cause irritability. Whether it leads to aggressive behavior depends on provocation, social skills and other aspects of the situation" (p. 147). Benton noted that there are marked individual differences in the response to diet.

In the case of ADHD, neither dietary challenge studies nor comparisons of hyperactive and normal children support the view that sugar plays a major role in these behaviors (Kanarek, 1994). Kanarek pointed out, however, that parents and teachers continue "to supply anecdotal reports of the deleterious consequences of sugar" (p. 530). He suggested that these parents and teachers misperceive a relation between sugar and behavior for a variety of reasons including the fact that hyperactive children have difficulties in modifying their behavior in response to different environmental demands, especially in group activities.

Studies on food intolerance and hostility have attracted much attention. Benton (1996) concluded that on the available evidence "it seems reasonable to assume that some cases of extreme violence reflect food intolerance" (p. 141). Courts in the United

States and the United Kingdom have accepted such pleas. Kanarek (1994) specifically looked at food additives and ADHD, an area popularized by Feingold (1975), who also concentrated on salicylates. Kanarek (1994) concluded that Feingold's claims were overstated and "at best, only a small percentage of hyperactive children may be adversely affected by food additives" (p. 533).

Kanarek (1994) also reviewed the claimed inverse relationship between blood cholesterol level and violent behavior. There is some intriguing evidence of an association between incidence of accident, suicide, or homicide, and lower cholesterol values, whether these values are achieved using drug treatment or by dietary manipulation but such relationships are not observed in all studies. Further, interpretation is often made difficult by failure to monitor diet adequately or to note levels of alcohol ingestion in the populations studied.

Kanarek (1994) clearly thought that the association between lead toxicity and antisocial behavior was worthy of serious consideration. Exposure to lead has been linked to ADHD and ADHD is a well-established risk factor for later antisocial behavior.

Benton (1996) reviewed the data concerning vitamin and mineral intake and antisocial behavior in institutionalized individuals. There is now an adequately controlled California double-blind, placebo-controlled study supporting the view that "correcting" dietary deficits with a multivitamin and mineral supplement significantly decreases the incidence of rule breaking.

Kanarek (1994) concluded that "it is important to remember that diet is but one of many factors that could contribute to violent behavior" (p. 535) and Benton (1996) maintained that "it is totally unreasonable to see diet as 'the' cause of aggressive behaviour" (p. 156). It can, however, under some circumstances, predispose.

Summary

There is obviously a wealth of information in the literature exploring various aspects of the biology of human aggression. Some of it is impressively documented and some overstates the enthusiasms of the authors. There are dangers in assuming that aggression is a unitary phenomenon on which easy agreement can be reached. The view that all aggression in humans and other animals is a uniformly negative attribute to be "cured" is difficult to maintain. Associations repeatedly have been found between some expressions of human aggression and genes, neurobiology, hormones, and diet but none provide easy answers so far as clinical treatment is concerned. Biological factors, if sensitively handled, may have some credibility as predictors of potential violence. Biology is clearly an important factor in the expression of hostile behaviors but it is (a) difficult to disentangle the effects of genes, neural circuits, hormones, and diet from the effects of accumulated experiences and situational determinants; (b) probably true that therapies based on biology alone will be appropriate only in a small minority of clinical cases; (c) not easy to estimate fairly the relative contribution of biological factors to events such as assault and homicide; and (d) true that many ethical dilemmas are raised by such areas. Having said this, it does look as if a more complex but realistic appreciation of the importance of biological variables in violent behavior is emerging. This will be of benefit, not only to improving our understanding of the concept of aggression but in abolishing some of the unhelpful, simplistic myths that abound in this area.

References

Benton, D. (1996), *Food for Thought*. Harmondsworth, England: Penguin.

Bock, G. R., & Goode, J. A. (1996). *Genetics of criminal and antisocial behaviour*. Chichester, England: Wiley.

Brain, P. F. (1984a). Biological explanations of human aggression and the resulting therapies offered by such approaches: A critical evaluation. In R. J. Blanchard and D. C. Blanchard (Eds.). *Advances in the study of aggression* (Vol. 1) (pp. 63–102). New York: Academic Press.

Brain, P. F. (1986). Multidisciplinary examinations of the "causes" of crime: The case of the link between alcohol and violence. *Alcohol and Alcoholism, 21,* 237–240.

Brain, P. F. (1990). *Mindless violence? The nature and biology of aggression.* Swansea, Wales: University College of Swansea Press.

Brain, P. F. (1994a). Biological explanations of human aggression and the resulting therapies offered by such approaches: A critical evaluation. In R. J. Blanchard & D. C. Blanchard (Eds.), *Advances in the Study of Aggression* (Vol. 1, pp. 63–102). New York: Academic Press.

Brain, P. F. (1994b). Biological-psychological. In M. Hersen, R. T. Ammerman, & L. A. Sisson (Eds.), *Handbook of aggressive and destructive behavior in psychiatric patients* (pp. 3–16). New York: Plenum.

Brain, P. F. (1994c). Hormonal aspects of aggression and violence. In A. J. Reiss, Jr., K. A. Miczek, & J. I. Roth (Eds.)., *Understanding and preventing violence: Vol. 2. Biobehavioral influences* (pp. 173–244). Washington, DC: National Academy Press.

Brain, P. F. (1994d). Neurotransmission, the individual and the alcohol/aggression link. Commentary on Miczek *et al.,* "Neuropharmacological characteristics of individual differences in alcohol effects on aggression in rodents and primates." *Behavioural Pharmacology, 5,* 422–424.

Brain, P. F., & Haug, M. (1992). Hormonal and neurochemical correlates of various forms of animal aggression. *Psychoneuroendocrinology, 17,* 537–551.

Brain, P. F., & Susman, E. J. (1997). Hormonal aspects of aggression and violence. In D. M. Stoff, J. Breiling, & J. D. Maser (Eds.)., *Handbook of antisocial behavior* (pp. 314–325). New York: Wiley.

Brunner, H. G. (1996). MAOA deficiency and abnormal behaviour: Perspectives on an association. In G. R. Bock & J. A. Goode (Eds.)., *Genetics of criminal and antisocial behaviour* (pp. 155–167). Chichester, England: Wiley.

Carey, G. (1994). Genetics and violence. In A. J. Reiss, K. A. Miczek, & J. A Roth (Eds.)., *Understanding and preventing violence: Vol. 2 Biobehavioral influences* (pp. 21–58). Washington, DC: National Academy Press.

Christiansen, K. O. (1978). The genesis of aggressive criminality: Implications of a study of crime in a Danish twin study. In W. W. Hartup & J. de Wit (Eds.)., *Origins of aggression* (pp. 99–120). The Hague, Netherlands: Mouton.

Denno, D. W. (1996). Legal implications of genetics and crime research. In G. R. Bock & J. A. Goode (Eds.). *Genetics of criminal and antisocial behaviour* (pp. 248–264). Chichester, England: Wiley.

Feingold, B. F. (1975). Hyperkinesis and learning disabilities linked to artificial food, flavors and colors. *American Journal of Nursing, 75,* 797–803.

Glover, J. (1996). The implications for responsibility of possible genetic factors in the explanation of violence. In G. R. Bock & J. A. Goode (Eds.)., *Genetics of criminal and antisocial behaviour* (pp. 237–247). Chichester, England: Wiley.

Hall, G. S. (1904). *Adolescence.* New York: Appleton.

Jacobs, P. A., Brunton, M., Melville, M. M. (1965). Aggressive behaviour, mental subnormality and the XYY males. *Nature* (London), *208,* 1351–1352.

Kanarek, R. B. (1994). Nutrition and violent behavior. In A. J. Reiss, K. A. Miczek, & J. A Roth (Eds.), *Understanding and preventing violence: Vol. 2. Biobehavioral influences* (pp. 515–539). Washington, DC: National Academy Press.

Kruttschnitt, C. (1994). Gender and interpersonal violence. In A. J. Reiss, Jr. & J. A. Roth (Eds.)., *Understanding and preventing violence: Vol. 3. Social influences* (pp. 293–376). Washington, DC: National Academy Press.

Langevin, R., Wortzman, G., Wright, P., & Handy, L. (1989). Studies of brain damage and dysfunction in sex offenders. *Annals of Sex Research, 2,* 163–179.

Maccoby, E. E., & Jacklin, C. N. (1974). *The psychology of sex differences.* Stanford, CA: Stanford University Press.

Mark, V. H., & Ervin, F. R. (1970). *Violence and the brain.* New York: Harper and Row.

Meyer-Bahlberg, H. F. L., Ehrhardt, A. A., Rosen, L. R., Gruen, R. S., Veridiano, N. P., Vann, F. H., & Neuwalder, H. F. (1995). Prenatal estrogens and the development of homosexual orientation. *Developmental Psychology, 31,* 12–21.

Miczek, K. A., Mirsky, A. F., Carey, G., DeBold, J., & Raine, A. (1994). An overview of biological influences on violent behavior. In A. J. Reiss, Jr., K. A. Miczek, & J. A. Roth (Eds.)., *Understanding and preventing violence: Vol. 2. Biobehavioral influences* (pp. 1–20). Washington, DC: National Academy Press.

Mirsky, A. F., & Siegel, A. (1994). The neurobiology of violence and aggression. In A. J. Reiss, K. A. Miczek, & J. A. Roth (Eds.)., *Understanding and preventing violence: Vol. 2. Biobehavioral influences* (pp. 59–172). Washington, DC: National Academy Press.

Rutter, M. (1996). Concluding remarks. In G. R. Bock, & J. A. Goode (Eds.)., *Genetics of criminal and antisocial behaviour* (pp. 265–271). Chichester, England: Wiley.

Virkkunen, M., Goldman, D., & Linnoila, M. (1996). Serotonin in alcoholic violent offenders. In G. R. Bock & J. A. Goode (Eds.)., *Genetics of criminal and antisocial behaviour* (pp. 168–182). Chichester, England: Wiley.

II

VIOLENT CRIME BY CHILDREN AND ADOLESCENTS

Firesetting in Children and Youth

David J. Kolko

Introduction

Children account for a significant proportion of the fires set in this country. Based on figures reported by the National Fire Protection Association (NFPA), children playing with fire committed 98,410 fires that were reported to U.S. fire departments, causing an estimated 408 civilian deaths and 3,130 civilian injuries (see Hall, 1995). And, for the first time ever, in 1994 juvenile firesetters accounted for a majority of the arrests for arson in this country (National Fire Protection Association [NFPA], 1995). An estimated $300.7 million in direct property damages was caused by children playing with fire. Fireplay was the leading cause of death among preschoolers. Tragically, most of the victims of child-set fires were under 5 years of age. Those victims who survive may suffer pediatric burn trauma and its serious medical (e.g., hospitalization) and psychological (e.g., posttraumatic stress, depression) sequellae (Cella, Perry, Kulchycky, & Goodwin, 1988; Stoddard, Norman, Murphy, & Beardslee, 1989).

Definitions

Child involvement with fire in a nonsanctioned and nonfunctional manner has been described using several types of behaviors. The most general behavior, fire interest, conveys the fact that some children show or report curiosity about fire, as demonstrated through questions, play activities, or collection of fire gear. Fireplay can mean actual experimentation or use of fire, frequently depicted as accidents and with a low level of recidivism. Firesetting is viewed as intentional firestarts or incidents involving fire, with some type of motive for causing the fire, the pursuit of firesetting materials, and an assumed high risk for recidivism. Arson represents an incident meeting the legal definition of firesetting, the definition for which varies by state regulation and penal code. Arson is charged as a felony offense if the offender is shown to have demonstrated maliciousness (wish to annoy, injure, or destroy) and willful in-

David J. Kolko • Director, Special Services Unit, Western Psychiatric Institute and Clinic; Associate Professor of Child Psychiatry and Psychology, University of Pittsburgh Medical Center, Pittsburgh, Pennsylvania 15213.

Handbook of Psychological Approaches with Violent Offenders: Contemporary Strategies and Issues, edited by Van Hasselt and Hersen. Kluwer Academic/Plenum Publishers, New York, 1999.

tent (awareness of potential consequences). Arson has a higher percentage of juvenile involvement than any other serious offense (Federal Bureau of Investigation [FBI], 1995). Empirical studies and clinical reports vary in their description and definition of childhood firesetting or firestarting (see Gaynor & Hatcher, 1987; Kolko, 1989). Because most studies do not differentiate fireplay and firesetting, the term firesetting will be used to reflect children's actual involvement with fire where no distinctions have been made.

Prevalence

Prevalence of childhood firesetting has been examined in a few studies. In a large community survey, 38% of the children (ages 6–14) surveyed reported ever having played with fire and 14% reported fireplay since the school year began (Grolnick, Cole, Laurenitis, & Schwartzman, 1990; Kafry, 1980). The highest percentage of recent fireplay (within the past 6 months) was reported by 12-year-old children (23%). Age was significantly related to several child (e.g., knowledge of fire destructiveness, perception of control), environmental (e.g., exposure, supervised experience, expectation of no parental response), and agent variables (e.g., access). Beyond child age, access to fire-related materials, expectations of no parental response, and fire responsibility predicted fireplay.

Among psychiatric samples, high prevalence rates have been found for firesetting and matchplay among outpatients (19.4%, 24.4%) and inpatients (34.6%, 52.0%), respectively, and for firesetting recidivism among inpatients (54.6%; Kolko & Kazdin, 1988b). Moderate rates of recurrent firesetting have been found among child referrals to community fire departments (65%; Parrish *et al.*, 1985) or psychiatric centers (23%–58%; Kolko & Kazdin, 1988b; Stewart & Culver, 1982).

Assessment and Evaluation

Screening and Classification

There are various methods for the assessment of firesetting children and their fire-related involvement. Perhaps the most common screening instruments used for this purpose are those published by the Federal Emergency Management Agency (Federal Emergency Management Agency [FEMA], 1979, 1983, 1987). The three interview guides, designed for children ages less than 7, 7–12, and 13 years and older, include several questions. Briefly, each interview is designed to screen cases into little, definite, and extreme risk for recidivism, primarily by evaluating the clinical severity of the child's and family's problems, and both the details and seriousness of the fire incident. Information is obtained at the level of the individual, social circumstances, and environmental conditions that support firesetting behavior.

In terms of the three categories of risk, little risk is characterized by no major individual problems or disorders, positive peer and family circumstances, and an intact family with no salient precipitants for fire activity. Definite risk children are described as having some psychological problems (e.g., abuse, learning disability), parental problems (e. g., poor discipline), other personal problems (social isolation e.g., school problems), and other family difficulties (single parent), whose single-incident fires are often set due to attention seeking. Extreme risk children are viewed as having more severe behavioral and emotional problems (e.g., disorders, impulsivity, aggression or violence), parental pathology, minimal family support, peer rejection, school failure, and family stressors. These children are believed to set multiple fires, influenced by peer pressure, and to receive few consequences for their fires.

Subgroups

As incorporated in the FEMA interviews, subgroups of children involved with fire are differentiated on the basis of their clinical characteristics and firesetting histories to reflect on the likelihood of (i.e., risk for) firesetting recidivism. Certainly, subgroups have been described or considered in several other clinical sources. Some children, often younger ones, have set a single, apparently accidental, fire at home due to curiosity or experimentation, which may be among the most common motives for children (Lewis & Yarnell, 1951). Such children are described as "curiosity" firesetters. Other children, commonly described as "pathological," appear to exhibit serious firesetting characterized by frequent, intentional, concealed, and destructive incidents (Fineman, 1980; Wooden & Berkey, 1984). Two other groups have been described that reflect the "cry for help" firesetter, whose firesetting is believed to reflect the need for attention or assistance in dealing with a recent stressor or crisis, and the "delinquent" firesetter, whose firesetting may reflect more generalized involvement in antisocial behavior, especially due to peer pressure and delinquency (Wooden & Berkey, 1984). Some practitioners also describe a group of severely disturbed firesetters (Humphreys, Kopet, & Lajoy, 1994). Recent research highlights aspects of all of these groups in different samples, but has not directly compared their clinical features (Bumpass, Fagelman, & Brix, 1983; Jacobson, 1985b; Kolko & Kazdin, 1986; Kuhnley *et al.*, 1982; Lewis & Yarnell, 1951; Stewart & Culver, 1982).

A recently reformulated model for understanding deviant fire behavior has differentiated eight types of firesetters that may help to delineate risk for future fire-related dangerous behavior. Fineman (1995) describes the following types in terms of their psychological state or diagnostic category, what was set on fire, or whether the fire was set in relation to the person's self-focus (bringing attention to self) or other-focus (directing attention away from self). There are two types of nonpathological firesetters (curiosity, accidental). The remaining six types are considered pathological (cry for help, delinquent or antisocial, severely disturbed, cognitively impaired, sociocultural, wildland). Pyromania is considered a subtype of the sensory reinforcement type that is classified within the severely disturbed type.

This revised model for understanding firesetting posits that firesetting is represented by the following characteristics: (1) dynamic historical factors predisposing the offender toward maladaptive and antisocial behaviors, (2) historical and current environmental factors that have taught and reinforced firesetting as acceptable behavior, and (3) immediate environmental contingencies that encourage firesetting behavior. The third is postulated to be composed of several components: crisis or trauma; characteristics of the fire; distortions before, during, and after the fire; feelings before, during, and after the fire; and both internal and external reinforcement for firesetting. These factors are rated in one of three levels of perceived risk using a firesetting sequence analysis and motive analysis. This revised model provides an organized approach to understanding a variety of assessment details regarding the firesetter and the fire incident in the hope of clarifying needed therapeutic directions and legal decision making regarding the level of dangerousness.

One report of firesetters in residential treatment reported general percentages for some of these various subgroups, as follows: (1) curiosity (15%), cry-for-help (25%), attention seeking (8%), pathological (30%–40%), and pyromaniacs (20%) (see Sakheim & Osborn, 1994). Another recent report based on fire department records indicates a much lower percentage of cases in the extreme risk group (4%), as compared with the definite (34%) or little risk (62%) groups (Porth, 1996). A related study compared 50 severe firesetters (more than one fire, intentional) with 50 minor firesetters (one fire, accidental) on psychological test data, psychiatric evaluations, and social histories (Sakheim, Osborn, & Abrams, 1991). The severe firesetters were characterized by more extreme scores on several child and family variables (e.g., sexual excitement, rage at insults, impulsivity, poor social judgment, neglect and abuse, identity confusion, lack of empathy, cruelty to animals, little guilt or remorse). When examined together, a larger sample consisting of these cases found that certain variables distinguished severe firesetters and nonfiresetters (defiance, physical violence, curiosity, limited guilt, poor parental supervision) (see Sakheim & Osborn, 1994, p. 13).

Limited social effectiveness and skill, often manifested by emotional (e.g., anger) expressiveness difficulties, also have been implicated in the motives for firesetting (see Kolko, 1989). Accordingly, use of fire may permit one to achieve interpersonal outcomes that could not have been easily produced through more direct expressive means. Unfortunately, though, few comparison studies have examined how these groups actually differ in the severity of the child's firesetting or other clinical problems. One study classified firesetters as high and low on each of two primary motives (Curiosity, Anger) and then compared them on measures of firesetting behavior and clinical dysfunction (Kolko & Kazdin, 1991c). Heightened (vs. low) curiosity was associated with greater psychopathology (externalizing and internalizing behavior problems, hostility, inappropriate social behavior), firesetting risk (curiosity, exposure to materials, community complaints, early experiences), and fire involvement (e.g., fire interest, matchplay, firesetting recidivism). Heightened (vs. low) anger was associated with certain firesetting risk measures (involvement in fire-related acts, knowledge about combustibles, exposure, complaints, use of mild punishment) and fire involvement (matchplay), but not increased behavioral or emotional problems.

Description and Parameters of Children's Firesetting Incidents

The FEMA screening instruments contain certain questions to evaluate characteristics of children's firesetting incidents. It is important to ascertain additional details of children's firesetting incidents, such as the child's involvement in the fire, intention, social context, reactions, and impact (R. Cole, Grolnick, & Schwartzman, 1993). These and other questions have been examined in structured interview studies. In one study, parents completed the Fire Incident Analysis (FIA) based on items from other measures (FEMA, 1979) and the general literature (see Kolko, 1989; Wooden & Berkey, 1984), to document parameters of their children's most serious incidents (Kolko & Kazdin, 1991c). The FIA-parent version included coded responses for several questions. Factor analysis of several items yielded three general motive factors (Curiosity, Anger, Attention/Help-seeking) and two other items (accident, peer pressure or destructiveness) designed to understand the presumed reason for the fire.

The FIA-P also evaluated details and characteristics of the firesetting incident (e.g., how materials were obtained, site of fire, type of property damage), levels of behavioral and emotional correlates just prior to the fire (e.g., aggression and defiance, depression and withdrawal, rule violations), and consequences following the fire, such as family and disciplinary (e.g., family discipline, child was talked to or counseled by someone outside the family), financial (e.g., value of damages), medical (i.e., injury, death), legal (e.g., criminal record, removal from home), and social and peer effects (e.g., peer acceptance, peer rejection or avoidance). The study provides descriptive details of the fires set by the children. Interestingly, in this study heightened (vs. low) curiosity was associated with greater fire involvement out of the house and less costly fire damages, whereas heightened (vs. low) anger was associated with greater aggression and defiance just prior to the fire and peer rejection following the fire.

A parallel study of 95 firesetters described the Fire Incident Analysis for Children based on this work (FIA-C; Kolko & Kazdin, 1994). The FIA-C consists of 21 questions that identified details and characteristics (e.g., how materials were obtained, site, severity of damages, forethought, planning), primary motives (curiosity or experimentation; anger, revenge, manipulation), and consequences as mediated by family members and friends (e.g., discipline, attention), reactions to the incident, and the impact of the incident on future firesetting. The FIA-C provides a structured approach to understanding the child's reports to questions regarding the incident. Among the study's findings, access to incendiaries, lack of child remorse and parental consequences, and motives of curiosity and fun were commonly reported characteristics. Four of the fire characteristics predicted children's overall severity of involvement in fire at follow-up (i.e., fire out of home, acknowledgment of being likely to set another fire, a neutral or positive reaction to the fire, no parental response to the fire). Such instruments may facilitate a quantitative evaluation of the details of an individual incident.

Measurement of Risk Factors for Firesetting

Other characteristics to be evaluated reflect factors that may increase the child's risk for subsequent firesetting and clarify the need or targets for intervention. An extension of some of the information in the FEMA (1979, 1983) interviews provides an operationalization of several risk factors that are evaluated in separate interview measures with parents (the Firesetting Risk Inventory or FRI; Kolko & Kazdin, 1989a) and children (the Children's Firesetting Inventory or CFI; Kolko & Kazdin, 1989b). The FRI examines several factors specific to fire (e.g., curiosity about fire, involvement in fire-related activities, early experiences with fire, exposure to peer or family models, knowledge of fire safety, fire skill or competence), and more general factors (e.g., positive and negative behavior, frequency and efficacy of harsh punishment). Compared with nonfiresetters, parents of firesetters acknowledged significantly higher scores on measures of firesetting contact (e.g., curiosity about fire, involvement in fire-related acts, exposure to peers or family fire models), general child and parent behavior (e.g., negative behavior), and family environment (e.g., use of harsh punishment, less effective mild punishment).

The CFI includes a smaller set of risk factors believed to be easiest for children to answer. The six factors included curiosity about fire (e.g., How much do you want to play with fire? How special or magical is fire to you?), involvement in fire-related activities (e.g., How many times did you pull a fire alarm?), knowledge about things that burn (e.g., Will clothes, like a shirt or pair of pants, burn?), fire competence (e.g., What steps would you follow to light a fire in a fireplace?), exposure to models and materials (e.g., How many of your friends have you seen playing with matches or lighting fire?), and supervision and discipline (e.g.,. How often are you disciplined at home?). Relative to nonfiresetters, firesetters acknowledged more attraction to fire, past fireplay, family interest in fire, exposure to friends or family who smoke, and, somewhat surprisingly, knowledge of things that burn, but tended to show less fire competence (skill) on role-plays than nonfiresetters.

Clinical Characteristics and Correlates of Child Firesetting

There is growing consensus as to the need to evaluate and understand the diverse clinical characteristics of children who set fires and their relationship to firesetting behavior. Just as fires may differ in terms of the ages of the children, frequency of firesetting, presence of property damages, and nature of children's motives, clinical context and level of family dysfunction, among other characteristics, may be quite variable and unique.

Child, Parent, and Family Dysfunction.

Several diagnostic and clinical characteristics have been documented among children who set fires. Empirical evidence in controlled studies has found a relationship between childhood firesetting and several forms of child dysfunction, such as heightened aggression, psychopathology, and social skills deficits (Kolko, Kazdin, & Meyer, 1985). In an extension of this study (Kolko & Kazdin, 1991a), firesetters were reported by parents to exhibit more covert behavior than both matchplayers and nonfiresetters. Firesetters and matchplayers received more extreme scores than nonfiresetters on measures of aggression, externalizing behaviors, impulsivity, emotionality, and hostility, but did not differ from one another. In contrast, child report measures revealed only a few differences associated with firesetting (e.g., aggression, unassertion, low self-esteem), relative to nonfiresetters.

Firesetters in residential treatment also have been distinguished from their nonfiresetting peers on several related features based on projective assessments (e.g., sexual excitement, anger at mother and father, rage and fantasies of revenge, sexual conflicts or dysfunction, poor social judgment, difficulty verbalizing anger, a diagnosis of Conduct Disorder; see Sakheim & Osborn, 1986). Many of these adolescents gained power over adults by setting fires. Related findings have been reported for inpatient firesetters versus other inpatients in terms of their history of sexual abuse and level of dysfunction on scales of the MMPI (e.g., schizophrenia, mania) (Moore, Thompson-Pope, & Whited, 1994).

Firesetting has also been associated with heightened parental psychiatric distress, marital disagreement, and exposure to stressful life events, and less child acceptance, monitoring, discipline, and involvement in activities that enhance the child's personal development and family relationships (Kazdin & Kolko, 1986; Kolko & Kazdin , 1990, 1991b). Firesetters have characterized their parents' child-rearing practices as involving greater lax discipline, nonenforcement, and anxiety induction, with scores for matchplayers generally falling between firesetters and controls.

These findings reflect a diffuse pattern of psychological and family characteristics of firesetters, relative to their nonfiresetting peers. Several characteristics, then, may merit evaluation in cases where children have been implicated in a fire, among other behavioral and emotional qualities such as whether the child has a psychiatric diagnosis (e.g., Attention-Deficit/Hyperactivity Disorder, Conduct Disorder), has developmental limitations or shows poor judgment or contact with reality, receives medication, has interpersonal or emotional expressiveness difficulties, or has delinquent or deviant peers. Areas of parental or family dysfunction that bear consideration are parental monitoring, supervision, effectiveness, and involvement with the child, parental drug or alcohol use or abuse, the presence of abuse or neglect, level of child stimulation and family structure, and the safety of the home environment.

Recidivism and Follow-up

There is surprisingly little information about the likelihood and predictors of recidivism based on empirical studies. One prospective study that followed a sample of 138 children for 1 year showed that 14 of 78 nonfiresetters (18%) later had set a fire, and that 21 of 60 firesetters (35%) had set an additional fire by follow-up (Kolko & Kazdin, 1992). Late starting was associated only with limited family sociability, whereas recidivism was associated with child knowledge about combustibles and involvement in fire-related activities, community complaints about fire contact, child hostility, lax discipline, family conflict, and limited parental acceptance, family affiliation, and organization. Some of these variables parallel certain characteristics that have been associated with adult arson (Rice & Harris, 1991). Recent fire department statistics indicate a recidivism rate of 6.2% (4 out of 65) based on a mailing or phone contact procedure, though the time interval was unspecified (Porth, 1996).

Summary of Risk Factors and Psychological Correlates

Individual factors associated with the onset and continuation of firesetting based on these studies reflect two general domains. The first, involvement with, interest in, and awareness of fire, includes experiences or conditions that support fireplay (e.g., exposure to fire models), idiosyncratic causes (e.g., curiosity, motive resolution), and limited fire competence (see R. E. Cole et al., 1983; R. E. Cole et al., 1986; Kafry, 1980; Kolko & Kazdin, 1989a, 1989b). The second domain, general behavioral-environmental dysfunction or conditions, reflects variables such as the use of indirect forms of aggression other antisocial behaviors and parental or family dysfunction (R. E. Cole et al., 1986; 1993; Gaynor & Hatcher, 1987; Jacobson, 1985a, 1985b; Kolko et al., 1985; Showers & Pickrell, 1987; Stewart & Culver, 1982). Some of these youth may exhibit symptoms of Conduct Disorder (see American Psychiatric Association, 1987; Heath, Hardesty, Goldfine, & Walker, 1985; Kelso & Stewart, 1986), with some exceptions (Kolko et al., 1985; Kolko & Kazdin, 1989a, 1989b). Some of these characteristics have been described in adult arsonists (see Geller, 1987; Kolko, 1989).

While motives and antecedent characteristics are important to understand, it is plausible that certain children may set additional fires due to the absence of any swift parental consequences or referral for services, because unsanctioned fireplay has gotten out of control (Kafry, 1980), or both, but these explanations have not been well examined empirically (Kolko, 1988). In our research, children who acknowledge or whose parents acknowledge any unsanctioned use of fire that produces at least some damage to property have been classified as firesetters (Kolko & Kazdin, 1988a). Some evidence described in a later section has suggested that children who simply play with matches are more similar to firesetters than nonfiresetters. Absence of prospective, empirical studies makes it difficult to determine which children have clinically significant problems with fire and are likely to set additional ones, and what interventions they should receive. Other aspects of these cases make them challenging to the practitioner, such as the difficulty in predicting who is likely to set another fire and under what circumstances and in knowing whether psychological problems or more benign environmental factors underlie firesetting behavior and should be targeted during intervention, what individual and family characteristics should be targeted during treatment, and what to look for in terms of clinical response or improvement.

Intervention and Treatment

Background on Approaches and Procedures

Intervention methods vary in the degree to which they target fire-specific experiences or more general behavioral-environmental characteristics (Gaynor & Hatcher, 1987; Kolko, 1989, Wooden & Berkey, 1984). This may reflect the fact that fire education is conducted primarily by the fire service, whereas psychological treatment is conducted primarily by mental health practitioners. Programs in the fire department have documented the importance of several program components: (1) developing interventions based on conceptual models and empirically supported procedures, (2) assessing child and family variables associated with firesetting, (3) teaching fire safety skills and making psychosocial intervention available, and (4) conducting a formal follow-up to assess outcome and evaluate its predictors (Kolko, 1988). Attention to various evaluation and intervention tasks may facilitate the effective administration of community-based programs (see Table 6.1). Indeed, integration of these approaches in comprehensive programs is one of the more important program developments in this area that is reflected in numerous settings across the country.

Fire Safety Skills and Prevention Education

Much more attention has been paid in recent years to characteristics, functions, and service delivery issues associated with community treatment of firesetting. Fire safety or prevention education consisting of instruction in fire safety skills and prac-

TABLE 6.1
Tasks for Implementation in Community Programs

Educate parents on effective prevention and intervention methods
Consider child's family role and motives (functions of fire)
Attend to parent's and family's resources and stressors
Screen for behavioral and emotional problems and consider mental health referral or involvement
Carefully examine and evaluate fire safety training materials, and provide skills training
Evaluate program operations and outcomes

tices (e.g., stop-drop-roll) is perhaps the most common procedure conducted by community programs (Cook, Hersch, Gaynor, & Roehl, 1989). Technical materials include risk interviews and manuals for use in intervention (Interviewing and Counseling Juvenile Firesetter Program [ICJF]; Federal Emergency Management Agency [FEMA], 1979, 1983). Among didactic presentations, the Learn Not To Burn [LNTB] program (NFPA, 1979) emphasizes protection (e.g., fire drills), prevention (e.g., using matches safely), and persuasion (e.g., practicing safe smoking), and may be the only prevention program that has demonstrated its impact on fire safety knowledge, relative to controls (NFPA, 1978).

Studies of instruction in fire safety skills are rare, despite the ubiquitousness of this approach. Early work by Jones and his colleagues has described and evaluated training procedures to enhance fire evacuation and assistance skills in young children, some of whom were developmentally delayed (see Jones, Kazdin, & Haney, 1981; Jones, Ollendick, & Shinske, 1989). A noteworthy feature of these studies was their articulation of a sequence of evacuation skills that could be trained systematically. Follow-up studies incorporated methods to train these skills, to reduce children's fear, and to teach children to respond to a fire when necessary. For example, Williams and Jones (1989) found improvements in behavioral performance on fire emergency responding and less fear of fire for a fire safety skills training group and a combined fire safety and fear reduction group, relative to two control groups. The combined group performed at a higher level at 5-month follow-up than the other groups. Elaborated rehearsal strategies have been found to add to behavioral rehearsal in the acquisition of fire emergency skills and the reduction of fear of fire (Jones, Ollendick, McLaughlin, & Williams, 1989). Such information may be applied in cases of children who have developed posttraumatic stress disorder following their involvement in a serious fire incident.

Another study documented the benefit of intervention with hospitalized firesetters who were randomly assigned to Group Fire Safety/Prevention Skills Training (FSST) or Individual Fire Awareness/Discussion (FAD) (Kolko, Watson, & Faust, 1991). FSST was associated with a reduction in contact with fire-related toys and matches in an analogue task, and an increase in fire safety knowledge, relative to FAD children. Parent-report measures at 6-month follow-up showed that FSST children were less frequently engaged in all four forms of involvement with fire than PSD children (16.7% vs. 58.3%). Although this study offered preliminary empirical findings to support FSST, relative to certain similar standard practices, further expansion and evaluation of this educational approach is clearly needed. Other similar work has applied fire safety and prevention education with children in inpatient or residential treatment settings using the "Smokey the Bear" theme (DeSalvatore & Hornstein, 1991). Concepts taught included the fire triangle, hazards, campfires, match safety, and reporting fires. Only 1 of 35 of the children followed was found to have set another fire at 1-year follow-up. A novelty of this program was its use of parents to extend training activities to the home.

Fire safety skills training is not always conducted in a systematic and formal manner. Fire departments commonly provide the family with a firehouse orientation and tour for the typical "young and curious" firesetter to heighten the child's awareness of the dangers of fire. These meetings may be followed by an occasional follow-up visit or call (Gaynor, McLaughlin, & Hatcher, 1984) or a home visit to review safety precautions and provide information to children and their parents. Brief but focused interventions may be effective depending on the content or skills to be reviewed, the care with which the material is conveyed, and the level of motivation and interest on the part of parents.

Psychological Intervention and Treatment

Treatment designed to alter the child's cognitive-behavioral repertoire is an alternative intervention with psychiatrically disturbed or behavior problem children that has been described in this literature for some time. Case reports and empirical studies have described various approaches and procedures. For example, one of the earliest methods involved using negative practice (repeatedly lighting matches) to satiate and then extinguish a child's interest in fire (Holland, 1969; Kolko, 1983; McGrath, Marshall, & Prior, 1979), though fewer recent reports include this procedure. A few early cases also employed structural and behavioral family therapies (Eisler, 1974; Madanes, 1981; Minuchin, 1974). Contingency management procedures are commonly used to discourage involvement with fire and reinforce contact with nonfire materials (R. G. Adler, Nunn, Laverick, & Ross, 1988; Stawar, 1976). Beyond use of consequences, prosocial skills training in the expression of anger and emotional arousal has been employed to address the motives for setting fires (Kolko & Ammerman, 1988; McGrath *et al.*, 1979) or to enhance cognitive-behavioral skills that promote assertive, nondestructive problem solving (DeSalvatore & Hornstein, 1991). Certain applications offer related services, such as graphs that represent the personal and environmental context of a fire (Bumpass, Fagelman, & Brix, 1983) and individual and family psychotherapy (Bumpass, Brix, & Preston, 1985). Most interventions have incorporated several procedures (e.g., contingencies, behavioral training skills) and reported reduced firesetting at follow-up, though few controlled data have been noted. These reports highlight the need to consider the behavioral-functional context of firesetting and its relationship to the child's interpersonal repertoire, and the use of punishment and reinforcement procedures. Information about specific content and operations of various intervention procedures or treatment programs is available elsewhere (R. Cole *et al.*, 1993; Gaynor & Hatcher, 1987; Kolko, 1989, 1996).

There are very few studies or empirical reports of behavioral or psychological procedures. Applications by the author have examined specialized cognitive-behavioral and contingency management procedures with clinically referred children, including home-based reinforcement and response–cost contingencies (Kolko, 1983), graphing of prior incidents and psychological skills training (Kolko & Ammerman, 1988), and fire safety assessment–skills training combined with medication and parent management training (Cox-Jones, Lubetsky, Fultz, & Kolko, 1990). These interventions were associated with reduced firesetting behavior and improved behavioral adjustment at follow-up. One implication of these reports is the potential benefit of targeting child behavior, environmental contingencies in the home, or both. Another recent report highlights the benefit of providing comprehensive psychological services to a young adult that integrated cognitive-behavioral assessment information (e.g., functional analysis) and treatment (e.g., social skills, coping and relaxation, assertion training, covert sensitization), with facial surgery (Clare, Murphy, Cox, & Chaplin, 1992). At 4-month follow-up, no further firesetting or related behavior had been reported.

Combined and Collaborative Programs

An important advance in intervention is the integration of multiple approaches within one network or program. One of the earliest reports integrating mental health and fire department services in the city of Dallas was reported by Bumpass and colleagues (1985). The program incorporated use of a graphing technique to depict the child's firesetting incident, fire safety films and slides, and promotion of involvement in community-based activities. The authors reported several changes from before to after treatment in percentage of recidivist cases (32% vs. 2%), number of reported juvenile fires (204 vs. 141), and fire costs ($1,031,606 vs. $536,102). Integrated community-based services also have extended the use of fire department and mental health screening evaluations in order to identify appropriate interventions (Webb, Sakheim, Towns-Miranda, & Wagner, 1990). Beyond assessment of risk, this interagency program incorporates strategies to facilitate engagement, liaison, and outreach, and provides a range of services that reflect primary (school-based education), secondary (education and mental health), and tertiary prevention (intensive treatment).

The National Juvenile Firesetter/Arson Control and Prevention Program (JFACPP) was sponsored by the Office of Juvenile Justice and Delinquency Prevention (OJJDP) and U.S. Fire Administration (USFA) to assess, develop, evaluate, and disseminate information on promising approaches for the control and prevention of juvenile firesetting and arson. The program operated in stages (assessment of problem, development of comprehensive approach and training and technical materials, testing and dissemination of materials). One primary product of this work was the development of a modular or components model for a juvenile firesetter program emphasizing seven components: program management, screening and evaluation, intervention services, referral mechanisms, publicity and outreach, monitoring systems, and developing relationships with juvenile justice. Among the products were several materials such as a user's guide (FEMA, 1994, FA-145), guidelines for setting up early intervention programs (FEMA, 1994, FA-146), general guidelines for implementation (FEMA, 1994, FA-147), an executive summary (FEMA, 1994, FA-148), and a trainer's guide (FEMA, 1994, FA-149). These materials offer a comprehensive perspective on all aspects of program development and design, including lists of resource materials, evaluation tools, and considerations in the packaging and funding of a program.

The JFACCP material offers one of the first systematic approaches to the application of field-tested concepts and methods in the organization of multiple services for juvenile firesetters. The executive summary, for example, highlighted certain program linkages to mental health and juvenile justice made by the three test sites, but also noted difficulties with extending the program throughout targeted areas and maintaining an efficient monitoring system. Interestingly, about two thirds of the cases referred to two of the sites were rated as needing a mental health evaluation. Suggestions were made to take advantage of agencies with leadership functions in the area and to draw upon regional programs that can integrate multiple services and resources. The implications of this program development initiative must await attempts at replication as these materials are disseminated.

Recommendations for dealing with different types of firesetting children clearly merit integration of various intervention components, such as fire safety education, conducting checks for fire-related materials, providing assistance to express strong affect, working with parents to establish structure and consequences at home, family therapy, and installing smoke alarms (Humphreys *et al.*, 1994). Humphreys and colleagues offer several practical suggestions for parents to help them monitor, instruct, and manage their firesetting children (e.g., remove matches, monitor television habits, discuss consequences in advance, forbid fireplay).

Another advance in the service delivery area concerns the development of comprehensive and coordinated clinical assessment and treatment methods. The Oregon Office of State Fire Marshal has coordinated several work groups devoted to expanding a model of evaluation and treatment. In conjunction with the treatment strategies task force, a needs assessment protocol was developed to assess mental health needs, take an accurate firesetter history, determine precipitating stressors and a firesetter typology, and make appropriate treatment and supervision recommendations (Humphreys & Kopet, 1996). The protocol was devised as a needs assessment, rather than a risk assessment, with implications for treatment planning. For example, interview questions are surveyed in various domains (e.g., family, social, trauma, mental health, fire), used to develop typology scores (e.g., curiosity, delinquent), and then aggregated to form an impression of diagnosis, prognosis, and treatment. A strength of this method is its specification of relevant questions in an organized assessment protocol and inclusion of an explanatory manual.

A companion model to expedite mental health treatment was also developed by this task force of the Oregon Treatment Strategies Task Force (1996). The model recognizes the importance of understanding the various subtypes of firesetters just noted and incorporates a description of cyclic patterns often shown by families of juvenile firesetters and the community, and describes the behavioral and cognitive cycles that may contribute to the risk for recidivism. There are four overlapping cycles or rings, each representing a dimension that may influence a child's behavior, stated as the emotional-cognitive (e.g., thinking errors, belief that life is unfair, boredom, anger), the behavioral (e.g., limit testing, power struggles, covert behaviors), family (e.g., initial response to fire, stressors, ineffective discipline), and community-social (e.g., special services, institutional conflicts, community resources).

Based on this assessment, a practitioner can estimate the likelihood of recidivism and take steps to address these problems using specific intervention procedures, including child (e.g., elimination of negative peer influences, restitution, anger management), family (communication training, logical discipline, fire safety education), and fire department interventions (education, contract), as well as referral and backup plans. A related asset to this approach is the well-coordinated network of agencies involved in serving firesetting youth (e.g., school, law enforcement, mental health). Of course, this model is preliminary and, thus, will benefit from clinical examination in terms of its scope and overall utility.

Newer program materials also merit consideration. Johnston (1996) has described an approach to group treatment and fire safety education in the context of an eight-session manual for primarily younger children. The manual includes novel lesson plans that address key principles that focus on feelings and behaviors, and on peer pressure and how to make appropriate choices in response to it. Various fire-related concepts are addressed using worksheets and group activities (e.g., understanding fire's destructive capability, conducting home fire safety checks, describing fire interventions for the home) similar to the presentation of more general psychological or behavioral strategies for self-control (e.g., relaxation, understanding feelings, problem solving, assertion).

Delinquent firesetters have also been targeted by a group program developed by Campbell and Elliot (1996). The program includes 14 lessons that cover many of the concepts commonly found in cognitive-behavioral treatments, such as communication, assertion, and anger-control. Certain lessons provide novel attention to communication and listening, conscience and thinking errors, relapse prevention plans, and working with parents. The program is strengthened by the inclusion of discussion questions for evaluating participant perceptions of certain principles and homework exercises, concrete examples of skills to be trained, and a posttest.

Parents and other adults are infrequently targeted by training programs to address the child firesetter, but are clearly appropriate as recipients of fire awareness and preparation information. Pinsonneault (1996) describes a fire awareness curriculum for foster parents or child protective services workers that seeks to help them understand the reasons for firesetting and the types of firesetters. Helpful strategies for creating a safe environment that may help to minimize the family's risk for fire and other supportive interventions to enhance positive relationships, home safety, and ways to talk about fire in the news also are described. This program is well written and incorporates several forms that make discussion of fire safety clear and constructive. The accumulation of program evaluation data and consumer satisfaction data will help to evaluate the overall utility of all three of these new programs.

A recent study from Australia provides one of the few controlled evaluations of alternative approaches to working with children 5–16 years of age who were classified as either curiosity or pathological firesetters (R. Adler, Nunn, Northam, Lebnan, & Ross, 1994). Curious and nondysfunctional firesetters were randomly assigned to either education (fire safety information to child and parents, discussion of fire awareness) or a combined condition (education, satiation, response cost for fires, graphing of fire) with both being conducted by a firefighter at home, whereas pathological cases were offered psychiatric referral and treatment by a specialist in a children's hospital clinic and then randomized either to the same education alone or to the combined condition.

Findings showed a significant reduction in the frequency of firesetting when comparing the year prior to and then following the intervention, but no difference as a function of the home-specialist or the education-combined comparisons. Overall mean rates of firesetting were 7.1 and 1.5 at each of these two respective time periods. There was also a reduction in the severity of firesetting. Of 80 children considered improved, 59 children (42.8%) set no fires during the 12-month posttreatment period and an additional 21 (15.2%) no longer met the referral criterion as they set less than three fires during that period. Home-based (vs. specialist) cases tended to have a higher proportion of improvement (73% vs. 52%) and a lower percentage of dropout (20% vs. 35%). The combined (vs. education only) group also tended to have a higher dropout rate (35% vs. 21%). The overall 28% dropout rate and absence of data on treatment integrity and general child behavior notwithstanding, this study is the first controlled outcome study of its kind, and is important in showing that even minimal intervention may be effective in reducing firesetting over a long interval.

A separate but related study conducted in the United States examines relative efficacy of fire service and mental health intervention conducted in a clinic setting in comparison with a brief home visit from a firefighter (Kolko, 1996). Firesetting boys ages 5–13 were randomly assigned to either Fire Safety Education (FSE) or Psychosocial Treatment (PT) and compared with boys who were assigned to a brief and routine condition that was designed to reflect contemporary educational practices in the fire service (Home Visit from a Firefighter, FHV). Intervention was designed to be short-term, executed by trained specialists using program manuals, monitored to ensure therapeutic integrity, and evaluated using multiple measures from multiple sources.

FSE involves primarily training in fire safety education principles and tasks that teach fire safety practices, and fire protection and evacuation strategies (e.g., stop-drop-roll, emergency phone calls, exiting a burning house, declining an invitation to engage in matchplay), whereas PT involves teaching generalized self-control and problem-solving skills, establishing environmental conditions (consequences) that encourage behaviors other than firesetting, and altering the motive for using fire. FHV includes learning about the danger of fires and functions of firefighters, asking children to promise not to get involved again with unsanctioned fireplay ("no-fire contract"), and distributing program materials to serve as a reminder to avoid using fire (e.g., coloring book on fire safety, plastic fire helmet, NFPA, 1982). Thus, two intensive programs are being compared with one another and then with a third, minimal contact condition. Both children and their parents are targeted in each intervention.

The study evaluates program impact on the frequency of involvement with fire and related activities, and, secondarily, specific psychosocial correlates or firesetting risk factors, such as interpersonal repertoire, antisocial behavior, and parent-family stress. Pre–post comparisons are being supplemented with 1-year follow-up data. This study will determine whether brief exposure to a firefighter is as effective as active participation in more intensive skills training procedures derived from firesetting research findings and will identify predictors of treatment outcome (e.g., firesetting recidivism, severity).

Of course, there are still many obstacles to developing and maintaining an effective collaborative program in most communities. A task force on juvenile firesetting convened by the NFPA in 1993 reported on several impediments and some potential solutions (NFPA, 1993). To address lack of public and professional awareness of the problem of firesetting, several suggestions were made to train juvenile firesetter professionals in community coalition building strategies, educate media professionals, develop fire science information and parent education materials in the area, enlist fire service leaders in juvenile programs, and train mental health professionals in intervention techniques. The need to access existing resources was also emphasized by suggestions to establish a national clearinghouse and document the ways in which programs assure their long-term stability. Finally, using data effectively was considered important in terms of describing, planning, and revising program components. Such suggestions illustrate the broad array of potential solutions to improving the field and the multidisciplinary makeup of those who may contribute to these solutions.

Summary of Intervention Procedures

The aforementioned anecdotal, clinical, and limited empirical evidence highlight the role of two primary domains targeted by firesetting interventions: children's experience with, exposure to, and interest in fire (fire-specific involvement), and the individual and family conditions that influence child behavior (behavioral-environmental control). In general, fire safety education targets the former, while psychosocial intervention targets the latter, such that each approach addresses specific characteristics associated with increased firesetting risk (Cook *et al.,* 1989). There exists only anecdotal or limited empirical support for the utility of these approaches. Thus, a comparative evaluation of both interventions would advance the treatment of childhood firesetters. An evaluation of the separate and combined effects of these two complementary interventions is justified when considering that there is a sizable population of firesetters who may set multiple fires and exhibit psychosocial maladjustment, firesetters are referred to both fire service and mental health systems for services, and elements of these two risk factor domains can be effectively translated into procedures applied to reduce firesetting behavior.

Summary and Future Directions

Multidisciplinary collaboration in the administration of services for firesetting youth has become an important advance in this area and, in recent years, represents more the rule than the exception. This is due, in part, to accumulation of evidence suggesting the relevance of fire safety and mental health considerations in understanding the problem of juvenile firesetting, and to the recognition of the roles being played by professionals in the juvenile justice, burn care, and other medical, educational, and social service systems. At the same time, there is a strong need to expand the scope and comprehensiveness of intervention programs in this area and the level of regional support and resources received by various programs to assure their long-term viability. Efficient delivery and coordination of service is one of the most critical elements in promoting the maintenance of multidisciplinary team efforts. Table 6.2 presents some of the program components that should be considered in the development of a services network. Although it is too early to develop a clinical pathway in this area, one might consider how the following intervention components could be organized and then invoked based on screening and evaluation findings: (1) brief fire brochure on dangers of fire, (2) training in fire safety and prevention skills, (3) parental management of fire and use of behavioral consequences, (4) training in cognitive-behavioral skills , (5) parental counseling, family treatment, or both, (6) juvenile justice involvement, (7) restitution, and 8) hospitalization or residential program.

Given this expansion, there is a compelling need to disseminate relevant multidisciplinary information to professionals working with any aspect of the childhood firesetting problem. A newsletter published by the Oregon Office of the State Fire Marshal, *Hot Issues* and the Massachusetts Coalition for Juvenile Firesetter

TABLE 6.2
Potential Program Components

Type	Characteristic or goal
Referral and screening	Centralized
Publicity and outreach	Public awareness
Services and format	Types, sequence
Treatment planning	What to assess, how serious, what treatment options?
Networking	Coordination
Evaluation and outcomes	Clients, services, systems, impact

TABLE 6.3
Content Domain for Staff Training

Area	Issue
Preparation	Review of cases and literature
	Staffings, shared cases
Liability	Reporting laws; duty to warn
	Laws and statutes
Standards of care	Knowledge, skills, safety and protection
Networking	Cooperative operations

Programs (The Strike Zone) has served this function for several years. This newsletter includes news, announcements, articles, resources, and program descriptions evaluation data and has developed a national distribution list. One of the other functions in this regard is to promote "best practice" concepts, procedures, and programs by highlighting information on cost-effectiveness. Training of staff generally requires attention to several content domains, some of which are listed in Table 6.3. Beyond implementation of routine staff training based on advanced curricula, there may be some benefit to organizing a national registry of service providers in this area. An updated list of providers across disciplines could serve an important resource procurement function and allow practitioners to easily identify referral sources in different areas. Further, such a network could encourage the development of private–public partnerships in the maintenance of regional centers devoted to working with firesetting youth.

There is also a need to better understand the nature of firesetting in children and youth. For example, studies must begin to evaluate whether a continuum of fire behavior exists and to describe paths in the progression to more serious forms of the behavior. Addressing the relationship among these behaviors (fire interest, fireplay, firesetting, arson) would be important in order to identify predictors of more serious fire involvement (Hersch, 1989). Further, examination of methods of evaluating firesetting history and other important psychosocial characteristics, as in the Oregon model, would shed light on the clinical utility of novel assessment instruments in this area. Other areas of evaluation for consideration during assessment can be found in Table 6.4. Finally, follow-up studies of firesetting behavior are needed to understand the natural course or history of children's involvement with fire. Because only one

TABLE 6.4
Areas Worthy of Evaluation

Focus	Content
Child	Details of fire and motive
	Firesetting history (interest, exposure, involvement)
	Emotional and behavior dysfunction; general adjustment
Parent	Effectiveness/pathology, monitoring and discipline
	Depression, substance abuse, poor judgment
Family	Safety, relationships, activities
	Cohesion and support, conflict, service involvement
	Abuse and neglect
Community	Fire safety and therapeutic resources; programs

TABLE 6.5
Common Intervention Strategies for Different Domains

Target Domain	Content/form
Child	Functional analysis
	Knowledge of dangers, contingencies
	Relaxation, problem-solving skills
	Anger-control, social and expressiveness skills
Parent	Behavior management, monitoring, consistency
	Restitution, anger-control
Family	Monitoring, contingencies, home programs
	Communication
Court system	Contact with fire department and police
	Probation, restitution, commun. service, facility

prospective study has been reported (Kolko & Kazdin, 1992), there is limited information regarding the prevalence and predictors of recidivism or cessation.

Data as to the feasibility and effectiveness of alternative interventions are just beginning to appear, but we still know little about the impact of services on children's contact with and use of fire, and their level of behavioral dysfunction. For example, is training in fire safety skills more effective for curious children, and is psychosocial treatment more useful with behaviorally dysfunctional children? Such information must be collected to provide the field with clear directions for initiating intervention. Relatedly, an evaluation of the relative efficacy and long-term impact of comprehensive (multimodal) interventions that combine various approaches, such as fire safety and psychological counseling, versus very specific and focused interventions is needed, especially those than can be easily and inexpensively delivered (e.g., groups, films). Common psychosocial and fire safety intervention approaches are listed in Table 6.5.

Another area worth exploring is the development of methods to minimize children's heightened attraction to and interest in fire. Most practitioners can identify cases of children and youth who appear to be excessively fascinated by fire and expend considerable energy in making contact with fire, even in the face of parental restrictions and punishment. These cases raise significant questions about treatment strategy and concerns about public safety. At the other extreme are those children whose fear of fire and associated symptoms have developed following a serious fire (e.g., posttraumatic stress disorder). Such children, whose firesetting results in significant avoidance of fire-related stimuli and heightened anxiety when encountering these stimuli, may benefit from exposure-based treatments similar to ones evaluated by Jones and colleagues (e.g., Jones et al., 1989). Certainly, more information is needed to better understand the etiology of firesetting, including both the interest in and fear of fire, and the methods that are most likely to modify the expression of these troublesome behaviors.

ACKNOWLEDGMENTS

Preparation of this chapter was supported, in part, by a renewal of grant MH-39976 to the author from the National Institute of Mental Health. The author acknowledges the contribution of the following staff associated with Project SAFETY (Services Aimed at Fire Education and Treatment for Youth): Karen Ankrom, Dr.

Oscar Bukstein, Brian Day, Karen Drudy, Audrey Fincher, Evelyn Savido, Dana Schei-dhauer, Patricia Stewart, and Valerie Newell, and Dr. D. Scott Wood. The author would also like to thank Catherine Rich for her assistance in the preparation of this chapter. Many of the background studies reviewed herein were conducted in collaboration with Alan E. Kazdin, Ph.D., in the original grant application. Reprint requests can be obtained from David J. Kolko, Director, Child & Parent Behavior Clinic, Western Psychiatric Institute and Clinic, 3811 O'Hara St., Pittsburgh, PA 15213.

References

Abidin, R. R. (1983, August). *Parenting Stress Index: Research update*. Poster presented at the American Psychological Association Conference.

Achenbach, T. M., & Edelbrock , C. (1983). *Manual for the Child Behavior Checklist and revised child behavior profile*. Burlington, VT: Queen City Publishers.

Achenbach, T. M., & Edelbrock , C. (1989). *Manual for the Youth Self Report*. City, VT: Queen City Publishers.

Adler, R. , Nunn, R., Northam, E., Lebnan, V., & Ross, R. (1994). Secondary prevention of childhood firesetting. *Journal of the American Academy of Child and Adolescent Psychiatry, 33*, 1194–1202.

Adler, R. G., Nunn, R. J., Laverick, J., & Ross, R. (1988, October). *Royal Children's Hospital/Metropolitan Fire Brigade juvenile fire awareness & intervention program: Research and intervention protocol*. Unpublished paper. Parkville, Victoria, Australia.

American Psychiatric Association. (1987). *Diagnostic and statistical manual of mental disorders* (3rd ed., rev.). Washington, DC: Author.

Bumpass, E. R., Fagelman, F. D., & Brix, R. J. (1983). Intervention with children who set fires. *American Journal of Psychotherapy, 37*, 328–345.

Bumpass, E. R., Brix, R. J., & Preston, D. (1985). A community-based program for juvenile firesetters. *Hospital and Community Psychiatry, 36*, 529–533.

Campbell, C., & Elliot, E. J. (1996). *Skills curriculum for intervening with firesetters (ages 13–18)*. Salem, OR: Office of State Fire Marshal.

Cella, D. F., Perry, S.W., Kulchycky, S., & Goodwin, C. (1988). Stress and coping in relatives of burn patients: A longitudinal study. *Hospital and Community Psychiatry, 39*, 159–166.

Clare, I. C. H., Murphy, G. H., Cox, D., & Chaplin, E. H. (1992). Assessment and treatment of firesetting: A single-case investigation using a cognitive-behavioral model. *Criminal Behavior, 2*, 253–268.

Cole, R., Grolnick, W., & Schwartzman, P. (1993). Fire setting. In R. T. Ammerman, C. Last, & M. Hersen (Eds.), *Handbook of prescriptive treatments for children and adolescents* (pp. 332–346). Boston: Allyn & Bacon.

Cole, R. E., Laurenitis, L. R., McCandrews, M. M., McKeever, J. M., & Schwartzman, P. I. (1983). *Final report of the 1983 Fire-Related Youth Program Development Project*. Rochester, NY: New York State Office of Fire Prevention and Control.

Cole, R. E., Grolnick, W. S., McCandrews, M. M., Matkoski, K. M., & Schwartzman, P. I. (1986). *Rochester Fire-Related Youth Project, progress report* (Vol. 2). Rochester, NY: New York State Office of Fire Prevention and Control.

Cook, R., Hersch, R., Gaynor, J., & Roehl, J. (1989, April). *The National Juvenile Firesetter/Arson Control and Prevention Program: Assessment report, Executive summary*. Washington, DC: Institute for Social Analysis.

Cox-Jones, C., Lubetsky, M., Fultz, S. A., & Kolko, D. J. (1990). Inpatient treatment of a young recidivist firesetter. *Journal of the American Academy of Child Psychiatry, 29*, 936–941.

DeSalvatore, G., & Hornstein, R. (1991). Juvenile firesetting: Assessment and treatment in psychiatric hospitalization and residential placement. *Child & Youth Care Forum, 20*, 03-114.

Eisler, R. M. (1974). Crisis intervention in the family of a firesetter. *Psychotherapy: Theory, Research and Practice, 9*, 76–79.

Federal Bureau of Investigation (1995). *Uniform Crime Reports*. Washington, DC.: Author.

Federal Emergency Management Agency. (1979). *Interviewing and counseling juvenile firesetters*. Washington, DC: U.S. Goverment Printing Office.

Federal Emergency Management Agency. (1983). *Juvenile firesetter handbook: Dealing with children Ages 7 to 14*. Washington, DC: U.S. Goverment Printing Office.

Federal Emergency Management Agency (1987). *Juvenile Firesetter Handbook: Dealing with Adolescents Ages 14 to 18.* Washington, DC: U.S. Government Printing Office.

Federal Emergency Management Agency (1994). *Controlling Juvenile Firesetting: An Evoluation of the Three Regional Pilot Programs*; Executive summary. (Fire Administration No. 148), Washington, D.C.: Author.

Fineman, K. R. (1980). Firesetting in childhood and adolescence. *Psychiatric Clinics of North America, 3,* 483–500.

Fineman, K. R. (1995). A model for the qualitative analysis of child and adult fire deviant behavior. *American Journal of Forensic Psychology, 13,* 31–59.

Gaynor, J., & Hatcher, C. (1987). *The psychology of child firesetting: Detection and intervention.* New York: Brunner/Mazel.

Gaynor, J., McLaughlin, P. M., & Hatcher, C. (1984). *The Firehawk Children's Program: A working manual.* San Francisco: National Firehawk Foundation.

Geller, J. L. (1987). Firesetting in the adult psychiatric population. *Hospital and Community Psychiatry, 38,* 501–510.

Grolnick, W. S., Cole, R. E., Laurenitis, L., & Schwartzman, P. I. (1990). Playing with fire: A developmental assessment of children's fire understanding and experience. *Journal of Clinical Child Psychology, 19,* 128–135.

Hall, J. R. (1995, August). *Children playing with fire: U.S. experience, 1980–1993.* Quincy, MA: National Fire Protection Association.

Heath, G. A., Hardesty, V. A., Goldfine, P. E., & Walker, A. M. (1985). Diagnosis and childhood firesetting. *Journal of Clinical Psychology, 41,* 571–575.

Hersch, R. K. (1989, May). A look at juvenile firesetter programs. *Juvenile Justice Bulletin,* Washington, D.C: U.S. Department of Justice.

Holland, C.J. (1969). Elimination by the parents of firesetting behaviour in a 7-year old boy. *Behaviour Research & Therapy, 7,* 135–137.

Humphreys, J., & Kopet, T. (1996, March). *Manual for juvenile firesetter needs assessment protocol.* Office of State Fire Marshal, Salem, OR.

Humphreys, J., Kopet, T., & Lajoy, R. (1994). Clinical considerations in the treatment of juvenile firesetters. *Behavior Therapist, 17,* 13–15.

Jacobson, R. R. (1985a). Child firesetters: A clinical investigation. *Journal of Child Psychology and Psychiatry, 26,* 759–768.

Jacobson, R. R. (1985b). The subclassification of child firesetters. *Journal of Child Psychology and Psychiatry, 26,* 769–775.

Johnston, K. (1996). *A step by step approach to group treatment and fire safety education: An eight session intervention program for child firesetters.* Salem, OR: Office of State Fire Marshal.

Jones, R. T., Ollendick, T. H., McLaughlin, K. J., & Williams, C. E. (1989). Elaborative and behavioral rehearsal in the acquisition of fire emergency skills and the reduction of fear of fire. *Behavior Therapy, 20,* 93–101.

Jones, R. T., Ollendick, T. H., & Shinske, F. K. (1989). The role of behavioral versus cognitive variables in skill acquisition. *Behavior Therapy, 20,* 293–302.

Kafry, D. (1980). Playing with matches: Children and fire. In D. Canter (Ed.), *Fires and human behaviour* (pp. 41–60). Chichester, England: Wiley.

Kazdin, A. E., & Kolko, D. J. (1986). Parent psychopathology and family functioning among childhood firesetters. *Journal of Abnormal Child Psychology, 14,* 315–329.

Kelso, J., & Stewart, M. A. (1986). Factors which predict the persistence of aggressive conduct disorder. *Journal of Child Psychology and Psychiatry, 27,* 77–86.

Kolko, D. J. (1983). Multicomponent parental treatment of firesetting in a developmentally-disabled boy. *Journal of Behavior Therapy and Experimental Psychiatry, 14,* 349–353.

Kolko, D. J. (1985). Juvenile firesetting: A review and critique. *Clinical Psychology Review, 5,* 345–376.

Kolko, D. J. (1988). Community interventions for childhood firesetters: A comparison of two national programs. *Hospital and Community Psychiatry, 39,* 973–979.

Kolko, D. J. (1989). Fire setting and pyromania. In C. Last & M. Hersen (Eds.), *Handbook of child psychiatric diagnosis* (pp. 443–459). New York: Wiley.

Kolko, D. J. (1996). Education and counseling for child firesetters: A comparison of skills training programs with standard practice. In E. D. Hibbs and P. S. Jensen (Eds.), *Psychosocial treatments for child and adolescent disorders: Empirically based strategies for clinical practice,* pp. 409–433. Washington, DC: American Psychological Association.

Kolko, D. J., & Ammerman, R. T. (1988). Firesetting. In M. Hersen & C. Last (Eds.), *Child behavior therapy casebook* (pp. 243–262). New York: Plenum.

Kolko, D. J., & Kazdin, A. E. (1986). A conceptualization of firesetting in children and adolescents. *Journal of Abnormal Child Psychology, 14,* 49–62.

Kolko, D. J., & Kazdin, A. E. (1988a). Parent–child correspondence in identification of firesetting among child psychiatric patients. *Journal of Child Psychology and Psychiatry, 29,* 175–184.

Kolko, D. J. & Kazdin, A. E. (1988b). Prevalence of firesetting and related behaviors in child psychiatric inpatients. *Journal of Consulting and Clinical Psychology, 56,* 628-630.

Kolko, D. J., & Kazdin, A. E. (1989a). Assessment of dimensions of childhood firesetting among child psychiatric patients and nonpatients. *Journal of Abnormal Child Psychology, 17,* 157–176.

Kolko, D. J., & Kazdin, A. E. (1989b). The Children's Firesetting Interview with psychiatrically referred and nonreferred children. *Journal of Abnormal Child Psychology, 17,* 609–624.

Kolko, D. J., & Kazdin, A. E. (1990). Matchplay and firesetting in children: Relationship to parent, marital, and family dysfunction. *Journal of Clinical Child Psychology, 19,* 229–238.

Kolko, D. J., & Kazdin, A. E. (1991a). Aggression and psychopathology in matchplaying and firesetting children: A replication and extension. *Journal of Clinical Child Psychology, 20,* 191–201.

Kolko, D. J., & Kazdin, A. E. (1991b). Matchplaying and firesetting in children: Relationship to parent, marital, and family dysfunction. *Journal of Clinical Child Psychology, 19,* 229–238.

Kolko, D. J., & Kazdin, A. E. (1991c). Motives of childhood firesetters: Firesetting characteristics and psychological correlates. *Journal of Child Psychology and Psychiatry, 32,* 535–550.

Kolko, D. J., & Kazdin, A. E. (1992). The emergence and recurrence of child firesetting: A one-year prospective study. *Journal of Abnormal Child Psychology, 20,* 17–37.

Kolko, D. J., & Kazdin, A. E. (1994). Children's descriptions of their firesetting incidents: Characteristics and relationships to recidivism. *Journal of the American Academy of Child & Adolescent Psychiatry, 33,* 114–122.

Kolko, D. J., Kazdin, A. E., & Meyer, E. C. (1985). Aggression and psychopathology in childhood firesetters: Parent and child reports. *Journal of Consulting and Clinical Psychology, 53,* 377–385.

Kolko, D. J., Watson, S., & Faust, J. (1991). Fire safety/prevention skills training to reduce involvement with fire in young psychiatric inpatients: Preliminary findings. *Behavior Therapy, 22,* 269–284.

Kuhnley, E. J., Hendren, R. L., & Quinlan, D. M. (1982). Firesetting by children. *Journal of the American Academy of Child Psychiatry, 21,* 560–563.

Lewis, N. O. C., & Yarnell, H. (1951). Pathological firesetting (pyromania). *Nervous & Mental Disease, Monograph No. 82.* Nicholasville, KY: Coolidge Foundation.

Madanes, C. (1981). *Strategic family therapy.* San Fransisco: Jossey-Bass.

McGrath, P., Marshall, P. T., & Prior, K. (1979). A comprehensive treatment program for a firesetting child. *Journal of Behavior Therapy and Experimental Psychiatry, 10,* 69–72.

Minuchin, S. (1974). *Families and family therapy.* San Fransisco: Jossey-Bass.

Moore, J. M., Thompson, S. K., & Whited, R. M. (1994, May). *MMPI-A profiles of adolescent males with a history of firesetting.* Paper presented at the 29th annual symposium on recent developments in the use of the MMPI. Minneapolis, MN.

National Fire Protection Association. (1978). *Executive summary report of the Learn Not to Burn Curriculum.* Quincy, MA: Author.

National Fire Protection Association. (1979). *Learn Not to Burn Curriculum.* Quincy, MA: Author.

National Fire Protection Association. (1982). *Sparky's coloring book.* Quincy, MA: Author.

National Fire Protection Association. (1987). *United States arson trends and patterns.* Quincy, MA: Author.

National Fire Protection Association. (1993, October). *Report of the NFPA Task Force on Juvenile Firesetting.* Inaugural meeting, Norwood, MA.

National Fire Protection Association. (1995, September). *Report of the NFPA firesetter practitioners' forum.* Braintree, MA.

Office of Juvenile Justice and Delinquency Prevention & U.S. Fire Administration. (1994). *National Juvenile Firesetter/Arson Control and Prevention Program.* Washington, DC: U.S. Government Printing Office.

Oregon Treatment Strategies Task Force (1996). *The cycles of firesetting: An Oregon model.* Salem, OR: Oregon Office of the State Fire Marshal.

Parrish, J. M., Capriotti, R. M., Warzak, W. J., Handen, B. L., Wells, T. J., Phillipson, S. J., & Porter, C. A. (1985, November). *Multivariate analysis of juvenile firesetting.* Paper presented at the annual meeting of the Association for the Advancement of Behavior Therapy, Houston, TX.

Pinsonneault, I. (1996). *Fire awareness: Training for foster parents.* Fall River, MA: F.I.R.E. Solutions.

Porth, D. (1996). A report on the juvenile firesetting problem. In *The Portland Report '95*. Portland, OR: Portland Fire Bureau.

Rice, M. E., & Harris, G. T. (1991). Firesetters admitted to a maximum security psychiatric institution: Offenders and offenses. *Journal of Interpersonal Violence, 6,* 461–475.

Sakheim, G. A., & Osborn, E. (1986). A psychological profile of juvenile firesetters in residential treatment: A replication study. *Child Welfare, 65,* 495–503.

Sakheim, G. A., & Osborn, E. (1994). *Firesetting children: Risk assessment and treatment*. Washington, D.C: Child Welfare League of America.

Sakheim, G. A., Osborn, E., & Abrams, D. (1991). Toward a clearer differentiation of high-risk from low-risk fire-setters. *Child Welfare, 70,* 489–502.

Showers, J., & Pickrell, E.P. (1987). Child firesetters: A study of three populations. *Hospital and Community Psychiatry, 38,* 495–501.

Soltys, S. M. (1992). Pyromania and firesetting behaviors. *Psychiatric Annals, 22,* 79–83.

Stawar, T. L. (1976). Fable mod: Operantly structured fantasies as an adjunct in the modification of firesetting behavior. *Journal of Behavior Therapy and Experimental Psychiatry, 7,* 285–287.

Stewart, M. A., & Culver, K.W. (1982). Children who set fires: The clinical picture and a follow-up. *British Journal of Psychiatry, 140,* 357–363.

Stoddard, F. J., Norman, D. K., Murphy, J. M., & Beardslee, W. R. (1989). Psychiatric outcome of burned children and adolescents. *Journal of the American Academy of Child and Adolescent Psychiatry, 28,* 589–505.

Webb, N. B., Sakheim, G. A., Towns-Miranda, L., & Wagner, C. R. (1990). Collaborative treatment of juvenile firesetters: Assessment and outreach. *American Journal of Orthopsychiatry, 60,* 305–310.

Williams, C. E., & Jones, R. (1989). Impact of self-instructions on response maintenance and children's fear of fire. *Journal of Clinical Psychology, 18,* 84–89.

Wooden, W., & Berkey, M. L. (1984). *Children and arson: America's middle class nightmare*. New York: Plenum.

Adolescent Sex Offenders

John A. Hunter, Jr.

Introduction

Youth-perpetrated violence is a problem of growing concern in today's society. Data reflect that the incident rate of violent and deadly assaults by juveniles is dramatically higher than at any previous time in American history (Blumstein, 1995). Consistent with the trend of increased violence perpetrated by youths over the past decade, there has been a steady increase in the number of youths arrested for sexual offenses (Snyder & Stickmund, 1995).

Current estimates are that juveniles account for 20%–30% of the rapes committed in this country each year, and 30%–60% of the cases of child sexual abuse (Brown, Flanagan, & McLeod, 1984; Fehrenbach, Smith, Monastersky, & Deishner, 1986). Although clinical data suggest that an ever growing number of prepubescent youths and juvenile females are identified as having committed sexual crimes, the preponderance of cases of sexual assault committed by juveniles are accounted for by adolescent males (Davis & Leitenberg, 1987).

Concern about the problem of juvenile sexual offending is accentuated by data that suggest that, left untreated, many juveniles progress to more serious and chronic patterns of offending. The study of adult male sex offenders reveals that up to 60% report a juvenile onset of the behavior (Abel *et al.*, 1987). With reference to child molestation, a juvenile onset of the offending behavior has been found to be most often associated with adult patterns of pedophilia, particularly those involving selection of victims of the same gender (Marshall, Barbaree, & Eccles, 1991). Recent data suggest that rape may also have a developmental onset prior to adulthood (Elliott, 1994).

Etiology

The study of juvenile sexual offending has led to an exploration of its etiology and an attempt to identify developmental experiences that may accentuate the risk

John A. Hunter, Jr. • University of Virginia Department of Health Evaluation Sciences, Health Sciences Center, Charlottesville, Virginia, 22908.

Handbook of Psychological Approaches with Violent Offenders: Contemporary Strategies and Issues, edited by Van Hasselt and Hersen. Kluwer Academic/Plenum Publishers, New York, 1999.

of a juvenile's engaging in such behavior. Most professional attention to date has focused on the observed association between juvenile sexual offending and a prior history of childhood maltreatment. It has been found that 40%–80% of male juvenile sex offenders report a prior history of sexual victimization and 25%–50% a history of physical abuse (Hunter, Goodwin, & Becker, 1994; Kahn & Chambers, 1991). Rates of sexual victimization appear even higher in samples of prepubescent male and adolescent female sexual perpetrators (Hunter & Becker, 1994; Hunter & Mathews, 1997).

The role of sexual victimization in the etiology of juvenile sexual offending has been the subject of considerable theoretical discussion. Evolutionary and social learning theorists have cited the potential negative influence of the modeling of aggressive behavior on young children, particularly by individuals of the same gender (Hunter & Becker, 1999). Psychodynamically oriented theorists have commented on the manner in which early victimization experiences may induce deficits in self-esteem and a sense of loss of personal control which may trigger subsequent compensatory reactions (Ryan, Lane, Davis, & Isaac, 1987; Steele, 1985). Theorists working from a number of perspectives have commented on the finding of Posttraumatic Stress Disorder (PTSD; American Psychiatric Association, 1994) symptomatology in juvenile sexual offenders, particularly prepubescent male and adolescent female offenders, and have suggested that the sexual acting-out of such youth may be associated with repetition compulsion and re-enactment phenomena (Gil & Johnson, 1992).

In addition to maltreatment experiences, the risk of juvenile sexual offending may be heightened through exposure to peer and domestic violence and pornography, and by drug and alcohol abuse. Empirical support for these risk factors is beginning to emerge. Kobayashi, Sales, Becker, Figueredo, and Kaplan (1995) found increased sexual aggression in juvenile sex offenders to be associated with a history of physical abuse by the father and sexual abuse by males. Hunter and Figueredo (in press) found that a younger age at time of sexual victimization, a greater number of incidents of abuse, delayed reporting, and perceptions of less familial support postrevelation of the abuse differentiated adolescent sex offenders with a history of childhood sexual victimization from youths who had been victimized, but had never perpetrated sexual offenses. Ford and Linney (1995) and Becker and Stein (1991) found support for the potential role of pornography in juvenile sexual offending. Studies of the association between alcohol and drug abuse and sexual aggression are currently under way, with criminologic data reflecting parallels with rises in juvenile arrests for homicide and drug violations (Blumstein, 1995).

Characteristics of the Offender

Adolescent male sex offenders have been clinically described as suffering from a number of psychosocial and behavioral problems, including poor impulse control and disinhibition, low self-esteem and social skill deficits, deviant sexual arousal and interests, tendencies to endorse beliefs that are associated with minimizing the seriousness of sexual perpetration or justifying the behaviors, generalized psychopathy and antisocial attitudes, and deficits in empathy and sexual knowledge (Becker, Harris, & Sales, 1993; Davis & Leitenburg, 1987). The incidence of psychiatric comorbidity in juvenile sex offenders samples appears relatively high, particularly in those drawn from residential treatment settings. Frequently detected coexistent conditions include: Conduct Disorder, depressive symptomatology, academic dysfunction and Attention-Deficit/Hyperactivity Disorder, and substance abuse (Awad & Saunders, 1991; Becker, Kaplan, Tenke, & Tartaglini, 1991; Becker, Johnson, & Hunter, 1995).

Recent empirical studies have suggested that juvenile child molesters as a group may be less distinguishable based on their sexual characteristics and psychopathy than the deficits that they manifest in self-esteem and social competencies (Hunter & Figueredo, in press). To date, studies have not provided strong support for the assumption that the majority of these youths manifest more pronounced deviant sexual arousal and interest than nonsexually offending youths, are more apt to endorse distorted sexual cognitions, or are highly antisocial or psychopathic in their personality makeup.

The presence of relatively strong deviant to nondeviant arousal in juvenile male child molesters appears to be associated with exclusively sexually offending against young males, and thus may be an indicator of early-onset same-gender pedophilia (Hunter *et al.*, 1994). Indications of nonsexual delinquency and generalized antisocial tendencies have been found most frequently in the backgrounds of juveniles who have engaged in "hands-on" and aggressive sexual offending (Becker *et al.*, 1993). While paraphilic interest and high levels of psychopathy may be a characteristic of only a subset of adolescent child molesters, these youths as a group appear deficient in competencies associated with successful relationship formation and maintenance (Hunter & Figueredo, in press). In this regard, many adolescent sex offenders appear to be lacking in self-confidence, ability to be assertive, and skills relating to self-sufficiency. Future studies will determine whether there are significant differences in the clinical characteristics of those juveniles who rape as opposed to those who molest younger children.

Assessment Issues and Methodologies

The careful assessment of adolescent sex offenders is critical to formulating recommendations regarding disposition. These recommendations should involve consideration of several factors, including (1) the youth's judged amenability to treatment, (2) the type and level of care required given the nature of the adolescent's sexual and nonsexual problems, (3) the assessed level of risk that he represents for engaging in sexual and nonsexual recidivism, and (4) the familial and community resources available to meet the client's needs. Dispositional recommendations can range from placement in a community-based treatment program to referral to a secure and highly structured residential program. Alternatively, youths who are not judged to be likely to benefit from treatment may be recommended for placement in a correctional setting. The mental health professional should remain cognizant that he or she is typically functioning in an advisory capacity and that the authority for determining final disposition rests with the referring agency. For adjudicated youths, final determinations are made by the court. Ideally, dispositional recommendations should reflect the collaborative thinking of the mental health professional, the youth and his family, and the other agencies involved in his care.

It is recommended that mental health evaluations generally be conducted postadjudication and presentencing for all youths who have pending legal charges. Preadjudication evaluations are typically complicated by issues associated with the admissibility of statements made by the alleged offender to the ensuant court proceeding. Under such circumstances, clients should be advised that any and all information provided to the evaluator may be used against him in court. It is also very important for both the clinician and referral agencies to understand that determination of innocence or guilt is a legal matter and not a valid function of the clinical assessment process. In this regard, it is the consensus of most experts in the field that judgments of innocence or guilt based on psychometric or psychophysiological assessment are without sufficient scientific merit and should be avoided (Murphy & Peters, 1992).

Evaluations should be comprehensive and directed at not only assessing the nature of the youth's psychosexual problem, but also identifying coexistent psychiatric conditions and issues that need to be addressed in order for the youth to achieve long-term behavioral and psychosocial stability. This should include assessment of the viability and advisability of the youth's remaining in his current living environment.

Prior to meeting with the adolescent offender and his family, the clinician should peruse all available records, including police reports, criminal record files, results of polygraph examinations, social history information, previously conducted psychological and psychiatric evaluations, educational records, and treatment reports. Particularly helpful when available are victim statements derived from police or social services investigations. Such victim accounts can be used to improve the accuracy of the youth's self-report given the observed tendency of many juvenile offenders to minimize the extent of their sexual transgressions.

Clinical Interview

The clinical interview provides the foundation for the assessment process and should be conducted with sensitivity to both process and content issues. It is important that the evaluator establish a working relationship with the youth that conveys the purpose of the evaluation, the manner in which the gathered information will be used, and the importance of the youth's full cooperation. It is especially important that an emotional environment be created that is conducive to the youth's discussing his or her sexual issues without feeling subjected to shame, humiliation, or fear of reprisal. It is important that the evaluator demonstrate the capacity to process the youth's report of sexual acting-out, and any prior history of maltreatment, without the loss of emotional composure or professional objectivity. Any indications of emotional shock, embarrassment, or condemnation on the part of the evaluator will likely impede full divulgence of the extent of the youth's offending and compromise the validity of the information obtained.

Inclusion of the family of the youth in the assessment process is generally helpful, and is imperative when the youth will continue to reside in the home during the course of treatment. It is generally advisable for the evaluator to interview the youth and his parents separately so as to provide both parties with the opportunity to openly discuss relevant issues. Although the youth may feel more comfortable discussing the sexual acting-out privately, it is important that he or she understand that the evaluator will not withhold important information from the parents or referral agency. It is often useful to meet conjointly with the youth and parents following the evaluation to discuss treatment recommendations.

The clinical interview should be structured so as to ensure that critical information is elicited. This information should include a comprehensive review of the chronology of the youth's sexual experiences, including those related to victimization, perpetration, and consensual peer activity. It is noted that victimization data are best elicited in the context of a comprehensive review of the youth's sexual experiences, as many youths define victimization as being limited to experiences with males and where coercion was involved. Similarly, sexual experiences described by the youth as consensual may in fact meet legal definitions of sexual offending. For these reasons, it is usually wise to avoid labels for the behavior during the initial interview.

In gathering data relevant to sexual offending, the evaluator will benefit from first attempting to get an accurate behavioral description of events, and later information related to the offender's cognitions and affect. Focusing on the offender's thinking patterns and feelings about the sexual acting-out too early in the interview may induce the provision of responses that are judged by the youth to be socially acceptable. In gathering a behavioral description, it is important that the interviewer avoid technical jargon and permit the youth to use language with which he or she is comfortable.

The gathering of data relevant to offending behavior should include a detailed account of events, including identification of the following: the victim's age, gender, and relationship to the perpetrator; the age of the perpetrator at the time of the sexual acting-out; a description of where the offense occurred; and a description of what the offender said and did to the victim, and what the victim in turn said and did. This information should include a review of issues related to the modus operandi of the offender, including an exploration of issues associated with victim selection, methods of gaining victim compliance, and means of maintaining victim silence postcommission of the offense. It is especially important to attempt to determine whether the offender used threat, force, or weapons in the commission of the offense.

Following the gathering of detailed behavioral data, the clinician should explore cognitions and fantasies associated with the behavior and inquire about the extent to which the youth experiences sexual arousal to such thoughts. With regard to the latter, the evaluator should inquire as to the nature of the youth's masturbatory fantasy and attempt to assess the extent to which such fantasy reflects emerging paraphilic interests. Finally, it is important to assess the offender's affect before, during, and following the sexual acting-out, and whether he or she appears capable of experiencing remorse and empathy for the victim.

In additional to a thorough exploration of the youth's sexual experiences, the interviewer should also inquire as to the following: history of academic performance, relationships with family and peers, history of substance abuse and nonsexual delinquencies, evidence of exposure to pornography and violence, and psychiatric history and current mental status. This information is critical to understanding the overall personality and environmental context in which the sexual acting-out has occurred and to identifying coexistent conditions that should be addressed over the course of treatment.

The clinical interview should be supplemented by psychometric assessment of sexual attitudes and adjustment and general personality functioning. Intelligence and educational testing may be warranted in cases where there is a long history of academic dysfunction, evidence of intellectual impairment, or both. It is recommended that all youths be administered a personality assessment inventory, such as the MMPI-A, to screen for the presence of non-sexually related psychological disturbances. Individuals who show evidence of the presence of more generalized psychological dysfunction should be referred for more extensive psychological or psychiatric evaluation.

Psychometric Assessments

A number of specialized assessment instruments can be used to aid in the assessment of juvenile sex offenders. Selected instruments are briefly described here.

- *Multiphasic Sex Inventory (Juvenile version) (Nichols & Molinder, 1984).* This instrument contains 21 scales that are designed to measure various aspects of sexual functioning relevant to juvenile sexual offending. Included are scales that assess sexual knowledge and beliefs, sexual obsessions, feelings of sexual inadequacy, cognitive distortions and immaturity, and justifications for sexual acting-out. The authors report moderate to high internal consistency for the scales appropriate to such analysis. Scales from the adult version of the test have been demonstrated to differentiate sex offenders from normal controls.
- *Adolescent Cognition Scale (Becker & Kaplan, 1985).* This scale was designed to identify thinking errors in juvenile sex offenders associated with a tendency to rationalize or minimize the significance of the offending behavior, or project blame for its occurrence onto the victim. The scale appears to have fair internal consistency and test–retest reliability, but may contain a social desirability response bias that compromises its validity (Hunter, Becker, Kaplan, Goodwin, 1991). It is recommended that this instrument be used cautiously and with the awareness of its potential vulnerability to producing false-negative response sets.
- *Adolescent Sexual Interest Card Sort (ASIC) (Becker & Kaplan, 1988).* This instrument was designed to help identify paraphilic patterns of arousal and interest in adolescent sex offenders. Respondents are directed to rate their interest in various deviant and nondeviant sexual activities on a 3-point Likert-type scale. The scale has been found to have relatively good internal consistency and test–retest reliability: However, responses provided on this instrument were not found to correlate significantly with phallometrically measured sexual arousal across most common categories of interest (only 4 of 14) (Hunter, Becker, & Kaplan, 1995). As with other self-report measures, this instrument is subject to dissimulation.
- *Multidimensional Assessment of Sex and Aggression (MASA) (Knight, Prentky, & Cerce, 1994).* This instrument was developed for the assessment of sexual and aggressive thoughts, fantasies, and behaviors in adults. Preliminary reliability and validity data appear favorable. Its authors are standardizing an adolescent version of the test.
- *Phallometric Assessment* (plethysmographic assessment of penile tumescence) has been used with older adolescent males to supplement self-report of sexual interest and arousal. Assessments employing auditory stimuli developed specifically for the evaluation of juvenile sex offenders have been found to have satisfactory test–retest reliability and to produce discriminable profile patterns (Becker, Hunter, Goodwin, Kaplan, & Martinez, 1992; Becker, Stein, Kaplan, & Cunningham-Rathner, 1992). Assessments of juveniles should be conducted consistent with guidelines established by the National Task Force on Juvenile Sexual Offending (1993) and the Association for the Treatment of Sexual Abusers ([ATSA], 1993). These guidelines include recommendations that assessments be conducted only on pubescent males (14 years of age or

older), and only with the full informed consent of the youth, his parent or guardian, and his referral agency.

Data from the sources described should be interpreted in an integrated manner for the purpose of formulating recommendations regarding amenability to treatment, required level of care, and prognosis. While risk profiling criteria for juvenile sex offenders awaits empirical validation, consideration of the following factors may be helpful: (1) the individual's past criminal record for sexual and nonsexual offense, (2) the nature and severity of his psychosexual disturbance, (3) his demonstrated attitude toward treatment and motivation for change, (4) the degree of manifest psychopathy, (5) the extent of concomitant psychiatric impairment, and (6) the availability of famil-ial and community resources.

Individuals who are typically referred for more intensive residential treatment are those who manifest a relatively long-standing pattern of repeated and serious sex-ual offending in the context of more broad-based emotional and behavioral problems. Individuals who are referred for community-based treatment typically are those less chronically and severely sexually and emotionally maladjusted youths who do not represent an imminent threat to self or others, and who with reasonable environmen-tal support and treatment can successfully maintain control over their behavior. Juve-niles who may be most appropriately referred for correctional placement are those who evidence a relatively high level of psychopathy and those who do not appear to have benefited from past treatment efforts. This category should also include those youths who profess to have no motivation for change.

Treatment

Given that juvenile sex offenders are a relatively heterogeneous population re-flecting an array of psychosexual and nonsexual problems and levels of disturbance, a continuum of care is required to successfully meet their treatment needs. The fol-lowing discussion is directed at identifying key components of both community-based and intensive residential treatment programs.

Establishment of a Context for Treatment

The criminal justice system can be of invaluable support to the treatment provider in maintaining client accountability and compliance with therapeutic directives. In many cases, the youth can be referred to the treatment program with a legal sentence that has been suspended contingent upon successful completion of treatment. Such contingencies are optimal in providing needed leverage to the treatment provider in ensuring that the client remains motivated and therapeutically diligent. Under such circumstances, the treatment provider can convincingly convey to the youth and his family the importance of viewing treatment as an opportunity to get help for a prob-lem that, untreated, can lead to a series of increasingly more severe legal repercussions.

Of equal importance to the establishment of accountability is the infusion of hope and optimism in the adolescent and his family. Many juvenile sex offenders lack self-confidence, suffer from poor self-esteem, and are generally pessimistic about their ability to alter their life circumstances. It is helpful for the treating clinician to educate the adolescent and his or her family about the positive outcome associated with successful completion of treatment programs, and to communicate confidence that the youth is capable of making positive life changes, if he and his family remain committed to this endeavor.

Community-Based Services

The majority of juvenile sex offenders can be safely and effectively treated on a community-based level if specialized and comprehensive services are developed, and if detection occurs prior to the emergence of more serious sexual and characterological impairment. The planning and implementation of these services should reflect the collaborative involvement of the youth, the family, and the agencies involved. Often, this is best accomplished by the treatment provider or agency's forming an advisory board consisting of representatives from the referral agencies and other public institutions providing case oversight (e.g., prosecutor's effice). The advisory board can ensure that the referral program is operating in a maximally effective and efficient manner and fully serving the needs of sexually troubled youths and the community at large.

Community-based treatment efforts are most effective when a variety of "wrap-around" services can be developed to supplement more traditional individual, group, and family therapy efforts. While less disturbed youths from more intact families may require only outpatient counseling, other youths and families may achieve stability only with the provision of additional support services. Such services can range from "in-home" counseling by professionals and paraprofessionals to the creation of specialized therapeutic foster and group homes. The latter may be necessary when the youth has victimized a younger sibling in the home, or the home environment does not provide the youth with the degree of structure and support that he or she requires. It is important that these alternative environments not contain younger children or other youth vulnerable to sexual expolitation.

Youths placed in community-based treatment programs should receive therapeutic attention in the areas delineated in the "Areas of Therapeutic Focus" section. Typically, most youths are able to complete programs of treatment in 12–16 months. Upon completion of the active phase of treatment, it is advisable that the youth enter aftercare phase. This typically involves "check-ups" with the treating therapist, at decreasing frequency, over a period of 6–12 months.

Intensive Residential Treatment

Intensive residential treatment is appropriate for the more psychosexually, behaviorally, and psychiatrically disturbed youth. Such programs provide 24-hour-a-day care, and comprehensive clinical, educational-vocational, medical, recreational-adjunctive, and milieu services. Because the youths requiring this level of care typically manifest a multitude of emotional and behavioral problems, it is important that their treatment be approached in a holistic manner and that all of their relevant service needs be identified in a comprehensive plan of intervention.

Treatment in a residential setting requires careful planning and collaboration between members of the multidisciplinary treatment team, the youth and his family, and the referring agency. Clinical staff should remain cognizant of the importance of properly educating direct-care and ancillary staff as to the nature and treatment of juvenile sexual offending and should provide them with ongoing training, supervision, and support. The effectiveness of the program in attenuating patterns of sexual offending in juveniles likely rests as much on the uniformity of staff effort as on the sophistication of the clinical program per se.

Careful attention should be given to the establishment of a safe and therapeutic environment wherein residents can explore and adopt values to live by, and acquire self-control and prosocial living skills. All staff should view themselves as role models and make every attempt to conduct themselves in a manner consistent with the principles of the program in their interactions with residents and one another. Living areas should be closely supervised and structured so as to minimize the risk of sexual acting-out or physical assault. In this regard, it is advisable that youths be grouped on units according to age, gender, and level of disturbance. It is not recommended that adolescent male sex offenders be placed on units with nonoffending youths because of the risk of sexual offense, and the general inhibitory effect that mixed clinical populations can have on open discussion of issues of sexual perpetration.

Most youths are able to complete intensive residential treatment programs in 12–24 months; however, more pervasively and severely disturbed youths may require a longer period of care. Residential treatment programs should be designed so that youths transition from highly structured environments to less structured ones as they make therapeutic gains and near readiness for discharge. It is important that staff and family members have an opportunity to observe the extent to which the youth is able to utilize the skills acquired in treatment in interactions with others and in coping with the stresses of everyday life. It is strongly recommended that all youths enter a period of aftercare following completion of a residential program. This aftercare typically is 12 months or more in duration and focuses on the client's ability to successfully adhere to a relapse prevention plan.

Areas of Therapeutic Focus

The following provides a description of issues believed to be particularly relevant to the treatment of juvenile sex offenders. The extensiveness of interventions in each area depends on the setting in which the services are being rendered and the degree of dysfunction the youth manifests. These issues can be addressed in *individual* or *group* therapies, or both, but should be reinforced in all realms in which the youth functions.

Juvenile sex offenders benefit from *clarification of values* as they relate to a respect for self and others, and the need to curb expressions of violence in our society. Programming in this domain may fruitfully be presented in a context of promoting a sense of healthy male and female identity, egalitarian male–female relationships, and a respect for cultural diversity.

Related to the teaching of values is the provision of *sex education* and an understanding of healthy human sexuality. This may involve review of a number of issues, including human anatomy and physiology, psychological and physiological changes associated with puberty, birth control, prevention of venereal disease, and correction of distorted sexual cognitions.

Juvenile sex offenders also appear to benefit from programming directed at developing greater self-confidence and social competency. It appears that the adolescent's ability to refrain from future sexual acting-out is contingent not only on the possession of self-control skills, but also the ability to form and maintain healthy relationships with peers and successfully function in a variety of social contexts. Given the manifest deficits that most adolescent sex offenders evidence in this realm, it is important that they receive *social skills training*. These skills may range from the basic (e.g., how to introduce oneself to others), to those that are more advanced (e.g., how to express feelings of insecurity or jealousy). It has been the author's experience that these skills are best taught in a group setting using modeling and behavior rehearsal. The effectiveness of feedback to the youth may be enhanced by the use of video equipment that allows the youth to view himself practicing these skills.

The teaching of *impulse control* and *coping skills* is also an essential component of clinical programming for juvenile sex offenders. Most of these youths exhibit difficulty delaying gratification and have a low tolerance for frustration. This is especially true for those youths who also suffer from Attention-Deficit/Hyperactivity Disorder, those who are more conduct disordered, and those who experience persistent deviant sexual arousal. It has been found helpful to employ cognitive-behavioral methodologies, such as covert sensitization, which help youths understand the cognitive, affective, and environmental precursors of their acting-out behavior and learn to anticipate the consequences of the behavior. Youths also frequently benefit from the teaching of *assertiveness skills* and *conflict resolution* in learning to resolve interpersonal conflicts and manage feelings of anger.

Another vital area of programming is the *enhancement of empathy* and promotion of an understanding of the negative impact that sexual acting-out has on victims and their families. The empathy deficits that many of these youths manifest appear to be related to the lack of support that they received as children in coping with difficult life circumstances, including maltreatment experiences. It is helpful to support these youths in identifying and recognizing the adverse affect that maltreatment had on their lives prior to having them examine the pain and suffering that they have caused others. Empathy work may be enhanced by having the perpetrator write an "empathy letter" to the victim and their family, and engage in role-playing exercises. Such empathy letters are typically used only in the context of the treatment program and not actually mailed. However, in cases of sibling incest, it may be appropriate for the letter to be read in a family therapy session at a time when the perpetrator and victim have been judged to be ready for such a meeting.

All treatment programs should provide for the development of an individualized *relapse prevention* plan. This plan should reflect the client's understanding of the cycle of thoughts, feelings, and events that triggered the sexual acting-out, and identification of environmental circumstances and thinking patterns that should be avoided because they increase the risk of re-offending. Relapse prevention should also include identifying and practicing the use of coping and self-control skills for dealing with stressful situations.

In addition to individual and group therapies, when viable, *family therapy* should be provided to juvenile sexual offenders. It is imperative that the family of the youth be involved in his or her treatment, and have a full understanding of the relapse prevention plan, when youth is to return home after discharge. As previously mentioned, family work may involve focusing on issues of reparation and restoring trust in cases where a member of the family has been victimized. Occasionally, family work results in identification of family systems issues (e.g., marital problems) which are beyond the scope of the treatment program, but which indirectly impact the youth.

Under such circumstances, the family therapist can work with the referring agency in identifying community resources that can assist the family.

Adjunctive Therapies

A number of adjunctive psychiatric and psychological therapies may be appropriate depending on the particular needs of the youth. Some youths, including those who suffer from major affective disorders, disturbances in thinking, or impulse regulatory problems (e.g., ADHD) may benefit from pharmacologic treatment. Youths who are identified as experiencing persistent deviant sexual arousal may benefit from specialized cognitive-behavioral techniques, such as satiation therapy (Hunter & Goodwin, 1992). There is also an emerging literature on the use of pharmacologic agents in attenuating deviant sexual arousal, including the use of selective serotonin reuptake inhibitors, and the use of hormonal therapies with offenders 18 years of age or older (Hunter and Lexier, 1998). It is noted that the use of hormonal therapies is typically limited to those offenders who remain refractory to psychologically based therapies and who appear to be at high risk for sexually re-offending. Other useful adjunctive services may include the provision of substance abuse counseling and remedial educational and vocational programming.

Treatment Outcome

As the treatment of juvenile sex offenders is a relatively recent phenomenon, large, well-controlled outcome studies have yet to be completed. However, initial efforts at assessing the effectiveness of specialized programming for adolescent sex offenders provide reason for optimism about the treatability of the majority of these youths. In the only controlled outcome study conducted to date, Borduin, Henggeler, Blaske, and Stein (1990) found that 8 adolescent sex offenders treated with specialized "multisystemic" therapy had sexual recidivism rates of 12.5% at a 3-year follow-up interval, in contrast to a recidivism rate of 75% for the 8 youths who received more generic individual therapy. Becker (1990) reported a sexual recidivism rate of 8% (follow-up period of up to 2 years) for 80 juvenile sex offenders treated in an outpatient setting, while Bremer (1992) found that only 11% of residentially treated juvenile sex offenders sexually recidivated following discharge (follow-up period of 6 months to 8.5 years). Similarly, low rates of sexual recidivism in treated juvenile sex offenders were reported by Kahn and Chambers (1991) (7.5%) and Schram, Milloy, and Rowe (1991) (12.2%). A number of these studies indicated that the nonsexual recidivism rate in their samples was generally higher (25%–50%), suggesting that the therapeutic effect may be specific to the sexual offending behavior.

Future Directions

The study and treatment of juvenile sex offenders is a rapidly growing field. It is expected that significant advances will be made in the future that will enable clinicians to more accurately predict the likelihood of a positive treatment outcome for particular clients, and refine treatment protocols to meet the differential needs of various subtypes of offenders.

The accomplishment of such goals will depend on the development of improved assessment instruments and ultimately on the development of an empirically validated typology of juvenile sex offenders. The creation of a typology would potentially permit delineation of major subtypes of juvenile sex offenders based on clinical characteristics, response to treatment, and long-term risk of recidivism. This work could also aid in identifying developmental pathways associated with various types of offending behavior in juveniles. Advances in understanding the etiology of juvenile sexual offending, particularly the role of prior maltreatment, should facilitate the development of prevention programs for high risk populations, and make more efficient efforts to identify youths who are developing sexual behavior problems.

References

Abel, G. G., Becker, J. V., Cunningham-Rathner, J., Mittelman, M. S., Murphy, W. D., & Rouleau, J. L. (1987). Self-reported sex crimes of nonincarcerated paraphiliacs. *Journal of Interpersonal Violence, 2,* 3–25.

American Psychiatric Association. (1994). *Diagnostic and statistical manual of mental disorders* (4th ed.). Washington, DC: Author.

Association for the Treatment of Sexual Abusers. (1993). Standards for the use of phallometric assessment. OR: Author. (For information, write ATSA, 10700 SW Beavaerton-Hillsdale Hwy., Suite 26, Beaverton, OR 97005-3035.)

Awad, G. A., & Saunders, E. B. (1991). Male adolescent sexual assaulters: Clinical observations. *Journal of Interpersonal Violence, 6*(4), 446–460.

Becker, J. V. (1990). Treating adolescent sexual offenders. *Professional Psychology: Research and Practice, 21*(5), 362–265.

Becker, J. V., & Kaplan, M. (1985). *Adolescent Cognition Scale.* (Available from Judith V. Becker, Department of Psychology Building, University of Arizona, Tucson, Arizona 85721.)

Becker, J. V., & Kaplan, M. S. (1988). The assessment of sexual offenders. In R. J. Printz (Ed.), *Advances in behavioral assessment of children and families* (Vol. 4, pp. 97–118). Greenwich, CT: JAI Press.

Becker, J. V., & Stein, R. M. (1991). Is sexual erotica associated with sexual deviance in adolescent males? *International Journal of Law and Psychiatry, 14,* 85–95.

Becker, J. V., Kaplan, M. S., Tenke, C. E., & Tartaglini, A. (1991). The incidence of depressive symptomatology in juvenile sex offenders with a history of abuse. *Child Abuse and Neglect, 15,* 531–536.

Becker, J. V., Hunter, J. A., Goodwin, D. W., Kaplan, M. S., & Martinez, D. (1992). Test–retest reliability of audio-taped phallometric stimuli with adolescent sexual offenders. *Annals of Sex Research, 5,* 45–51.

Becker, J. V., Stein, R. M., Kaplan, M. S., & Cunningham-Rathner, J. (1992). Erection response characteristics of adolescent sex offenders. *Annals of Sex Research, 5,* 81–86.

Becker, J. V., Harris, C. D., & Sales, B. D. (1993). Juveniles who commit sexual offenses: A critical review of research. In G. C. N. Hall, R. Hirschman, J. Graham, & M. Zaragoza (Eds.), *Sexual aggression: Issues in etiology and assessment, treatment, and policy,* (pp. 215–228). Washington, DC: Taylor and Francis.

Becker, J. V., Johnson, B. R., & Hunter, J. A. (1995). Adolescent sex offenders. In C. Hollins & K. Howells (Eds.), *Clinical approaches to working with young offenders.* Sussex, England: Wiley.

Blumstein, A. (1995). Violence by young people: Why the deadly nexus? *National Institute of Justice Journal, 229,* 2–9.

Borduin, C.M., Henggeler, S. W., Blaske, D. M., & Stein, R. J., (1990). Multisystemic treatment of adolescent sexual offenders. *International Journal of Offender Therapy and Comparative Criminology, 34*(2), 105–114.

Bremer, J. F. (1992). Serious juvenile sex offenders: Treatment and long-term follow-up. *Psychiatric Annals, 22,* 326–332.

Brown, F., Flanagan, T., & McLeod, M. (Eds.). (1984). *Sourcebook of criminal justice statistics.* Washington, DC: Bureau of Justice Statistics.

Davis, G. E., & Leitenberg H. (1987). Adolescent sex offenders, *Psychological Bulletin, 101,* 417–427.

Elliott, D. S. (1994, November). *The developmental course of sexual and non-sexual violence: Resulting from a national longitudinal study.* Paper presented at the meeting of the Association for the Treatment of Sexual Abusers 13th annual Research and Treatment Conference, San Francisco.

Fehrenbach, P. A., Smith, W., Monastersky, C., & Deishner, R. W. (1986). Adolescent sexual offenders: Offender and offense characteristics. *American Journal of Orthopsychiatry, 56,* 225–233.

Ford, M. E., & Linney, J. A. (1995). Comparative analysis of juvenile sexual offenders, violent nonsexual offenders, and status offenders. *Journal of Interpersonal Violence, 10,* 56–70.

Gil, E., & Johnson, T. C. (1992). *Assessment and treatment of sexualized children and children who molest.* Rockville, MD: Launch Press.

Hunter, J. A., & Becker, J. V. (1994). The role of deviant sexual arousal in juvenile sexual offending: Etiology, evaluation, and treatment. *Criminal Justice and Behavior, 21,* 132–149.

Hunter, J. A., & Becker, J. V. (1999). Motivators of adolescent sex offenders and treatment perspectives. In J. Shaw (Ed.), *Sexual aggression.* Washington, DC: American Psychiatric Press.

Hunter, J. A. & Figueredo, A. J. (in press). *The influence of personality and history of sexual victimization in the prediction of juvenile perpetrated child molestation.* San Francisco: Sage.

Hunter, J. A., & Goodwin, D. W. (1992). The utility of satiation therapy in the treatment of juvenile sexual offenders: Variations and efficacy. *Annals of Sex Research, 5,* 71–80.

Hunter, J. A., & Mathews, R. (1997). Sexual deviance in females: Psychopathology, theory, assessment and treatment. In W. O'Donohue & R. Laws (Eds.), *Handbook of sexual deviance: Theory and application* (pp. 465–480). New York: Guilford.

Hunter, J. A., & Lexier, L. T. (1998). Ethical and legal issues in the assessment and treatment of juvenile sex offenders: *Child Maltreatment, 3,* 337–348.

Hunter, J. A., Becker, J. V., Kaplan, M., & Goodwin, D. W. (1991). The reliability and discriminative utility of the Adolescent Cognition Scale for juvenile sexual offenses. *Annals of Sex Research, 4,* 281–286.

Hunter, J. A., Goodwin, D. W., & Becker, J. V. (1994). The relationship between phallometrically measured deviant sexual arousal and clinical characteristics in juvenile sexual offenders. *Behavior Research and Therapy, 32,* 533–538.

Hunter, J. A., Becker, J. V., & Kaplan, M. S. (1995). The Adolescent Sexual Interest Card Sort: Test–retest reliability and concurrent validity in relation to phallometric assessment. *Archives of Sexual Behavior, 24,* 555–561.

Kahn, T. J., & Chambers, H. J. (1991). Assessing reoffense risk with juvenile sexual offenders. *Child Welfare, 19,* 333–345.

Knight, R. A., Prentky, R. A., & Cerce, D. D. (1994). The development, reliability, and validity of an inventory for the multidimensional assessment of sex and aggression. *Criminal Justice and Behavior, 21,* 72–94.

Kobayashi, J., Sales, B. D., Becker, J. V., Figueredo, A. J., & Kaplan, M. S. (1995). Perceived parental deviance, parental–child bonding, child abuse, and child sexual aggression. *Sexual Abuse: A Journal of Research and Treatment, 7,* 25–44.

Marshall, W. L., Barbaree, H. E., & Eccles, A. (1991). Early onset and deviant sexuality in child molesters. *Journal of Interpersonal Violence, 6,* 323–336.

Murphy, W. D., & Peters, J. M. (1992). Profiling child sexual abusers: Psychological considerations. *Criminal Justice and Behavior, 19,* 24–27.

National Task Force on Juvenile Sexual Offending. (1993). *Final report.* Denver: National Adolescent Perpetrator Network, C. H. Kempe National Center, University of Colorado Health Sciences Center.

Nichols, H. R., & Molinder, M. A. (1984). *Multiphasic Sex Inventory manual.* (Available from H.R. Nichols and M. A. Molinder, 437 Bowes Drive, Tacoma, WA 98466.)

Ryan, G., Lane, S., Davis, J., & Isaac, C. (1987). Juvenile sex offenders: Development and correction. *Child Abuse and Neglect, 11,* 385–395.

Schram, D. D., Milloy, C. D., & Rowe, W. E. (1991). *Juvenile sex offenders: A follow-up study of reoffense behavior.* Unpublished manuscript.

Snyder, H. N., & Sickmund, M. (1995). *Juvenile offenders and victims: A focus on violence.* Pittsburgh, PA: National Center for Juvenile Justice.

Steele, B. (1985). Notes on the lasting effects of early childhood abuse throughout the life cycle. *Child Abuse and Neglect, 10,* 283–291.

Child and Adolescent Homicide

Dewey G. Cornell

Description of the Problem

Murders committed by children invariably arouse feelings of shock and dismay, and elicit probing questions about the social, psychological, or even biological factors that might account for such a tragic phenomenon. Yet, efforts to characterize "*the* adolescent murderer" or "*the* child killer" reflect lack of familiarity with the diversity of homicidal youth as well as inappropriate expectations about the scientific status of a legal category. Apart from the victim's fatality and the youthfulness of the perpetrator, homicides by juveniles defy a single common explanation or explication. Consider the following case examples:

> 17 year-old Fred goes cruising with friends through a poor urban neighborhood, looking for persons to rob. It is winter and the youth needs a new coat. They confront a young man wearing an attractive leather coat. When the man refuses to give up his coat, a struggle ensues, and Fred pulls out a pistol and shoots him.

> 15 year-old Alice has been sexually molested and forcibly raped by her stepfather regularly for nearly a year. Her mother has been physically and emotionally abusive for as long as she can remember. One night after an argument with her parents, Alice creeps into their bedroom and shoots them both in their sleep.

> 13-year-old Jackie lures a 4-year-old child away from the sidewalk and into a garage. Jackie sexually molests and then strangles the child.

It is difficult to imagine a psychosocial profile that would shelter Fred, Alice, and Jackie under a common explanatory umbrella. Their circumstances, motives, and behaviors are diverse, but their actions are united by the common fatal outcome for each of their victims. Were it not for the legal categorization of these behaviors as murder, it is unlikely that behavioral scientists would make an effort to find underlying common factors in their actions, or even that they would choose to describe them in the

Dewey G. Cornell • Curry Programs in Clinical and School Psychology, School of Education, University of Virginia, Charlottesville, Virginia 22903-2495.

Handbook of Psychological Approaches with Violent Offenders: Contemporary Strategies and Issues, edited by Van Hasselt and Hersen. Kluwer Academic/Plenum Publishers, New York, 1999.

same book chapter. Fred is much more like the thousands of teenage robbers who never kill anyone than he is like the girl who killed her parents or the boy who molested a young child. Moreover, homicides by youth are not readily distinguishable from homicides by adults, so that the arbitrary, albeit justifiable, distinctions of law impose an unnatural boundary across a developmental continuum.

Nevertheless, appropriately conceptualized, study of homicide by children and adolescents can further efforts to understand the varieties of circumstances and psychological conditions under which juveniles as well as young adults engage in lethal or potentially lethal acts of violence. Study of juvenile homicide represents an unequivocal and compelling means of contributing to the understanding of juvenile violence and, ultimately, larger efforts to understand human violence and aggression.

Perhaps the most critical and perplexing problem is to understand the decision-making process that leads to violent behavior. An enraged youth might well act impulsively with little forethought, but all youth experience feelings of anger and rage, and even consider some form of violent response in certain situations. Yet, few ever take the final step of engaging in potentially lethal actions. What distinguishes those youth who act upon their homicidal rage from the many more who consider such action, but choose some alternative? Are there differences in the nature and quality of the young person's anger, or perhaps the person's tolerance for anger? Or, are the differences merely a matter of circumstance, such as the ready availability of a weapon or peer encouragement during a moment of crisis?

Perhaps most troubling are the stark cases of premeditated murder wherein the youth considered the possibility of murder for hours, if not days or weeks, before taking action. Here the decision-making process presents multiple opportunities for more adaptive outcomes. Cognitively, the youth might generate more benign alternatives to violence. Affectively, he or she might experience prohibitory feelings of empathy and concern for the victim. Or from a practical perspective, the youth might reject a course of action so likely to lead to arrest, public shame, and years of imprisonment. Across the variety of youth who have committed homicide, one can observe a multiplicity of psychological deficits and stressful circumstances adversely affecting the decision-making process.

Historical Background

Juvenile homicide has long been the subject of case reports and descriptive studies based on small clinical samples (e.g., Bender, Keiser, & Schilder, 1937; Stearns, 1957). Not surprisingly, clinicians in psychiatric settings (Lewis, Shanok, Grant, & Ritvo, 1983; Pfeffer, 1980; Sendi & Blomgren, 1975) have emphasized the presence of major psychopathology while clinicians in correctional or forensic settings (Sorrells, 1977; Yates, Beutler, & Crago, 1984; Zenoff & Zients, 1979) have drawn attention to personality disorders or character problems. Offenders who exhibit unusual psychopathology (Medlicott, 1955) or who commit murders for unusual reasons (Stearns, 1957) receive disproportionate attention. Researchers have examined offender characteristics ranging from EEG patterns (Scherl & Mack, 1966) to astrological sign (Sorrells, 1977) as an explanation for violent behavior. Unfortunately, the attention to unusual cases makes it difficult to identify general trends and common characteristics of any group.

Historically, theorists have favored explanatory factors that seem commensurate with the severity and seriousness of the juvenile's crime: schizophrenia, brain damage, dissociative conditions, severe sexual and physical abuse (see reviews by Adams, 1974; Benedek & Cornell, 1989; Ewing, 1990). Certainly, there is clinical evidence to support these factors in some cases, but no profile encompasses the full range of youthful homicide cases. For every generalization about juvenile homicide there are multiple exceptions; for every characterization of a juvenile murderer in the literature there seem to be distinctive features and unique circumstances.

There is ample documentation of the diversity of juvenile homicide offenders (Benedek & Cornell, 1989; Ewing, 1990; Heide, 1992; Mones, 1990). More recent studies have made use of national data bases or records drawn from regional catchment areas that are less vulnerable to selection bias (Cornell, 1990, 1993; Heide, 1994; Loper & Cornell, 1996; Rowley, Ewing, & Singer, 1987). Not coincidentally, there has been more attention directed to distinguishing among groups of juvenile homicide offenders and identifying developmental pathways, personality profiles, and environmental factors that increase the risk of violent outcomes, as will be emphasized in this chapter. Major points will be illustrated with case examples of youth evaluated by the author.

Epidemiology

Murder, more technically termed "criminal homicide," can be defined as the willful killing of one human being by another, excluding deaths caused by negligence, accident, or legally justifiable actions, such as self-defense (Federal Bureau of Investigation [FBI], 1995). Epidemiological knowledge of juvenile homicide is based primarily on arrest statistics, especially the FBI's annual Uniform Crime Reports and the separate database comprising the annual Supplemental Homicide Reports. Arrest statistics have some well-known limitations: They represent only persons apprehended for a crime and they do not contain detailed clinical and circumstantial information. Yet, arrest statistics for murder are more representative of actual incidence than arrest statistics for other crimes, since murders are much more likely to be reported, intensively investigated, and cleared by an arrest. In 1994, approximately 64% of known murders were cleared by an arrest, compared to 56% of aggravated assaults, 52% of forcible rapes, and just 24% or robberies (FBI, 1995). Other sources of information are more selective than arrest data and are less likely to tap the breadth of cases necessary to avoid inappropriate generalizations.

Although juvenile homicide garners great public attention, the overwhelming majority of homicides are committed by adults, and the most dangerous age period for homicidal violence occurs in early adulthood—the late teens and early twenties. For example, according to the FBI's national arrest statistics for 1994 (FBI, 1995), there were 15,395 adults (ages 18 and over) compared to 3,102 juveniles arrested for murder; more than 83% of the 18,497 identified homicide perpetrators were adults. Most of the adult offenders were young: 7,519 (41%) were between the ages of 18 and 25 and 10,057 (54%) were between 18 and 29. The frequency of homicide begins to climb in the early teens, peaks in the late teens, and declines steadily thereafter.

Juvenile Homicide Trends

A more legitimate cause for concern is the rapid increase in juvenile homicide over the past decade (Cornell, 1993). As indicated in Figure 8.1, arrests of juveniles for homicide tripled from 1984 to 1994. There are similar but less dramatic increases

ARRESTS

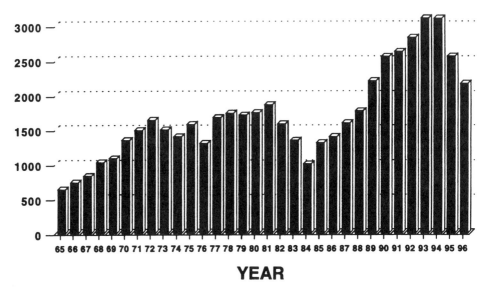

FIGURE 8.1. Juveniles arrested for homicide: 1965–1997. From FBI *Uniform Crime Reports,* by the Federal Bureau of Investigation, Washington, DC: U.S. Government Printing Office.

in other violent crimes by juveniles, and juvenile crime has increased more than adult crime. From 1985 to 1994, aggravated assault increased 97% among juveniles, but 71% among adults; robbery increased 57% among juveniles, but 11.9% among adults; and forcible rape increased 5.6% among juveniles compared to a 5.1% decrease among adults.

The rapid growth in juvenile violence cannot be attributed to changes in the size of the juvenile population; on the contrary, large increases occurred during years when the teenage population was *declining.* The homicide rate per 100,000 persons has actually increased among persons more than 16 years of age (Pierce & Fox, 1992). Although there has been a welcome drop in juvenile homicide arrests since 1994, demographic trends indicate that the juvenile population is now growing at a rate that will further boost the incidence of juvenile homicide. A 1995 report of the Office of Juvenile Justice and Delinquency Prevention (Snyder & Sickmund, 1995) asserted that if trends of the past 10 years continue, juvenile arrests for violent crime will double by the year 2010 and arrests for murder will exceed 8,000.

Cornell (1993) characterized 1,668 juveniles arrested for homicide in 1991, using data from the FBI's Supplemental Homicide Reports. The overwhelming majority of juveniles arrested for murder were male (93.6%), and a disproportionate percentage were African American (73.9%), with relatively smaller proportions of White non-Hispanics (22.4%), Hispanics (1.8%), and other groups (1.9%). A majority of offenders (58.5%) acted without an accomplice, most commonly using a handgun (61.2%) or other firearm (14.7%) to commit the homicide, and less often using a knife (12.6%), some other weapon (7.6%), or their bare hands (3.8%). Most homicide victims were acquaintances (56.8%), some were strangers (34.3%), and few were family members

(8.9%). Excluding unclear cases, just over half (51.7%) of the homicides could be characterized as resulting from interpersonal conflicts and the remainder (48.3%) were associated with some other crime such as a robbery or burglary.

Compared with adults, juvenile homicide offenders are more likely to be male and African American; they are more likely to act with an accomplice, to use a handgun, and to kill a stranger. Juveniles were more likely than adults to kill someone in the course of another crime rather than during an interpersonal conflict (Cornell, 1993).

The 162% increase in juvenile homicide from 1984 to 1991 was almost entirely an increase in deaths by firearms, especially handguns (Cornell, 1993). This finding prompts speculation that increased availability of guns to youth may have transformed otherwise nonlethal confrontations into homicides. Although there was little change in the number of family member victims, the number of stranger and acquaintance victims more than doubled. The largest increases were among African American males.

Gender Differences

Female juveniles commit just 2.7% of violent crimes and only 1% of homicides (FBI, 1995). Yet, their actions draw substantial media attention and public interest. When 18-year-old Amy Fisher attempted to kill the wife of her middle-aged lover, the news media made her the focus of national attention, and the entertainment industry produced three television dramas based on her story. When information was leaked to the media that an 18-year old high school honors student named Gina Grant had killed her abusive mother at age 14, Harvard University withdrew its offer of admission, prompting a national debate about policies toward juvenile offenders.

From 1985 to 1994, female juvenile arrests for violent crime increased 128.3% and arrests for homicide increased 64.2% (FBI, 1995). A comparison of 121 girls and 1,939 boys arrested for homicide in 1993 revealed a series of gender differences in offense characteristics (Loper & Cornell, 1996). Girls were far less likely to use a firearm (32%) than were boys (83%); however, girls were more likely to use a knife (35%) than were boys (8%). Most of the homicides committed by girls were associated with an interpersonal conflict with the victim (79%), whereas most homicides by boys (57%) were crime-related offenses.

There were striking gender differences in the victims of homicide by girls and boys (Loper & Cornell, 1996). Girls were more likely to kill family members (32%) than strangers (10%), but boys were more likely to kill strangers (36%) than family members (8%). Boys were more likely to kill victims of the same gender (86%) than were girls (42%). Finally, girls were more likely to kill younger victims. In fact, 24% of the girls' victims were under the age of 3, in contrast to less than 1% of the boys' victims.

These gender differences suggest that homicides by girls are much more often the product of interpersonal conflict between the girl and a familiar person, often a family member. A relatively large proportion of cases involved homicides of younger children, notably infants. Such offenses may involve girls who are frustrated by caretaking responsibilities, either as mothers or babysitters to young children. Peer disputes leading to homicide also are common. Other offenses may involve girls aggressing against abusive parents or boyfriends. In contrast to boys, girls are infrequently involved in more instrumental homicides associated with a robbery or burglary.

Characteristics of the Offender

Main Groups

A series of studies demonstrated the viability of sorting juvenile homicide offenders into three groups: psychotic, crime, and conflict offenders (Benedek & Cornell, 1989; Cornell, Benedek, & Benedek, 1987). Offenders in these three groups differed in the nature and circumstances of their offense as well as their prior adjustment, including previous delinquency and violence, substance abuse, family problems, and school adjustment. This typology was developed with a sample of 72 adolescents charged with murder in Michigan (Cornell et al., 1987) and supported by a second study of 71 juveniles convicted of murder in Virginia (Cornell, 1990). A replication study by an independent researcher (Toupin, 1993) studying precrime adjustment of 63 Canadian adolescent homicide offenders found "strikingly similar" (p. 147) results in support of the typology.

Although some authors (Lewis, Shanok, Pincus, & Glaser, 1979; Lewis et al., 1985; Lewis et al., 1988; Sendi & Blomgren, 1975) have emphasized the role of psychotic symptoms in juvenile homicide cases, the preponderance of studies demonstrates that only a small group of offenders, probably less than 5%, have psychotic disorders (Ewing, 1990; Myers & Kemph, 1990; Sorrells, 1977). Psychotic homicide offenders typically have a history of psychiatric hospitalization, fail to maintain a remission of symptoms, and act under the influence of delusions or hallucinations.

The crime group offenders commit homicides in the course of some other criminal activity, such as a robbery or burglary, rape, drug deal, or gang-related dispute. Their behavior is motivated largely by instrumental purposes, although they may be angry with their victims. Crime group offenders tend to have a significant history of prior delinquent activity, most notably stealing and fighting. These youth often have abused multiple substances, especially alcohol and marijuana, with an early (often preteen) age of onset. They have a history of poor school adjustment and may no longer be attending school by the time of the offense.

The MMPI profiles of crime group youth typically contain high elevations on multiple clinical scales, most frequently scales 1, 6, 7, and 8 (Cornell, Miller, & Benedek, 1988). Their profiles do not differ substantially from those of nonviolent, serious juvenile offenders, but they are significantly elevated in comparison with the conflict group, particularly on scales F, 1, 3, and 8. The Rorschach protocols of crime group youth are noteworthy for their sparse content and the primitive quality of their human responses, which generally indicate a low level of object relations or interpersonal maturity, often with poor form quality and in some cases depicting a victim of aggression (Greco & Cornell, 1992).

Juvenile homicide offenders in the conflict group typically kill friends or family members in the context of an ongoing dispute or conflict. The homicide is motivated by hostility rather than instrumental goals. The unexpected violence of these offenders may seem surprising and out of character to persons familiar with the youth. Conflict group offenders are less likely than crime group offenders to have a history of prior criminal activity, although some have a history of petty theft or minor fights. Their substance use, if present, is more limited and consistent with that of their nonhomicidal peers. Socially, these youth are often described as shy, introverted, and especially sensitive to insult or humiliation. Their infrequent expression of anger suggests a pattern of overcontrolled hostility. They generally have an adequate school adjustment, and some may have been regarded as very good students.

Additional Subgroups

The three juvenile homicide groups can be further subdivided. Within the crime group there may be critical differences between youth who participate in gang-related acts of violence and those who act more independently (Ewing, 1990; Rogers, 1993). Ewing used the term "senseless homicides" to describe groups of youth who participate in thrill killings of strangers or who attack individuals because of their membership in a different racial or ethnic group. Myers (1994) suggested that sexual homicide demands separate attention.

The conflict group in particular contains some distinctive subgroups, such as juveniles who killed parents or relatives versus those who killed peers. Most parricide offenders fall into the conflict group (Heide, 1992; Mones, 1991). There are some cases of youth who have killed family members for monetary gain associated with property inheritance or life insurance, so that both instrumental and hostile motives are present. Nevertheless, the typical parricide offender acts in response to a long pattern of parental abuse (Heide, 1992, 1994; Mones, 1991). Extensive physical abuse need not be present, although often it is threatened and may be reflected in milder forms of corporal punishment and by slapping and pushing. Sexual abuse may be easily overlooked, both because the abuser may have a flawless reputation that casts doubt on any allegations, and because the youth is unable to overcome feelings of shame and guilt to acknowledge the abuse (Gardiner, 1985; Mones, 1991).

More commonly, however, the parricidal youth has experienced prolonged and consistent emotional abuse in the form of repetitive derogatory and rancorous remarks (Benedek & Cornell, 1989, Ewing, 1990; Heide, 1992; Mones, 1991). The perjorative and malicious quality of verbal abuse has a devastating effect on the youth's self-image and fuels a deep and abiding resentment. The offender's abusive parent tends to be a controlling and dominating individual who restricts the youth from typical adolescent activities and privileges (Heide, 1992; Mones, 1990; Post, 1982). Sometimes the conflict precipitating the homicide concerns a relatively minor matter of driving the family car or attending a social event. The offense itself may not take place during the heat of an argument; the youth may act in anticipation of a disciplinary confrontation or in order to free himself or herself from the abusive situation. Ironically, the juveniles most frightened and intimidated by their abusers are, consequently, more likely to ambush their victims and therefore to be prosecuted for the more serious charge of first-degree murder.

Many authors attribute primary responsibility for the act of parricide to family conflict and dysfunction, especially parent psychopathology and substance abuse (Cormier, Angliker, Gagné, & Markus, 1978; Heide, 1992; Post, 1982). Sargent (1962) described several cases of juveniles who committed homicide with the implicit or explicit encouragement of other family members, especially abused spouses. In addition to child abuse, many authors describe multiple family problems including parental substance abuse and psychopathology, marital instability and father absence, and multiple changes in residence, child custody, or both.

Homicide committed by preteenage children is rare. National arrest statistics indicate that 33 children under the age of 13 were arrested for murder in 1994, including only three under the age of 10. These numbers include children who merely participated in homicides committed by a group or carried out actions at the direction of older youth. It is questionable whether children under the age of 10 adequately comprehend the permanency of death or the gravity of their aggressive intentions. Their actions chiefly represent unintended tragic outcomes of acts of aggression expressing their frustration and anger, and are meant to hurt, but not kill, their victims. Such children usually kill a younger child in the course of an argument that escalates and leads to a fatal act of rage. Several case reports (Carek & Watson, 1964; Paluszny & McNabb, 1975) described young children left to babysit defiant siblings. Adelson (1972) documented cases of children as young as 2 years old who inflicted fatal injuries on infants in an angry attempt to stop them from crying. Other studies characterized highly aggressive children whose assaults on peers might well have resulted in death (Lewis *et al.*, 1983; Petti & Davidman, 1981; Pfeffer, 1980, Tooley, 1975).

Family Patterns

There is widespread agreement that many juvenile homicide offenders were exposed to violent criminal offenders in their family environment and were socialized to engage in similar behavior (Adams, 1974; Busch, Zagar, Hughes, Arbit, & Bussell, 1990; Lewis *et al.*, 1983; Sorrells, 1977; Zagar, Arbit, Sylvies, Busch, & Hughes, 1990). Either parent may have a history of violent or criminal behavior or both, often in association with substance abuse. In many cases the juvenile had little if any contact with a biological father, and may have experienced abusive treatment by a series of men living with the mother. There is a well-established link between ineffective parenting and the development of increasingly antisocial and aggressive behavior (Kazdin, 1994; Patterson, 1986).

Yet, it should be acknowledged that there are cases in which well-intentioned and seemingly capable parents are faced with the nightmarish scenario of a youth who has engaged in seemingly inexplicable homicidal violence. In one case evaluated by the author, the son of a prominent minister killed his pregnant girlfriend when it became clear to him that she would bring public shame and humiliation to him, his much-admired father, and his entire family. In another case, the son of a well-regarded school principal became angry and despondent when his parents insisted he attend college rather than join the military. When it became apparent his parents would discover that he had secretly squandered his college tuition money, he carried out a methodical plan to ambush and kill both mother and father in succession. In both of these tragic cases, there was ample information from siblings that the parents were devoted, caring, and not abusive. It is noteworthy that the siblings were the more favored, high-achieving, and successful children in the family, while the murdering sons had long suffered by comparison and felt they could not measure up to their parents' expectations. In neither case did the son have a history of violent behavior, although both had a fascination with guns and bolstered their self-images with narcissistic and aggressive fantasies.

One important factor in the upsurge in youth violence may be children's exposure to increasing levels of violence in the entertainment media. Parents often question the need to limit their children's exposure of media violence. There is voluminous evidence, through both laboratory experiments and observational field studies, that children who watch violent television shows are stimulated to engage in aggressive behavior and also grow more aggressive over time (Berkowitz, 1993; Huesmann & Miller, 1994). There is considerable reluctance by the television industry, as well as the general public, to recognize and respond to the implications of these conclusions. The mechanisms by which exposure to media violence can increase aggressiveness include desensitization to violence, increased expectations of violence by others, role modeling of violent behavior, and the development of internalized cognitive scripts that guide decision making in social conflict situations (Berkowitz, 1993; Huesmann & Miller, 1994). The author evaluated a 16-year-old boy who decided that he could prevent his stepfather from administering a beating by pulling a shotgun on him, similar to a scene he had witnessed in a movie. When his stepfather decided to leap forward and grab the gun, the boy inadvertently pulled the trigger and killed him.

Other forms of media violence have not been extensively studied, but may have similar effects. The author has evaluated juvenile homicide offenders who describe great interest in movies that depict reckless violence and sadistic killing. They enjoy music advocating homicidal behavior and they are enthralled by video games that permit them to shoot, stab, or otherwise mutilate their adversaries. Some are avid participants in fantasy games that also involve killing their opponents.

> One lamentable case involved a 15-year-old boy who was regarded as both the local expert at the Mortal Kombat video game and the reigning champion of his Dungeons & Dragons fantasy game club at school. His obsession with fantasy violence dated back to the horror movies he began watching with his father at age 7; he became desensitized to the point that he preferred gruesomely violent videos that even his father could not bear to watch. One evening he became furious when his grandmother accused him of stealing money from her purse. He retreated to his room for several hours, spending the time listening to violent rock music and reading a Stephen King novel called *The Shining* which depicts a madman who assaulted his family with an ax. The boy came out of his room, armed himself with an ax and a knife, and proceeded to murder his grandmother. The boy had no history of prior violence, substance abuse, or other delinquent activity. He presented no significant symptoms of psychopathology or neuropsychological impairment. He was not a victim of child abuse, and expressed substantial remorse for the loss of his grandmother.

Certainly there is need for more research to determine personality and family characteristics that increase the vulnerability of some juveniles to media violence (e.g., Gadow & Sprafkin, 1987). Children reared in dysfunctional families, with parents who approve or support aggressive behavior, and who otherwise lack positive and supportive role models that discourage violence, may be particularly at risk. Psychoanalytic clinicians (McCarthy, 1978; Miller & Looney, 1974) theorized that homicidal youth have severe narcissistic deficits and associated omnipotent fantasies that permit them to dehumanize victims, particularly in the context of intense personal conflict and threats to their sense of self. Perhaps media violence fuels narcissistic, grandiose fantasies and supports a superficial and unempathic conception of others.

Assessment and Diagnosis

General Issues

Legal authorities and clinicians alike find it disconcerting that a homicide was committed by a youth who looks and acts like a typical teenager. The youth may suppress or deny feelings of concern about the homicide, and present little overt sign of either significant distress or major psychopatholoy. Some defiant, defensive youth may even feign a lack of concern for their victim or their present legal circumstances. There is an understandable expectation that there must be some hidden gross abnormality to account for murder by someone whose very youth and immaturity we so commonly associate with innocence. Consequently, it is particularly important to conduct a thorough, comprehensive diagnostic evaluation that rules out psychosis or severe neuropsychological impairment. Conduct Disorder and substance abuse appear to be the most common diagnoses assigned to juvenile homicide offenders, although a variety of disorders have been observed (Myers & Kemph, 1990). Malmquist (1990) reported that major affective disorder was pervasive among his sample of 44 homicidal adolescents.

A comprehensive evaluation would include thorough diagnostic interviewing along with a developmental and social history. The youth's self-report should be corroborated and supplemented with interviews of family members or witnesses, and a review of medical, school, and legal records. The clinician should be persistent in seeking all available records, especially any documentation of the offense from witnesses, investigators, and defendant statements.

Psychological tests are appropriate to address specific issues, such as the juvenile's level of intellectual functioning, presence of psychiatric symptoms including depression and thought disturbance, and personality characteristics associated with antisocial or psychopathic development. Both projective tests such as the Rorschach and TAT, and structured tests, such as the Millon Adolescent Clinical Inventory (MACI) and the Minnesota Multiphasic Personality Inventory—Adolescent form (MMPI-A), can be useful. Clinicians are advised to follow standard administration and scoring procedures for these tests, and to be prepared to defend the conclusions drawn from these tests in court should they be reviewed by a skeptical expert hired by an opposing attorney. Clinicians should not rely on the interpretive statements from computer-generated reports, which to date have not been validated for forensic application with juvenile offenders.

There has been considerable attention to the possibility of brain damage in violent juvenile offenders (Busch et al., 1990; Lewis et al., 1983; Lewis et al., 1985; Martinius, 1983; Zagar et al., 1990). Neuropsychological impairment may be overlooked in some rare cases. For example, Martinius (1983) reported that a chronically aggressive 14-year-old boy, who killed an 8-year-old during an argument, was later found to have a right temporal lesion. Restifo and Lewis (1985) noted that two published case reports of the same juvenile offender failed to mention the youth's history of delivery difficulties and multiple head trauma. Nevertheless, most cases do not present compelling evidence of neurological impairment, although clinicians and defense attorneys alike may be tempted to seek neurological evaluations and sophisticated brain studies in hopes of identifying a rare abnormality.

Brain damage or impairment refers to a continuum of abnormality that might include youth with soft neurological signs not associated with any discernible physical abnormality. And of course even the presence of gross brain abnormality does not necessarily provide an explanation for violent behavior or indicate that the youth was not criminally responsible for his behavior at a specific time.

Brain impairment might serve as a contributing factor that increases the likelihood of aggressive behavior without being a necessary or sufficient cause of violence. For example, there is a high incidence of learning and attention problems among violent and homicidal youth which often rise to the level of a diagnosis of Attention-Deficit/Hyperactivity Disorder or Specific Learning Disability (Busch *et al.*, 1990; Zagar *et al.*, 1990). Many studies find that a disproportionate percentage of juvenile offenders have a verbal–performance discrepancy on intelligence testing that reflects verbal or language-based impairment (although nonviolent delinquents show similar deficits—see Cornell & Wilson, 1992; Hays, Solway, & Schreiner, 1978). Cognitive and learning problems may contribute to school failure, poor self-esteem, deficits in moral reasoning, poor social skills and difficulties resolving interpersonal conflicts, or other negative outcomes that directly or indirectly increase the risk for violent behavior.

Clinicians should be exceedingly careful in diagnosing rare or unusual conditions, such as dissociative disorders or seizure-related syndromes speculatively linked to violent behavior, particularly when the evidence for such diagnoses is limited to criminal behavior. Diagnostic criteria for such conditions rely heavily on clinical inference and interpretation of the youth's subjective experience, which cannot be readily verified. Youth who claim amnesia or describe dissociative-like experiences during the offense should not on this basis be considered psychotic, and of course all criminal defendants claiming psychotic symptoms should be evaluated carefully for malingering. The clinician must resist the temptation to explain away behavior that can be more parsimoniously attributed to interpersonal conflict or antisocial personality characteristics.

Persons frequently describe their recollection for homicidal acts as dreamlike or hazy, and claim that they did not feel like themselves. They may describe a subjective loss of control associated with rage that serves to disclaim personal responsibility for their actions. The phenomenological sensation of giving in to one's angry impulses, which most persons experience to varying degrees from time to time, is not equivalent to a loss of capacity for intentional behavior. Moreover, the observation that murderous violence seems inconsistent with the youth's mild-mannered, submissive presentation during the diagnostic interview, or the commonplace assertion of family members that "he is not the kind of child to do this sort of thing," should be given little weight in diagnostic formulations.

Forensic Issues

A variety of mental health professionals may be involved in a single juvenile homicide case. Clinicians working for the incarcerating institution will assume the front-line clinical management responsibilities, while outside professionals may be assigned to conduct forensic evaluations to address a number of legal issues. Because of the potential for role conflict and compromised confidentiality, the duties of treatment provision and forensic evaluation should be undertaken by different professionals. Forensic evaluation requires specialized training and experience, and legal standards and requirements vary by jurisdiction, so the forensic issues addressed in juvenile evaluations will be reviewed only briefly here.

Transfer to Adult Court

Usually the first forensic issue to be addressed is the juvenile's transfer to adult court. In an increasing number of states a juvenile charged with murder is tried as an adult automatically, while in others there are hearings to determine whether the case is suitable for transfer from juvenile to adult court (Bonnie, 1989; Snyder & Sickmund, 1995). A forensic evaluation for transfer purposes (sometimes called a waiver evaluation) typically includes consideration of the juvenile's amenability to treatment and competency to stand trial. The juvenile court's traditional emphasis on rehabilitation leads logically to the issue of amenability to treatment, while the adult court's greater emphasis on punishment and incapacitation heightens concern for the juvenile's competency to stand trial.

Amenability to treatment is not well defined, but involves consideration of several related questions. Perhaps the basic underlying question is whether the juvenile's offense can be considered the product of a persistent antisocial orientation that is likely to lead to further criminal behavior. Obviously this is a complex question that requires inferences about the juvenile's motives and behavior at the time of the offense, a conceptualization of antisocial personality development in adolescence, and the difficult issue of recidivism prediction. Further questions concern whether the juvenile has a treatable mental disorder and is sufficiently motivated to engage in treatment. Of course, amenability to treatment also begs the question that there are effective treatments available, and clinicians should be knowledgeable concerning current treatment and prevention approaches for youth violence (Eron, Gentry, & Schlegel, 1994). Moreover, in evaluating amenability to treatment, the court also will consider the practical issue of the availability and efficacy of treatment resources in the community.

Competency to Stand Trial

The juvenile's competency to stand trial is certainly an issue in adult court, but similar concerns also may be a consideration in juvenile court. As the punitive nature of juvenile court has increased over the years, the issue of competency to participate in legal proceedings would seem to be more salient than in the past, but it is often overlooked (Fitch, 1989). Competency to stand trial concerns the defendant's present mental state, not his or her behavior at the time of the offense. Competency to stand trial is usually considered to require that the defendant, "has sufficient present ability to consult with his attorney with a reasonable degree of rational understanding and a rational as well as factual understanding of the proceedings against him" (*Dusky v United States*, 362 U.S. 402, 1960).

Waiver of Miranda Rights

Most juveniles detained for a crime will waive their Miranda rights and give a statement to the police without benefit of counsel (Grisso, 1981). Even when parents are available to the juvenile, in most cases, parents will assume a passive role or encourage the juvenile to give a statement (Grisso, 1981). With prolonged questioning, many juveniles can be prodded, cajoled, or beguiled into giving the police incriminating statements. Adolescents often surrender to the appeal of an investigator who assumes a supportive, sympathetic attitude and offers fatherly advice and encouragement to confess. In one case known to the author, a sleep-deprived juvenile who had been detained for many hours agreed to give a statement essentially in exchange for a soft drink and potato chips.

It is difficult to distinguish when the poor judgment of a nervous, immature adolescent should be regarded as competent in such a momentous matter as deciding to confess to murder. In general, a competent decision must be knowing, intelligent, and voluntary (Grisso, 1986). In his landmark studies of juvenile competence to waive Miranda rights, Grisso (1981) investigated the ability of juveniles to respond to a series of questions concerning their understanding of key elements of the Miranda warning as well as their ability to apply the warning to hypothetical situations. Compared with adults, most juveniles under the age of 17 displayed noteworthy gaps in their understanding of their Miranda rights, particularly their right to remain silent. Grisso (1981) concluded that juveniles under age 15, as well as 15- to 16-year-olds with IQs below 80, generally did not understand their rights as well as adults, so that their competence should be of special concern. African American youth also tended to evidence greater misunderstanding of their rights. However, in clinical practice, each juvenile's capacity to understand his or her rights should be carefully evaluated.

Mental State at Offense

When evidence of the adolescent's incrimination is unequivocal, the defense attorney may consider an insanity defense, prompting an evaluation of the youth's criminal responsibility, less provocatively termed a mental state at offense (MSO) evaluation. An MSO evaluation requires a detailed, painstaking review of all available evidence bearing on the juvenile's state of mind and behavior during the time period bracketing the alleged offense. Legal standards for insanity vary from state to state. However, most commonly require that the defendant meet the threshold condition of a mental disease or defect, followed by the secondary condition of either a cognitive or volitional impairment directly linked to the offense (Melton, Petrila, Poythress, & Slobogin, 1987). These conditions all contain ambiguous and controversial language that is subject to interpretation and debate—matters that go well beyond the scope of this chapter.

A mental disease or defect is usually considered to be a severe mental disorder or mental retardation that substantially impairs the youth's understanding of reality (Melton *et al.*, 1987). The mental state associated with this mental disease or defect cannot be merely the product of voluntary intoxication, and is best exemplified by psychotic disorders such as schizophrenia or bipolar disorder. Second, the mental state must involve a cognitive impairment such that the juvenile did not understand the nature and quality of the criminal act or did not understand that the act was wrong. An example might be someone with schizophrenic delusions who killed a person whom he or she believed to be a threatening demon. Some jurisdictions permit volitional impairment as an alternative to cognitive impairment. In these cases, the person might have a cognitive understanding of his or her actions, but nevertheless be unable to resist the impulse to commit the violent act.

Disposition

Mental health professionals frequently are asked to provide information that would assist the court in deciding the juvenile's legal disposition. Most often, the clinician offers treatment recommendations and identifies educational or vocational needs. The court may be interested in the juvenile's remorsefulness and acceptance of responsibility for his or her crime. More generally, the court may request information concerning the juvenile's prospects for rehabilitation and capacity for change.

Implicit or explicit in court requests will be the question of the juvenile's potential for future acts of violence. Clinicians are well advised to defer making unqualified or categorical predictive statements that exceed the bounds of current knowledge and professional expertise (Grisso & Applebaum, 1992; Melton *et al.*, 1987). Nevertheless, clinicians should be aware of the substantial literature and knowledge base on risk factors for criminal recidivism, especially psychopathy and mental disorder (Monahan & Steadman, 1994; Rice & Harris, 1995), that can be used to frame appropriately qualified dispositional recommendations.

Course, Prognosis, and Recidivism

We know little about the long-term course for juvenile homicide offenders, but the available evidence is surprisingly optimistic. First, it should be noted that criminal recidivism for adult homicide offenders is relatively low in comparison with other adult offenders. For example, a study by the Virginia Department of Criminal Justice Services (1989) examined several indices of recidivism during the 5-year period after parole. For 237 homicide parolees, recidivism rates were as follows: felony arrest, 28.7%; violent felony arrest, 12.7%; violent felony conviction, 6.3%; and new identical violent felony conviction, 3.4%. For 238 aggravated assault parolees, recidivism rates were approximately twice as high: felony arrest, 47.5%; violent felony arrest, 26.5%; violent felony conviction, 15.1%; and new identical violent felony conviction, 10.9%. For 239 robbery parolees, recidivism was even higher: felony arrest, 50.2%; violent felony arrest, 23.8%; violent felony conviction, 32.6%; and new identical violent felony conviction, 11.7%.

Even capital murderers evidence a much lower risk of future violence than would be anticipated based on the nature of their offense. Follow-up studies of several hundred capital murderers whose death sentences were set aside by the Supreme Court's 1972 Furman decision revealed that capital murderers moved from death row to the general prison population were far less likely than other inmates to engage in violent behavior in prison (Bohm, 1991; Marquart & Sorensen, 1989). Moreover, those former death row inmates who eventually were paroled and released to the community did not exhibit recidivism levels as high as nonhomicide comparison offenders (Bohm, 1991; Marquart & Sorensen, 1989). Of course, one reason for the comparatively lower recidivism rate of homicide offenders may be their relatively greater age and increased maturity by the time they were released from incarceration.

There are few studies of recidivism among juvenile homicide offenders. Case reports and studies of small samples depict surprisingly positive treatment outcomes and low recidivism rates among juvenile homicide offenders (Cormier & Markus, 1980; Gardiner, 1985; Hellsten & Katila, 1965). Corder, Ball, Haislip, Rollins, and Beaumont (1976) reported especially good outcomes among 10 adolescents convicted of parricide (see also Cormier *et al.*, 1978).

Toupin (1993) conducted a follow-up study of 43 Canadian juvenile homicide offenders an average of 83.5 months after release to the community. Recidivism was documented from federal police records. Toupin classified homicide offenders using the crime and conflict group distinction (Cornell *et al.,* 1987) and compared the homicide groups to a property offender group. He found that crime homicide and property offenders committed similar levels of violent and nonviolent crimes after release to the community, but that conflict group offenders committed significantly lower numbers of violent offenses than either of those two groups. Crime group offenders committed an average of .15 violent offenses per year, while conflict group offenders committed approximately .004 violent offenses per year. Property offenders committed .31 violent offenses per year, and an index of offense seriousness indicated that their crimes were more serious than those of the conflict group offenders.

Reyes (1990, 1996) conducted outcome research on a structured group therapy program for juvenile homicide offenders at a Texas correctional facility. The program made use of psychodrama, homework assignments, and video presentations to help youth explore their life experiences, crime stories, and future goals. After completion of the 4-month program, homicide offenders demonstrated a significant decline in self-reported hostility-aggression in comparison with a control group of offenders incarcerated for aggravated assault. No significant treatment effects were found for self-reported empathy, although empathy specifically for crime victims was not directly assessed. These findings are promising in light of the relatively short-term nature of the program, but more comprehensive assessment of offender changes would be desirable. Reyes (personal communication, February 17, 1993, see also Reyes, 1996) subsequently examined 1-year recidivism data for 85 youth released from the program and found that 17% were rearrested for any offense, compared to a 33% rearrest rate for homicide offenders who had not been included in the program because of resource limitations.

Clinical Management

Clinicians working in jail or juvenile detention settings have primary responsibility for clinical management of juvenile homicide offenders. The clinician's first task is to assess the youth's mental state, with particular attention to suicide risk. Although suicide attempts are rare, the youth may be struggling with feelings of shame, guilt, and grief that lead to suicidal ideation and warrant careful monitoring.

A second concern is the youth's potential for further violent behavior directed at others. Security staff may be inclined to judge the youth's potential for problem behavior based on the seriousness of the offense; on the contrary, predictions should give heavy consideration to a review of his or her prior behavior under relatively structured conditions such as school. In cases known to the author, youth with little history of fighting or aggressive behavior prior to the homicide tend to return to this pattern following the offense. Surprisingly, in most cases, youth charged with homicide conform to institutional requirements and often are described by security staff as compliant, well-behaved inmates. Depending on jurisdictional laws and policies, when juveniles are transferred to adult court, they may be removed from a juvenile detention center and placed in a jail to await trial.

A third clinical management issue is preparation for a long period of incarceration prior to trial. Juvenile homicide cases are rarely tried promptly, and the youth must deal with a long period of uncertainty over his or her legal status and eventual disposition. This uncertainty makes it extremely difficult for the youth to engage in a psychotherapy process or to begin to come to terms with the horror and tragedy of the homicide. Clinical work is largely supportive and educational, and focused on day-to-day adjustment to the institution and preparation for trial. Given that the pretrial period is so lengthy, it may be desirable to seek judicial authority to maintain the youth in a juvenile setting. In any event, the youth should be involved in a daily educational program working toward high school completion or the equivalent.

A fourth issue throughout pretrial confinement is the youth's relationship with family members and close friends. There will be painful initial meetings with friends or family members who now see the teenager as a "killer" or "murderer." There often are dramatic splits in family attitudes and reactions to the homicide. Some family members will vehemently condemn the youth and break off contact, while others will dedicate themselves to providing emotional support and reassurance. Some family members will testify at trial or at sentencing, so that their attitudes toward the youth have legal as well as emotional consequences. In some cases, it can be helpful for the counselor clinician to hold one or two joint meetings with the youth and a supportive family member. Youth may be more willing to discuss conflictual family relationships with the encouragement and prompting of a supportive relative, and new information about the youth often comes to light. At the same time, the clinician can assist the youth in communicating painful feelings.

Treatment

The juvenile offender's treatment needs will change markedly as he or she moves through the justice system and into long-term confinement. The immediate challenges of adapting to incarceration and preparing for prosecution take precedence over longer-term objectives such as coming to terms with the offense and repairing deficiencies in identity and maturity. A supportive counselor can be most effective in guiding the youth through the initial adjustment period, which includes the following tasks: (1) acceptance of incarceration and institutional routine; (2) development of a working relationship with the defense attorney; and (3) tolerating the stress of legal proceedings. Typical among the stages of legal proceedings are transfer to adult court, arraignment, and numerous trial delays and postponements, culminating in the trial itself with possible testimony, followed by sentencing.

Initially, the juvenile may cope with the shock and disruption associated with arrest and incarceration by focusing on seemingly insignificant matters, such as the daily jail schedule and access to favorite television programs. In counseling sessions, many youth manifest such a detached and wooden presentation that they appear cold and indifferent. This defensive facade is usually associated with denial of the significance of the offense and a massive effort to control and contain emotions. One youth, who had confessed to shooting his father, continued for months to speak of his aspirations to play football for his high school team when he returned home. Nevertheless, even the most detached youth usually acknowledge considerable preoccupation with the offense and, in unguarded moments, they may display intense anxiety, grief, and guilt. All juvenile homicide offenders should be evaluated for suicidality and monitored accordingly.

More ambitious therapeutic goals can be pursued after the juvenile is sentenced. However, this means that the youth begins treatment with a new clinician, who must begin again the slow and uncertain process of establishing rapport and trust. Because many youth continue to harbor unrealistic hopes about the possibility of acquittal or a light sentence, the convicted youthful offender may be especially demoralized and discouraged, and less than optimally motivated for treatment. And in adult institutions where therapist resources are limited, offenders may receive attention restricted to acute needs and behavior management rather than their potential for growth and maturity over the course of intensive psychotherapy.

Myers (1992) argued for the use of psychiatric hospitalization and therapeutically oriented juvenile offender institutions for homicide offenders. In many respects, treatment for juvenile homicide offenders should be similar to treatment for other aggressive and antisocial youth (Goldstein, 1994; Kazdin, 1994). Group therapy can be useful in helping youth overcome resistance to acknowledging their behavior and accepting responsibility for their actions. Groups also can provide a context for improving social skills and problem-solving capacities. Educational and vocational programs are important components of any rehabilitative effort.

Treatment of juvenile homicide offenders differs from that for other aggressive youth when it comes to dealing with the crime. The unalterable tragedy and permanency of death, and its devastating effect on loved ones, make homicide a singularly demanding therapeutic challenge, one likely to require long-term individual psychotherapy. Eventually the youth must come to terms with his or her crime in all of its complexity and horror. This process would include examining motivations, alternatives, and decisions that led to the offense, and is likely to entail intense grief and remorse as the youth fully accepts responsibility for his or her actions. The process might culminate in some act of dedication to an expiatory goal. The length and complexity of this process is illustrated by Leopold's (1957) first-person account of his incarceration for the murder of a young boy. After years of defensive denial, Leopold went through a period of depression and despondency evolving into a gradual acceptance of responsibility for his crime. There are structured therapy programs, such as the psychodrama program described by Reyes (1990, 1996), that attempt to overcome offender denial and accelerate the process of coming to terms with the offense. The long-term results of these experimental treatment efforts will be a valuable contribution to the field.

For those incarcerated youth who eventually will be released, it is particularly important to prevent further development of antisocial and psychopathic characteristics. Juveniles who must cope with a prison environment may be inclined to develop the attitudes and values of their associates, and to overcome feelings of vulnerability by hardening themselves against anxiety or dependency. Institutions should minimize juvenile exposure to the most corruptive adult offenders, and facilitate involvement in a more prosocial peer environment, with access to therapeutic role models. Family members can and should play an important role by preserving positive ties to the youth, maintaining morale, and providing a source of hope for the future.

References

Adams, K. A. (1974). The child who murders: A review of theory and research. *Criminal Justice and Behavior* 1, 51–61.
Adelson, L. (1972). The battering child. *Journal of the American Medical Association*, 222, 159–161.

Bender, L., Keiser, S., & Schilder, P. (1937). *Studies in aggressiveness* (Genetic Psychology Monographs No. 15). Worester, MA: Clark University.

Benedek, E., & Cornell, D. (Eds.) (1989). *Juvenile homicide*. Washington, DC: American Psychiatric Press.

Berkowitz, L. (1993). *Aggression: Its causes, consequences, and control*. Philadelphia: Temple University Press.

Bohm, R. M. (Ed.). (1991). *The death penalty in America: Current research*. Cincinnati, OH: Anderson.

Bonnie, R. J. (1989). Juvenile homicide: A study in legal ambivalence. In E. P. Benedek & D. G. Cornell (Eds.) *Juvenile homicide* (pp. 183–218). Washington, DC: American Psychiatric Press.

Busch, K. G., Zagar, R., Hughes, J. R., Arbit, J., & Bussell, R. E. (1990). Adolescents who kill. *Journal of Clinical Psychology, 46*, 472–485.

Carek, D. J., & Watson, A. S. (1964). Treatment of a family involved in fratricide. *Archives of General Psychiatry, 11*, 533–542.

Corder, B. F., Ball, B. C., Haizlip, T .M., Rollins, R., & Beaumont, R. (1976). Adolescent parricide: A comparison with other adolescent murder. *American Journal of Psychiatry, 133*, 957–961.

Cormier, B. M., & Markus, B. (1980). A longitudinal study of adolescent murderers. *Bulletin of the American Association of Psychology and Law, 8*, 240–260.

Cormier, B. M., Angliker, C. C. J., Gagné, P. W., & Markus, B. (1978). Adolescents who kill a member of the family. In J. M. Eekelaar & S. N. Katz (Eds.), *Family violence: An international and interdisciplinary study* (pp. 466–r78). Toronto, Ontario, Canada: Butterworth.

Cornell, D. (1990). Prior adjustment of violent juvenile offenders. *Law and Human Behavior, 14*, 569–578.

Cornell, D. (1993). Juvenile homicide: A growing national problem. *Behavioral Sciences and the Law, 11*, 389–396.

Cornell, D., & Wilson, L. (1992). The PIQ > VIQ discrepancy in violent and nonviolent delinquents. *Journal of Clinical Psychology, 48*, 256–261.

Cornell, D., Benedek, E., & Benedek, D. (1987). Juvenile homicide: Prior adjustment and a proposed typology. *American Journal of Orthopsychiatry, 57*, 383–393.

Cornell, D., Miller, C., & Benedek, E. (1988). MMPI profiles of adolescents charged with homicide. *Behavioral Sciences and the Law, 6*, 401–407.

Eron, L. D., Gentry, J. H., & Schlegel, P. (Eds.) (1994). *Reason to hope: A psychosocial perspective on violence and youth*. Washington, DC: American Psychological Association.

Ewing, C. P. (1990). *When children kill: The dynamics of juvenile homicide*. Lexington, MA: Lexington Books.

Federal Bureau of Investigation. (1995). *Uniform crime reports for the United States 1994*. Washington, DC: U.S. Government Printing Office.

Fitch, W. L. (1989). Competency to stand trial and criminal responsibility in juvenile court. In E. P. Benedek & D. G. Cornell (Eds.) *Juvenile homicide* (pp. 143–162). Washington, DC: American Psychiatric Press.

Gadow, K., & Sprafkin, J. (1987). Effects of viewing high versus low aggression cartoons on emotionally disturbed children. *Journal of Pediatric Psychology, 12*, 413–427.

Gardiner, M. (1985). *The deadly innocents: Portraits of children who kill*. New Haven, CT: Yale University Press.

Goldstein, A. P. (1994). *Student aggression: Prevention, management, and replacement training*. New York: Guilford.

Greco, C., & Cornell, D. (1992). Rorschach object relations of adolescents who committed homicide. *Journal of Personality Assessment, 59*, 574–583.

Grisso, T. (1981). *Juveniles' waiver of rights: Legal and psychological competence*. New York: Plenum.

Grisso, T. (1986). *Evaluating competencies: Forensic assessments and instruments*. New York: Plenum.

Grisso, T., & Applebaum, P. S. (1992). Is it unethical to offer predictions of future violence? *Law and Human Behavior, 16*, 621–634.

Hays, J. R., Solway, K. S., & Schreiner, D. (1978). Intellectual characteristics of juvenile murderers versus status offenders. *Psychological Reports, 43*, 80–82.

Heide, K. M. (1992). *Why kids kill parents: Child abuse and adolescent homicide*. Columbus: Ohio State University Press.

Heide, K. M. (1994). Evidence of child maltreatment among adolescent parricide offenders. *International Journal of Offender Therapy and Comparative Criminology, 38*, 151–162.

Hellsten, P., & Katila, O. (1965). Murder and other homicide by children under 15 in Finland. *Psychiatry Quarterly, 39* (Suppl.), 54–74

Huesmann, L. R., & Miller, L. S. (1994). Long-term effects of repeated exposure to media violence in childhood. In L. R. Huesmann (Ed.), *Aggressive behavior: Current perspectives* (pp. 153–180). New York: Plenum.

Kazdin, A. E. (1994). Interventions for aggressive and antisocial children. In L. D. Eron, J. H. Gentry, & P. Schlegel (Eds.), *Reason to hope: A psychosocial perspective on violence and youth* (pp. 341–382). Washington, DC: American Psychological Association.

Leopold, N. F., Jr. (1957). *Life plus 99 years*. Garden City, NY: Doubleday.

Lewis, D. O., Shanok, S. S., Pincus, J. H., & Glaser, G. H. (1979). Violent juvenile delinquents: Psychiatric, neurological, psychological and abuse factors. *Journal of the American Academy of Child Psychiatry, 18*, 307–319.

Lewis, D. O., Shanok, S. S., Grant, M., & Ritvo, E. (1983). Homicidally aggressive young children: Neuropsychiatric and experiential correlates. *American Journal of Psychiatry, 140*, 148–153.

Lewis, D. O., Moy, E., Jackson, L. D., Aaronson, R., Restifo, N., Serra, S., & Simos, A. (1985). Biopsychosocial characteristics of children who later murder: A prospective study. *American Journal of Psychiatry, 142*, 1161–1167.

Lewis, D. O., Pincus, J. H., Bard, B., Richardson, E., Feldman, M., Prichep, L. S., & Yeager, C. (1988). Neuropsychiatric, psychoeducational, and family characteristics of 14 juveniles condemned to death in the United States. *American Journal of Psychiatry, 145*, 584–589.

Loper, A., & Cornell, D. G. (1996). Homicide by adolescent girls. *Journal of Child and Family Studies*.

Malmquist, C. P. (1990). Depression in homicidal adolescents. *Bulletin of the American Academy of Psychiatry and the Law, 18*, 23–36.

Marquart, J. W., & Sorensen, J. R. (1989). A national study of the Furman-commuted inmates: Assessing the threat to society from capital offenders. *Loyola of Los Angeles Law Review, 23*, 5–28.

Martinius, J. (1983). Homicide of an aggressive adolescent boy with right temporal lesion: A case report. *Neuroscience and Biobehavioral Reviews, 7*, 419–422.

McCarthy, J. (1978). Narcissism and the self in homicidal adolescents. *American Journal of Psychoanalysis, 38*, 19–29.

Medlicott, R. W. (1955). Paranoia of the exalted type in a setting of folie à deux: A study of two adolescent homicides. *British Journal of Medical Psychology, 28*, 205–223.

Melton, G. B., Petrila, J., Poythress, N. G., & Slobogin, C. (1987). *Psychological evaluations for the courts: A handbook for mental health professionals and lawyers*. New York: Guilford.

Miller, D., & Looney, J. (1974). The prediction of adolescent homicide: Episodic dyscontrol and dehumanization. *American Journal of Psychoanalysis, 34*, 187–198.

Monahan, J., & Steadman, H. J. (1994). *Violence and mental disorder: Developments in risk assessment*. Chicago: University of Chicago Press.

Mones, P. (1991). *When a child kills: Abused children who kill their parents*. New York: Pocket Books.

Myers, W. C. (1992). What treatments do we have for children and adolescents who have killed? *Bulletin of the American Academy of Psychiatry and the Law, 20*, 47–58.

Myers, W. C. (1994). Sexual homicide by adolescents. *Journal of the American Academy of Child and Adolescent Psychiatry, 33*, 962–969.

Myers, W. C., & Kemph, J. P. (1990). DSM-III-R classification of murderous youth: Help or hindrance? *Journal of Clinical Psychiatry, 51*, 239–242.

Paluszny, M., & McNabb, M. (1975). Therapy of a six-year-old who committed fratricide. *Journal of American Academy of Child Psychiatry, 14*, 319–336.

Patterson, G. R. (1986). Performance models for antisocial boys. *American Psychologist, 41*, 432–444.

Petti, T. A., & Davidman, L. (1981). Homicidal school-age children: Cognitive style and demographic features. *Child Psychiatry Human Development, 12*, 82–89.

Pfeffer, C. R. (1980). Psychiatric hospital treatment of assaultive homicidal children. *American Journal of Psychotherapy, 34*, 197–207.

Pierce, G. L., & Fox, J. A. (1992). *Recent trends in violent crime: A closer look*. Unpublished report, National Crime Analysis Program, Northeastern University, Boston.

Post, S. (1982). Adolescent parricide in abusive families. *Child Welfare, 61*, 445–455.

Restifo, N., & Lewis, D. O. (1985). Three case reports of a single homicidal adolescent. *American Journal of Psychiatry, 142*, 388.

Reyes, L. S. (1990). *A treatment program for juvenile homicide offenders: Impact on hostility-aggression, empathy, and locus of control*. Unpublished doctoral dissertation, University of Texas at Austin.

Reyes, L. S. (1996, August). *Juvenile violence: Trends, social response, and the efficacy of treatment*. Paper presented at the meeting of the American Psychological Association, Toronto, Ontario, Canada.

Rice, M. E., & Harris, G. T. (1995). Violent recidivism: Assessing predictive validity. *Journal of Consulting and Clinical Psychology, 63*, 737–748.

Rogers, C. (1993). Gang-related homicides in Los Angeles County. *Journal of Forensic Sciences, 38*, 831–834.

Rowley, J. C., Ewing, C. P., & Singer, S. I. (1987). Juvenile homicide: The need for an interdisciplinary approach. *Behavioral Sciences and the Law, 5*, 1–10.

Sargent, D. (1962). Children who kill—A family conspiracy? *Social Work, 7,* 35–42.

Scherl, D. J., & Mack, J. E. (1966). A study of adolescent matricide. *Journal of American Academy of Child Psychiatry, 5,* 559–593.

Sendi, I. B., & Blomgren, P. G. (1975). A comparative study of predictive criteria in the predisposition of homicidal adolescents. *American Journal of Psychiatry, 132,* 423–428.

Snyder, H. N., & Sickmund, M. (1995). *Juvenile offenders and victims: A national report.* Washington, DC: Office of Juvenile Justice and Delinquency Prevention.

Sorrells, J. M. (1977). Kids who kill. *Crime and Delinquency, 23,* 312–320.

Stearns, A. (1957). Murder by adolescents with obscure motivation. *American Journal of Psychiatry, 114,* 303–305.

Tooley, K. (1975). The small assassins: Clinical notes on a subgroup of murderous children. *Journal of American Academy of Child Psychiatry, 14,* 306–336.

Toupin, J. (1993). Adolescent murderers: Validation of a typology and study of their recidivism. In A. V. Wilson (Ed.), *Homicide: The victim/offender connection* (pp. 135–156). Cincinnati, OH: Anderson.

Virginia Department of Criminal Justice Services. (1989). *Violent crime in Virginia.* Richmond, VA: Author.

Yates, A., Beutler, L. E., & Crago, M. (1984). Characteristics of young, violent offenders. *Journal of Psychiatry and Law, 11,* 137–149.

Zagar, R., Arbit, J., Sylvies, R., Busch, K. G., & Hughes, J. R. (1990). Homicidal adolescents: A replication. *Psychological Reports, 67,* 1235–1242.

Zenoff, E. H., & Zients, A. B. (1979). Juvenile murderers: Should the punishment fit the crime? *International Journal of Law and Psychiatry, 2,* 533–553.

III

HOMICIDE

Serial Murder and Sexual Homicide

Wade C. Myers, Ann W. Burgess, Allen G. Burgess,
and John E. Douglas

The crimes of serial and sexual murderers regularly attract the attention of the lay press, and the response of the public on learning of these acts is typically outrage and disgust. Paradoxically, a number of recent box office hits have been based on serial killers (e.g., *Copycat, Seven, Heat*), suggesting at the same time a certain fascination by many people with this form of violence. Adding to the macabre and mysterious quality of these violent crimes is the limited scientific literature available to explain them. This void is slowly being filled by the combined effort of workers in the fields of law enforcement, mental health, and sociology.

Definitions

To proceed in describing the phenomena of serial murder and sexual homicide, it is first necessary to define these separate, yet related, terms. From a historical perspective, a variety of terms, including lust murderer, sadistic murderer, compulsive murderer, sexually sadistic murderer, and erotophonophilia have been applied to this type of criminal.

Sexual homicide refers to murders with evidence demonstrating a sexual component to the crime (Burgess, Hartman, Ressler, Douglas, & McCormack, 1986; Ressler, Burgess, & Douglas, 1988). Observations at the crime scene to suggest sexual interest or sadistic fantasy may include removal of the victim's clothing, exposure of the victim's sexual organs, sexual positioning of the body, evidence of oral, vaginal, or anal intercourse, or other signs of sexual exploitation. This sexual component may involve penile penetration of the victim, or a sexually symbolic act, such as the insertion of a foreign object into one of the victim's orifices (Douglas, Burgess, Burgess, & Ressler, 1992). The elements of power, brutality, and callousness in the offender's personality are often revealed through psychological clues available at the crime scene.

Wade C. Myers • Department of Psychiatry, Health Sciences Center, University of Florida, Gainesville, Florida 32610. *Ann W. Burgess* • School of Nursing, University of Pennsylvania, Philadelphia, Pennsylvania 19104-6096. *Allen G. Burgess* • School of Business, Northeastern University, Boston, Massachusetts 02115-5096. *John E. Douglas* • Midhunters, Inc., Box 1957, Vienna, Virginia 22183.

Handbook of Psychological Approaches with Violent Offenders: Contemporary Strategies and Issues, edited by Van Hasselt and Hersen. Kluwer Academic/Plenum Publishers, New York, 1999.

There are varying definitions of *serial murder*. Douglas and Burgess (1986) succinctly define serial murder as three or more separate homicidal events in three or more separate locations with a "cooling off" period between. This cooling off period can last for days, weeks, or months, and is the key feature that distinguishes the serial killer from other multiple killers. Egger (1990) provides a more restrictive definition, stating that serial murder occurs when one or more individuals, typically male, commit a second, unrelated murder of an unknown victim at a different time and geographical location. The motive is not for material gain, but instead the murderer's aim is to exert power over his vulnerable victim.

This latter definition implies that two murders are sufficient. Other sources believe there should be a minimum of three or more victims to definitively establish the occurrence of serial murder (Douglas & Burgess, 1986; Hickey, 1991; Jenkins, 1988). A minimum of three victims is certainly a more convincing demonstration of a serial pattern. Furthermore, some disagree that serial murderers kill only strangers, or that nearly all offenders are male (Hickey, 1991). In a review of serial murders over almost 200 years, Hickey found that 17% were female.

A confounding factor in the literature, particularly in earlier works, was the use of nonspecific classification schemes, leading to a failure to make a distinction between the terms serial murder and sexual homicide. Yet, as the preceding definitions show, there can be significant overlap between sexual homicide and serial murder. For example, someone who commits a series of sexual murders becomes a serial murderer. On the other hand, not all serial murderers commit murders that are sexual in nature, although the majority do (Ressler *et al.*, 1988).

It is also important to make a distinction between serial murder, spree serial murder, and mass murder. The National Center for the Analysis of Violent Crime (1992b) divides serial murder into *spree* and *classic* types. Spree serial killings involve two or more murders at separate locations with no cooling off period between acts. The time period between spree murders can be minutes or days; the offender tends to have a high excitation level and may be a fugitive.

In contrast, mass murder involves the killing of multiple victims by one offender during a single episode at one location. The time period for the mass killings may cover minutes, hours, or even days. The prototype of a classic mass murderer is a mentally disordered individual whose problems have increased to the point that he acts out against groups of people who are unrelated to him or his problems, unleashing his hostility through shootings and stabbings. Other mass murderers direct their deadly hostility at their own family members.

There are other differences that distinguish the mass, spree, and serial murderer. In addition to the number of events and locations, and the presence or absence of a cooling-off period, the classic mass murderer and the spree murderer are not concerned with who their victims are. They will indiscriminately kill anyone who crosses their path. In contrast, the serial murderer usually selects a preferred type of victim, and commonly stalks his victims in a predatory fashion. He believes he will not be caught, and carefully monitors his behaviors to avoid detection.

Classification Efforts

The few studies that specifically address homicidal aggression suggest the existence of two types of sex murderers: the vindictive, or displaced anger, murderer (Cohen *et al.*, 1971; Groth, Burgess, & Holmstrom, 1977; Knight & Prentky, 1990;

Prentky, Burgess, & Carter, 1986; Rada, 1978) and the sadistic, or lust, murderer (Becker & Abel, 1978; Bromberg & Coyle, 1974; Cohen *et al.*, 1971; Guttmacher & Wei-hofen, 1952; Groth, Burgess, & Holmstrom, 1977; Knight & Prentky 1990; Podolsky, 1966; Prentky, Burgess, & Carter, 1986; Rada, 1978; Ressler, 1985; Scully & Marolla, 1985). Podolsky notes that the former, the rape murderers, kill after raping their victims, primarily to escape detection. These murderers, according to Rada, rarely report sexual satisfaction from their murders or perform postmortem sexual acts with their victims. In contrast, the sadistic murderer kills as part of a ritualized, sadistic fantasy (Groth *et al.*, 1977). For this murderer, aggression and sexuality become fused into a single psychological experience—sadism—in which aggression is eroticized. According to Brittain (1970), subjugation of the victim is of importance to this type of sexual killer; cruelty and infliction of pain are merely the means to effect subjugation.

The most notable classification system to date for serial murder and sexual homicide was developed by Ressler and colleagues (1988). They defined four categories of sexual homicide: organized, disorganized, mixed, and sadistic. Organized crimes are planned, conscious, methodical acts in which the victim is typically not known. Disorganized crimes are spontaneous, unplanned, acts often against a known victim. Mixed crimes contain elements of these two categories. Sadistic crimes are marked by the offender's satisfaction gained from causing suffering and pain through torture. This classification system has been expanded in the FBI's *Crime Classification Manual* (Douglas *et al.*, 1992), a pioneering work that seeks to classify all types of homicide, as well as arson and sexual assault, by motive.

Historical Background

Historical Case Examples

Serial homicide is not a new phenomenon. Gilles de Rais, a 15th-century French nobleman, is believed to have tortured, raped, and killed hundreds of children (Hickey, 1991). He practiced necrophilia on his victims, and also reportedly decapitated victims in order to later use their heads for sexual activities. Another serial killer from the 15th century, was Countess Elizabeth Bathory, who tortured and killed young girls. She also washed herself with their blood to keep her complexion fair (Hickey, 1991). In 16th century Germany, a "werewolf" named Peter Stubb murdered numerous men and women. He also raped, sexually tortured, and murdered a number of girls and women before cannibalizing them (Hill & Williams, 1967). Fritz Haarman, "The Ogre of Hanover," sodomized, murdered, and cannibalized scores of young boys in 19th-century Germany. Part of his sexual gratification may have been obtained from ripping out the throats of his victims (Holmes & DeBurger, 1985). Perhaps the most infamous of all serial murderers throughout history is Jack the Ripper. He terrorized England in 1888 by killing and mutilating five or six prostitutes. Similar cases have occurred in 20th-century England.

Evolution of FBI Research on Serial and Sexual Killers

Recognizing the need for national crime statistics in the 1920s, the International Association of Police formed a committee to develop a system of uniform violent crime statistics. The Uniform Crime Report (UCR) was the first official system developed for the classification of homicide in the United States. The UCR, prepared annually by the FBI in conjunction with the U.S. Department of Justice, presents statistics for crimes committed in the United States within a given year. Originally, seven offenses were chosen: murder, non-negligent manslaughter, forcible rape, robbery, aggravated assault, and the property crimes of burglary, larceny theft, and motor vehicle theft. Arson was added in 1979. The Uniform Crime Report provides information about age, race, sex of victims and offenders, types of weapons used, and situations in which the killings took place. There are no specific categories for serial or sexual murder in these statistics. Such crimes are placed under the rubric "Other motives or circumstances" or "Unknown motives" categories.

The FBI Academy's Behavioral Science Unit at Quantico, Virginia, first published a system for typing lust murder approximately 15 years ago (Hazelwood & Douglas, 1980). The typology delineated two categories, the organized nonsocial category and the disorganized asocial category. This early work on lust murder evolved into a programmatic effort to devise a classification system for serial sexual murder (Ressler *et al.*, 1988).

In the late 1980s, FBI Academy agents from the Investigative Support Unit teamed up with the Behavioral Science Unit to begin working on a crime classification manual. An advisory committee representing federal and private associations was formed. This endeavor was modeled on the format of the American Psychiatric Association's *Diagnostic and Statistical Manual of Mental Disorders (DSM)*, and covers the major crime categories of murder, arson, and sexual assault. Sexual homicide has its own section in the results of this collaboration, the *Crime Classification Manual (CCM)* (Douglas *et al.*, 1992). The other three major categories for homicide are Criminal Enterprise, Personal Cause, and Group Cause.

The purpose of the *CCM* is fourfold: (1) to standardize terminology in the criminal justice field, (2) to facilitate communication with the criminal justice field and between criminal justice and mental health, (3) to educate the criminal justice system and the public at large about the types of crimes being committed, and (4) to develop a database for investigative research (Douglas *et al.*, 1992). Efforts are under way to expand the classification of additional crimes. For example, a typology of interpersonal stalking has been proposed by Wright *et al.* (1996).

Epidemiology

The number of serial and sexual murderers currently operating in American society is unknown, and estimates vary (Egger, 1990). Many variables make it difficult to arrive at confident prevalence figures. For example, a percentage of serial murder victims are never identified as such. Serial murderers sometimes kill in different geographic regions, thus preventing the establishment of a connection between victims. Law enforcement may not detect the linkage between homicides, and at other times it is difficult to determine the sexual element in a homicide (Ressler *et al.*, 1988). And some offenders may escape apprehension altogether. As an illustration, the "Green River Killer" has killed as many as 30 victims in Washington state over the past decade, yet remains at large despite an intensive investigation that has cost millions of dollars. Thus, no interview can take place to help determine the crimes for which he is actually responsible. The linkage of deaths to one killer can be especially difficult to establish when the offender's modus operandi changes along with the geographic locations of his crimes. More readily identified is the killer who follows a consistent modus operandi in the same locale. For example, a serial killer has recently been identified in Miami (Staff, 1996). He has been targeting homeless female crack cocaine addicts in a poverty stricken area of the city called Mean Streets. The victims are beaten and set ablaze.

The FBI has calculated that there are about 35 to 70 of these killers active in the United States (Egger, 1990). Others place the number as high as 100 or more (Egger, 1990; Hickey, 1991; Holmes & Holmes, 1994; Wilson, 1988). As many as 3,500 to 5,000 Americans each year may be victims of serial killers (Holmes & DeBurger, 1988; Norris, 1988). Egger (1990) criticized this estimate as being too high, explaining that it is a gross misrepresentation of the available data on homicide.

Hickey (1991) estimates that there has been an almost 10-fold increase in the number of U.S. serial murder cases in the past two decades in comparison with the previous two centuries. Most serial killings are stranger-to-stranger crimes. It is hypothesized that the steady increase since the 1960s in the category of unknown motive murders, into which most stranger to stranger killings fall, reflects an increase in serial killings (Egger, 1990). Percentages for other categories of murder (e.g., intimate, family, and acquaintance killings) have remained relatively stable or dropped over the past few decades (Block, 1987). Critics of these figures reason that the prevalence of serial murder is stable, and the supposed increase is simply the result of enhanced reporting procedures by the media.

As of 1990, 47 U.S. states have had one or more serial killers active in their territory (Hickey, 1991). Only Hawaii, Iowa, and Maine are believed to have been spared. Serial murderers have been active in other countries as well (Holmes & Holmes, 1994; Jenkins, 1988; Myers, Recoppa, Burton, & McElroy, 1993; Smith, 1987).

Characteristics of the Offender

General Offender and Victim Findings

Different from other violent criminals, the great majority of serial murderers, as well as their victims, are white (Ressler et al., 1988). The offenders are generally male, less than 35 years old, and first begin killing in their 20s (National Center for the Analysis of Violent Crime, 1992b; Ressler et al., 1988). They typically commit their offenses while alone, although up to one third may have one or more partners. Although there have been a number of documented cases of female serial killers (Hickey, 1991), only equivocal evidence exists for there having been a female lust murderer (Holmes & Holmes, 1994; Myers et al., 1993). One possibility was Carol Wuornos; while working as a prostitute in Florida, she fatally shot five men during the course of having sex for hire with them.

Data on 222 classic serial murderers collected by the National Center for the Analysis of Violent Crime (1992b) revealed that the mean age of their first murder was 27.5 years, and their last murder 30.1 years. For the period of approximately 1960 though 1990, the Center identified 357 serial killers. Their careers spanned years on average, and they are responsible for or suspected of killing 3,100 victims, an average of 9 victims each. Sexual murderers sometimes commit their first sex killings as juveniles

(Myers, 1994). Indeed, Burgess and colleagues (1986) found that 10 out of 36 (28%) sexual homicide offenders first committed murder as juveniles.

Some serial killers are far more prolific in numbers of victims than this average of 9. Henry Lee Lucas, arguably the most prolific serial murderer in U.S. history, is reputed to have murdered more than 140 victims in the United States between 1976 and 1982, although this figure ranges from 40 to 600 victims (Hickey, 1991). Others give this distinction to Theodore Bundy, who by his own questionable report may have killed hundreds of young women.

Usually, serial killer victims share the characteristics of being vulnerable and easy to control (Egger, 1984; Levin & Fox, 1985). Young women, children, prostitutes, hitchhikers, and vagrants are frequently targeted (Egger, 1984). Favorite hunting grounds of serial killers include red-light districts, places where men engage in casual homosexual contacts, skid row areas, and college campuses (Jenkins & Donovan, 1987).

Most serial killers engage in some sort of sexual activity with their victims. This activity may include sexual intercourse, masturbation, necrophilia, or other acts. Unlike the average murder victim, serial homicide victims are often mutilated. Bite marks, even signs of cannibalism, may be discovered. Body areas commonly disfigured include the breasts, genitals, rectum, and stomach (Geberth, 1993). While firearms are the most common weapon in most murders, serial killers more often kill by such "hands-on" methods as mutilation, asphyxiation, strangulation, beating, or bludgeoning (Holmes & DeBurger, 1985; Ressler *et al.*, 1988). It is hypothesized that firearms are too impersonal, and do not allow the murderer to experience the psychosexual gratification he could otherwise obtain during a close-range, personal-contact killing. As in adult sexual murderers (Douglas *et al.*, 1992), Myers, Scott, Burgess, and Burgess (1995) found that use of a knife, being armed beforehand, and overkill (excessive trauma or injury beyond that necessary to cause death) was significantly more common in juvenile sexual murderers than in nonsexual murderers.

Another common characteristic found at the crime scene is evidence of bondage. Dietz, Hazelwood, and Warren (1990) noted that three quarters of a series of sexually sadistic offenders had used bondage with their victims. Also present in this sample were the use of staging, props, costumes, and sometimes a script to be followed for the sadistic activities.

Some offenders will arrange the victim's body apparently in an effort to shock discoverers of the crime (Douglas & Olshaker, 1995). Danny Rollings, the serial murderer who killed five college students in Gainesville in 1991, decapitated one of his victims, and then placed the head on a shelf so anyone coming into the residence would be startled on seeing.

Eckert, Katchis, and Donovan (1991), writing from the perspective of forensic pathology, provided a classification of sexually related injuries and deaths, one of which covers serial murderers. This work brings to attention the need to be careful of labeling a death a sexual homicide in the face of bondage, asphyxiation, anorectal injuries, or other signs of sexual aberrance. Some cases prove to be accidental deaths during consensual sexual activity, despite appearances to the contrary, such as the rare participant who dies during anal or vaginal fisting, or the victim of erotic asphyxiation.

In Hickey's (1991) review of serial murderers since 1795, 34 female offenders were identified, or 17% of his total sample. These women, generally in their early 30s, murdered an average of 11 victims each. Their killing careers lasted just over 9 years.

Many tended to fall into the "black widow" or nurse category. Unlike male serial killers, sexual gratification was rarely found to be an aspect of these women's crimes. Poisoning was the most common method of death for their victims, with money and "enjoyment" being the two most often cited motives. One example of a female serial killer was Nanny Doss, the "Giggling Grandma," who apparently took pleasure in killing people. Over a two-decade killing career, she used rat poison and arsenic to kill four husbands, her mother, two sisters, two children, and two other relatives.

Organized Versus Disorganized Crimes

The organized versus disorganized crime scene characterization of sexual homicide offenders is a useful concept in understanding these crimes (Ressler, Burgess, Douglas, Hartman, & D'Agostino, 1986). The organized crime scene reveals a well-planned and executed act, as distinguished from the spontaneous, chaotic behavior evident at the disorganized murder site. When the time is right for the organized serial killer, and he has cooled off from his last homicide, he selects his next victim and proceeds with his plan. Conversely, the disorganized killer acts impulsively; a blitz attack may be used to overwhelm the victim. Organized murders appear to be nearly twice as common as disorganized murders. In a study by Prentky, Burgess, and colleagues (1989), crime scenes were significantly more likely to be organized for serial murderers than for single murderers (68% vs 24%).

The organized offender appears to take pride in his planning and staging of the murderous act and is typically driven by fantasy. In addition to premeditating the act, the organized offender is more likely to commit sexual acts with live victims, show or display control of the victim, use restraints, and drive to the crime scene. Disorganized offenders are more likely to perform sexual acts with the corpse, leave weapons at the scene, position the dead body, and possibly even keep it. Disorganized crimes more often exhibit depersonalization of the body. This refers to actions taken to obscure the identity of the victim, as through mutilation or covering of the face.

With time, the career of organized killers will sometimes drift toward more disorganized crimes. This may reflect growing confidences in their ability to avoid detection or an acceleration of their withdrawal into an idiosyncratic world further removed from reality.

Mobility Classification of Serial Murderers

Another feature of serial killers to consider is whether they are geographically stable or transient (Holmes & DeBurger, 1985) or, in Hickey's (1991) terms, "local," "place-specific," or "traveling." The geographically stable or local murderer lives and kills in one particular area, usually urban. An example of this type of offender is Wayne Williams, who murdered up to 30 young Black males in the Atlanta area over the course of 2 years before being arrested.

John Wayne Gacy is an example of a place-specific killer, someone who carries out murders in one location, such as at home or a place of employment. He lured 33 young male victims back to his Chicago home where he tortured and murdered them. Many of the bodies were hidden in a crawl space under his home. Another example of the place-specific killer was registered nurse Terri Rachals. She was charged in the deaths of six surgical intensive care unit hospital patients in the 1980s, and was implicated in many other mysterious hospital deaths. Her murder method was to inject potassium chloride into her victim's intravenous line, causing cardiac arrest, supposedly to relieve their suffering (Hickey, 1991).

The geographically transient or traveling offender covers wide areas in committing his crimes. In the 1920s, serial killer Earle Nelson committed 21 murders in nine states and two countries, ranging from California to New York to Canada. Ted Bundy murdered people in at least six states, spanning the width of the country from the state of Washington to Florida.

Social Background Characteristics

In their study of 36 men who had committed at least one sexual homicide (four fifths had killed more than 1 victim for a total of 109 known murders, or an average of 3 victims per offender), Ressler and colleagues (1988) found that these men had the native intelligence to perform well in school, yet academic failure was the norm. The majority had to repeat elementary grades and did not finish high school. In addition, school failure was frequently mentioned by the men as an early fortifier of their sense of inadequacy. The men also had the ability to perform skilled jobs. In reality, however, most offenders had poor work histories in unskilled jobs, and only 20 had ever held steady jobs. Examination of performance behavior of these murderers reveals another paradox. Despite reasonably high intelligence and potential in many areas, performance in school, employment, social relationships, and military service was often poor. In all of these areas, performance fell far short of potential.

The sadistic offender often will gain employment at jobs that have the qualities of offering control over others or connections with suffering and death. Work as a security guard, or at hospitals, correctional facilities, mortuaries, and butcher shops can fill this niche (Holmes & DeBurger, 1985). Relatedly, a history of extreme cruelty to animals is common; a strong interest in horror movies, violent pornography, weapons, and police paraphernalia is also common.

In an interesting study with offenders in England, Grubin (1994) compared those who had committed sexual murders with rapists. One of the most robust findings he discovered was the social isolation and lack of sexual relationships in the sexual murderers. Even as children, many of them had experienced trouble fitting into peer groups.

Most sexual murderers are heterosexual, but sexual dysfunction, discomfort with ordinary sexual relations, and paraphilias of a nonsadistic nature (i.e., voyeurism, fetishism, exhibitionism, transvestism) are frequently present (Gratzer & Bradford, 1995; Prentky, Burgess, *et al.*, 1989: Ressler *et al.*, 1988). Prentky, Burgess, and colleagues (1989), in comparing serial sexual murderers with sexual murderers who committed only one offense, found that the former had significantly higher paraphilias, especially fetishism and cross-dressing. In another study of sexual homicide offenders, more than three quarters of the group rated pornography as their top sexual interest (Burgess *et al.*, 1986). A high rate of paraphilias in sexually sadistic offenders appears to be common.

Etiology

There is as yet no clear answer to what causes a person to commit serial or sexual homicide. Theories addressing this question offer sociocultural, psychologic, psychodynamic, and biological explanations (Hickey, 1991).

From a sociocultural perspective, a number of investigators who have studied serial murder cases believe that violent pornography may be contributory in the vulnerable. (Douglas & Olshaker, 1995). Others feel that the widespread societal bombardment by and acceptance of mass media violence plays a role in sexual violence. Inundation by violence and the devaluation of life, with the resultant message that violence is acceptable, seems to create a climate of apathy in society. This in turn may lower individuals' resistance to aggressive and sexual drives. Ted Bundy, shortly before his execution, pointed to media violence and pornography as spawning his career of murder.

The acts of the serial killer can be viewed as compulsive behavior. Revitch (1980) described the need to commit the sexually murderous act as compelling and likely to be repeated. Resisting this need purportedly brings on severe anxiety in the offender, akin to the feeling that those with obsessive-compulsive disorder experience when their compulsions are blocked. Other types of sexual offenses also have been described by some as a compulsive disorder.

Liebert (1985) offered a psychodynamic explanation for serial murder, noting that most killers of this type have a borderline or narcissistic personality structure. The destructive elements of the early mother–child relationship remain in the unconscious. These aggressive, dissociated elements are eventually split from the self and projected onto the female victim. In another psychodynamic view, Weinshel and Calet (1972) hypothesized that the mutilations associated with serial killing represent a wish to reenter and explore the mother's womb.

There is a modicum of literature on the biological basis of sexual and serial killers. Money (1990) looks at this behavior as a disease. The diseased brain is postulated to send messages of attack along with messages of sexual arousal and mating behavior simultaneously, perhaps in a fashion similar to the psychomotor seizures in temporal lobe epilepsy. No studies have examined the role of hormones and neurotransmitters in sexual killers. One study found that subjects who had killed a sexual partner had significantly lower cerebrospinal fluid levels of 5-HIAA, a metabolite of serotonin (Lidberg, Tuck, Asberg, Scalia-Tomba, & Bertilsson, 1985). There are scattered case reports in which sexual homicide perpetrators are found to have histories of serious head trauma and abnormalities on CT head scans, EEGs, and neuropsychological testing. However, such findings are nonspecific and common in other populations of nonsexual murderers.

Role of Fantasy

A relatively consistent psychological finding in many studies of serial and sexual murderers is the presence of violent fantasy. This is believed to play a critical role in these types of crimes (Brittain, 1970; MacCulloch, Snowden, Wood, & Mills, 1983; Ressler *et al.*, 1988).

Prentky, Burgess, and colleagues (1989), in examining the role of fantasy, compared serial sexual killers with subjects who had killed a single victim. Significantly more serial murderers had violent fantasies (86% vs. 23%). Classical conditioning may help explain the power of fantasy in serial murders. Many sexual murderers are believed to masturbate to sexually sadistic themes (MacCulloch *et al.*, 1983). As with other sexual offenders, it is hypothesized that the selective reinforcement of deviant fantasies through paired association with repeated masturbation contributes to sexual homicide, particularly the organized type.

MacCulloch and colleagues (1983) evaluated the presence of sadistic fantasy in 16 forensic hospital patients with psychopathic personality disorder who had committed violent sexual crimes. Most of these offenders' crimes were specifically linked to preceding fantasies. Progressively more sadistic behavioral "try-outs" linked to fantasy were conducted by these offenders, stopping only when they were apprehended.

Burgess and colleagues (1986) advanced a motivational model for sexual homicide based on the role of fantasy. Five factors in this model include impaired early attachments, early psychologic trauma, patterned responses that generate fantasy, a violent fantasy life, and a "feedback filter" that nourishes repetitive thinking patterns. In this study, many of the murderers described the central role of fantasy in their early development, expressed in part through a variety of paraphilias. When asked to rank their sexual interests, the highest ranking activity was pornography (81%), followed by compulsive masturbation (79%), fetishism (72%), and voyeurism (71%). These fantasies were often violent and sadistic in nature. Twenty offenders had rape fantasies prior to the age of 18, and 7 of these men acted out these fantasies within a year of being consciously aware of them. There was evidence of physical and sexual abuse in nearly half of the killers and a higher percentage of emotional neglect. In general, it is interesting to note the isolated pattern of these deviant sexual expressions. The men seemed either to engage in paraphilias that were solitary in practice or in sexually violent activities, neither of which reflected any degree of interpersonal contact.

In addition, when questioned about the murders themselves and their preparations for the murders, the men identified the importance of fantasy in the crimes. After the first murder, the men found themselves deeply preoccupied and sometimes stimulated by the memories of the act, all of which contributed to and nurtured fantasies about subsequent murders.

One begins to see how an early pattern used to cope with a markedly deficient and abusive family life might turn a child away from that reality and into his own private world of violence where he can not only exert control, but can exact retribution for the physical and emotional injuries inflicted on him. The control evidenced in these fantasies appears to be crucial not only to the child, but later to the adult. Importantly, these are not fantasies of escape to a better life, as one often sees in children recovering from sexual assaults and abusive treatment. These men did not compensate by retreating to a fantasy world in which love reigned and abuse was unheard of. Rather, their fantasies were fueled by feelings of aggression and mastery over those who were abusing them, suggesting a projected repetition of their own abuse and identification with the aggressor. As one murderer put it, "Nobody bothered to find out what my problem was and nobody knew about the fantasy world."

Family Patterns

It is often argued that the structure and quality of family interaction is an important factor in the development of a child, especially in the way the child perceives family members and their interaction with him (and with each other). For children growing up, the quality of their attachments to parents and other members of the family is critical to how these children relate to and value other members of society. From developmental and social learning perspectives, these early life attachments evolve into detailed architectural plans for how the child will interact with his or her world.

In a study of 81 sexual offenders (54 rapists and 27 child molesters) incarcerated at the Massachusetts Treatment Center (Prentky *et al.*, 1989), three noteworthy findings were obtained. First, sexual and nonsexual aggression in adulthood each were related to distinct aspects of developmental history. Specifically, caregiver inconstancy and sexual deviation in the family were related to the amount of sexual aggression, whereas childhood and juvenile institutional history and physical abuse and neglect were associated with the amount of nonsexual aggression. Second, contrary to previous studies of other criminal populations, the amount of aggression rather than the frequency of crimes was predicted by developmental history. Third, the presence of caregiver inconsistency and family sexual deviation accounted for 87.5% of all cases of extreme sexual aggression in adulthood. The presence of an institutional history and physical abuse and neglect accounted for 81.2% of all cases of extreme nonsexual aggression in adulthood. Results of this study suggest that the quality of early interpersonal attachments and the experience of sexual abuse as a child may be important to understanding sexual aggression in adulthood. Given these rather compelling findings, we were especially interested in looking at factors that best addressed level of interpersonal attachment in a sample of serial murderers.

Data from the most extensive study to date on sexual murderers reveal multiple problems in the family histories of the 36 who were studied (Ressler *et al.*, 1986). For example, one half of the offenders' families had members with criminal histories and over one half of the families had members with psychiatric problems, suggesting, at the very least, inconsistent contact between some family members and the offender as a child. In addition, however, there was evidence of irresponsible and maladaptive parenting in a large number of cases. Nearly 70% of the families had histories of alcohol abuse, and one third of the families had histories of drug abuse. Sexual deviance among family members was present or suspected in almost half of the cases. Abuse of these subjects was also prevalent, as 74% had been emotionally abused, 42% physically abused, and 43% sexually abused. Thus, the likelihood that these offenders experienced a high quality of family life as children is remote.

When examining the child-rearing patterns described by the murderers, one is most impressed by the high degree of family instability and by the poor quality of attachment among family members. Only one third of the men reported growing up in one location. The majority said they experienced occasional instability, and six reported chronic instability or frequent moving. More than 40% lived outside the family (e.g., in foster homes, state homes, detention centers, mental hospitals) before age 18. Twenty-five of the men for whom data were available had histories of early psychiatric difficulties. In general, these families were bereft not only of internal or nuclear attachments, but external or community attachments as well. Consequently, the children in these families had no opportunities to develop stable, healthy attachments within the community, thus reducing the child's opportunities to develop positive, stable relationships outside the family, relationships that might otherwise have compensated for family instability.

These data suggest that most of the 36 murderers, as children, had little or no attachment to family members. Further, they felt a high degree of uninvolvement with their fathers, ambivalence toward their mothers, and little attachment to siblings. Their parents were preoccupied with their own problems of substance abuse, psychiatric disturbance, and criminality. They tended to engage in aberrant sexual behavior and often argued and fought with each other. Although the parents offered little constructive guidance, it appears that they did offer ample role modeling of deviant behavior.

Revitch (1980) also pointed out the presence of disturbed family functioning in sexually violent men, particularly centered around the mother. Such problems as maternal overprotection, infantilization, seductive behaviors toward the son, and even outright rejection of the son were noted. Maternal promiscuity, real or not, and a cold, distant, authoritarian, and punitive father are also cited as contributory factors (Brittain, 1970; Revitch, 1980).

Assessment and Diagnosis

In any criminal assessment, the interviewer must assess the intelligence of the offender in order to begin to make sense of who they are and what their unlawful actions represent. Certain studies have shown that the majority of serial killers have an average to superior level of intelligence (Burgess *et al.*, 1986; Prentky, Burgess, *et al.*, 1989). While organized serial murderers often have average to above average intelligence, disorganized sexual murderers tend to be below average in intelligence (National Center for the Analysis of Violent Crime, 1990). It has been suggested, however, that these offenders' ability to escape apprehension during their killing careers is a sign of cunning and deceit rather than intellectual capacity (Hickey, 1991).

Only about one fifth of serial murderers have had psychiatric treatment at some point in their lives (Hickey, 1991). Burgess and colleagues (1986), in their series of sexual murderers, found that 70% of them had undergone psychiatric assessment or institutional placement as children.

Diagnostic Issues and Findings

It is generally believed that most serial murderers are not psychotic. The point has been raised that if they were truly psychotic, then they would not have the mental resources to escape apprehension (Dietz, 1986). In an early study, Revitch (1965) diagnosed "clinical schizophrenia" in one fifth of 43 male gynocidal offenders, some of whom had committed more than one murder. However, schizophrenia covered a broader spectrum of psychopathology at the time of the study, and it is unlikely that these 9 offenders would meet *DSM-IV* criteria for schizophrenia. Psychotic symptoms seen in this population after arrest may often represent malingering rather than true psychosis.

Generally, mental health professionals diagnose serial and sexual murderers as psychopaths, with corresponding qualities of inability to feel guilt, evidence of callousness, and demonstrated irresponsibility, to name a few. Another common diagnostic finding in these offenders is sexual sadism, that is, the need to control others through domination, humiliation, or the infliction of pain to obtain sexual arousal (MacCulloch *et al.*, 1983): Levin and Fox (1985) explain that these murderers are usually sociopathic personalities without guilt who have a powerful need to control and dominate others: "Though their crimes may be sickening, they are not sick in either a medical or a legal sense." Clifford Olson, Canada's most notorious serial murderer, was sentenced to life imprisonment for the torture and killing of at least 11 male and female children. A personality assessment following his arrest was consistent with that of a typical psychopath (Hare, Forth, & Hart, 1989).

Occasionally the diagnosis of multiple personality disorder (MPD) will be raised in the serial murderer, and there may be an association between criminality and MPD (Coons, Bowman, & Milstein, 1988). Kenneth Bianchi, the "Hillside Strangler," killed at least 10 women in the Los Angeles area two decades ago, and attributed his actions to MPD. His clinical presentation of MPD was contradictory, the corroborating evidence was equivocal, and experts were split over his diagnosis (Watkin, 1984). Ultimately, the court did not accept the diagnosis of MPD. To date, there are no well-documented cases of MPD in serial murder, and the possibility of malingering in such cases must be seriously considered (Hickey, 1991; Orne, Dinges, & Orne, 1984).

Although several lust murderers equate their acts to overwhelming compulsions with repetitive, ritualistic features, and describe severe anxiety on attempts to resist these needs, these activities are not bona fide compulsions because the offender experiences pleasure from the sadistic behavior and he resists merely because it places his freedom at jeopardy if he is caught. Professionals with a more analytical approach have been prone to consider severe borderline or narcissistic personality disorders in these cases due to specific abnormalities in the personality functioning of these individuals.

Yarvis (1990) has brought attention to the point that research findings in the extant literature on the relevance of psychopathology in murderers are discordant and contradictory. For example, he noted that rates of psychosis range from 4% to 83%, substance abuse from 3% to 40%, antisocial personality disorder from 8% to 28%, dissociative reactions from less than 1% to almost 70%, and no psychiatric disorder from 0% to almost 90%. In his examination of 100 murderers, 10 were classified in the homicide-rape category. These sexual murderers were characterized by substance abuse (40%), all other diagnoses (40%), and no diagnosis (20%) on Axis I, and antisocial personality disorder (90%) on Axis II. This is consistent with the presumed high rate of antisocial personality and substance abuse in sexual murderers. Substance abuse may approach 50% in some samples of sexual murderers (Grubin, 1994; Ressler *et al.*, 1988).

Diagnoses in Juvenile Sexual Homicide Offenders

Myers & Blashfield (1998), and Myers, Burgess, and Nelson (1998) evaluated 14 incarcerated juvenile sexual murderers in an ongoing study using standardized psychological instruments, record review, and clinical interview. The sample's mean age at the time of the offenses was 15 years. All victims were female, and averaged 24 years of age. One half of the sample had violent sexual fantasies.

The most common *DSM-III-R* diagnosis present at the time of the crimes was conduct disorder (86%), bringing to light their preceding pattern of serious antisocial behavior. Personality disorders at follow-up (mean age 19) were common (62%) with schizoid, schizotypal, and sadistic personality disorder each found in roughly one third of the sample. A measure quantifying psychopathy, the Psychopathy Checklist—Revised (Hare, 1990), found the sample to score in the general range of incarcerated young offenders. The group tended to come from chaotic, abusive backgrounds, and all were having serious school problems at arrest.

Course, Prognosis, and Recidivism

Sexual murderers often have a history of antisocial behaviors as youths. Conduct disorder symptoms in adolescence, such as assaultiveness toward adults (84%), stealing (81%), and lying (75%), were noted in the study by Ressler and colleagues (1988). These antisocial behaviors continued into adulthood for many of this group, as assaultiveness toward other adults (86%), stealing (56%), and lying (68%) continued to be commonplace. Most serial murderers have a criminal history prior to their commission of sadistic acts, and nearly one half have committed other sex offenses (Hickey, 1991).

Once imprisoned, these offenders are often easy to manage. However, they may not fit into the prison population, and other inmates may regard them with contempt or disgust, making their safety from other prisoners' attacks an issue. Albert DeSalvo, the "Boston Strangler," was stabbed to death by another inmate (Levin & Fox, 1985). Jeffrey Dahmer, who killed 17 men and boys, met a similar fate in a Wisconsin prison when he was bludgeoned to death.

The serial murderer has a strong psychological need to have absolute control, dominance, and power over his victims. The infliction of torture, pain, and ultimately death is carried out to meet this need (Levin & Fox, 1985). A psychological structure supports this manner of thinking and feeling is believed to be deeply ingrained in their personalities. Personality disorders are "enduring patterns of inner experience and behavior that deviates markedly from the expectations of the individual's culture, are pervasive and inflexible, have an onset in adolescence or early adulthood are stable over time, and lead to distress or impairment" (American Psychiatric Association, 1994, p. 629). In conceptualizing the occurrence of serial murder within the framework of an antisocial, sadistic personality, one would predict them to be highly recidivistic. That is what we find. More than one serial killer has warned authorities that he would reoffend if released back into society.

Clinical Management and Treatment

There are different ways to think about the management and treatment of an offender who has committed serial or sexual murder. Initially, there is the management and treatment of the societal problem created by the offenders' crimes through law enforcement and the judicial system. Energies of various agencies are vigorously focused on apprehending the murderer as rapidly as possible due to the high risk of repeated offenses. Next, the campaign of the opposing attorneys' offices begins in trying to establish guilt or innocence, and sometimes legal culpability— the insanity defense. Upon sentencing, the sexual murderer will usually receive a maximum sentence, often life imprisonment or the death penalty. There remains little room in this process for the application of classical psychological treatments. Perhaps guilty of hyperbole, Liebert (1985) has postulated that no lust murderers are psychologically capable of intensive psychotherapy because of their inability for intimacy.

However, the occasional sexual homicide offender will receive a limited sentence in prison, and thus will be released back into the community with a significant portion of his life remaining. In fact, the majority of juveniles who commit sexual homicide will eventually be released (Myers, Scott, Burgess, & Burgess, 1995). Recidivism is a serious concern with regard to these offenders. Perhaps intensive community-based services, broader in scope and contact than parole measures, should be considered for the released sexual homicide offender to help lower the risk of recidivism.

Such "wraparound" care services that assist and monitor psychological, social, and occupational aspects of offenders' lives might be enlisted. Wraparound care has been used with limited early success with young sexual offenders released back to the community (Santarcangelo & Mandelkorn, 1995).

The Insanity Defense

A successful insanity defense for serial murders is a rarity. Even in cases where the defendant has a history of psychosis, and expert witnesses to testify to its existence, the court is rarely swayed (Jenkins, 1988, 1989). For example, Albert Fish, who murdered many children in the 1920s and 1930s, was diagnosed with paranoid psychosis (Jenkins, 1989). He was subsequently found sane and executed. Two others who may well have had paranoid schizophrenia, John George Haigh in 1949 and Peter Sutcliffe in 1980 (the "Yorkshire Ripper"), were found to be responsible for their actions (Jenkins, 1988). The difficulty for the defense team is in convincing the jury that the sadistic acts of murder are the product of psychotic thinking to the degree that the defendant did not know the nature and quality of his acts or their wrongfulness, or was unable to conform his conduct to the requirements of the law. It is especially difficult for the defense to prove an ongoing, consistent psychotic state in an offender who commits serial killings separated by long periods of time.

The National Center for the Analysis of Violent Crime

The National Center for the Analysis of Violent Crime (NCAVC), located at the FBI Academy in Quantico, Virginia, has been in existence now for over a decade. This organization seeks to assist law enforcement agencies confronted with unusual, bizarre, or repetitive crimes by providing expertise in the areas of research, training, and investigative support (National Center for the Analysis of Violent Crime, 1992a).

One component of the NCAVC is the Violent Criminal Apprehension Program (VICAP). This program receives and distributes criminal reports from the United States and other countries in an attempt to link murders committed by serial violent offenders. VICAP requires all homicides to be reported to the NCAVC where the data are entered into a computer system and cross-checked to see whether they match other reported homicides. To date, thousands of cases have been entered into the VICAP system.

Another component of NCAVC is the Criminal Investigative Analysis Program (CIAP). One of the functions of this subunit is criminal profiling, previously referred to by the term "psychological profile" (Douglas & Burgess, 1986). The profiling process seeks to identify major personality and behavioral characteristics of the offender based on crime analysis. These techniques require an in-depth knowledge of the "criminal personality," an area until recently researched partly by psychiatrists or psychologists (Yochelson & Samenow, 1977), who examined criminals in a psychological framework, or by sociologists and criminologists, who studied the demographics and social stratification of crime. Missing from these areas of inquiry were critical aspects of offender apprehension important to the law enforcement community. Thus, researchers with a law enforcement perspective began to shift the focus to the investigative process of crime scene inquiry and victimology.

Investigative Profiling

Investigative profiling is best viewed as a strategy enabling law enforcement to narrow the field of options and generate "educated guesses" about the perpetrator. It has been described as a collection of leads (Rossi, 1982), as an informed attempt to provide detailed information about a certain type of criminal (Geberth, 1981), and as a biographical sketch of behavioral patterns, trends, and tendencies. (Vorpagel, 1982). Geberth (1981) has noted that the investigative profile is particularly useful when the criminal has demonstrated some clearly identifiable form of psychopathology. In such a case, the crime scene is presumed to reflect the murderer's behavior and personality in much the same way as furnishings reveal the home-owner's character. The process of profiling involves evaluating the original act, crime scene specifics, victim characteristics, police reports, and medical examiner's autopsy results. Then, a profile is developed with critical offender characteristics and investigative suggestions based on construction of the profile (Douglas & Burgess, 1986). At present, there have been no systematic efforts to validate these profile-derived classifications.

Community Issues

There is also a need to develop ways to treat society for the negative impact serial murderers exert. From a practical standpoint, serial murders are extremely expensive for local and state governments. The financial burden of investigations and the subsequent trial and appeals processes easily run into millions of dollars. It is estimated that Ted Bundy's trial and appeals cost $9 million (Hickey, 1991). The costs of the legal defense alone for serial killer Danny Rollings was almost $1 million.

Then, there are the psychological effects of the serial murders on a community. It has been said that the community anxiety and excitement caused by the discovery of a serial murderer rival the risks of the murders themselves (Liebert, 1985). Herkov (1992), in an assessment of the psychological impact of a serial homicide on Gainesville, Florida, surveyed area resident adults and children (Herkov, Myers, & Burket, 1994) to determine the community's response to violent acts by a serial murderer. Over several days, the news was gradually released that the mutilated bodies of five college students had been discovered. Almost half of the residents reported moderate to severe disruption of their daily lives. One third felt panicked or frightened in the weeks following the murders. Many residents, adults and children alike, also experienced posttraumatic stress disorder symptoms, including an increased startle response, distressing thoughts, sleep difficulties, and trouble concentrating. Understandably, the most disturbed were female students living close to the murder sites. Of concern was the finding that a number of citizens purchased and began carrying firearms for protection; this certainly raised the probability of innocent people being maimed or killed by firearms in the hands of the inexperienced.

Case Study: Organized Sexual Homicide

Instead of going to school that morning, Skip got into his car and drove across town to the home of a female classmate. He was 17 years old and in his senior year.

He knew where this girl lived because they had carpooled with other students to several school functions in the past. Although they were only acquaintances, Skip knew that she would be home from school that day. She was recovering from an illness that had kept her out of school for 2 weeks already. He was also aware that her parents would be away at work that morning. In his coat pocket were several lengths of rope and a knife.

Upon arriving at her neighborhood, he parked his car around the block from her house so that his location would not be betrayed. He broke into her residence through the back door. Once inside, he cut the phone lines and checked to make sure that all the doors to the house were locked. He then headed toward the rear of the home where her bedroom was located.

He found her still asleep as he entered her bedroom. As he approached her, she startled. She resisted him as he came over to the bed, grabbed her breast, and tried to remove her nightgown. To gain her submission he began choking her with his hands from behind. He then informed her that she had better comply "or else." At this point, he attempted to bind her wrists with the rope he had brought, but the pieces were too short. However, she was lying there petrified with fear, so he abandoned his plan to tie her up. He then tore her clothing off and vaginally raped her. After the sexual assault, he was feeling nervous, and forgot he had brought a knife with him. He left her temporarily in the room, and warned her not to move. Out in the garage he found a suitable garden instrument and returned to her room. He then bludgeoned her to death.

Skip had been arrested twice before for sexual battery. These earlier crimes both occurred in his neighborhood. The first time, he grabbed a young girl's buttocks while she walked down a sidewalk in broad daylight. He did the same thing to an adult female a year later, although this time he grabbed the victim's breast. After the sexual homicide, Skip admitted to rape but not murder fantasies. Yet, he knew he would kill the victim, and felt a sense of "commitment" in his plans to go through with it while driving to the victim's home. When asked what drove him to decide to take her life, he responded, "Dead men tell no tales."

Summary

A review of the clinical and research literature on the crimes of serial and sexual murders suggests the importance of early detection and treatment of offenders, both juvenile and adult. Studies specific to sexual homicide suggest the importance of formative life events in the development of homicidal fantasies that are subsequently acted out. Further study is needed to determine clinical interventions that can assist in early detection and prevention.

References

American Psychiatric Association. (1994). *Diagnostic and statistical manual of mental disorders* (4th ed.). Washington, DC: American Psychiatric Association.

Becker, J. V., & Abel, G. G. (1978). Men and the victimization of women. In J. R. Chapman & M. R. Gates (Eds), *Victimization of Women*. Beverly Hills, CA: Sage.

Block, C. R. (1987). *Homicide in Chicago*. Chicago: Loyola University of Chicago.

Brittain, R. P. (1970). The sadistic murderer. *Medical Science and the Law, 10*, 148–207.

Bromberg W., & Coyle, E. (1974, April). Rape! A compulsion to destroy. *Medical Insight*, 21–25

Burgess, A. W., Hartman, C. R., Ressler, R. K., Douglas, J. E., & McCormack, A. (1986). Sexual homicide: A motivational model. *Journal of Interpersonal Violence, 1,* 251–272.

Cohen, M. L., Garofalo, R. F., Boucher, R., & Seghorn, T. (1971). The psychology of rapists. *Seminars in Psychiatry, 3,* 307–327.

Coons, P. M., Bowman, E. S., & Milstein, V. (1988). Multiple personality disorder: A clinical investigation of 50 cases. *Journal of Nervous Mental Disease, 176,* 519–527.

Dietz, P. E. (1986). Mass, serial and sensational homicides. *Bulletin of the New York Academy of Medicine, 62,* 477–491.

Diets, P. E, Hazelwood, R. R., & Warren, J. (1990). The sexually sadistic criminal and his offenses. *Bulletin of the American Academy of Psychiatry and the Law, 18,* 163–178.

Douglas, J., & Olshaker, M. (1995). *Mindhunter: Inside the FBI's Elite Serial Crime Unit.* New York: Scribner.

Douglas, J. E., & Burgess, A. E. (1986). Criminal profiling: A viable investigative tool against violent crime. *FBI Law Enforcement Bulletin, December, 55,* 9–13.

Douglas, J. E., Burgess, A. W., Burgess, A. G., & Ressler, R. K. (1992). *Crime classification manual.* New York: Lexington Books of Macmillan.

Eckert, W. G., Katchis, S., & Donovan W. (1991). The pathology and medicolegal aspects of sexual activity. *American Journal of Forensic Medicine and Pathology, 12,* 3–15.

Egger, S. A. (1984). A working definition of serial murder and the reduction of linkage blindness. *Journal of Police Science and Administration, 12,* 348–356.

Egger, S. A. (1990). *Serial murder: An elusive phenomenon.* Westport, CT.: Praeger.

Geberth, V. J. (1981, September). Psychological profiling. *Law and Order,* 46–49.

Geberth, V. J. (1993). *Practical homicide investigation: Tactics, procedures, and forensic techniques.* Boca Raton, FL: CRC.

Gratzer, T., & Bradford, J. M. W. (1995). Offender and offense characteristics of sexual sadists: A comparative study. *Journal of Forensic Sciences, 40,* 450–455.

Groth, A. N., Burgess, A. W., & Holstrom, L. L. (1977). Rape: power, anger and sexuality. *American Journal of Psychiatry, 134,* 1239–1243.

Grubin, D. (1994). Sexual murder. *British Journal of Psychiatry, 165,* 624–629.

Guttmacher, M. S., & Weihofen, H. (1952). *Psychiatry and the Law.* New York: Norton.

Hare, R. D. (1990). *The Revised Psychopathy Checklist.* Vancouver, British Columbia, Canada: University of British Columbia, Department of Psychology.

Hare, R. D., Forth, AE, & Hart, S. D. (1989). The psychopath as prototype for pathological lying and deception. In J. C. Yuille, M. A. Hingham (Eds) *Credibility Assessment.* Kluwer Academic Publishers.

Hazelwood, R. R., & Douglas, J. E. (1980). The lust murderer. *FBI Law Enforcement Bulletin, April,* 18–22.

Herkov, M. J. (1992). *Community reactions to serial murder: A guide for law enforcement* (National Institute of Justice Contract, Grant No. 90-IJ-R035). Washington, DC: National Institute of Justice.

Herkov, M. J., Myers, W. C., & Burket, R. (1994). Children's reactions to serial murder in a community. *Behavioral Sciences and the Law, 12,* 251–259.

Hickey, E. W. (1991). *Serial murderers and their victims.* Pacific Grove, CA: Brooks/Cole.

Hill, D., & Williams, P. (1967). *The supernatural.* New York: Signet Books.

Holmes, R. M., & DeBurger, J. E. (1985). Profiles in terror: The serial murderer. *Federal Probation, 49,* 29–34.

Holmes, R. M., & DeBurger, J. E. (1988). *Serial murder.* Newbury Park, CA: Sage.

Holmes, R. M. & Holmes, S. T. (1994). *Murder in America.* Thousand Oaks, CA: Sage.

Jenkins, P. (1988). Serial murder in England 1940–1985. *Journal of Criminal Justice, 6,* 1–15.

Jenkins, P. (1989). Serial murder in the United States 1900–1940: A historical perspective. *Journal of Criminal Justice, 17,* 377–391.

Jenkins, P., & Donovan, E. (1987). Serial murder on campus. *Campus Law Enforcement Journal, July–August,* 42–44.

Knight, R. A., & Prentky, R. A. (1990). Classifying sexual offenders: The development and corroboration of taxonomic models. In W. L. Marshall, D. R. Laws, & H. E. Barbaree (Eds), *Handbook of Sexual Assault.* New York: Plenum.

Levin, J., & Fox, J. A. (1985). *Mass murder: America's growing menace.* New York: Plenum.

Lidberg, L., Tuck, J. R., Asberg, M., Scalia-Tomba, B. P., & Bertilsson, L. (1985). Homicide, suicide and CSF 5-HIAA. *Acta Psychiatric, 71,* 230–236.

Liebert, J. A. (1985). Contributions of psychiatric consultation in the investigation of serial murder. *International Journal of Offender Therapy and Comparative Criminology, 29,* 187–200.

MacCulloch, M. J., Snowden, P. R., Wood, P. J. W., & Mills, H. E. (1983). Sadistic fantasy, sadistic behavior and offending. *British Journal of Psychiatry, 143,* 20–29.

Money, J. (1990). Forensic sexology: Paraphiliac serial rape (biastophilia) and lust murder (erotophono-philia). *American Journal of Psychotherapy, 44,* 26–36.

Myers, W. C. (1994). Sexual homicide by adolescents. *Journal of the American Academy of Child and Adolescent Psychiatry, 33,* 962–969.

Myers, W. C., & Blashfield, R. (1998). Psychopathology and personality in juvenile sexual homicide offenders. *Journal of the American Academy of Psychiatry and the Law, 25,* 497–508.

Myers, W. C., Burgess, A. W., Nelson, J. A. (1998). Criminal and behavioral characteristics of juvenile sexual homicide. *Journal of Forensic Sciences, 43,* 340–347.

Myers, W. C., Recoppa, L., Burton, K., & McElroy, R. (1993). Malignant sex and aggression: An overview of serial sexual homicide. *Bulletin of the American Academy of Psychiatry and the Law, 34,* 1483–1489.

Myers, W. C., Scott, K., Burgess, A. W., & Burgess, A. G. (1995). Psychopathology, biopsychosocial factors, crime characteristics, and classification of 25 homicidal youths. *Journal of the American Academy of Child and Adolescent Psychiatry, 34,* 1483–1489.

National Center for the Analysis of Violent Crime. (1990). *Criminal investigative analysis/sexual homicide* (FBI Report). Washington, DC: U.S. Department of Justice.

National Center for the Analysis of Violent Crime. (1992a). *1992 annual report* (FBI Report). Washington, DC: U.S. Department of Justice.

National Center for the Analysis of Violent Crime. (1992b, October). *Serial, mass and spree murderers in the United States: Search of major wire services and publications on offenders operating from 1960 to the present* (FBI Report). Washington, DC: U.S. Department of Justice.

Norris, J. (1988). *Serial killers: The growing menace.* New York: Doubleday.

Orne, M. T., Dinges, D. F., & Orne, E. C. C. (1984). On the differential diagnosis of multiple personality in the forensic context. *International Journal of Clinical and Experimental Hypnosis, 32,* 118–169.

Podolsky, E. (1966). Sexual violence, *Medical Digest, 34,* 60–63.

Prentky, R. A., Burgess, A. W., & Carter, D. L. (1986). Victim responses by rapist type: An empirical and clinical analysis. *Journal of Interpersonal Violence, 1,* 73–98.

Prentky, R. A., Burgess, A. W., Rokous, F., Lee, A., Hartman, C., Ressler, R., & Douglas, J. (1989). Presumptive role of fantasy in serial sexual homicide. *American Journal of Psychiatry, 146,* 887–891.

Prentky, R. A., Knight, P. A. Sims-Knight J. E., Straus, H. (1989). Developmental antecedents of sexual aggression. *Development and Psychopathology, 1,* 153–169.

Rada, R. T. (1978). *Clinical Aspects of the Rapist.* New York: Grune & Stratton.

Ressler, R. K., & Burgess, A. W. (1985). Violent crimes. *FBI Law Enforcement Bulletin, 54,* 1–31.

Ressler, R. K., Burgess, A. W., Douglas, J. E., Hartman, C. R., & D'Agostino, R. B. (1986). Sexual killers and their victims: Identifying patterns through crime scene analysis. *Journal of Interpersonal Violence, 1,* 288–308.

Ressler, R., Burgess, A. W., & Douglas, J. E. (1988). *Sexual homicide: Patterns and motives.* Lexington, MA: Lexington Books.

Revitch, E. (1965). Sex murderer and the potential sex murderer. *Diseases of the Nervous System, 26,* 640–648.

Revitch, E. (1980). Gynocide and unprovoked attacks on women. *Corrective and Social Psychiatry, 26,* 6–11.

Rossi, D. (1982). Crime scene behavioral analysis: Another tool for the law enforcement investigator, *The Police Chief,* 152–155.

Santarcangelo, S., & Mandelkorn, D. (1995). Wraparound care approaches for youth with sexual offending behaviors and their families. In C. R. Ellis & N. N. Singh (Eds.), *Children and adolescents with emotional and behavioral disorders: Proceedings of the fifth annual Virginia Beach Conference* (p. 141). Richmond, VA: Medical College of Virginia, Virginia Commonwealth University.

Scully, D. & Marolla, J. (1985). "Riding the bull at Gilley's: Convicted rapists describe the rewards of rape. *Social Problems, 5,* 344–362.

Smith, H. E. (1987). Serial killers. *Criminal Justice International, 3,* 1–4.

Staff. (1996, January 27). Miami may have new serial killer. *The Gainesville Sun,* p. 4B

Vorpagel, R. E. (1982). Painting psychological profiles: Charlatanism, charisma, or a new science? *The Police Chief,* 156–159.

Watkin, J. G. (1984). The Bianchi (L.A. Hillside Strangler) case: Sociopath or multiple personality? *International Journal of Clinical and Experimental Hypnosis, 2,* 67–101.

Weinshel, E., & Calet, V. (1972). On certain neurotic equivalents of necrophilia. *International Journal of Psychoanalysis, 53,* 67–75.

Wilson, P. R. (1988). "Stranger" child murder: Issues relating to causes and controls. *Forensic Science International, 36*, 267–277.

Wright J. A., Burgess, A. G., Burgess, A. W., & Lasco, A. T. (1966). A typology of interpersonal stalking. *Journal of Interpersonal Violence, 11*, 487–502.

Yarvis, R. M. (1990). Axis I and Axis II diagnostic parameters of homicide. *Bulletin of the American Academy of Psychiatry and the Law, 18*, 249–269.

Yochelson, S., & Samenow, S.S. (1977). *The criminal personality.* New York: Aronson.

Making Sense of Mass Murder

Jack Levin and James Alan Fox

Introduction

The execution-style murder of 14 family members by a rejected and controlling middle-aged man in rural Arkansas, the vengeful slayings of six coworkers by a disgruntled postal worker in a Royal Oak, Michigan, post office, and the indiscriminate slaughter of 23 customers at a Luby's Cafeteria in Killeen, Texas, by a gunman apparently gone berserk are dramatic examples of the large and growing number of mass killings that have captured the attention and anxiety of Americans over the past two decades. Mass murders or massacres—the killing of four or more victims during a single event—are both frightening and tragic. They are frightening because they could happen to anyone, anytime, anyplace. Unlike other crimes, they are as likely to occur in a suburban shopping mall as in an urban slum, as likely in a small southern town as in a big city. They are tragic because so many innocent people die.

Despite the widespread concern, however, mass murder has received very little attention outside the popular press. Indeed, there have been few systematic studies of the circumstances under which such crimes are committed or the conditions that give rise to them. In a review of the limited available literature, Busch and Cavanaugh (1986) suggested that quantitative studies are needed to draw valid conclusions about multiple murder. Indeed, their search through the literature produced only 11 clinical studies, 9 of which were single case histories.

Indeed, the psychiatric literature consists primarily of case studies and analyses of highly unrepresentative samples of multiple killers whose biographies are based on courtroom testimony and psychiatric interviews before trial; most of these psychiatric studies, furthermore, have focused on serial killings rather than on offenders who have committed massacres (see Banay, 1956; Berne, 1950; Bruch, 1967; Evseeff & Wisniewski, 1972; Galvin & Macdonald, 1959; Kahn, 1960; Lunde, 1976; by contrast, see Dietz, 1986).

Social scientists have similarly ignored the study of mass murder (for exceptions, see Fox & Levin 1994; Holmes & Holmes, 1994; Levin & Fox, 1985; Leyton, 1986).

Jack Levin • Department of Sociology and Anthropology, College of Arts and Sciences, Northeastern University, Boston, Massachusetts 02115. *James Alan Fox* • College of Criminal Justice, Northeastern University, Boston, Massachusetts 02115.

Handbook of Psychological Approaches with Violent Offenders: Contemporary Strategies and Issues, edited by Van Hasselt and Hersen. Kluwer Academic/Plenum Publishers, New York, 1999.

Some may have regarded massacres as merely a special case of homicide, explainable by the same criminological theories they have previously applied to single-victim murder. Others may have seen massacres as essentially a psychiatric phenomenon, apparently perpetrated by individuals who possess a severe mental disorder (i.e., psychosis) best understood at a psychiatric level of analysis.

Lack of attention to mass murder may stem in part from the difficulty in acquiring data. Most mass killers do not survive their crimes. Although they may leave diaries or notes that help us understand their motivation, most of the answers to our questions remain in doubt. Another reason for the paucity of research may have more to do with the immediacy with which these cases are closed by law enforcement. Unlike other forms of homicide, massacres generally do not pose much of a challenge to the police. A person who massacres is typically found at the crime scene, slain by his own hand, shot by police, or alive and ready to surrender. Finally, and perhaps most important, scholars may regard mass murder with some lack of interest because of a perception, not necessarily accurate, that mass murder is so rare that it is not a worthy research focus.

Patterns of Mass Murder

One of the purposes of this study is to examine systematically the characteristics and circumstances of massacres and to compare massacres with their single-victim and double- or triple-victim counterparts. In particular, we set out to test the hypothesis, often supported by psychiatric observation, that victims of massacres are usually strangers to their killer, who selects them on a random basis after he "goes berserk" (see Westermeyer, 1982). At the same time, we hope to determine whether massacres differ enough from single-victim homicides that they ought to be regarded as a distinct and separate phenomenon deserving of their own theoretical framework.

Our data set consisted of the Supplementary Homicide Reports (SHR) of the Federal Bureau of Investigation for the years 1976–1994 (Fox, 1996). These data include the age, race, and sex of offenders and victims, weapon use, victim–offender relationship, circumstances, and location for all homicides including those that involve multiple victims.

For an incident to be classified as a mass murder, the criminal homicide must have involved four or more victims. Furthermore, to concern ourselves with only those cases most closely representative of mass "murder," we removed any incident considered "manslaughter by negligence." Finally, we accepted into the study only those incidents where the motive underlying the crime was, in all probability, death to the victims. Thus, events occurring strictly as a result of arson, where the specific intent of the perpetrator may be to destroy property rather than lives, were also removed from data analysis. Even after removing incidents classified as arson, there remained a large number of cases with four or more victims in which the weapon was fire. So as not to distort the analysis by using cases for which the circumstance of arson may have been missed, we eliminated all cases in which fire was used. This will produce a small distortion in the prevalence of mass murder (as there are a few mass killers who specifically select fire), but the potential for large distortion by inclusion of cases in which the murder may not have been planned is avoided.

TABLE 10.1
Mass Murder Incidents, Offenders and Victims, 1976–94

Year	Incidents	Offenders	Victims
1976	24	27	105
1977	32	36	133
1978	19	25	84
1979	36	43	155
1980	29	45	124
1981	18	27	82
1982	30	36	143
1983	20	23	91
1984	21	23	114
1985	14	15	59
1986	19	25	91
1987	19	21	105
1988	22	26	96
1989	24	34	103
1990	22	33	89
1991	30	37	137
1992	28	42	121
1993	32	49	146
1994	17	29	70
Total	456	596	2048

We examined massacres in comparison with single-victim homicides and double and triple homicides. As shown in Table 10.1, the data set contained 456 massacres (i.e., simultaneous killings of at least four victims), involving more than 596 offenders and more than 2,000 victims for the period 1976–1994. The data revealed that, on average, two incidents of mass murder had occurred every month in the United States claiming over 100 victims annually. This suggests that the phenomenon of the massacre, although hardly of epidemic proportions, is not the rare occurrence that it is sometimes assumed to be.

Tables 10.2 through 10.5 display situational, incident, offender, and victim characteristics by type of homicide. Although these tables classify homicide type into single-victim, double-victim, triple-victim, and mass murder, we focus primarily on the differences between the two extremes, that is, single-victim homicide versus mass murder.

As shown by the situational data in Table 10.2, differences in season are modest, with mass murders more prevalent in summer (28.9%). More noteworthy is the fact that mass murders do not tend to cluster in large cities as do single-victim crimes; instead, massacres are most likely to occur in small town or rural settings (44.3% compared to 34.3% for single-victim incidents). The most striking differences are those associated with region. While the South (and the deep South in particular) is known for its high rates of murder, this does not hold for mass murder (only 30.9% of massacres but 42.1% of single-victim homicides occurred in the South).

Table 10.3 shows incident characteristics—weapon use, victim–offender relationship, and circumstance—by type of homicide. As one would expect, the firearm is the weapon of choice in mass murder incidents (77.6%), even more than in single-victim

TABLE 10.2
Situational Characteristics by Homicide Type

	Single murder (N = 343,111)	Double murder (N = 9,598)	Triple murder (N = 1,198)	Mass murder (N = 456)
Season				
Winter	24.3%	25.9%	26.0%	24.6%
Spring	24.3%	24.4%	25.8%	22.6%
Summer	26.5%	25.7%	24.1%	28.9%
Fall	24.9%	24.0%	24.1%	23.9%
Total	100.0%	100.0%	100.0%	100.0%
Urbanness				
Large city	39.0%	32.9%	28.5%	32.7%
Medium city	26.7%	25.0%	27.1%	23.0%
Small town	34.3%	42.2%	44.4%	44.3%
Total	100.0%	100.0%	100.0%	100.0%
Region				
East	17.5%	15.4%	16.1%	22.1%
Midwest	18.8%	19.6%	22.9%	24.6%
South	42.1%	37.9%	33.7%	30.9%
West	21.6%	27.1%	27.3%	22.4%
Total	100.0%	100.0%	100.0%	100.0%

TABLE 10.3
Incident Characteristics by Homicide Type

	Single murder (N = 343,111)	Double murder (N = 9,598)	Triple murder (N = 1,198)	Mass murder (N = 456)
Weapon				
Firearm	65.4%	79.0%	76.5%	77.6%
Knife	19.6%	12.5%	12.6%	11.3%
Blunt object	5.6%	3.5%	4.1%	3.6%
Other	9.4%	4.9%	6.8%	7.5%
Total	100.0%	100.0%	100.0%	100.0%
Victim/offender relationship				
Family	22.3%	28.0%	42.3%	40.1%
Other known	56.9%	51.9%	42.4%	38.6%
Stranger	20.9%	20.1%	15.3%	21.3%
Total	100.0%	100.0%	100.0%	100.0%
Circumstances				
Felony	26.2%	35.9%	33.8%	37.1%
Argument	53.5%	38.0%	30.8%	23.0%
Other	20.3%	26.1%	35.4%	39.9%
Total	100.0%	100.0%	100.0%	100.0%

crimes (65.4%). Clearly, a handgun or rifle is the most effective means of mass destruction. By contrast, it is difficult to kill large numbers of people simultaneously with physical force or even a knife.

Findings regarding victim–offender relationship are as counterintuitive as the weapon-use results were obvious. Contrary to popular belief, mass murderers infrequently attack strangers (21.3%) who just happen to be in the wrong place at the wrong time. In fact, 40% of these crimes are committed against family members. While it is well known that murder often involves family members, this is even more often the case in massacres.

The differences in circumstance underlying these crimes are dramatic. While more than half of all single-victim homicides occur during an argument between the victim and offender, it is relatively rare for a dispute to escalate into mass murder (23.0%). As suggested by the results, massacres are often committed to cover up other felonies (37.1%), for example, armed robberies. The largest category of mass murder circumstance is unidentified in this table primarily because of limitations in the SHR classification scheme. These crimes involve a wide array of motivations, including revenge, love and hate, as we discuss later.

Some of the most fascinating differences between homicide types emerge in the offender data in Table 10.4. Compared with those offenders who kill but one, mass murderers are far more likely to be male (93.8%), are more likely to be white (63.1%), and are somewhat older (36.7% are in their 30s or 40s and only 15.9% are less than 20 years of age). Typically, the single-victim offender is a young male, either Black or White, whereas the massacrer is more often a middle-aged White male.

Prevalence of older mass killers is especially pronounced among those who target family members or fellow workers. By contrast, the more indiscriminate slaughters

TABLE 10.4
Offender Characteristics by Homicide Type

	Single murder (N = 392,451)	Double murder (N = 12,248)	Triple murder (N = 1,490)	Mass murder (N = 956)
Offender age				
Under 20	20.2%	18.9%	16.6%	15.9%
20–29	40.6%	41.7%	37.7%	42.8%
30–49	31.0%	32.6%	39.8%	36.7%
50+	8.2%	6.9%	5.9%	4.6%
Total	100.0%	100.0%	100.0%	100.0%
Offender sex				
Male	87.0%	94.2%	93.1%	93.8%
Female	13.0%	5.8%	6.9%	6.2%
Total	100.0%	100.0%	100.0%	100.0%
Offender race				
White	46.5%	59.5%	60.2%	63.1%
Black	51.7%	37.2%	34.4%	33.3%
Other	1.8%	3.2%	5.4%	3.6%
Total	100.0%	100.0%	100.05	100.0%

TABLE 10.5
Victim Characteristics by Homicide Type

	Single murder (N = 343,111)	Double murder (N = 19,196)	Triple murder (N = 3,594)	Mass murder (N = 2,048)
Victim age				
Under 20	14.2%	18.7%	32.5%	34.3%
20–29	34.4%	32.0%	25.9%	23.7%
30–49	36.2%	30.9%	27.0%	28.7%
50+	15.2%	18.4%	14.6%	13.4%
Total	100.0%	100.0%	100.0%	100.0%
Victim sex				
Male	77.6%	64.1%	57.5%	57.4%
Female	22.4%	35.9%	42.5%	42.6%
Total	100.0%	100.0%	100.0%	100.0%
Victim race				
White	50.5%	65.9%	67.7%	71.5%
Black	47.5%	31.1%	27.9%	24.6%
Other	2.0%	3.0%	4.4%	3.9%
Total	100.0%	100.0%	100.0%	100.0%

often involve younger perpetrators, who may be driven more by profound mental disorder than by the long-term accumulation of situational exigencies. For these mass murderer data (table not shown), 54.4% of family annihilators are over 30 years of age, while 63.7% of mass killers of strangers are under 30 years of age.

The victim characteristics contained in Table 10.5 are, of course, largely a function of the offender characteristics just discussed, indicating that mass killers generally do not select their victims on a random basis. That is, for example, the victims of mass murder are usually White (71.5%) simply because the perpetrators to whom they may be related are White. Similarly, the youthfulness (34.3% are under 20 years of age) and greater representation of females (42.6%) among the victims of mass murder stem from the fact that a typical mass killing involves the breadwinner of a household who wipes out the whole family—his wife and his children.

A Typology of Mass Murder

In an early typology of multiple murder, we (Levin & Fox, 1985) distinguished between family massacres, mass killings for profit, and slaughters motivated by sex or sadism (most of which were serial killings). Besides the obvious fact that this classification scheme includes both serial and mass killings, more importantly, it confounds victim–offender relationship with motive.

We propose the revised and enhanced typology of exclusively mass murder, shown in Table 10.6, based on motivation alone. This typology presents four major forms of motive, the most predominant of which is subdivided into three subcategories. These types, furthermore, are distinguished and compared in terms of vic-

TABLE 10.6
Mass Murder Typology

Type of Mass Murder	Known victim	Planned	Random	Psychotic
		Characteristics		
Revenge				
Individual-specific	Y	Y	N	N
Category-specific	N	Y	N	M
Nonspecific	N	Y	Y	Y
Love	Y	Y	N	N
Profit	M	Y	Y	N
Terror	N	Y	N	N

Y = Typically Yes; M - Maybe; N = Typically No

tim–offender relationship, degree of planning and randomness, and state of mind of the perpetrator.

Most mass killings are motivated by revenge against either specific individuals, particular categories or groups of individuals, or society at large. Most commonly, the mass murderer seeks to get even with his estranged wife and all her children or the boss and all his employees.

As an attempt to explain family annihilation, Frazier (1975) has identified the phenomenon of "murder by proxy" in which family members are victimized because they are associated with a primary target of revenge. According to this view, a husband-father may murder all of his children because he perceives them to be an extension of his estranged spouse.

This notion can be applied to understand the motivation underlying crimes perpetrated by R. Gene Simmons, who in 1987 massacred his entire family, including infants and young children. Simmons hoped to even the score against his wife and an older daughter, with whom he had had an incestuous relationship, because they both had rejected him.

The concept of murder by proxy can be generalized to crimes outside the family setting, particularly the workplace. For example, on the fateful day when former pressman Joseph Wesbecker showed up at work to get even, the boss was out of town, but there were still plenty of his subordinates around. Seeing other employees as an extension of management, Wesbecker murdered them as revenge against the Standard Gravure printing plant. In a sense, Wesbecker was trying "to kill the company" in the same way that an estranged husband-father may kill the family.

Both these crimes involve specific victims chosen for specific reasons. Some revenge mass killings are motivated by a grudge against an entire category of individuals, such as all Blacks, all women, or all Southeast Asians, who are viewed as responsible for the killer's difficulties in life. He seeks to get even, not with specific people whom he knows, but with anyone who fits his single criterion for hate. In fact, these are hate crimes (Levin & McDevitt, 1993).

In 1989, for example, antifeminism ignited Marc Lepine's murderous rampage at the University of Montreal, which resulted in the violent deaths of 14 female students. Twenty-five-year-old Lepine blamed feminists for all of his woes, including his inability to gain admission to the highly respected engineering program at the university. Rather than "staying in the kitchen where they belonged," these "overambitious and aggressive women" had the audacity to take *his* seat in the class.

A few revenge-motivated mass murders arise from the killer's paranoid view of society. He suspects that there is a complex and expansive web of conspiracy involving family, friends, and strangers who wish him harm and are out to get him. Thirty-five-year-old George Hennard, for example, imagined that the whole world was against him. Unlike Marc Lepine's somewhat focused disdain, Hennard hated all of humanity—men and women alike. In October 1991, Hennard crashed his pickup truck through the plate glass window of the Luby's Cafeteria in Killeen, Texas, and indiscriminately fired on lunchtime customers, killing 23, before taking his own life.

As shown in Table 10.6, the more specific and focused the element of revenge, the more likely that the outburst is planned and methodical rather than spontaneous and random. Also, the more specific the targets of revenge, the less likely it is that the killer's rage stems from the extreme mental illness known as psychosis.

At one extreme, R. Gene Simmons's crime spree was a cold-blooded execution, which he had been planning for 6 months. After killing his 14 family members, he toured the town of Russellville, Arkansas, seeking out former bosses and a woman who had spurned his romantic advances—in his words, "all those who had hurt me." Far from psychotic, Simmons was declared sane and rational by several court-appointed psychiatrists. Indeed, Simmons was disillusioned, despondent, disappointed, and dejected, but hardly deranged.

James Oliver Huberty, known for his 1984 massacre of 21 people in a McDonald's restaurant in San Ysidro, California, represents the other extreme. Bitter and fed up with life after having lost his job as a security guard at a nearby apartment complex, Huberty babbled to his wife that he was going hunting, walked into the McDonald's, and shot indiscriminately at customers, employees, and pedestrians—anything or anybody that moved. Huberty had been experiencing extreme psychological problems, including hallucinations. He may not have even known that he was killing people.

Whereas most mass murders are motivated by hate, whether or not directed at specific targets, a few family massacrers are inspired to kill by a warped sense of love, essentially what Frazier (1975) describes as "suicide by proxy." Typically, a husband-father is despondent over the fate of the family unit and takes not only his own life, but also those of his children and sometimes his wife, in order to save them all from pain and suffering.

For example, by May 1990, Hermino Elizalde, described by friends as a devoted father, had become hopelessly despondent over his recent firing from his job as a welder's helper and deeply concerned that his estranged wife might take custody of his five children. Rather than losing his beloved children, he decided to keep them together at all cost . . . at least spiritually. According to police, Elizalde said he would rather kill his children than "let them go." Before taking his own life, Elizalde doused his sleeping children with gasoline and set them afire one at a time. When he was sure they were dead, he set himself on fire. By killing them all, Elizalde felt assured that they would be reunited in a better life after death.

As illustrated in the case of Elizalde, the mass killer motivated by love knows his victims well; in fact, they are his family. As in cases of suicide generally, suicide by proxy should not be assumed to result from insanity. The killer may be depressed or despondent, but not necessarily deranged. He feels personal responsibility for the well-being of his children and sees no other way out of their predicament.

We should note that many cases of family mass murder appear to involve at least some degree of ambivalence between hate or revenge, on the one hand, and love or devotion, on the other. Even where the motivation is apparently love, as in the case of Hermino Elizalde, one can still find a shred of anger directed against the victims. Elizalde may have sought to keep his family together in the hereafter, but he also chose an extremely painful method for killing them (i.e., fire).

Similar mixed feelings can be seen in the 1991 case of 39-year-old James Colbert of Concord, New Hampshire, who kissed his wife after strangling her. He said that he loved her, but could not stand to see her with another man. In his words, "She's not going to take my kids away. We're all going to die tonight." Colbert made the sign of the cross over his three daughters before killing them, too. Planning to commit suicide, Colbert reasoned that he was doing his children a favor. In this way, they would not have to grow up without parents.

Unlike mass murder for revenge and love, the last two forms of mass killing are more instrumental than expressive. Some mass murders are committed for profit. Specifically, they are designed to eliminate witnesses to a crime, usually robbery. For example, in 1983, three men crashed the Wah Mee Club in Seattle's Chinatown, robbed each patron, and then methodically executed all 13 victims by shooting them in the head. Although still unsolved, robbery clearly appears to be the motive in the 1993 massacre of seven employees of the Brown's Chicken restaurant in Palatine, Illinois, a suburb of Chicago.

Some instrumental massacres can be interpreted as terrorist acts in which the assailants attempt to "send a message" through violence. In August 1969, Charles Manson and his followers scrawled the message "Death to Pigs" in blood on the walls of actress Sharon Tate's Beverly Hills home, in the hope of precipitating a war between Blacks and Whites. Similarly, in 1978, the Johnston brothers of Chester County, Pennsylvania, reinforced their multimillion-dollar family crime ring by executing those gang members they suspected would snitch to a federal grand jury investigating their operations. To the many remaining gang members, the message was clear: "Be disloyal and the same thing will happen to you." There was, of course, an element of profit in the Johnston brothers' crime ring, but their central objective in murdering gang members was to create terror, that is, to remind everyone of just how powerful they were.

Both forms of instrumental mass murder—that for profit and that for terror—are clearly well planned by perpetrators who know exactly what they are doing. They differ, however, in whether the victims are chosen with purpose in mind. Terrorist acts generally require victim selection that is sure to make the point. For example, Manson's choice of wealthy and famous victims maximized the publicity that the crimes would receive.

Factors Contributing to Mass Murder

Most people stereotype the mass murderer as someone who suddenly "goes berserk" or "runs amok." They may recall James Huberty, the unemployed security guard who strolled into a McDonald's restaurant and fatally gunned down 21 victims at random. They may think of Pat Sherrill, who killed 14 fellow postal employees in

Edmond, Oklahoma, in 1986. Those old enough to remember may think of Charles Whitman, the ex-marine who in 1966 opened fire from atop a tower on the campus at the University of Texas, killing 14 and wounding 30 others; or they may think of Howard Unruh, a former World War II hero who, in 1949, wandered down a street in Camden, New Jersey, killing 13 people in 13 minutes.

Fortunately, these sudden, seemingly episodic and random incidents of violence are as unusual as they are extreme. As we have discussed, most mass killers have clear-cut motives, such as profit or revenge, and their victims are specially chosen, not just because they are at the wrong place at the wrong time. Thus, the indiscriminate slaughter of strangers by a "crazed" killer is the exception to the rule.

Why, then, would a 31-year-old former postal worker, Thomas McIlvane, go on a rampage in Royal Oak, Michigan, killing four fellow postal workers before shooting himself in the head? What would cause a 28-year-old graduate student, Gang Lu, to execute five others at the University of Iowa before taking his own life? Finally, why would a 55-year-old Missourian, Neil Schatz, fatally shoot his wife, two children, and two grandchildren before committing suicide?

The need to make sense of seemingly senseless acts of mass destruction has led some observers to examine simplistic biological explanations, as in the long-standing debate over the causation in the infamous Texas tower massacre (Lavergne, 1997). On August 1, 1966, Charles Whitman positioned himself atop the 307-foot tower on the campus of the University of Texas in Austin and opened fire on students below, killing 14 and wounding 30 more. Whitman's autopsy revealed a walnut-size malignant tumor of the brain, which has often been blamed for his "sudden episodic attack." As Valenstein (1976) notes, however, Whitman's violent behavior was anything but episodic or sudden. In fact, he had planned the massacre far in advance and had begun killing deliberately the night before the tower sniping. Moreover, no one can say with certainty what role the tumor may have played, because its location in the brain was obscured by the gunshots that ended his life. While the debate over Whitman's behavior may never be resolved, the assumption that the tumor was responsible is clearly not justified.

A similar and more recent biological controversy surrounds the role of the antidepressant drug Prozac in the 1989 mass murder at a Louisville printing plant by former pressman Joseph Wesbecker. On medical disability for chronic depression, Wesbecker had been taking the popular prescription medication for weeks prior to killing 8 employees and wounding 12 others. Surviving victims questioned in an unsuccessful lawsuit against Eli Lilly Pharmaceutical whether Wesbecker's actions were a side effect of Prozac. Of course, one must be cautious in attributing a causal role to any drug that is designed to combat major depression. More important, Wesbecker made several threats against a number of coworkers on his hit list long before he commenced taking the antidepressant.

Leaving aside the few cases in which biological factors may, by themselves, produce "out of character" episodic outbursts (see Fishbein, 1990), we believe that most acts of mass murder can be understood with the help of the six contributing factors shown in Table 10.7. These factors cluster into three types: (1) *predisposers*, long-term and stable preconditions that become incorporated into the personality of the killer, which are nearly always present in his biography; (2) *precipitants*, short-term and acute triggers, i.e., catalysts; and (3) *facilitators*, conditions, usually situational, that increase the likelihood of a violent outburst but are not necessary to produce that response.

TABLE 10.7
Factors Contributing to Mass Murder

Class	Factor	Explanation
Predisposers *(Both are necessary)*	Long-term frustration Externalization of blame	Failures at work, military, and home Tendency to blame others for problems
Precipitants *(Either is necessary)*	Catastrophic loss External cue	Loss of job or relationship Obedience to authority, or copycat behavior
Facilitators *(Neither is necessary)*	Social, psychological or situational isolation Access to weapon of mass destruction	Live alone, unable to share problems with others, cut off from support Training in and access to firearms

The first group of contributors predisposes the mass murderer to respond violently. These factors include *frustration* and *externalization of blame.*

The mass killer suffers from a long history of frustration and failure, concomitant with a diminishing ability to cope. As a result, he may also develop a condition of profound and unrelenting depression, although not necessarily at the level of psychosis. This helps to explain why it is that so many family and workplace mass killers are middle-aged; it takes years to amass sufficient childhood and adulthood disappointments that culminate in a profound and overwhelming sense of frustration. Forty-one-year-old James Ruppert, for example, massacred his 11 relatives in Hamilton, Ohio, on Easter Sunday, 1975, to avenge a lifetime of failure and disappointment. Ruppert had fared poorly throughout his youth in school, friendships, and sports, had lost his father at an early age, and had suffered from debilitating asthma and spinal meningitis. As an adult, he was so uncomfortable around women that he never experienced a sexual relationship, and was unable to hold a steady job.

Of course, many people who suffer from frustration and depression over an extended period of time may commit suicide without physically harming anyone else. Part of the problem is that they perceive themselves as worthless, and that they are in fact responsible for their failures in life. Their aggression is intropunitive, that is, turned inward.

Thus, an important precondition for frustration to result in extrapunitive aggression (that is, aggression turned outward) is that the subject perceives others to be blameworthy. As a learned response style, the mass murderer sees himself never as the culprit but always as the victim. More specifically, he externalizes blame; his problems are invariably someone else's fault. He reasons, "my boss is unfair," "my wife doesn't understand my needs," "my girlfriend doesn't appreciate my good deeds," "my coworkers take credit for my accomplishments," and "while we're on the subject . . . the whole stinkin' company is corrupt," "women are out to destroy men's rightful position in society," "immigrants are taking all the jobs," and "now the government wants to take guns away from all us decent, law-abiding, red-blooded Americans."

In January 1989, 24-year-old Patrick Edward Purdy murdered 5 children and wounded 30 others at the Cleveland Elementary School in Stockton, California. He intended to get even with those elements in society that he believed were responsible for his inability to get a decent job and to escape his impoverished lifestyle.

It is no accident that Purdy chose a school to carry out his plan of attack. In his way of thinking, society was corrupt and unfair to him. So, he targeted society's most cherished members, its schoolchildren . . . but not just *any* children nor *any* school. Purdy deliberately directed his anger at the Cleveland School, which had an overwhelming majority of students of Cambodian, Laotian, or Vietnamese descent. Purdy despised Southeast Asian immigrants, feeling that they were taking away the opportunities that he never had. Purdy also blamed, albeit indirectly, the teachers and pupils at the Cleveland Elementary School for his own miserable childhood. Ironically, he had spent an unhappy four years at the Cleveland School, from kindergarten through the third grade.

Given both long-term frustration and an angry, blameful mind-set, certain situations or events can precipitate or trigger a violent rage. In most instances, the killer experiences a *sudden loss* or the threat of a loss, which from his point of view is catastrophic. The loss typically involves an unwanted separation from loved ones or termination from employment.

For example, James Colbert of Concord, New Hampshire, killed his estranged wife and three daughters. Learning that his wife had started a new relationship, Colbert reasoned, "If I can't have her and the kids, then no one can." James Ruppert, by contrast, was about to be kicked out of the family house by his disgusted mother. She had repeatedly warned him to stop his drinking and pay his debts, or he would have to go.

Work-related problems are even more frequently found to precipitate mass murder. Just prior to his murderous rampage, for example, 31-year-old Thomas McIlvane was fired from his job at the Royal Oak post office and subsequently lost his appeal for reinstatement. Similarly, Joseph Wesbecker's employment problems came to a head when his request for an exemption from a particularly stressful task was denied, and he was forced to take long-term disability.

The disproportionate prevalence of men among mass killers, even more than among murderers generally, is in part because men are more likely to suffer the kind of catastrophic losses typically associated with mass murder. It is usually the husband-father who is ousted from the family home in the wake of a separation or divorce. Despite advances in the status of women, moreover, males more than females continue to define themselves through their occupational roles ("what they do" determines "who they are") and, therefore, have a greater tendency to suffer psychologically from the loss of a job.

In a few cases, external cues or models have served as catalysts for mass murder, even in the absence of some profound loss. Although the so-called "copycat" phenomenon is difficult to document scientifically, anecdotal evidence is suggestive. For example, the clustering of several schoolyard slayings in a matter of months—beginning with Laurie Dann's May 1988 shooting at a Winnetka, Illinois, elementary school and ending with Patrick Purdy's January 1989 attack in Stockton, California—suggests the possibility that mass killers inspire one another. A telling and tragic episode was the case of James Wilson of Greenwood, South Carolina, a "fan" of Laurie Dann. In September 1988, Wilson, much like his mentor, sprayed a local elementary school with gunfire, killing two children. When police searched Wilson's apartment, they found the *People* magazine cover photo of Laurie Dann taped to his wall. They also discovered from speaking with those who knew the gunman, that Wilson had talked about Dann incessantly. Finally, Joseph Wesbecker, although not himself a schoolyard sniper, was clearly influenced by one. After his workplace rampage, the police found at Wesbecker's home an 8-month-old news magazine opened to an article featuring Patrick Purdy's assault on schoolchildren in Stockton.

More powerful than media inspiration, charismatic authority figures can serve as catalysts for extreme violence. For example, members of the Manson "family" and followers of cultists Jim Jones and David Koresh were clearly inspired to kill by self-proclaimed messiahs. These "father figures" provided the excuse or justification for murder by making their "disciples" feel special and then convincing them that "death was love."

The final category of contributory factors consists of facilitators. Social, psychological or situational isolation as well as access to weapons of mass destruction are not necessary for mass murder to occur, but they increase both the likelihood and extent of violence.

Mass murderers are often characterized in the popular press as "loners." Many of them are indeed removed from sources of encouragement and guidance, from the very people who could have supported them through difficult times. Some mass killers have lived alone for extended periods of time. For example, Patrick Sherrill, who massacred 14 coworkers at the Edmond, Oklahoma, post office, had been living alone in his mother's home for 8 years following her death. Other mass killers move great distances away from home, experiencing a sense of anomie or normlessness. They lose their sources of emotional support. William Cruse had abandoned his roots in Lexington, Kentucky, to start a new life in Florida, where in 1987 he shot to death 6 and wounded 12 at the Palm Bay Shopping Center. After losing his job in Massillon, Ohio, James Huberty traveled thousands of miles to San Ysidro, California, as his "last resort," leaving behind his friends and relatives. When he lost his job there, too, he felt alone. There was no place to turn for support and guidance. Instead, he vented his anger through mass murder at the neighborhood McDonald's.

The isolation is not always physical. Although surrounded by family members, family killer R. Gene Simmons was also very much alone. He often retreated from his wife and children. Feeling like the "Commander-in-Chief" in the family, he simply could not share the burden of decision making or his problems with his "foot soldiers." For an authoritarian type like Simmons, it was "lonely at the top."

Finally, many Americans feel angry, hopeless, and isolated, yet they do not commit mass murder. Some simply don't have the means for widespread bloodshed. It is almost impossible to commit a massacre with a knife or a hammer. Such weapons are potentially destructive, but are not *mass* destructive. Mass murderers James Ruppert and James Huberty, for example, had particular expertise in the use of firearms and had assembled large collections of guns and ammunition. In his spare time, Ruppert went target shooting on the banks of a nearby river; Huberty practiced at his own firing range located in the basement. Moreover, both men were armed with loaded firearms at the very moment they felt angry enough to kill.

Summary

This study examined characteristics and circumstances of mass murder—the slaughter of four or more victims during the same episode. Using FBI homicide data for the years 1976–1994, we assessed patterns in 456 incidents of mass murder in the United States and compared them with cases claiming fewer lives. Overall, we found that the mass murderer tends to be a White male adult who methodically kills family members or other victims he knows well with a gun or rifle; by contrast, the single-victim murderer tends to be a young, Black male who is more likely to kill during an argument. A typology was also advanced in which motivations for mass murder are interpreted typically as revenge against particular individuals, against a particular category of individuals, or against society in general. In addition to revenge, other motivations include love, profit, and terror. Finally, we offered six factors that can be used to explain the often deliberate actions of the mass murderer. These include long-term frustration, externalization of blame, catastrophic loss, external cues, isolation, and access to weapons of mass destruction.

It is important to emphasize that none of the conditions or factors outlined here, even in combination, is sufficient to produce mass homicide. In other words, there may be thousands of Americans who fit the profile contained in the model but never kill anyone, let alone large numbers of people. Some of the inability of this six-factor model to predict or identify potential mass killers in a reliable way may stem, of course, from inadequacies in the model itself. Certainly, empirical research is needed to test, refine, or refute components of the model. The infancy of multiple murder research notwithstanding, however, we will likely never be in a position to apply explanatory models to the task of future prediction of this kind of homicidal behavior. The problem is one of false positives in predicting rare events. In a country of a quarter of a billion people, it is virtually impossible to predict incidents that occur only twice per month, no matter how advanced and sophisticated our understanding of mass murder.

References

Banay, R. S. (1956). Psychology of a mass murderer. *Journal of Forensic Science, 1,* 1.
Berne, E. (1950). Cultural aspects of multiple murder. *Psychiatric Quarterly, 24,* 250.
Bruch, H. (1967). Mass murder: The Wagner case. *American Journal of Psychiatry, 124,* 693–698.
Busch, K. A., & Cavanaugh, J. L. (1986). A study of multiple murder: Preliminary examination of the interface between epistemology and methodology. *Journal of Interpersonal Violence, 1,* 5–23.
Dietz, P. E. (1986). Mass, serial and sensational homicides. *Bulletin of the New York Academy of Medicine, 62,* 477–491.
Evseeff, G. S., & Wisniewski, E. M. (1972). A psychiatric study of a violent mass murderer. *Journal of Forensic Science, 17,* 371–376.
Fishbein, D. H. (1990). "Biological Perspectives in Criminology." *Criminology 28,* 27–72.
Fox, J. A. (1996). *Supplementary Homicide Reports, 1976–1994.* Ann Arbor, MI: Inter-University Consortium for Political and Social Research, Univesity of Michigan.
Fox, J. A., & Levin, J. (1994). *Overkill: Mass murder and serial killing exposed.* New York: Plenum.
Frazier, S. H. (1975). Violence and social Impact." In J. C. Schoolar & C. M. Gaitz (Eds.), *Research and the psychiatric patient.* New York: Brunner/Mazel.
Galvin, A. V., & Macdonald, J. M. (1959). Psychiatric study of a mass murderer. *American Journal of Psychiatry, 115,* 1057–1061.
Holmes, R. M., & Holmes, S. (1994). *Murder in America.* Newbury Park, CA: Sage.
Kahn, M. W. (1960). Psychological test study of a mass murderer." *Journal of Projective Techniques, 24,* 148.
Lavergne, G. (1997). *A sniper in the tower: The Charles Whitman murders.* Denton: University of North Texas Press.
Levin, J., & Fox, J. A. (1985). *Mass murder: America's growing menace.* New York: Plenum.

Levin, J., & McDevitt, J. (1993). *Hate crimes.* New York: Plenum.

Leyton, E. (1986). *Compulsive killers: The story of modern multiple murderers.* New York: New York University Press.

Lunde, D. T. (1976). *Murder and madness.* San Francisco: San Francisco Book.

Valenstein, E. S. (1976). Brain stimulation and the origin of violent behavior. In W. L. Smith & A. Kling (Eds.), *Issues in brain/behavior control* (pp. 43–48). New York: Spectrum.

Westermeyer, J. (1982). Amok. In C. T. H. Friedmann & R. A. Faguet (Eds.), *Extraordinary disorders of human behavior* (pp. 173–190). New York: Plenum.

11

Women Who Kill

Janet I. Warren and Jeff Kovnick

Introduction

Over the past 20 years, there has been a significant increase in the overall rate of crime attributable to women. In 1975, women were responsible for 16% of the crime that occurred in the United States; in 1994 they were responsible for 20% of the crime. This change has been attributed, by some authors, to the liberation of women over the past 30 years, women's increasing involvement in the drug culture, the growth of poverty among some segments of society, and the emergence of psychopathy in some female populations. Over this same period, however, the rate of murder perpetrated by women dropped from 16% in 1976 to 10% in 1991 (U.S. Department of Justice 1981–1992).

The 10% of murders perpetrated by women are substantially different in their interpersonal context than those perpetrated by men. While men are more likely to murder strangers or acquaintances in some type of instrumental altercation, women use lethal violence almost exclusively in the context of their intimate and familial relationships. They tend to murder their children, their lovers, and their spouses. As Rosenblatt and Greenland (1974) contend that "it is this very attempt to fulfill her culturally defined role as wife and mother on our society, which is often at the core of much of the violence" (p. 12).

In order to more fully understand this lethal violence, both as it most commonly occurs and its exceptions, three categories of murder are examined in some detail: (1) the killing of a child by the mother; (2) the killing of a spouse or partner; and (3) the less common forms of instrumental violence perpetrated by women against acquaintances or strangers.

Janet I. Warren • Clinical Psychiatric Medicine, University of Virginia, and Institute of Law, Psychiatry, and Public Policy, Charlottesville, Virginia 22908.   *Jeff Kovnick* • Department of Psychiatry, Neuropsychiatry Institute, University of Utah School of Medicine, Salt Lake City, Utah 84103.

Handbook of Psychological Approaches with Violent Offenders: Contemporary Strategies and Issues, edited by Van Hasselt and Hersen. Kluwer Academic/Plenum Publishers, New York, 1999.

Maternal Filicide

Alternative terms are used to describe the act of a parent murdering a child. Filicide is a general term for the killing of a child by his or her parent. Neonaticide, a term coined by Resnick (1969), refers to the killing of a child less than 24 hours old. Infanticide is a general term used in American research that generally refers to the killing of an infant (Bourget & Bradford, 1990). In British law, the Infanticide Act of 1938 refers to a mother killing her child under the age of one year by a "wilful act or omission." It implies a lesser degree of culpability in that the mother's mind "was disturbed by reason of her not having fully recovered from the effect of giving birth to the child or by reasons of the effect of lactation consequent on the birth of the child" (Infanticide Act of 1938). As the age of the child victim decreases, there is increasing likelihood that its killer is the parent (Jason, Gilliland, & Tyler, 1983).

Filicide has occurred throughout history and in a multitude of cultures. Archaeological evidence for child sacrifice dates to 7000 B.C. Infanticide was also well documented in ancient Rome and Greece. Children with congenital anomalies or who were otherwise weak were killed, both for eugenic reasons and so that they would not become a burden on the state. These practices were reflected in laws that treated these deaths differently from other types of killing. For example, early Roman law contained a doctrine called *patrias potestas*, which referred to a father's right to kill his children (Resnick, 1969). Only in 300 A.D. did Christianity, heavily influenced by Judaic law, begin to regard the killing of children by their parents as a crime. Still, under church and state laws, mothers who killed their newborns or infants received lesser sentences than did parents who killed older children (Kaye, Bornstein, & Donnell, 1990). In England from the 17th through the 19th centuries, there was frequent killing of infants by their parents. (Kellet, 1992). In the late 1870s, children less than one year old comprised less than 3% of the population, but represented about 50% of the murders (Rose, 1986).

Filicide is also culturally determined. Native Americans of the Mojave tribe regularly killed all mixed-race children at birth (Devereux, 1948). Eskimos also routinely killed infants with congenital anomalies and one child from sets of twins, thus improving collective survival when resources were scarce (Garber, 1947). Japanese girls born in 1966, the "year of the fire-horse," were thought to carry bad luck; the female neonatal mortality rate was 57% higher in that year than in the years before and afterward (Kaku, 1975).

Various investigators have developed classification schemes of filicide for the purposes of understanding motives, aiding in prevention, and assessing culpability for the crime. Resnick (1970), Scott (1973), D'Orban (1979), and Bourget and Bradford (1990) are major researchers who have offered slightly different classification schemes. By integrating these prior studies, we can identify five types of maternal filicide: neonaticide, mental illness, maltreatment, psychopathic killing, and mercy killing.

Neonaticide

Women who commit neonaticide fit the characteristic profile as defined by Resnick (1969) and confirmed by D'Orban (1979). The mother is usually young, unmarried, and financially dependent, but rarely mentally ill. The child is usually her first, and the mother is often in denial of the pregnancy throughout much, if not all, of her term. If not in denial, the mother typically tries to conceal her pregnancy. Frequently, the mother gives birth alone, fearing the stigma of being unmarried. The means of death are usually by drowning (in the toilet or tub), suffocation, exposure, or skull fracture, but the killing is rarely premeditated (D'Orban, 1979; Resnick, 1969). It can be anticipated that increases in teenage pregnancy, coupled with increases in drug abuse, may contribute to higher rates of neonaticide (Grayson, 1990).

Mentally Ill

This category includes filicidal women suffering from such psychopathology as psychosis and mood disorders of all etiologies, including those associated with postpartum onset. Rates of psychosis in filicidal women range from 16% to 88% (Daniel & Harris, 1982; D'Orban, 1979; Myers, 1970; Resnick, 1970). Women in this category are generally older, married, and tend to kill more than one child in a single incident (Bourget & Bradford, 1990; Daniel & Harris, 1982; D'Orban, 1979). The symptomatology that contributes to the killing is usually delusional. In some instances, the woman may feel persecuted by her children and believe them to have special powers of destruction (Daniel & Harris, 1982; Husain & Daniel, 1984). In others, the mother may kill out of a desire to save her child from a delusory fate (Myers, 1970). Depression is also related to filicide. Many depressed or psychotic mothers feel pathologically bonded to their children, believe that the children are extensions of themselves, and, as a result, may kill the children and commit suicide. In these instances, the suicidal mother believes the child cannot survive without her and, therefore, should not be abandoned, or that the world is heinous and hostile and that the child would be better off dead than left to suffer in life. Women in this category generally do not try to hide their deeds (D'Orban, 1979; Myers, 1970; Resnick, 1970).

Compared with children of other ages, children under 12 months are at particular risk for maternal filicide (D'Orban, 1979; Resnick, 1970). This coincides with the period when mothers are most likely to develop a postpartum mental illness. The incidence of postpartum depression is approximately 10% (Casiano & Hawkins, 1987; Harding, 1989), and its onset is typically 2 weeks to 1 year after delivery (Harding, 1989). It is characterized by all of the symptoms of Major Depression, as well as fearfulness, hypochondriasis, extreme self-denigration, and emotional lability. In addition, its etiology is multifactorial (Sturner, Sweeney, Callery, & Haley, 1991). Steiner (1990) noted that despite its incidence rate, postpartum depression is identified relatively infrequently, and suggested that this occurs for a number of different reasons. He observed that women and their families tend to believe that they should experience and express only happiness at having a child, and that families and friends often are preoccupied with the new baby and are relatively less attentive to the mother. Steiner adds that this disorder is also often mistaken for the more benign "baby blues." Postpartum psychosis, on the other hand, has an incidence of 1–2 per 1000 (Kendall, 1985). Its onset is usually from day four to one month after delivery (Hamilton, 1982). Symptoms are delusions, hallucinations, cognitive disorganization, delirium, agitation, and a markedly labile affect (Hamilton, 1982; Kaye *et al.*, 1990; Resnick, 1969; Wisner, Peindl, & Hanusa, 1994). The speed at which symptoms fluctuate and the unpredictable nature of its course has led one author to describe this psychosis as "mercurial" (Hamilton, 1989). The risk of recurrence with future pregnancies increases dramatically, and has been estimated to range from 20% to 50% (Hamilton, 1989; Harding, 1989).

Controversy exists over whether obsessions of wishing a child to be dead are a risk factor for filicide. McDermaid and Winkler (1995) reported on 11 cases of maternal filicide, 6 of whom were depressed and had some type of obsessional thinking. In only 1 of these cases was the obsession centered on killing the child. Button and Reivich (1972) reviewed the literature and reported on 36 mothers who had "obsessions" of killing their preadolescent child but had not carried out the act. They separated the mothers into three diagnostic groups and found that 14% had an "obsessive-compulsive reaction," 16% had depression, and 42% were schizophrenic. A recent study by Sichel, Cohen, Dimmock, and Rosenbaum (1993) reported on the retrospective review of 15 women who had postpartum onset of obsessive-compulsive disorder. All of the women had ego-dystonic intrusive thoughts of harming their baby and did not have concomitant compulsions. Sixty percent developed a secondary depression. None actually attempted to harm the child.

Child Abuse and Neglect

This category is composed of women who, without homicidal intent, kill their children as a result of impulsive rage or loss of temper. Some authors suggest including parental neglect in this category. Husain and Daniel (1984) found significant differences when comparing 8 mothers accused of filicide with 52 mothers accused of child abuse, all of whom had a pretrial psychiatric examination. In their sample, all the filicidal mothers were psychotic, had a past history of mental illness, rarely abused the children before they were killed, and, less frequently, had a childhood history of being abused themselves. In contrast, the abusive mothers had little history of mental illness but were previously reported for abusing their children and were themselves abused by their parents. Studies of mothers whose abuse eventually ended in their child's death found most of the women to be in their mid 20s, living in poverty, poorly educated, and married or living with another adult. Frequently, they have themselves been victims of spousal or parental abuse. The killing often occurs in times of high distress, such as financial strain, and may occur soon after a difficult reunion between a mother and child who have been separated (Husain & Daniel, 1984; Korbin, 1989; U.S. Department of Health and Human Services, 1995).

Condon (1986) reported on a phenomenon he termed fetal abuse, which is evidenced by a pregnant woman's physical assault on her abdominal wall or vagina, or her failure to protect the fetus from excessive alcohol or drug use. Fetal abuse is a likely antecedent to child maltreatment. A related phenomenon is the death of infants born to drug-dependent mothers. Some maternity hospitals have reported that, upon admission, up to 40% of mothers screen positive for drugs of abuse. These babies are at risk for death from abruptio placentae and from drug withdrawal (Sturner et al., 1991).

Related to maltreatment is the controversy currently surrounding SIDS death. In 1993, the U.S. Department of Health and Human Services issued the following definition of Sudden Infant Death Syndrome (SIDS): "The sudden death of an infant under one year of age which remains unexplained after the performance of a complete postmortem investigation, including an autopsy, an examination of the scene of death and review of the case history" (National Sudden Infant Death Resource Center, 1993, p. 15). In the United States, the rate of SIDS is 1.4 per 1,000 live births (Reece, 1993). Emery (1993) notes that 10% to 20% of SIDS deaths may be due to unnatural causes.

Since Steinschneider (1972) first described five cases of SIDS occurring in the same family, many have concluded that mechanisms responsible for the occurrence of SIDS could run in families. More recently, controlled studies have dispelled the notion that having one SIDS baby increases the likelihood that a sibling will die of SIDS (Reece, 1993; Wolkind, Taylor, Wait, Dalton, & Emery, 1993). However, there is still controversy not only over whether a propensity to die from SIDS is inherited, but also as to the actual prevalence of the syndrome itself. It has long been recognized that many children who purportedly die from SIDS may indeed have died from child abuse or other types of filicide. (Emery, 1993; Wolkind *et al.*, 1993). In 1994, 22 years after Steinschneider first reported that Waneta Hoyt's five children died of SIDS, Hoyt was convicted of the murder of those same children.

Neglect deaths can be due to a variety of factors, such as malnutrition, drowning in a bathtub, and dying in a house fire when a parent is absent from the home. The U.S. Advisory Board on Child Abuse and Neglect estimates that 2,000 children in the United States die each year as a result of all maltreatment. According to the National Committee for the Prevention of Child Abuse, 42% of these are a result of neglect alone.

Psychopathy

This category of maternal filicide includes women who have the core features of instrumental violence associated with psychopathy. These mothers kill their children by active aggression as opposed to the impulsive aggression of battering mothers. Often these women have severe personality disorders, attempt suicide, and are involved in chaotic hostile marital relationships (D'Orban, 1979). For example, they may displace their anger and kill their children as a means of partner retaliation or spousal revenge, and often perceive their children as a hindrance and lacking autonomy. They commit filicide purposefully, and often go to great lengths to conceal the act.

Mercy Killing

The final category involves the maternal killing of a seriously ill or deformed child. This category is often referred to as "altruistic" filicide. Mothers in this category kill to relieve the suffering of their child. They are not delusional about the child's suffering, and the killing is done out of compassion without any secondary gain on the part of the mother (Bourget & Bradford, 1990; Resnick, 1970; Scott, 1973).

In thinking of these various categories of murder, it is interesting to note that Resnick contended that 40% of women charged with non-neonaticide homicide were seen shortly before the murder by a psychiatrist (Resnick, 1969).

Spousal Homicide

Research indicates that some kind of physical aggression occurs in one fourth to one third of all marital, cohabiting or dating couples (Frieze & Browne, 1989; Gelles, 1974, 1991; O'Leary, 1988; Straus, 1971; Straus, Gelles, & Steinmetz, 1980; Hotaling & Sugarman, 1986). Angela Browne (1986), commenting on some of the earlier research, made the following observation: "The percent of serious assaults by husbands against wives in the Straus study would mean that 1.84 million women are beaten by their husbands each year, and would suggest that, at least in this country, a woman's chances of being assaulted at home by her partner, are greater than that of a police officer being assaulted on the job" (p. 61).

A more recent study in Kentucky of 1,793 women found that 21% of married women reported being abused by a partner and over two thirds of the women reported being separated or divorced in the previous year (Harris, 1979).

Of these abused women, only a very small number actually murder their partners. Wilson and Daly (1993), in examining all spousal homicides known to the police in Canada between 1974 and 1990; in New South Wales, Australia, between 1968 and 1986; and in Chicago between 1965 and 1990, found that the rate of spousal homicide in these three samples ranged from 47 per million registered married spouses per year in New South Wales to 150 per million registered married spouses per year in Chicago. The ratio of victimized women to that of victimized men was approximately 3:1 in Canada and New South Wales and approximately 1:1 in Chicago.

In a recent Bureau of Justice Statistics Report, Zawitz (1994) described the murder of intimates occurring in the United States in 1992. Citing the FBI's Crime in the United States report, she noted that 22,540 murders were committed nationwide in 1992. The relationship between the victim and the offender was known in 61% of the murders, and of these, 15% involved murders between intimates. Of these, 70% involved the murder of a woman and 30% the murder of a man. This ratio, however, was found to differ for Blacks and Whites: 59% of the Black victims were females, while 74% of the White victims were females.

In perhaps the first large-scale empirical study of murder, Marvin Wolfgang (1958) studied 588 murders that occurred in Philadelphia between January 1948 and December 1952. One hundred of these were spousal murders in which 53 women were killed by their husbands and 47 men by their wives. Despite this comparable rate of spouse killing, Wolfgang found that women were responsible for only 105 or 19% of the 588 murders and that in 45% of these, the victim was the woman's husband. In contrast, only 12% of the murders committed by men involved the murder of a spouse. Wolfgang observed that these female homicides tended to occur in the kitchen using a knife, were often associated with alcohol, and were generally explained in terms of self-defense. Wolfgang further reported that 34% of the women were acquitted compared to 4% of the men. The difference was attributed to provocation on the part of the husband.

Some years later, Barnard, Vera, Vera, and Newman (1982) studied 34 murderers referred for psychiatric evaluation following the murder of a spouse. They found that the 23 men in this investigation tended to be older and less educated, and often had histories of previous arrests and alcohol abuse. The majority reported incidents of "intolerable desertion, rejection and abandonment" (p. 274) and 13 of the 23 murders occurred after a separation. In contrast, the 11 women described histories of psychiatric treatment and suicide attempts. They reported being victims of physical and verbal abuse, and described chronic alcohol abuse by their husbands. Only one of the women was separated from her husband at the time of the murder. Both sexes tended to use handguns to murder their victims. However, 82% of the men were found guilty of murder, while only 54% of the women were found guilty of the crime.

By the 1980s, it was widely accepted that women who killed their partners were typically victims of prolonged and sustained abuse at the hands of those partners. In an influential study, Walker (1984) examined the predisposing characteristics and interpersonal dynamics of 400 abusive relationships. From this, she formulated the "Battered Woman Syndrome" characterized by a "violence prone personality" in the men, learned helplessness in the women, and a cycle of violence that involved mounting tension and an acute battering incident followed by reconciliation and contrition. Following the development of this syndrome concept, Walker (1989) examined 50 battered women who murdered their spouses and compared these with the 400 batterred women who had not. She concluded that the women who murdered felt that no one took them seriously, that they alone had to protect themselves, and, that because of some change in their spouse's mental or physical state, they believed that he was going to kill them. Walker suggests that certain factors increase the level of risk for lethal violence: increased involvement of children in the abuse, recent threats to kill the woman, weapons in the home, alcohol and drug abuse, triangulated relationships, and an increase in either the frequency or severity of the abuse.

Browne (1987), building on the earlier work by Walker, compared 42 homicidal women with 42 matched controls. The homicidal group was drawn from 15 states, while the controls were drawn from a self-referred sample used in a previous study that covered 6 states, including both urban and rural areas. The majority of women in each group reported being married to their abusers for an average of 6.9 to 7.7 years; 65%–71% reported that they had been the victims of or witnessed physical abuse in their families of origin. The men came from lower- or working-class families with 84%–91% also having experienced abuse in their families of origin. In the homicide group, the women tended to come from higher class backgrounds than their mates.

Using a discriminant function analysis, Browne (1987) found six factors that, in linear combination, best differentiated the homicidal group from the nonhomicidal group:

- *Severity of the woman's injury*: Women in the homicidal group received more injuries and more severe injuries than the nonhomicidal group. Injuries included bruises, cuts, broken bones, partial loss of hearing, and severe scarring.
- *Extent of partner's drug use and frequency of intoxication*: In the homicidal group, 29% of the men were reported to have been using street drugs every day or almost every day, and 80% reported being intoxicated every day or almost every day.
- *Frequency with which abuse occurred*: In the homicidal group, 40% reported that abusive incidents occurred more than once a week; 13% of the nonhomicidal group reported this frequency of abuse.
- *Force or threatened sexual acts by the men*: Of the homicidal group, 75% reported being forced to have sex or perform sexual acts against their will. This was true of only 37% of the nonhomicidal group.
- *Suicidal threats by the woman*: Almost half of the homicidal group had threatened to commit suicide compared to 31% of the nonhomicidal group.
- *Threats to kill by the man*: Of the men in the homicidal group, 83% threatened to kill someone other than themselves, while only 59% of the nonhomicidal group made such threats.

According to Browne (1987), the qualitative data of the study suggest that the women in the homicidal group experienced an acute sense of desperation, believing that the man no longer cared what he did to her and that his escalating use of drugs and alcohol, and his increasingly violent behavior, indicated that he was losing control. In describing the sample, Browne noted that, of the women who went to trial after the interview, 9 were acquitted, 11 received probation or a suspended sentence, and 20 received jail terms ranging from 6 months to 25 years.

Dutton, Hohnecker, Halle, and Burghardt (1994) compared 33 woman charged with murder or attempted murder with women seeking treatment from a family violence center. They found that the women who killed their abusive partners were more likely to have been hit with an object or forced to have sex. Blount, Silverman, Seller, and Seese (1994) found that higher levels of alcohol and drug use differentiated a group of women who killed their abusers from those who did not, even when the level of violence was comparable.

Focusing on racial differences, Mann (1990) studied 296 female homicides that occurred in Chicago, Houston, Los Angeles, New York, Atlanta, and Baltimore in 1979 and 1983, and found that Black women killed nearly four times more often than White or Hispanic women. She observed that Black women tended to murder male partners in the home, during the week, using guns, in a planned act, and while alone with the victim. Rejecting the applicability of a battered woman syndrome for most of these Black women, Mann suggested that "[p]rior arrest records, particularly for violent crimes, and careful analyses of the case narratives suggest that enough of the black homicide offenders were sufficiently 'tough' and were armed to hold their own in victim–offender interaction" (p. 190). In terms of disposition of the cases, Mann observed that less than half of these women ended up going to prison and most of these for only a few years.

Maguigan (1991), in a proposal to reform the standards for defining procedural requirements for a self-defense instruction, reviewed 394 appellate opinions that involved a woman convicted of killing an abusive partner. Dividing the sample into confrontational and nonconfrontational groups, she found that 223 murders met the criteria for battered woman homicide, and of these, 75% occurred during a direct confrontation with the abuser. Of the 20% that did not involve a direct confrontation, 8% were "sleeping-man" cases, 8% occurred during a lull in the initial violence, and 4% involved the hiring of a hit man. Maguigan concluded that these findings supported her thesis that most homicides by abused women do not occur in a nonconfrontational setting, as often assumed by legal scholars. Rather, given a fair application of substantive law and evidentiary rule by judges, the majority are shown to be instances of self-defense.

Finally, Campell (1995) has attempted to integrate some of this rudimentary research into a statistical risk factor assessment that can be used clinically to help women identify and be aware of factors that might increase their risk either of becoming lethally violent or of becoming the victim of lethal violence in their abusive relationships. The instrument is composed of 15 yes–no questions, including three demographic risk factors: age, minority status, and poverty. In completing the instrument, the woman is asked to mark a calendar indicating each date during the past year when she was abused, how long the incident lasted, and the relative seriousness of the incident on a 5-point scale (ranging from slapping to use of a weapon). The woman is then asked to answer 15 questions: (1) whether the violence has increased in frequency over the past year; (2) whether the violence has increased in frequency over the past year and the threat of or use of a weapon has occurred; (3) whether the man has tried to choke the woman; (4) whether there is a gun in the house; (5) whether the man has forced the woman into sex; (6) whether the man uses drugs such as speed, cocaine, heroin, or angel dust; (7) whether the man has threatened to kill the woman; (8) whether the man is drunk every day or almost every day; (9) whether the man is a binge drinker; (10) whether the man controls most of the woman's daily activities; (11) whether the man has ever beaten the woman while she was pregnant; (12) whether the man is violently jealous of the woman; (13) whether the woman has ever threatened or attempted suicide; (14) whether the man has ever attempted suicide; and (15) whether the man is violent outside of the home. Campell tested the instrument using three different abused populations, one recruited from the community, a second from a wife abuse shelter, and a third from a large urban hospital. Most recently, it has been used in a Center for Disease Control–funded prospective study of abuse during pregnancy. Campbell, reflecting on its marginal internal consistency, added that it is now being used in a longitudinal study of women's responses to abuse that will yield further reliability and construct validity information.

Recently, the Bureau of Justice Statistics examined the legal outcome of cases in which the defendant was charged with killing his or her spouse. In their report, *Spouse Murder Defendants in Large Urban Counties,* they reviewed 540 spousal murder cases that had occurred in 1988 in the 75 largest counties of the United States. Of the 540 cases, 59% were husband defendants and 41% were wife defendants. There were racial differences in the percentage of wife and husband defendants: Among husband defendants, 51% were Black and 45% were White; among wife defendants 61% were Black and 39% were White. In terms of the arrest charge, 70% of the defendants were charged with first-degree murder, 24% with second-degree murder, and 6% with nonnegligent manslaughter. Of the 540 spouse murder defendants, 80% were ultimately convicted of murdering their spouses. Of these, 52% were convicted of negligent or nonnegligent manslaughter. In terms of sentencing, 10% of the defendants were sentenced to probation, 89% to prison, and 1% to a county jail. The average length of prison sentences was 13 years. The female defendants, however, received both a higher rate of acquittal and average prison sentences than were 10 years shorter than those received by the males. The report noted that there was a relatively high rate of victim precipitation characteristic of the wife defendant cases. However, even in comparable cases, in which there was no victim precipitation, wife defendants received sentences that were 10 years shorter than those imposed on the husband defendants.

The Psychopathic Female Murderer

Unlike the interpersonally motivated murders discussed previously, the female psychopath murders for instrumental purposes and is primarily motivated by personal gain. The victims are more likely to be strangers or at least individuals with less personal significance to her, and the purpose is usually clearly defined (e.g., money, revenge, drugs). In support of this contention, McClain (1983), Goetting (1988), and Mercy and Saltzman (1989) found a decline in the number of women killing their spouses and an increase in the number of women killing strangers, while Weisheit (1984) found that an increasing number of female homicides involved other criminal activities such as robbery. In an earlier study, Mann (1984) also found that female murderers increasingly had criminal records.

In contrast to the burgeoning attention devoted to psychopathy in men, this type of personality structure in women has received little attention. Research by Robert Hare of Simon Fraser University over the past 30 years (Hare, 1965, 1968, 1970) has culminated in the development of the Psychopathy Checklist–Revised, a 12-item instrument that relies on a face-to-face interview and the review of collateral information. Factor analytic research using the PCL-R has shown it to contain a two-component factor structure: one made of the selfish, callous, and remorseless personality traits, and the other of either a chronically unstable and criminal lifestyle; or an aimless, unpredictable, and parasitic lifestyle (Harpur, Hakstein, & Hare, 1988). Research concerning the criminal careers of male psychopaths has shown that, as compared with nonpsychopathic offenders, they spend more time in prison between the ages of 16 and 40 years, offend with consistency throughout their 20s and 30s, and commit fewer property, but not violent, crimes after age 40 (Hare, McPherson, & Forth, 1984). Risk prediction research has also demonstrated that psychopaths are far more likely to violate conditions of release and are approximately three times more likely to become involved in some type of violent recidivism (Forth, Hart and Hare, 1990; Hart, Kropp, & Hare, 1988; Harris, Rice, & Quinsey, 1993).

Robertson, Bankier, and Schwartz (1987) studied 100 consecutive female admissions to the Remand Prison for Women in Winnipeg, Canada, in order to ascertain characteristics of Adler's assertions regarding the "new female criminal." Using a questionnaire, they collected extensive information on the personal history, family background, psychological factors, and mental health of the women. Twenty-four percent of the women were involved in violent crime. When these women were compared with the remaining 76% of the women charged primarily with theft, they were found to have a higher incidence of past violence, greater illicit drug use, more problems with alcohol, family histories of crime, low education, low socioeconomic status (SES), and childhoods that were replete with divorce, child abuse, alcoholism, and domestic disruptions. Twenty-one percent of the women reported head injuries, and 60% met the criteria for antisocial personality disorder as defined by the *Diagnostic and Statistical Manual of Mental Disorders*, third edition (*DSM-III;* American Psychiatric Association, 1980). According to the authors, the most common symptoms of the disorder were the initiation of fights, low school grades, thefts, repeated drunkenness, and delinquency. The majority of the women were repeat offenders (73%) and were observed to offend in the same type of crime category.

Brownstein, Spunt, Crimmins, Goldstein, and Langley (1994) conducted a study of 268 inmates charged with murder in New York State prisons in 1989. From these interviews, they analyzed the information provided by 9 of the 13 females included in the study. They report that two of the murders involved abuse by a partner, but note that the remaining seven cases involved an assortment of factors including heavy alcohol use, prostitution, and immersion in a criminal lifestyle. The following are case illustrations:

> She and her 17-year-old brother were in the basement of their mother's house smoking crack. By her recollection, they had shared about 50 to 60 vials. She may have had 40 herself. They got into an argument over who would smoke the last vial. He punched her. She grabbed a knife and probably stabbed him, though she could not remember for sure. He died from stab wounds, and she was arrested. Since she was a parole violator, she was returned to prison. (p. 106)

Another case reads:

> In one case the woman and man were friends. For three or four years, she would regularly "give him sex" in exchange for money, first for groceries then for crack. One night after she had repeatedly returned to his house to turn tricks in exchange for money for crack, they got into an argument. He had been drinking and she wanted her money to buy more crack. He resisted. She "went into a frenzy" and stabbed him. (p. 106)

In a third case, the authors report:

> . . . a woman was taking money for sex. . . . It was planned as a robbery. Two nights earlier, while they were both doing crack and thinking about the money they needed to buy more, she and her "running mate," a male associate, decided to rob one of her clients. She was supposed to set up the appointment and then leave the door unlocked when she got there. Her associate would push his way in, rob the "john" and take his things without any violence. But that night her associate had smoked a joint with PCP. At the time he walked in, she was performing oral sex on the client and the man had his back to the door. Her associate saw him and shot him in the back of the head. (p.107)

In discussing these cases, Brownstein and colleagues (1994) observe that studies of women who kill do not generally identify women whose violent actions are associated with cocaine or crack use. However, recent drug testing has demonstrated that the percentage of women arrested who test positive for cocaine is comparable to that of men (i.e., 64% to 65% in New York City). Commenting on the patriarchal structure of most drug organizations, the authors suggest that "crack appears to have opened opportunities for women in the drug business . . . and to reach the higher levels of that business, women would have to be as violent as their male counterparts" (p. 113).

In their characterization of the robberies and aggravated assaults of 65 women arraigned in New York City between January and June, 1990, Sommers and Baskin (1993) examined the motive, victim precipitation, victim–offender relationship, accomplices, precipitating circumstances, preparation, and use of weapons. Of those charged with robbery or assault and robbery, 28% reported a past history of homicide as well as numerous other offenses including drug sales, forgery, prostitution, and weapon possession and use. Sommers and Baskin noted that while the robbery and assault incidents involved a variety of factors, there were many similarities in the women's lifestyles: They focused largely on obtaining money and often did so illegally in order to support a drug habit. One of their respondents stated:

> When I first started it was for fun. I was 15. I wanted to be down with the group. We'd just take things. If I saw it I took it: chains, jewelry, stuff like that. Now, it is to take care of my habit. It is money for drugs, drugs. I was shooting morphine-based dope. I would use a bundle and half of dime bags. So that's like $150, that was just on the heroin. I would do a speedball with it so I had to get cocaine, that was about $80. Then I would have to have my methadone because I would have to come down. Than that was maybe $20 to $25. (p. 144)

Sommers and Baskin (1993) noted that the majority of robberies perpetrated by this type of offender involved relatively little planning, although the women often worked with accomplices, generally targeted a particular type of victim, and frequently used a weapon for intimidation. In describing one of the assaults, the authors report:

> I can recall, OK, I was walking home with my friend. There was this big fat girl who was arguing with another friend. I put my two cents in it. . . . Well, the next day, I'm sitting in the laundry room—inside the projects—folding my clothes. So she came up to me and I look up and she's taking off her earrings. So I say what's up? So she says, yeah from last night. So I wheel my son over to my girlfriend on the next bench and the Clorox is right there. Right, so, I stand up and open the Clorox and I keep throwing it at her. It's all over her eyes and she's still coming. She grabs the shopping cart, right and I see a big stick. I pull the cart from her and I constantly beat her with the stick and can't nobody stop me when I get at it, except the police. The police was called. (pp. 150–151)

Sommers and Baskin (1993) indicated that the majority of the assaults were also characteristically unplanned, largely unorganized, and frequently carried out while the woman was intoxicated. A minority of the incidents also involved drug dealing either in terms of retaliating against other dealers or trying to resolve disputes while under the influence of the drugs.

Perhaps the most extreme example of this type of psychopathic offender is the female serial killer. In her book, *Women Who Kill*, Jones (1981) describes several women who qualify as serial killers. One is Lydia Sherman who, in 1871, was convicted and sentenced to life imprisonment for killing each of her three husbands and six of her children with arsenic. She stated that her motivation for killing was despair over her inability to provide for her children and her wish to regain control over her life from the exploitative husbands. In 1886, Jane Robinson was sentenced to death for killing seven of her family members with arsenic in order to collect on their insurance policies. And, in 1908, Belle Gunness was killed in a fire that burned down her farm in Indiana, where 10 dismembered bodies were found buried. She had apparently poisoned the victims, who included farmhands and her children.

More recently, nurses have been found guilty of killing a number of their patients (Stross, Shasby, & Harlan, 1976). Dorothy Puente was also found guilty in 1995 of killing seven tenants of her boarding house in Sacramento, California. Apparently, she would kill tenants after convincing them to sign over to her their Social Security, SSI, pensions, and tax refunds. The boarders, who had been poisoned, were found buried in the yard of her boarding house (Norton, 1994).

Unlike male serial killings, these murders were not primarily sexual in nature, did not involve extreme forms of face to face violence, and were typically motivated by financial gain. An exception to this characterization is the case of Aillen Wournos, a 35-year-old prostitute who killed seven middle-aged men in Florida, victims she picked up while hitchhiking. She shot all of them either in their torsos or heads multiple times and stole their rings, cameras, and money. The bodies were found naked in the woods along a highway in Florida. According to Wournos, these men all tried to rape her and she killed in self defense. The jury concluded, however, that Wournos lured the men into the woods with the intent to kill them.

Wournos's life history is replete with developmental trauma. Her father was convicted of raping a child and hanged himself in prison. Her mother left one evening for a date and never returned, leaving Wournos to be raised by an alcoholic grandfather and passive grandmother. She was reportedly sexually abused as a child, badly burned at the age of 9, raped when she was 14, and attempted to kill herself six times (once shooting herself in the stomach) between the ages of 14 and 22. At her sentencing hearing, it was also reported that Wournos suffered from a cortical dysfunction, had an IQ that fell only one point above borderline retardation, and was reported to have vision and hearing problems that were never diagnosed or treated. Experts diagnosed Wournos as suffering from borderline personality disorder and attributed this diagnosis to her intense and unstable relationships, her impulsivity, her intense anger, her self-destructive behavior, and her extreme fears of abandonment. Coded on Hare's psychopathy checklist, Wournos scored a 32, suggesting that she not only met the criteria for psychopathy, but scored at the 86th percentile when compared with a male prison population.

This research suggests that there is an emerging category of violent female offenders who suffer from significant character pathology and whose criminal lifestyles involve prostitution, chronic drug addiction, and violence. Although various factors contribute to such a life, childhood trauma, poverty, and limited life opportunities appear to have significant effects.

Taken as a whole, this research suggests that the bonds of intimacy continue to hold the seeds of violence for the majority of female killers. They generally do not offend outside the family; when they do, the offending behavior is often preceded by drug addiction and a chaotic, crime-invested lifestyle. The most common forms of murder, the killing of a child or partner, are, in turn, generally associated with such traumas as severe mental illness, chronic abuse, deformity, and extreme poverty. These patterns, which differ significantly from those manifested by males, most likely reflect a complex blend of hormonal, physiological, social, and cultural influences that distinguish the lethal violence of women from that of men.

References

Barnard, G. W., Vera, H., Vera, M. I., & Newman, G. (1982). Til death do us part: A study of spouse murder. *American Academy of Psychiatry and Law, 271,* 274

Blount, W. R., Silverman, I. J., Seller, C. S., & Seese, R. A. (1994). Alcohol and drug use among abused women who kill, abused women who don't and their abusers. *Journal of Drug Issues, 24,* 165–177.

Bourget, D., & Bradford, J. M. W. (1990). Homicidal parents. *Canadian Journal of Psychiatry, 134,* 560–571.

Brown, S. L., Forth, A. B., Hart, S. D., & Hare, R. D. (1992). The assessment of psychopathy in a noncriminal population [Abstract]. *Canadian Psychology, 33,* 405.

Browne, A. (1986). Assault and homicide at home: When battered women kill. In M. Saks & L. Saxe (Eds.), *Advances in applied psychology* (Vol. 3, pp. 57–79). Hillsdale, NJ: Erlbaum.

Browne, A. (1987). *When battered women kill.* New York: Macmillan.

Browne, A., & Williams, K. R. (1993). Gender, intimacy, and lethal violence: Trends from 1976 through 1987. *Gender and Society, 7,* 78–98.

Brownstein, H. H., Spunt, B. J., Crimmins, S., Goldstein, P. J., & Langley, S. (1994). Changing patterns of lethal violence by women: A research note. *Women and Criminal Justice, 5*(2), 99–117.

Bureau of Justice Statistics. *Spouse Murder Defendants in Large Urban Communities.* Office of Justice Statistics, U.S. Department of Justice, September, 1995 (pp. 1–5).

Button, J. H., & Reivich, R. S. (1972). Obsessions of infanticide. *Archives of General Psychiatry, 27,* 235–240.

Campbell, J. C. (1995). Prediction of homicide of and by battered women. In J. Campbell & J. Milner (Eds.), *Assessing dangerousness: Potential for further violence of sexual offenders, batterers, and child abusers* (pp. 96–113). Newbury Park, CA: Sage.

Condon, J. T. (1986). The spectrum of fetal abuse in pregnant women, *Journal of Nervous and Mental Disease,* *174*(9), 509–516.

Daly, M., & Wilson, M. (1988). *Homicide.* New York: Aldine de Gruyter.

Daniel, A. E., & Harris, P. W. (1982). Female homicide offenders referred for pre-trial psychiatric examination: A descriptive study. *Bulletin of the American Academy of Psychiatry and Law, 10,* 261.

Devereux, G. (1948). Mojave Indian infanticide. *Psychoanalytic Review, 35,* 126–139.

D'Orban, P. T. (1979). Women who kill their children. *British Journal of Psychiatry, 134,* 560–571.

Dutton, M. A., Hohnecker, L.C., Halle, P.M., & Burghardt, K. J. (1994). Traumatic responses among battered women who kill. *Journal of Traumatic Stress, 7*(4), 549–564.

Emery, J. L. (1993). Child abuse, sudden infant death syndrome, and unexpected infant death. *American Journal of Diseases of Children, 147,* 1097–1100.

Forth, A. B., Kimlinger, T., Brown, S., & Harris, A. (1993). Precursors to psychopathic traits in a sample of male and female university students [Abstract]. *Canadian Psychology, 34,* 380.

Forth, A. E, Brown, S. L., Hart, S. D., & Hare, R. D. (1996). The assessment of psychopathy on male and female noncriminals: Reliability and validity. *Personality and Individual Differences.*

Frieze, I. H., & Browne, A. (1989). Violence in marriage, in family violence. *Crime and Justice—A Review of Research 163.*

Garber, C. M. (1947). Eskimo infanticide. *Scientific Monthly, 64,* 98–102.

Gelles, R.J. (1974). *The violent home: A study of physical aggression between husbands and wives.* Beverly Hills, CA: Sage.

Gelles, R. J. (1991). Physical violence, child abuse and child homicide: A continuum of violence or distinct behavior. *Human Nature, 2,* 59–72.

Gelles, R. J., & Cornell, C. P. (1985). *Intimate violence in families.* Beverly Hills, CA: Sage.

Goetting, A. (1988). Patterns of homicide among women. *Journal of Interpersonal Violence, 3,* 3–20.

Grayson, J. (1990). Child abuse fatalities. *Virginia Child Protection Newsletter, 32,* 1–16.

Hamberger, L. K., Saunders, D. G., & Hovey, M. (1992). The prevalence of domestic violence in community practice and rate of physician inquiry. *Family Medicine, 24,* 283–287.

Hamilton, J. A. (1982). The identity of postpartum psychosis. In I. F. Brockington & R. Kumar (Eds.), *Motherhood and mental illness* (pp. 1–17). New York: Academic Press.

Hamilton, J. A. (1989). Postpartum psychiatric syndromes. *Psychiatric Clinics of North America, 12*(1), 89–103.

Harding, J. J. (1989). Postpartum psychiatric disorders: A review. *Comprehensive Psychiatry, 30*(1), 109–112.

Hare, R. D. (1965). Temporal gradient of fear arousal in psychopaths, *Journal of Abnormal Psychology, 70,* 442–445.

Hare, R. D. (1968). Psychopathy, autonomic functioning, and the orientating response, *Journal of Abnormal Psychology,* Monograph Supplements, *73,* 1–24.

Hare, R. D. (1970). *Psychopathy: Theory and Research.* New York: Wiley

Hare, R. D., McPherson, L. M., & Forth, A. B. (1984). Psychopathy and perceptual asymmetry during verbal dichotic listening. *Journal of Abnormal Psychology, 93,* 140–149.

Hare, R. D., McPherson, L. M., and Forth, A. C. (1988). Male psychopaths and their criminal answers. *Journal of Clinical and Consulting Psychology, 56,* 710–714.

Hare, R. D., Strachen, C., & Forth, A. E. (1993). Psychopathy and crime: An overview. In C. R. Hollins & K. Howells (Eds.) *Clinical Approaches to the Mentally Disordered Offender* (pp. 165–178).

Hare, R. D., Williamson, S. B., & Harper, T. J. (1988). Psychopathy and language. In T. B. Moffitt & S. A. Mednick (Eds.), *Biological contributions to crime equation* (pp. 68–92). Dordrocht, The Netherlands: Martinus Nijhoff.

Hare, R. D., Strachen, C., & Forth, A. E. (1993). Psychopathy and crime: An overview. In C. R. Hollin & K. Howells (Eds.), *Clinical approaches to the mentally disordered offender* (pp. 165–178).

Harpur, T. J., Hakstein, R., & Hare, R. D. (1988). Factor structure of the Psychopathy Checklist. *Journal of Consulting and Clinical Psychology, 56,* 741–47.

Harris, L. (1979). *Survey of spousal violence against women in Kentucky* (Report No. 792701).

Harris, G. T., Rice, M. E., & Quinsey, V. L. (1993). Violent recidivism of mentally disordered offenders: The development of statistical prediction instruments. *Criminal Justice and Behavior, 20,* 315–335.

Hart, S. D., Kropp, P. R., & Hare, R. D. (1988). Performance of male psychopaths following constitutional release from prison. *Journal of Consulting and Clinical Psychology, 56,* 227–232.

Hotaling, G. T., & Sugarman, D. B. (1986). An analysis of risk markers in husband-to-wife violence: The current state of knowledge. *Violence and Victims, 1,* 101–124.

Husain, A., & Daniel, A. (1984). A comparative study of filicidal and abusive mothers. *Canadian Journal of Psychiatry, 29*, 596–598.

Infanticide Act (1938). 1 and 2 Ge. 6, C36, Sect. (1).

Jason, J., Gilliland, J. C., & Tyler, C. W. (1983). Homicide as a cause of pediatric mortality in the United States. *Pediatrics, 72*(2), 191–197.

Jones, A. (1980). *Women who kill.* New York: Holt, Rinehart and Winston.

Jurik, N. C., & Gregware, P. (1989). *A method for murder: An interactionist analysis of homicides by women.* Tempe: Arizona State University, School of Justice Studies.

Kaku, K. (1975). Were girl babies sacrificed to a fold superstition in 1966 in Japan? *Annals of Human Biology, 2*, 391–393.

Kaye, N. S., Bornstein, N. M., & Donnell, S. M. (1990). Families, murder, and insanity: A psychiatric review of paternal neonaticide. *Journal of Forensic Sciences, 35*(1), 133–139.

Kellet, R. J. (1992). Infanticide and child destruction—The historical, legal and pathological aspects. *Forensic Science International, 53*, 1–28.

Kendall, R. E. (1985). Emotional and physical factors in the genesis of puerperal mental disorders. *Journal of Psychosomatic Research, 29*(1), 3–11.

Korbin, J. E. (1986). Childhood histories of women imprisoned for fatal child maltreatment. *Child Abuse and Neglect, 10*, 331–338.

Korbin, J. E. (1989). Fatal maltreatment by mothers: A proposed framework. *Child Abuse and Neglect, 13*, 481–489.

Loucks, A. D., & Zamble, E. (1994). Criminal and violent behavior in incarcerated female federal offenders [Abstract]. *Canadian Psychology, 35*, 54.

Maguigan, H. (1991). Battered women and self-defense: Myths and misconceptions in current reform proposals. *University of Pennsylvania Law Review.*

Mann, C. R. (1984). Race and sentencing of female offenders: A field study. *International Journal of Women's Studies, 7*, 160–172.

Mann, C. R. (1990). Black female homicide in the United States. *Journal of Interpersonal Violence, 5*, 176–210.

McClain, P. D. (1983). Female homicide offenders and victims: Are they from the same population? *Death Education, 6*, 265–278.

McDermaid, G., & Winkler, E. G. (1995). Psychopathology of infanticide. *Journal of Clinical and Experimental Psychopathology, 16*(1), 22–41.

Mercy, J. A., & Saltzman, L. E. (1989). Fatal violence among spouses in the United States, 1976–85. *American Journal of Public Health, 79*, 595–599.

Myers, S. A. (1970). Maternal filicide. *American Journal of Diseases of Children, 120*, 534–536.

National Sudden Infant Death Resource Center (1993). SIDS Research: Analysis in Three Parts. U.S. Department of Health and Human Services, Maternal and Child Health Bureau.

Norton, C. (1995). *Disturbed Ground: The True Story of a Diabolical Killer.* New York: W. Morrow & Co.

O'Leary, K. D. (1988). Physical aggression between spouses: A social learning theory perspective,. In V. B. van Hasselt, R. L. Morrison, A. S. Bellack, & M. Hersen (Eds.), *Handbook of family violence,* (pp. 31–55). New York: Plenum.

Reece, R. M. (1993). Fatal child abuse and sudden infant death syndrome: A critical diagnostic decision. *Pediatrics, 91*(2), 423–429.

Resnick, P. (1969). Murder of the newborn: A psychiatric review of neonaticide. *American Journal of Psychiatry, 126*(10), 1414–1420.

Resnick, P. (1970). Child murder by parents: A psychiatric review of filicide. *American Journal of Psychiatry, 126*(3), 73–82.

Riggs, D. S., O'Leary, K. D., & Breslin, F. C. (1990). Multiple correlates of physical aggression in dating couples. *Journal of Interpersonal Violence, 5*, 61–73.

Robertson, R. G., Bankier, R. G., & Schwartz, L. (1987). The female offender: A Canadian study. *32*, 749–755.

Rose, L. (1986). *The massacre of the innocents: Infanticide in Britain 1800–1939.* Boston: Routledge and Kegan Paul.

Rosenblatt, E. M., & Greenland, C. (1974). Female crimes of violence. *Canadian Journal of Criminology, 16*, 1973–1980.

Rutherford, M. J., Cacciola, J. S., & Alterman, A. I. (1992). The Psychopathy Checklist–Revised with women. In *Problems of Drug Dependence 1991* (Research Monograph Series No. 119, p. 2). Rockville, MD: National Institute on Drug Abue.

Rutherford, M. J., Alterman, A. I., Cacciola, J. S., & Snyder, B. C. (1996). Gender differences in diagnosing antisocial personality disorder in methadone patients. *American Journal of Psychiatry, 152,* 1309–1316.

Scott, P. D. (1973). Parents who kill their children. *Medicine, Science, and the Law, 13*(2), 120–126.

Sichel, D. A., Cohen, L. S., Dimmock, J. A., & Rosenbaum, J. F. (1993). Postpartum obsessive compulsive disorder: A case series. *Journal of Clinical Psychiatry, 54*(4), 156–159.

Sommers, I., & Baskin, D. R. (1993). The situational context of violent female offending. *Journal of Research in Crime and Delinquency, 30*(2), 136–62.

Stanford, M., Ebner, D., Patton, J., & Williams, J. (1994). Multi-impulsivity within an adolescent psychiatric population. *Personality and Individual Differences, 16,* 395–402.

Steiner, M. (1990). Postpartum psychiatric disorders. *Canadian Journal of Psychiatry, 35,* 89–95.

Steinschneider, A. (1972). Prolonged apnea and the sudden infant death syndrome: Clinical and laboratory observations. *Pediatrics, 50*(4), 646–54.

Strachan, C. (1993). *Assessment of psychopathy in female offenders.* Unpublished doctoral dissertation, University of British Columbia, Vancouver, British Columbia, Canada.

Straus, M. A. (1971). Some social antecedents of physical punishment: A linkage theory interpretation. *Journal of Marriage and Family, 33,* 658–663.

Straus, M. A., Gelles, R. J., & Steinmetz, S. (1980). *Behind closed doors: Violence in the American Family.* Garden City, NY: Anchor.

Stross, J. K., Shasby, M., & Horlan, W. R. (1976). An epidemic of mysterious cardiopulmonary arrests. *New England Journal of Medicine, 20,* 1107–1120.

Sturner, W. Q., Sweeney, K. G., Callery, R. T., & Haley, N. R. (1991). Cocaine babies: The scourge of the 90's. *Journal of Forensic Sciences, 36*(1), 34–39.

U.S. Department of Justice (1981 to 1992). *Uniform Crime Reports.* Crime in the U.S. (1980 through 1991). Washington, D.C.: United States Government Printing Office.

Walker, L. E. (1989). *Terrifying Love: Why Battered Women Kill and How Society Responds.* New York: Harper-Collins.

Walker, L. E. (1984). *The battered woman syndrome.* New York: Springer.

Weisheit, R. A. (1984). Female homicide offenders: Trends over time in an institutionalized population. *Justice Quarterly, 1,* 471–489.

Wilson, M., and Daly, M. (1993). Spousal homicide risk and estrangement. *Violence and Victims, 8,* 3–16.

Wolfgang, M. E. (1958). *Patterns in criminal homicide.* Philadelphia: University of Pennsylvania Press.

Wolkind, S., Taylor, E. M., Wait, A. J., Dalton, M., & Emery, J. L. (1993). Recurrence of unexpected infant death. *Acta paediatrica, 82,* 873–876.

Zawitz, M. (1994). Violence between intimates. Bureau of Justice Statistics, U.S. Department of Justice, NCJ-149259.

IV

SEXUAL DEVIANCE AND ASSAULT

Paraphilias

Nathaniel McConaghy

Description of the Problem

An initial problem in providing a description of violent paraphilic criminal offenders is that rapists, one of the two major groups of violent sexual offenders commonly recognized (the other is child molesters) are not classified in the *DSM-IV* (American Psychiatric Association, 1994) as paraphiliacs. The *DSM-III-R* (American Psychiatric Association, 1987), allowed their inclusion as sexual sadists when the suffering inflicted on the victim was far in excess of that necessary to gain compliance, but added that, in most cases of rape, the rapist did not find the victim's suffering sexually arousing. Presumably, rape was excluded from the paraphilias in the *DSM-IV* to accommodate the theory cogently criticized by Palmer (1988) that rape is not sexually motivated; this theory appears totally implausible in view of the evidence that a significant percentage of normal men report experiencing sexually arousing rape fantasies, and in laboratory studies show genital arousal to descriptions of forceful rape (McConaghy, 1993). However there appears to be no empirical evidence to support the *DSM-III-R* distinction between sadistic and nonsadistic rapists and Knight and Prentky (1990) were unable to substantiate it in a prison population. Some rapists who did not inflict severe physical damage on victims nevertheless appeared motivated by sadistic or angry fantasies. Equally, there is no evidence that self-identified sadomasochists show any increased likelihood of raping nonconsenting subjects. It would seem appropriate that rape be classified as an independent paraphilia, and it is discussed here as such.

A further problem in definition is that violence in paraphilic offenses in the sense of the use of force resulting in some degree of physical harm, or indeed of the use of physical force at all, has largely been replaced in the discourse of these offenses by violence as an expression of power. This replacement is perhaps most explicit in feminist analyses: "[P]imps, procurers, members of syndicate and free-lance slavery gangs, operators of brothels and massage parlors, connected with sexual exploitation entertainment, pornography purveyors, wife beaters, child molesters, incest perpe-

Nathaniel McConaghy • Psychiatric Unit, The Prince of Wales Hospital, Randwick, New South Wales, Australia 2031.

Handbook of Psychological Approaches with Violent Offenders: Contemporary Strategies and Issues, edited by Van Hasselt and Hersen. Kluwer Academic/Plenum Publishers, New York, 1999.

trators, johns (tricks) and rapists, one cannot help be momentarily stunned by the enormous male population participating in female sexual slavery. The huge number of men engaged in these practices should be cause for declaration of a national and international emergency, a crisis in sexual violence" (Barry, 1979, p. 220). This passage was cited by Messerschmidt (1993) in his review of analyses in which heterosexuality was explicitly theorized as the underpinning essence of patriarchy and linked with violence against women. He cited Brownmiller as considering that all men are potential rapists; Dworkin, that sex and murder are fused in male consciousness, and the penis is the hidden symbol of terror even more significant than the gun, the knife, and the fist; and Caputi that serial sex murder is a previously unexamined sado-ritual. Sado-rituals are crimes of men against women previously identified by Daly, such as Indian suttee, Chinese footbinding, African genital mutilation, British witch burning, and U.S. gynecology, and are reenactments of goddess murder and the means by which men maintain a worldwide patriarchal system. Messerschmidt further pointed out that MacKinnon considered the universal system of patriarchy to be maintained through heterosexuality and sexual violence—rape, wife beating, wife rape, incestuous assault, sexual harassment, and pornography. She found it difficult to distinguish intercourse from rape under conditions of male dominance as heterosexuality is simply coercive and violent sex. Messerschmidt concluded that following the logic of MacKinnon's argument, all heterosexual women are victims and all heterosexual men are rapists. He pointed out that this concept of sexual violence obscures differences between men in terms of race, class, age, and sexual preference, focusing instead on an alleged typical male, and failing to consider how social differences between men create different types and degrees of violence against women.

Emphasis on violence as power rather than force in the area of sexual crime is an understandable reaction to the increased awareness that brutal and degrading sexual assaults do not necessarily involve force resulting in marked physical harm. Palmer (1988) cited evidence that 15% to 20% of victims of rape reported to the police required hospital treatment for physical injuries, and that severe, lasting physical injuries were rare. As discussed later, reported rapes constitute only a small percentage of total sexual assaults, but are likely to include most cases where significant physical injury was inflicted. Quinsey and Upfold (1985) investigated 95 completed rapes and 41 attempts made by 72 men referred to a maximum security psychiatric institution. Sixty-nine victims were not injured, 8 were treated in clinics and released, 7 were hospitalized overnight and 2 were killed.

Sanday (1990) recently provided an analysis of rapes that did not involve marked physical force but that were markedly degrading, the fraternity gang rapes that she considered to be part of a widespread sexual pattern found on college campuses throughout the United States. Because of the cloak of secrecy surrounding them, she pointed out that their incidence may have been much higher than indicated by the 75 cases documented in the previous 6 years. At one university, such rapes were reported to occur once or twice a month. The stereotypical pattern was that a vulnerable young woman "seeking acceptance or high on drugs or alcohol is taken to a room. She may or may not agree to having sex with one man. She then passes out, or she is too weak or scared to protest, and a 'train' of men have sex with her" (p. 91). Sanday reported four cases where the victims were either unconscious or at some stage made it clear that they were not consenting. Though the state law implied that regardless of a woman's past sexual history or provocative behavior, when she says no and asks a man or men to stop, they are legally bound to do so, and further stated that if a woman is incapable of consent, any sexual activity with her is legally classified as rape, district attorneys, despite their certainty of the men's guilt, did not charge the offenders as they felt there was little chance a jury would convict them. If the victim consented to sex with any man during the course of the evening, there was room for reasonable doubt as to whether she consented to all sexual activity. Presumably, had the force used resulted in significant physical harm the offenders would have been charged.

Los (1990) pointed out that stress on violence could send a message both to courts and the public that only really brutal rapes are criminal and that sexual imposition itself is not of much consequence. She cited a survey of several hundred sexual assault sentencing reports in the late 1980s that found that judges repeatedly commented on the absence of injury or damage to the victim: " '[N]o lasting and permanent damage to the complainant' was a comment made by the judge in a case where the victim was taken to a secluded area and raped. . . . The complainant struggled a great deal but the accused overpowered her" (p. 167). In her discussion of fraternity gang rapes, Sanday (1990) commented:

> Because she is a woman, weaker, and in the minority, the woman is triply disadvantaged and completely defenseless. Whether or not the woman agrees, acquiesces out of fear, or passes out, the inescapable fact remains that she is in the minority and the men in the majority. The whole scenario presents the classic case of victim and victimizer. . . . She is vulnerable, unable to retaliate, and there is unanimity within the group that she is the one at fault—e.g., "she drank too much"; "she wanted it"; "she was provocative"; "she didn't say no"; and so on. . . . Reasonable men who gang up sexually on one woman and honestly believe that she can physically withstand multiple sexual activity with many men are operating under the scapegoat delusion that she is more powerful than they. . . . The ritual reminds the brothers of their sexual dominance of women and at the same time it gives each a heterosexual stamp . . . by sharing the same sexual object, the brothers are having sex with each other as well. (pp. 108–110)

Kanin (1985) interviewed 71 self-disclosed college graduate date rapists and reported that, in every case, the rape followed a fairly intensive bout of sex play, the most common activity being orogenital. He had previously found (1969) that 87 of 341 unmarried male undergraduates stated that they had made a forceful attempt to obtain coitus that caused the female partner to show signs of offense. The maximum level of erotic activity preceding the attempt was kissing in 7%, breast fondling in 23%, and genital petting in 70%. Of course, victims may not have agreed with these accounts; the nature of the interaction preceding sexual coercion in date rape has been given little attention by other workers. If it commonly occurs when the couple are in an advanced state of mutual sexual interaction, the need to change community attitudes to emphasize that the issue of consent continues to remain paramount in states of high sexual arousal assumes a high priority. Goodchilds and Zellman (1984) found that their teenaged subjects considered as high on the list of items justifying male anger if sex was refused, the woman's behaviors of touching a man below the waist, or undressing herself or the man or allowing herself to be undressed. Refusal of a partner to proceed to coitus after orogenital sex would appear to be considered by many female and more male teenagers to justify ignoring the refusal, particularly if, as the rapists in Kanin's study reported was common, the partner (possibly out of guilt because of sharing the same value system) showed minimal physical resistance. This was consistent with Muehlenhard and Linton's (1987) findings that sexual assaults reported by women psychology students rarely involved violence or the threat of violence and that the most common method by which the male partners obtained unwanted sex was "just doing it" (p. 193). A further disturbing finding they reported was that women students who presented with scenarios describing men's asking them for unwanted intercourse, felt able to refuse comfortably in only 59% of these situations.

Comparison of cases of rape reported to police with those not reported, found that the more the features of rape were those of what was termed a classic case, the more likely it was to be reported (Holmstrom, 1985). In classic cases, the assailants broke into the victims' homes, attacked them in their automobiles, or abducted them from public places; the assailants were strangers or acquaintances rather than friends or relatives, and threatened the victims with weapons or seriously injured them. Such cases are markedly less frequent than are rapes of partners or dates, so that the term classic case could have the unfortunate effect of maintaining the stereotype that such rapes are typical rather than atypical. More appropriate terms are "blitz" and "confidence" rapes introduced by Burgess and Holmstrom (1980) on the basis of their study of female rape victims seen in an inner-city hospital emergency room setting during the course of 1 year. Bowie, Silverman, Kalick, and Edbril (1990) found the same two predominant types of rape in their study of 1,000 consecutive rape victims seen at a Boston rape crisis intervention program over a 10-year period. Blitz rapes were sudden surprise attacks by an unknown assailant. Confidence rapes involved some nonviolent interaction between the rapist and the victim before the attacker's intention to commit rape emerged. Incidents could be classified as blitz rapes in 60% of cases and confidence rapes in 36% (Silverman, Kalick, Bowie, & Edbril, 1988). Blitz rapes generally occurred in settings the victims assumed to be secure, significantly more occurring in their homes; and they were more likely to have involved threats to life. Use or threat of use of weapons were twice as likely as in confidence rapes. Blitz victims resisted their assailants less frequently than confidence victims and attempted to flee the situation only half as often. Bownes and O'Gorman (1991) reported that 10 of 50 victims of rape reported that their assailants experienced erectile insufficiency at some point during the assault and a further 6 reported that the assailants experienced retardation or failure to ejaculate. These men with sexual dysfunctions were more likely than the remainder to carry out intrarape violence and degrading sexual activity, which was related to onset of the dysfunction.

Confidence rape was more likely to have taken place in the rapist's home or automobile and to occur after the rapist has spent some time with the victim, who was more likely to have offered resistance, particularly attempts to flee. Some confidence rape victims, particularly victims of date rapes, were unclear that the assault or forced sexual encounter to which they were subjected constituted rape (Silverman *et al.*, 1988). Evidence that such rapes are rarely reported was provided by Koss (1985). Thirteen percent of women university students reported by questionnaire that they had experienced oral, anal, or vaginal intercourse against their will by force or threat of force, but only just over half acknowledged it as rape. Of those who did, 8% reported it to the police and 48% did not discuss it with anyone. Sixty percent, and all of those who had the experience but did not acknowledge it was rape, knew the assailant; 30% of those who acknowledged the rape and 76% of those who did not were romantically involved with him. Mean age at the time of the assault was 18.9 years for those who acknowledged it was rape and 17.3 years for the others. Earlier studies noting the prevalence of rape of women university students were carried out by Kanin and Parcell (1977) who repeated a 1957 study and found that, as in that study, about half the female students reported having experienced sexual coercion in the previous year, a quarter having been forced to have intercourse.

A separate dimension of rape from that of blitz or confidence was advanced by Groth, Burgess, and Holmstrom (1977). They distinguished anger and power rapes. In power rapes, which were more common, the rapist did not desire to harm but to control the victim. Anger rapists expressed anger, rage, contempt, and hatred for their victims by abusing them in profane language, beating them, sexually assaulting them, and forcing them to perform or submit to additional degrading acts. They used more force than was necessary simply to subdue the victims, who suffered physical violence to all parts of their bodies. Older or elderly women could be particular targets. Victims described a blitz style of attack or a sudden and dramatic switch in the rapist's behavior.

Finkelhor and Yllo (1985) found comparable forms of rape to those described by Groth and colleagues (1977) in their investigation of rape of women by their partners. In responding to a questionnaire, 10% of a probability sample of 323 Boston-area women with a child between 6 and 14 years of age living with them said that their husbands or male partners had used physical force or threat to try to have sex with them. A quarter were still living with the assaultive partner. Rape by partners along with that by dates (also reported by 10%) were the most common forms experienced. Further groups, each of 3%, reported the experience from strangers, from someone they knew slightly, and from friends, and 1% from a relative. Other studies have also found husbands to be the most common sexual assailants. In Russell's (1982) study of 50% of a probability sample of 930 adult women in San Francisco, more than twice as many reported being raped by a husband as by a stranger. D. G. Kilpatrick, Best, Saunders, and Veronen (1988) investigated 391 Charleston County women who participated in a study of lifetime victimization by sexual or physical assault, or robbery. Of the 91 who reported being raped, assailants were husbands in 24%, dates in 17%, and strangers in 21%. The women assaulted by husbands and boyfriends were more likely than the remainder to sustain physical injury, and to think they might be killed, though the difference was not statistically significant.

Finkelhor and Yllo (1985) obtained information concerning the nature of sexual assaults by partners from interviews with an independent sample of 50 victims, only 3 of whom were still living with the assailant. About half reported "battering rapes." These occurred during repeated physical attacks, often connected with drunkenness. They did not result from marital conflicts over sex, but were extensions of other violence perpetrated on the victims, and represented punishment and degradation for challenging the male partners' authority. In some cases, the hitting could continue throughout the sex, and the sex itself would be full of violence. In others, the men acted as though they were finished with beating and wanted to make up with sex. Finkelhor and Yllo pointed out that studies of battered women showed that from a third to a half were also victims of sexual assault from partners, and that among batterers, those who raped were among the most brutal and violent. In their study, twice as many battered women suffered from chronic rapes (20 times or more) than did the other raped women. "Force-only rapes" were reported by another approximate half the victims. In these, violence was unusual, and in some of the relationships was on both sides. They were more often prompted by sexual conflict over issues such as how often to have sex or what were acceptable sexual activities, which the male partner resolved by obtaining what he wanted by use of as much force as necessary; the goal was to obtain sex, not hurt the woman. Finkelhor and Yllo considered battering rapes and force-only rapes equivalent to the anger and power rapes described by Groth and colleagues (1977). A further 6 of the 50 women interviewed by Finkelhor and Yllo described what were classified as "obsessive" rapes, which had bizarre ritualistic elements, such as tying the victim up, inserting objects into her vagina, and photographing her.

Ageton (1983) reported the most representative study of the sexual assault of adolescent girls by men, based on interviews of 73% of a national probability sample of 2,360 subjects. Ageton concluded that in each year from 1978 to 1980, 5% to 7%, that is, 700,000 to 1 million of teenage women, were sexually assaulted in the U.S. One percent experienced assaults which involved physical violence, the use of a weapon, or both. Victims in Ageton's study reported that the offenders were mainly boyfriends or dates in their age range; less than 20% were unknown to them. The majority of victims were successful in deterring the assault. There were no significant race or social-class differences in the total sample of victims, although urban girls were more vulnerable. Those who reported violent sexual assaults were typically Black, lower-class, urban adolescents, characteristics of victims of reported rape. Only 5% of the assaults recorded in Ageton's study were reported to the police. These were primarily blitz rapes: those carried out by unknown or multiple assailants, and involving threats or employment of violence. More than half of those reported were completed assaults, compared with 20% of uncompleted assaults. Consistent with the features of confidence rapes discussed earlier, Ageton suggested that attempted nonviolent assaults by dates or boyfriends may not be defined by the victims as legitimate sexual assaults for purposes of reporting to officials. One third of the victims assaulted by their romantic partners reported no change in the relationship. Victims' reactions to date rapes had not changed from those reported by Kanin in 1959. The majority of university students he investigated who reported sexual aggression from a partner did not terminate the relationship. Alzenman and Kelley (1988) found that more than 50% of university students they studied reported continuance of a romantic relationship in which they considered they had been abused.

Most studies of rape take for granted that only women are victims. Ageton did not report the number of male victims or of homosexual assaults, stating that they were not typical and could result in misleading conclusions. As Finkelhor (1985) pointed out, concern about sexual assault originated in the women's movement of the 1960s and quickly coalesced around the model of father–daughter incest. Hence, little attention was initially given to the rarer situations where boys and men were the victims. Groth and Burgess (1980) combined data from offender and victim samples to describe 22 cases of male rape. Average age of the victim was 17.5 years. Groth and Burgess concluded that male subjects were at greater risk when engaged in solitary pursuits. In two thirds they were hitchhiking or engaged in out-of-doors activity. Most were intimidated by threat of physical harm or were suddenly hit or overpowered. Three were entrapped by the offender getting them drunk. The concepts of blitz and confidence rapes would seem equally applicable to rapes of of men as of women. The majority were sexually penetrated and, in half of the cases, the offenders attempted to make the victims ejaculate, in 7 cases performing fellatio on them. Half the offenders were known to the victims. Societal beliefs that men should be able to defend themselves, concern that their masculinity would be suspect, and embarrassment concerning the act of reporting, made male victims reluctant to report sexual assault.

Rapes reported by men resulted in more physical trauma than those reported by women (Kaufman, DiVasto, Jackson, Voorhees, & Christy, 1980). These workers found an increase of from 0% to 10% from 1975 to 1978 in percentage of male as compared to female victims of male sexual assault presenting to a sexual assault team in New Mexico. Five of the 14 males were over 18 years of age. Seven males and 23 of the 100 female victims had been attacked by more than one assailant. Eight male and 12 female victims were attacked multiple times. Nine male victims were beaten, 5 severely, so that they suffered more physical trauma than the 11 female victims who were beaten. All 14 male victims were sodomized and 9 were forced to commit fellatio. Five did not report their sexual assault during their initial contact with emergency department staff, preferring to seek treatment solely for their nongenital trauma. The authors speculated that a far smaller proportion of male as compared with female victims report their assault. Similar findings characterizd sexual assaults experienced by 22 male victims of mean age 26, who returned questionnaires in response to newspaper requests in the United Kingdom (King, 1992b). Ten self-identified as homosexual, 4 as bisexual, and 8 as heterosexual at the time of the assault. Forced anal intercourse was the principal assault in 17, and was attempted on a further 3. Five were injured to the extent of seeking medical attention and 1 lost blood clots from the rectum but was too embarrassed to seek medical help; 12 believed they were about to be killed by the attacker. Assailants of the 6 victims who were assaulted out of doors were unknown or 1–2-hour acquaintances and all 6 "were injured at least to some extent." The remainder were confidence rapes, 6 by someone well known, 3 by few-hour acquaintances, 3 by someone met for casual sex, 3 by homosexual lovers or ex-lovers and 1 by a family member. Five perpetrators attempted to masturbate the victims. Only 2 victims reported the assault to police and both were angry and disappointed that prison sentences imposed on their assailants were suspended.

One hundred male victims in London sought help from a volunteer-run service, "Survivors," after being sexually assaulted (Hillman, O'Mara, Taylor-Robinson, & Harris, 1990). Their mean age at the time of the assault was 14.5 years, and at presentation, 25.3 years, so that most were reporting past assaults. Of 37 for whom information was available, before the assault 38% considered themselves heterosexual, 51%, homosexual, and 11%, bisexual. This finding and that of King's study (1992b) suggests that predominantly homosexual rather than heterosexual adolescent males are more vulnerable to sexual assault or more willing to reveal it. The former possibility was supported by the finding that of 14 men who reported to a psychiatrist (Myers, 1989), they had been sexually abused earlier in life (in 11 after the age of 12), 8 were homosexual, 1 bisexual and 1 asexual. Male students aware of homosexual feelings were more likely to have been sexually coerced than those who were not (McConaghy & Zamir, 1995). Seventy-two of the 100 men investigated by Hillman and colleagues (1990) knew their assailant, who was in 28 cases a family member. Seventy-five victims had been assaulted on more than one occasion, 43 reported multiple assailants, and 15, women assailants, in 12 cases in combination with men. Assaults occurred most commonly in the home of the victim or assailant. Receptive anal intercourse was reported by 75% of the victims, receptive oral intercourse by 59%, insertive oral intercourse by 43%, masturbation by the assailant by 55%, and forced vaginal intercourse by 10%. In 88 cases the assailant ejaculated, as did 53 of the victims. Fifty-one victims felt their life had been endangered. Thirty-three suffered skin or mucosal damage, which the authors considered similar to the percentage reported in other studies of male victims and greater than that reported in studies of female victims. Seventeen sought medical help; 12 of the 17 revealed the sexual assault to the medical staff. Police were involved in 12 cases, but in only 2 did the victims feel they were helpful. Assailants were taken to court in 5 cases; however, only 2 were successfully prosecuted.

Sexual assaults of men by women are only rarely reported and the possibility treated dismissively by some workers. M. B. Harris (1992) stated that one aim of her study of aggressive behaviors carried out or experienced by 416 university students was to look at the effect of the sex of the aggressor and the victim separately. Being forced to have sex was reported by 8% of the men: in 2%, the aggressor was male and in 6%, female. Harris found the latter report surprising and commented that "it seems likely that most reflect either a grudging assent to unwanted sexual activity or a deliberate falsification in order to appear humorous" (p. 214). She raised no questions concerning the validity of the other aggressive behaviors reported by the subjects. Sarrel and Masters (1982) considered there was a widespread belief that it would be almost impossible for a man to achieve or maintain an erection when threatened or attacked by a woman, which belief meant that male victims of sexual assault have not been identified nor their psychotherapeutic needs met. They stated that most such sexual abuse was committed by older females on young males and that just as many women lubricate genitally and respond with orgasm when sexually molested, men can respond sexually to female assault even though their mental state is negative. They reported the sexual assault by women only, of 10 men; 3 in adulthood by more than one woman or by being threatened with a gun or scalpel and tied up or both. Three of the 100 men investigated by Hillman and colleagues (1990) were assaulted by women only; 1 of the 14 reported by Myers (1989) was fondled and fellated by his mother at age 13.

Other groups whose sexual abuse has been insufficiently emphasized so that they lack adequate protection and services are women in the workplace (Schneider, 1991), the handicapped (Rinear, 1985) and the mentally retarded (Tharinger, Horton, & Millea, 1990). The prevalence of sexual torture is beginning to be recognized. Torture has been widespread in one in three countries in the 1980s, affecting millions of people (Turner, 1992). Of 283 victims mainly from Europe, Turkey, and Latin America, 80% of the women and 56% of the men had experienced sexual torture, ranging from physical sexual assaults and violence against the sex organs to mental assaults including forced nakedness and witnessing others being sexually tortured (Lunde & Ortmann, 1990).

There appears to be little interest in the investigation and prevention of rapes of male prisoners. Judge Lois G. Foret, in her introduction to *Fraternity Gang Rape* (Sanday, 1990), stated, "Most street criminals get a graduate course in crime while in prison; many are raped by other inmates and abused by prison guards" (p. xxii). Nacci and Kane (1984) reported that 30 (9%) of 330 federal prison inmates randomly selected to be representative of the entire system reported having been sexually assaulted, including 7 of the 10 self-acknowledged homosexual or bisexual inmates. Sexual pressure attempts were potentially the most dangerous conflict situations in prison, involving use of weapons and damage to either or both inmates. They considered that the motivation of correctional officers to protect inmates could be improved.

Research investigating the sexual assault of children has also largely overlooked violence in the sense of use of physical force. This may be because apart from the fact that physical harm is relatively uncommon, studies reporting the use of force have found no consistent relationship between its use and the victims' long-term symptomatology (Browne & Finkelhor, 1986; Wyatt & Mickey, 1988). Objection to child–adult sexual activity has largely been based on evidence that it is followed by long-term psychopathology, rather than on its intrinsic unacceptability as an infringement of the human rights of children. Children are unable to make informed choices concerning their involvement in acts concerning which powerful discriminatory overt and covert social beliefs exist because the beliefs they will develop concerning these acts in later life are unpredictable (McConaghy, 1993).

Kincaid (1992), in his deconstruction of pedophilia, questioned the belief that large and older people are necessarily more powerful than small and younger people, pointing out that "anyone involved with the issue of pedophilia, even the police, admits that violence or physical force are almost never used by pedophiles" (p. 24) and that "the child may be further equipped with the power attached to the emotional vulnerability of the older partner and to the much blunter threat of exposure or blackmail" (pp. 24–25). In the paradoxical fashion common to postmodern analyses he added, "Perhaps power hates pedophilia so because it actually threatens to grant power to the child, placing the adult in a weakened, sometimes dependent position" (p. 25). He questioned the traditional view of pedophilia that "all sexual encounters between adults and children involve a self-evident power imbalance and are thus deeply coercive: the adult is larger; has invested in her or him psychological and cultural authority; is more experienced at manipulating the child. Through power, the narrative can only be told one way, as a story of rape, it being 'patently ridiculous' to suppose that the child can ever be the instigator in such relations. Furthermore, the damage to the child is inevitable and inevitably severe" (p. 187). Though the objection to adult–child sexual activity as an expression of an imbalance of power can be subverted in this way, the fundamental objection that it is an abuse of the child's inability to give informed consent would appear to be unassailable.

The major research studies of prevalence of child abuse classified acts as abusive which ranged from exposure and forced kissing to anal and vaginal penetration. As all child–adult sexual activities tended to be regarded as equally harmful, information was rarely provided concerning the degree of forcefulness of the various acts. This was the case when as part of the Los Angeles Epidemiologic Catchment Area Project (Stein, Golding, Siegel, Burnam, & Sorenson, 1988), reactions of 1,358 women and 1,325 men to pressure or force to have sexual contact were investigated; and when as part of a study funded by the National Center for the Prevention and Control of Rape at NIMH to describe the effects of sexual abuse on children (Conte & Schuetman, 1988), data were collected at or near the time of disclosure from contacts and the child, if over 12 years of age, for 369 children seen at a Sexual Assault Center. Herman (1985) reported that the abuse of daughters usually began when they were between the ages of 6 and 12, commencing with fondling and proceeding over time to masturbation and oral-genital activities; vaginal intercourse was not usually attempted until the child reached at least puberty. Physical violence was rare, the father's authority being sufficient to gain compliance. The sexual contact was repeated for years with secrecy ensured by threats of family breakup or expulsion of the child, so that the abuse ended only when the child found the resources to escape. In Russell's (1986) study of the incest victims among the San Francisco women investigated, in almost half the cases of abuse by stepfathers and a quarter of those by biological fathers, the abuse was in the category classified as very serious, which included activities ranging from forced penile-vaginal penetration to nonforceful attempted fellatio, cunnilingus, analingus, and anal intercourse. Male students molested before the age of 14, from an approximately representative national sample, reported the most serious experience was exhibitionism in a third, fondling in a third, and attempted or successful penetration in a third (Risin & Koss, 1987). In Becker's investigation (1988) of 139 adolescents accused of sexual crimes, of the 27 who indicated they were victims of sexual abuse, 11 reported they were physically coerced, 3 by aggression beyond that necessary to complete the abuse, and 1 required medical attention for assault-related injuries. Of 156 children sexually abused mainly by family members (Gomes-Schwartz, Horowitz, & Sauzier, 1990) 23% showed physical injuries, most of relatively minor bruises or irritations. Children's compliance was gained by emotional manipulation only in 32%, manipulation and threats in 19%, and manipulation, threats, and aggression in 28%. It was emphasized that family members were as likely to resort to violence as unrelated offenders. Freund, Heasman, and Roper (1982) noted the enormous discrepancy in reported incidence of the use of force in sexual abuse of children, ranging from 0% to 58%. They attributed the discrepancy to the different samples of victims studied. None of the 18,000 persons interviewed by the Kinsey group claimed to have been sadistically victimized as a child (Quinsey, 1986).

The widespread media attention, national and international, given violent sexually motivated acts resulting in death, masks the fact that they are extremely rare. A survey of child murders found that 3 of the 83 victims had been killed in a sexual assault (Quinsey, 1986). Most are committed by parents, more by neglect than physical abuse (Bourget & Bradford, 1990; A. C. Kilpatrick, 1992). Swigert, Farrell, and Yoels (1976) examined all cases of homicide in a jurisdiction in the northeastern United States from 1955 through 1973. Of 444 cases, 5 qualified as sexual homicides, and only 2 of these were considered cases of sexual sadism, 1 heterosexual and 1 homosexual. Two occurred in consensual sexual relationships, 1 heterosexual and 1 homosexual, and 1 from fear the victim of homosexual pedophilia would reveal the offense. Swigert and colleagues commented that all 5 cases received front-page newspaper coverage and weeks of follow-up reporting on their legal progress. The 350 cases of homicides that resulted from altercations among friends, relatives, and acquaintances received minimal newspaper attention.

On the basis of 20 years of experience in forensic psychiatry, Brittain (1970) described the typical sadistic murder as carefully planned and the method of killing as usually asphyxial, and more rarely by mutilating violence or multiple stabbing. Injuries were most commonly of the victim's breasts, genitalia, or rectum. There often appeared to be a deliberate attempt to offend modesty by the way the victim's body was arranged. Revitch (1965) reviewed accounts of 9 murders and 34 violent unprovoked assaults on women. They involved choking, inflicting multiple knife wounds, or battering with a heavy object. Erection and ejaculation may or may not have accompanied the aggressive acts. Rape and attempted rape were infrequent. Revitch commented that violence served as a substitute for it; consequently, the underlying sexual dynamics might be disregard.

Dietz, Hazelwood, and Warren (1990) selected 30 subjects as possibly sexually sadistic criminals from case files of subjects identified to the National Center for the

Analysis of Violent Crime (NCAVC) over 5 years on the basis that the 30 had been sexually aroused in response to images of suffering and humiliation on two or more occasions over at least 6 months. All were male. Seventy-three percent had murdered their victim, and 56% had murdered at least three, most often by strangulation, and next most often by shooting. Their crimes often involved careful planning, the selecting of strangers as victims, approaching the victim under a pretext, participation of a partner, restraining and beating victims, holding them captive, anal rape, forced fellatio, vaginal rape, foreign object penetration, and keeping records of offenses and personal items of victims. Seventy-three percent victimized only females, 17% only males, and 10% members of both sexes. Fifty-three percent victimized only adults and 17% only children. Lesieur and Welch (1991) pointed out in relation to serial murders that there was lack of community concern when victims were presumed to be prostitutes, and public anger was aroused only when this perception proved inaccurate.

When markedly violent rapes, such as sexual murders occur, they may attract significant media attention. The "Central Park Jogger Rape" in which a woman jogger was violently beaten and repeatedly raped by four 15–17-year-old African Americans, sustained multiple skull fractures, cuts and bruises, and was left unconscious and for dead (Messerschmidt, 1993) received worldwide publicity.

Historical Background

The current recognition of the importance of sexual violence in the United States resulted largely from the feminist politics of the 1960s with establishment of consciousness-raising groups and "speak outs" against rape. Burgess (1985) pointed out that at that time, almost all jurisdictions defined rape as "illicit carnal knowledge of a woman, forcibly and against her will" with "carnal knowledge" customarily interpreted as vaginal penetration by the penis. One of the first achievements of the anti-rape movement was the introduction of the Michigan Criminal Sexual Code which broadened the criteria of assaultive sexual acts, extended protection to separated spouses and males, eliminated requirements of resistance, and restricted use of the victim's sexual history. By 1976, 49 other states were revising or had revised their rape statutes. The U.S. federal government established the National Center for the Prevention and Control of Rape, broadening the definition to include criminal sexual assaults, heterosexual or homosexual, that involved the use or threat of force, and the coercion or bribery of children. Nevertheless, as discussed earlier, despite the change in legal definition, the community and even many victims' conception of rape appears to remain that of sexual assault involving penetration of a woman by a stranger, the form commonly reported to the authorities and in the media.

In relation to the debate over criminalizing marital rape when in most of the United States a husband could not be prosecuted for raping his wife, Finkelhor and Yllo (1985) quoted the opinion of public figures that it would involve relatively little of the psychological trauma incurred in rape by a stranger. They pointed out that in fact surveys showed more marital rape victims reported marked long-term effects than did victims of any other kind of rape, and commented, "When you are raped by a stranger you have to live with a frightening memory. When you are raped by your husband, you have to live with your rapist" (p. 138). They also countered the passionately held new argument that defining marital rape as a crime would lead to frivolous complaints by vindictive women. Forty-two cases of marital rape that came to the attention of the police or courts in the 2 years following the criminalization of marital rape in California in January 1980 were extremely brutal, with the use of knives and guns being common. One woman was raped with a crowbar; one forced to have sex with other men and dogs, and one was killed before her husband could be apprehended for her rape. Of the 72% of cases which went on to prosecution, 89% (25 out of 28) resulted in conviction, 17 of the offenders pleading guilty. Eight of the 11 who pleaded not guilty were convicted. Of the 25 found guilty, 14 went to prison, with the longest sentence for marital rape uncomplicated by other crimes and weapons violations being 3 years, when the maximal possible term for felony spousal rape was 8 years. Finkelhor and Yllo commented that if California's experience holds true elsewhere, rather than the cases dealt with legally being frivolous, they are the most blatant, brutal, and heinous.

As Messerschmidt (1993) pointed out, impressive gains influencing the law to limit sexual violence against women were also made in the last century. In the 1860s and 70s, feminists in the United States organized a campaign against state regulation of prostitution, arguing that such regulation forced alleged prostitutes into vaginal examinations. Only one city (St. Louis) introduced regulation and only for 4 years. Messerschmidt also cited Helen H. Gardner's comments in the Arena: "No being who is not degraded or too utterly, mentally and morally diseased to be a safe person to be at large, could wish that a little child, a baby girl fourteen, twelve, aye, ten years of age should be made, as is the case in many of our states, the legal and rightful prey of grown men" (p. 160). Representatives of the Women's Christian Temperance Union, the largest women's organization in the nation, from every state petitioned state legislatures to raise the age of sexual consent. In 1886, it was 10 for girls in many states; by 1900, only 2 states maintained it below 14, and 12 had raised it to 18 years.

To investigate the view advanced in the 1970s that rape should be regarded as on a continuum with normal male behavior, Koss and Oros (1982) developed the Sexual Experiences Survey, a questionnaire on which subjects reported their experiences of sexual intercourse associated with various degrees of coercion, threat, or force. It was administered in two parallel forms, one for men in which they reported acts of aggression, and one for women in which they reported acts of victimization. This apparently sexist approach was considered appropriate as women represented almost 100% of rape victims in U.S. Department of Justice investigations. Responses of a representative sample of 3,862 university students supported the dimensional concept. Thirty-three percent of women reported having intercourse when they did not want it because the man became so sexually aroused, and 23% of men reported becoming so sexually aroused they had intercourse with a woman who did not want it. Eight percent of women reported having intercourse when they did not want it because the man used some degree of force; 6% said they had been raped. A problem with this methodology was that it failed to explore the possibility that although most victims of forceful rape are women, less forceful coercion may be more equivalently used by both sexes. This was found to be the case when a modified form of the Sexual Experiences Survey in which men and women could report experiences both as aggressors and victims was completed by medical students (McConaghy & Zamir, 1995). Twenty percent of men and 14% of women reported making constant physical attempts to have sexual activity with an opposite-sex partner; 26% of men and 31% of women reported being victims of such attempts. Struckman-Johnson (1988) found 16% of male as compared to 22% of female university students reported at least one episode in which they were forced to engage in sexual intercourse on a date. Most men were coerced by psychological pressure and most women by force, but 28% of men were coerced by both. In a study of psychology students, more men (63%) than women (46%) reported experiencing unwanted sexual intercourse (Muehlenhard & Cook, 1988). McConaghy and Zamir found significant relationships between the degree of sexual coercion men and women reported carrying out and their masculinity scores on the Bem Sex Role Inventory (Bem, 1974). If the dimensional concept of rape has validity, it would seem that rape is on a continuum with masculine rather than male behavior, and that investigation of less forceful forms of sexual coercion requires a nonsexist approach.

Epidemiology

Burgess (1985) summarized prevalence figures for rape in national statistics. The Uniform Crime Reports defines forcible rape as "the carnal knowledge of a female forcibly and against her will. Assaults or attempts to commit rape by force or threat of force are also included; however, statutory rape (without force) and other sex offenses are excluded" (White & Koss, 1993). Reported rapes doubled from 1971 to 1981 to reach 34.4 of every 100,000 women, less than a hundredth of the prevalence revealed in community surveys. No male victims were included. The National Crime Survey (NCS), which attempts by a continuing survey of representative households to identify cases not disclosed to law enforcement agencies, reported rates that were several times higher, still substantially below those of community surveys (Burgess, 1985). Karmen (1991) pointed out that women told NCS interviewers that they failed to notify the authorities not because they were intimidated and feared reprisals, nor because they did not want to invest the time and effort to get involved in the criminal justice process. Rather, they believed the incidents were not serious enough or were personal matters, that nothing could be done, or that the police did not want to be bothered, or were inefficient, ineffective, or insensitive. In 1987 the number of reported rapes increased to 38 of every 100,000 women, while the number disclosed in the NCS decreased from a high of over 110 in 1979 to 71 in 100,000 women (Parker, 1991), suggesting that women have become less reluctant to report rape to the police. False allegations of rape present a further problem. Kanin (1994) found that over a 9-year period, an average of 41% of women's reports of completed forcible rapes to a police agency in the midwestern United States were officially declared false, one criterion of which was that the complainant admitted that no rape had occurred. Kanin provided data indicating that the women were not withdrawing accusations when rape had actually occurred, but pointed out that it was not possible to generalize from this finding to other police agencies. He found a comparable incidence (50%) of false allegations of forcible rape by women in the police records of two large midwestern state universities.

On the basis of the NCS figure, 11% of Black and 8% of White women will be victims of attempted or completed rape at least once during their lifetimes. As pointed out earlier, most rapes are not reported in these national surveys. The prevalence of rape makes totally understandable the finding cited by Warr (1991) that on a 10-point scale of fear, two thirds of a sample of Seattle women ages 19 to

35 indicated that their fear of being raped was over 5, and "a startling 31%" rated it 10. Correlates of rates of rape in standard metropolitan statistical areas were poverty, percentage Black, and percentage divorced, paralleling research on the correlates of homicide rates (Parker, 1991).

The 1,157 adult women participants in the NIMH North Carolina Epidemiologic Catchment Area (ECA) Program were questioned 1 year subsequently concerning experiences of sexual assault, defined as situations where someone pressured them against their will into forced contact with the sexual parts of their body or the offender's body (Winfield, George, Swartz, & Blazer, 1990). Seven percent of those 44 years of age or younger reported having experienced assault, compared with 3% of those 45 to 64 years of age. Sex of the offender was not reported. An earlier ECA study investigated male as well as female victims of assault as a supplement to the Los Angeles project (Sorenson, Stein, Siegel, Golding, & Burnam, 1987). Subjects were 1,480 men and 1,645 women, mainly Hispanics and non-Hispanic Whites. Sexual assault was any pressured or forced touching of the victim or offender's sexual parts or sexual intercourse. Thirteen percent of women reported having been sexually assaulted in adulthood (16 years or older) and 16% in their lifetime. Comparable percentages for men were 7% and 9%, respectively. Sexual assaults were reported more often by White non-Hispanics and by younger subjects and those with some college education. Age of victim at the time of first assault was 5 or younger in 6%, 6–10 in 13%, 11–15 in 19%, 16–20 in 34%, 21–25 in 15%, and 26 or older in 12%. Modal age of the victim at the time of assault was 18 years. One third reported one assault and two thirds, two or more. The most recent assault involved a male assailant in 75% of cases, who acted alone in 90% of cases, and was acquainted with but not related to the victim in 77% of cases. In 26% of the cases, the assailant was a spouse or lover, more being spouses in the case of women and lovers in the case of men. Verbal pressure was used with 62% of the male and 27% of the female victims, and harm or threat of harm in 37% of female and 9% of male victims. Eighty-three percent of the victims tried to resist, and the outcome was some form of intercourse in 50% of women and 39% of men. The sex of the victims of the 25% of female assailants was not reported.

Laumann, Gagnon, Michael, and Michaels (1994) reported of their 78.5% representative U.S. sample that in face-to-face interviews, 15% of women and 1.3% of men reported being forced after puberty by a person of the opposite sex to do anything sexually that they did not want to do. In anonymous questionnaires, 2.8% of men and 1.5% of women reported forcing an opposite sex person sexually, and 1.9% of men reported being forced by a man. The aggressor of the women was someone they were in love with, 46%; their spouse, 9%; someone they knew well, 22%; acquaintances, 19%; and strangers, 4%. Ten percent of the national sample of adolescent males interviewed by Ageton (1983) over 3 years reported having forced females into sexual behavior involving contact with the sexual parts of the body. Yearly over the same 3 years 1 adolescent male in 200 was arrested for forcible rape. Studies of college men have found that 4% to 7% report having perpetrated rape; a further 4% report attempted rape (White & Koss, 1993).

As Karmen (1991) pointed out, the most underreported crimes in the NCS are offenses committed by nonstrangers, especially intimates such as family members and lovers, as in acquaintance rape and the sexual abuse of children. Finkelhor, Hotaling, Lewis, and Smith (1990) reported the first national survey in which by use of a randomly generated sample of all residential phone numbers in the United States, 1,145 men and 1,481 women (76% of those requested) answered four questions concerning childhood (age 18 or younger) experiences that they would now consider sexual abuse. Someone trying or succeeding in having any kind of sexual intercourse, or anything similar was reported by 14.6% of women and 9.5% of men; touching, grabbing, kissing, or rubbing against their bodies, or anything similar, by 19.6% of women and 4.5% of men; having nude photos taken, being exhibited to or having a sex act performed in their presence, or anything similar, by 3.7% of women and 1.6% of men; and oral sex or sodomy, or anything similar, by .1% of women and .4% of men. Twenty-seven percent of women and 16% of men reported at least one of these experiences. Of the representative sample studied by Laumann and colleagues (1994), 17% of women and 12% of men reported they had been sexually touched before the age of 12 or 13 by someone over age 14. Perpetrators in the Finkelhor and colleagues study were men in 98% of the offenses against girls and 83% of those against boys; and in the Laumann and colleagues study were men only, women only, and both in 91%, 4%, and 4%, respectively of the offenses against girls; and 38%, 54%, and 7%, respectively, of the offenses against boys. The sexual behaviors reported to Laumann and colleagues, were vaginal intercourse in 14% of the women and 42% of the men, and anal sex in 18% of the men with male perpetrators. Oral sexual contact was reported by 30% of the men and 10% of the women with male perpetrators and 10% of the men with women perpetrators. In their study, the median age of abuse was 9.9 for boys and girls. Laumann and colleagues found that older men who touch girls or boys select a similar age profile, with modal age between 7 and 10; whereas women touched older boys and the touchers tended to be young. Perpetrators were relatives for 54% and strangers for 7% of the women and relatives for 20% and strangers for 4% of the men. In the study by Finkelhor and colleagues, perpetrators were relatives for 29% and strangers for 21% of the women and relatives for 11% and strangers for 40% of the men. Force was used in 15% of the incidents to boys and 19% of those to girls. Some marked disparities between these two studies of representative U.S. samples are discussed in relation to assessment. They agreed in finding that the prevalence of child–adult sexual experiences reported by subjects of different ages did not support the belief that there had been an increase in those growing up in the wake of the "sexual revolution" of the 1960s.

Community studies rarely question adult subjects concerning their sexual activities with children. About 15% of male and 2% of female university students in the United States and Australia reported some likelihood of having sexual activity with a prepubertal child if they could do so without risk (Malamuth, 1989; McConaghy, Zamir, & Manicavasagar, 1993). Homosexual male pedophiles commonly report molesting many hundreds of victims; heterosexual male pedophiles molest only a few. Since nearly half as many men as women report childhood victimization from men, there must be many more male offenders of female than of male children.

Characteristics of the Offender

Violent sex offenders most readily available for study are those who are convicted. However, as discussed earlier, they represent only a small proportion of sexually coercive subjects and child molesters in the community, constituting a highly skewed population, in which those who attack strangers, use extreme force, and lack the social skills to avoid detection are overrepresented (Herman, 1990). Factors leading to conviction independent of their sexual offenses would account for the findings of Knight, Rosenberg, and Schneider (1985) of marked similarities between convicted rapists, child molesters, and the general prison population. Findings that rapists and child molesters were deficient in social skills and accomplishments were not replicated when the offenders were compared with socioeconomically matched community controls (Stermac, Segal, & Gillis, 1990). Other similarities found by Knight and colleagues included low socioeconomic status, high rate of school failure or dropout, subsequent unstable employment record of an unskilled nature, previous convictions for nonsexual offenses, and poor and alcoholic family of origin. It seems likely that these features contributed to the detection and conviction of incarcerated sex offenders as they would to the rest of the prison population. Rapists and child molesters not convicted, as compared with those convicted for offenses carried out in adolescence (Knight & Prentky, 1993), showed less delinquent and antisocial behavior and aggressive responses to frustration. In regard to arrests for forcible rape, as with most arrests, Blacks are overrepresented. In 1986, when slightly over 12% of the U.S. population was counted as Black, 47% of those arrested for rape were Black. This overrepresentation did not appear due to police racism, as it was present in victims' reports in the NCS data of the perceived characteristics of their aggressors (A. R. Harris, 1991).

Bard and colleagues (1987) pointed out that a consistent difference in incarcerated rapists and child molesters was that the former were younger and the latter were more evenly distributed throughout the age span. U.S. Department of Justice studies were cited by Herman (1990) as consistently showing that about 25% of rapists were under 18 years of age. Knight and colleagues (1985) found that a number of studies reported a higher incidence of mental retardation and organic brain syndrome in child molesters. Not unexpectedly, rapists were more likely to show behavioral excesses, to be overassertive or explosive, and to have greater heterosexual experience. Clinical studies of nonincarcerated sex offenders seeking treatment have reported that subjects with evidence of congenital or acquired brain damage are overrepresented (Berlin & Meinecke, 1981; McConaghy, Blaszczynski, & Kidson, 1988).

Watkins and Bentovim (1992) cited evidence that a much higher percentage of pedophiles than rapists reported histories of childhood sexual victimization: 57% versus 23% in one study (Seghorn, Prentky, & Boucher, 1987) and 56% versus 5% in another (Pithers, Kashima, Cumming, & Beal, 1988). Adult sex offenders who carried out offenses in adolescence compared with those who had not were more likely to report having been sexually abused in childhood, the abuse being more serious and occurring at an earlier age (Knight & Prentky, 1993). The hypothesis that subjects sexually abused in their childhood become sex offenders through "identification with the aggressor" was criticized by Herman (1990) as based on retrospective reports of identified offenders who were not representative of the much larger undetected population of offenders. Also, most studies supporting the theory lacked appropriate comparison groups and employed vague definitions of childhood sexual abuse. It has also been argued that sex offenders, particularly child molesters, could report being victimized in childhood to obtain the sympathy of the interviewer or more lenient legal treatment, or unconsciously exaggerate remembered events to reduce feelings of guilt (Freund, Watson, & Dickey, 1990). The hypothesis is not applicable to all pedophiles; even when child molesters were excluded who did not show penile volume plethysmography evidence of an erotic preference for children, only a minority of the remaining pedophiles (43.9% and 49.4%) reported having been molested by an adult male or female (over 17 years) prior to ages of 12 and 16, respectively (Freund & Kuban, 1994). Significantly more sex offenders against adult women and control men with erotic preference for adult women reported having been seduced between ages 12 and 15 by a physically mature woman than did the pedophiles, a finding the authors considered should be pursued further. Evidence of an abused–abuser relationship in relation to adult sexual coercion was found in a study of medical students (McConaghy, Manicavasagar, & Zamir, 1995). Correlations of $r = 0.6$ were found in both men and women, between those coerced by men and coercing men, and those coerced by women and coercing women. With regard to the abused–abuser hypothesis, Watkins and Bentovim (1992) commented that the most extraordinary report was that of Chasnoff and colleagues (1986); of 3 baby boys whose maternal abuse stopped at 4, 9, and 18 months, respectively, 2 had begun before the age of 3 years to sexually molest other children

Increased exposure to pornography in childhood reported by sex offenders as compared with nonoffenders in several studies was attributed by Murrin and Laws (1990) to differences in the home life of the two groups. They also reviewed studies that found similar patterns of use by sex offenders and nonoffenders in adolescence, both reporting masturbating to pornography. In adulthood, the latter activity was more common in sex offenders, who also owned more pornography. The fact that the significant differences in use of pornography by sex offenders compared with controls was found in adulthood whereas, as discussed subsequently, most sexually deviant behavior appears established in adolescence, suggests that the use of pornography is not causal.

In reviewing classifications of incarcerated rapists, Knight and colleagues (1985) commented that few empirical data existed concerning their reliability or validity. However, that referred to in relation to the description of rape by Groth and colleagues (1977) has retained attention. They distinguished anger and power rapists. Power rapists were more common and did not desire to harm their victims, but to control them so that they had no say in the matter. Two subgroups were differentiated. Power-reassurance rapists used rape to alleviate doubts about their sexual adequacy and masculinity by placing their victim in a helpless, controlled position in which the victim could not refuse or reject the rapist. Power-assertive rapists' doubts were about their sense of identity and effectiveness. They used rape to display virility, mastery, and dominance. Anger rapists expressed anger, rage, contempt, and hatred for their victims by abusing them in profane language, beating them, sexually assaulting them, and forcing them to perform or submit to additional degrading acts. They used more force than was necessary simply to subdue the victim and she suffered physical violence to all parts of her body. Anger-retaliation rapists committed rape as an expression of their hostility and rage toward women. Anger-excitement rapists found pleasure, thrills, and excitement in the suffering of the victim. They were sadistic and aimed to punish, hurt, and torture the victim, so that their aggression was eroticized.

Yllo and Finkelhor (1985) found characteristics similar to those described by Groth and colleagues (1977) in sexually assaultive husbands, power motivating those who carried out nonbattering rape; anger, those who carried out battering rapes; and sadism, those who carried out obsessive rapes and appeared to require the ritualistic use of force to become sexually aroused. Sexual assaults of partners were more likely to be carried out by men from lower social-class backgrounds, battering rapes in response to what was seen as a challenge to their authority being twice as likely to be made by low-income and working-class as middle-class men, and three times as likely to be made by unemployed or part-time employed as fully employed men. This was attributed to the lower social-class perpetrators having a stronger traditional patriarchal gender division of labor and power (Messerschmidt, 1993). Perpetrators of force-only rape compared with battering rape were significantly more educated and more often middle-class, and believed it was their wives' duty to satisfy their sexual needs. Pointing out the paucity of information available from men who rape partners, Finkelhor and Yllo (1985) interviewed three who volunteered following community service group meetings. They were not typical of the husbands of women victims interviewed by the authors; none were chronic batterers and all three felt some degree of remorse. Finkelhor and Yllo commented: "They were not moral monsters, they talked about their problems and their fears in ways which seemed quite human. They explained and justified their behavior with attitudes that are probably shared by large segments of the male population. They made a convincing case for how normal marital rape can be" (p. 83).

Herman (1990), in outlining her feminist perspective, was critical of psychodynamic formulations such as those of Groth that describe rapists as committing their crimes in efforts to combat deep-seated feelings of insecurity and vulnerability or to express wishes for virility, masculinity, and dominance. She considered such formulations resulted in the victimizer being seen as a victim, no longer an object of fear but of pity. These euphemistic reformulations of the offender's behavior detoxified rape and made it more acceptable. She believed the would-be therapist ran the risk of credulously accepting the offender's rationalizations for his crimes as well as supplying him with new ones.

About half the noncharged rapists interviewed by Ageton (1983) had been drinking or taking drugs prior to the assault. They viewed their own sexual excitement and the behavior and physical appearance of the victim as instrumental in causing the assault, the largest proportion reporting their response included feeling satisfied, confused, guilty, and proud. About half indicated their friends knew about the assault and their reactions were overwhelmingly ones of approval. These reactions were predictable in the light of Ageton's comparison of the assaultive group with nonassaultive adolescents matched for age and class. The assaultive subjects were alienated from home and school, showed a wide variety of delinquent behaviors including physical[*] assaults, and greater exposure to delinquent peers who supported delinquent and sexually aggressive behaviors. Data obtained 2 years prior to the subjects' sexually assaultive behaviors revealed that they were then more committed to a delinquent peer group than were the controls. Ageton concluded that her results pointed to the fact that sexual assault offenders were basically delinquent youths. This conclusion is supported by the finding that delinquency, sexual promiscuity, hostile masculinity, social isolation, and attitudes supportive of violence predicted the sexual aggression reported by a national sample of college students (Malamuth, Sockloskie, Koss, & Tonaka, 1991). Sexually aggressive college students used alcohol and drugs at a significantly highly level than did the nonaggressive students (White & Koss, 1993).

The college date rapists studied by Kanin (1985) reported consensual heterosexual outlets averaging 1.5 per week as compared with 0.8 per month for nonrapist college graduate controls; they considered they needed more orgasms per week than the controls to feel sexually satisfied. It is possible some sex offenders have a biologically determined higher level of sexual interest. A number of studies have shown that self-reported aggressive college men and men who obtain high scores on the Attraction to Sexual Aggression Scale (Malamuth, 1989) show higher levels of physiological and self-reported sexual arousal to depictions of forced sex compared to sexually nonaggressive subjects; it was suggested that sexually coercive men, including acquaintance rapists, were generally more sexually arousable, whether to consenting or rape stimuli (White & Koss, 1993). Number of sexual partners (Koss, Leonard, Beezley, & Oros, 1985) and early age of sexual initiation (Koss & Dinero, 1988) predicted later-reported sexually aggressive behaviors in male university students. Kanin (1985) commented that date rapists' quests for heterosexual engagement bordered on the no-holds-barred, 93% as compared to 40% of controls employing at least one of such methods as trying to intoxicate their companions, falsely professing love, and promising "pinning," engagement, or marriage. White and Koss (1993) cited the finding of Kanin that the sexually assaultive behavior of young men was related to their fathers' attitude toward sexual aggression, and a further study that found a correlation between college men's reports of sexually aggressive behavior and their fathers' kissing, fondling, and forcing sexual activity with their mothers against the mothers' wishes.

Sanday (1990) considered that although the sexist attitudes and the phallocentric mentality associated with gang rapes in the form of "pulling train" have a long history in Western society, occurring in war and street gang activity, most on campus were associated with fraternities. The conception of rape held by the offenders was of forcing a woman to have sexual intercourse against her will, interpreting the lack of resistance of a woman drunk or high on drugs as willing acquiescence. "She could be unconscious and still be responsible because she has not said no and no force was applied. The brothers do not consider the possibility that their numbers may constitute force" (p. 65). From conversations with fraternity brothers, Sanday considered that in telling one another how to interpret sexual signals and how to act at parties, they encouraged one another in what can only be described as rape-prone behavior. She pointed out there was a very fine line between seduction and rape when they candidly admitted they did not take repeated "no's" for an answer. Sanday attributed a significant role in fraternity brothers' adopting these attitudes to initiation rituals in which as pledges they were initially abused and degraded as powerless and tied to their mothers, before power and manhood were conferred upon them by killing the inner woman. "The result . . . is a pattern of serious irresponsibility, sexism, racism, and homophobia (which) promotes the mutual mistrust and frequent incidents of sexual and racial violence that occurs at this university" (p. 155).

Koss and Gaines (1993) pointed out the recent focus of educators on fraternities and athletics as campus institutions encouraging sexual aggression through such behaviors as drinking and the abuse of women. They cited studies documenting the association of sexual aggression with use of alcohol, but were critical of those finding an association with membership in campus organizations on methodological grounds. In their study, 530 psychology students and football team members anonymously completed a modified version of the Sexual Experiences Survey in which questions were added which included standing in a line with other men to take a turn having sex with a "party girl." Stepwise multiple regression demonstrated nicotine use to account for 6% of the variance of the degrees of sexual aggression the men reported, drinking intensity for an additional 3%, and scores on a hostility to women scale and athletic involvement each for an additional 1%. The remaining variables including fraternity affiliation, failed to meet the criteria for inclusion in the prediction equation. A study of medical students (McConaghy, Manicavasagar, & Zamir, 1995) using the Sexual Experiences Survey, modified so that both men and women could report experiences as victims and as aggressors, found that although athletic involvement correlated with coercion of women (more so by women), it correlated more strongly in men and women with their being coerced by women.

The belief that sexually victimization of women and children by men results from the man's holding cognitions supportive of sexually assaultive behavior has not received strong empirical support. The sexually assaultive offenders in Ageton's study (1983) did not differ from the remainder in their beliefs concerning sex roles or their attitudes to sexual assault. Koss and Dinero (1988) investigated an approximately representative national sample of 2,972 male students at 32 U.S. institutions of higher education. Though the subjects' cognitions supportive of sexual aggression correlated with their reported sexually aggressive behaviors, Koss and Dinero found that the subjects' early exposure to family violence, childhood sexual abuse, and early age of sexual initiation, predicted their later sexually aggressive behaviors equally well, suggesting that the cognitions were not causing the sexual aggression, but like the aggression, were secondary to the childhood experiences, or variables associated with these experiences. These could include genetic determinants. Stermac and colleagues (1990) pointed out in regard to convicted rapists that although many investigators reported the clinical impression that they showed attitudes of hostility toward women, attempts to validate this by comparing rapists with other sex offenders, or men from similar socioeconomic groups, found no difference between the two groups.

With regard to characteristics of male rapists of men, 13 of the 22 male victims in the study by King (1992b) reported that their attackers had been drinking alcohol around the time of the assault and that alcohol use was suspected in a further five. Eleven believed the assailants were homosexual, 3 that they were bisexual, and 3 that they were heterosexual. They were described by their victims as angry, scornful, or sadistic in 14 assaults, and several verbally or physically humiliated the victims. The sexual orientation of the assailants of the 100 victims investigated by Hillman and colleagues (1990), was perceived by them to be heterosexual in 72%, homosexual in 16%, and bisexual in 12%, of the 69 in whom this information was available. In his review of male rape in institutional settings, King (1992a) pointed out the scarcity of research undertaken to delineate the nature and extent of the problem, a fact he attributed in part to the failure of authorities in charge to acknowledge the problem and allow research to proceed. A consistent finding has been of a disproportionate number of Black aggressors and White victims both in prisons and juvenile corrective training schools; it was suggested that coerced sexual assault in all-male institutions may be part of an ethnic power struggle taking place at a personalized level, and reflecting a deep-seated resentment harbored by lower-class Blacks against middle-class Whites. It was pointed out that this literature might be influenced by racial prejudice on the part of its writers. It could, of course, also reflect differences in the readiness of Black and White victims to report assaults. King also discussed the assaults occurring in the institutional life of military establishments stating that several involved groups of assailants in assaults that took on something of the nature of initiation ceremonies. King concluded that assaults in institutions were primarily an expression of anger and frustration in men who may be unable to achieve masculine identification and pride through avenues other than sex. Information concerning the perpetrators of the institutional sexual assault of victims of torture is also lacking; it is hoped that many acted unwillingly and under pressure. The United Nations definition made it clear that it was always carried out by or at the instigation of a public official (Turner, 1992).

Offenders of exclusively male and exclusively female children differ markedly. Groth and Birnbaum (1978) investigated 175 men convicted of pedophilia. Most homosexual pedophiles were single and had been exclusively attracted to male children since puberty. The victims were usually strangers or casual acquaintances. Their mean age was 10 years. Homosexual pedophiles (and hebephiles, men attracted to postpubertal adolescents) commonly seek victims in pinball parlors or other settings where young people congregate. Typically, they are of average intelligence or above, yet are uninterested in social or sexual relations with adults. Possibly to avoid detection, they rarely repeat an offense with the same victim unless they are able to form an emotional relationship with the boy, which many wish to do. Most give a history of stable employment. Their offenses usually commence in adolescence (McConaghy, 1993). The majority of convicted heterosexual pedophiles investigated by Groth and Birnbaum were predominantly attracted to adult women and were married. They had rarely shown evidence of pedophilic interest in adolescence and may have been sexually deprived at the time of the offense. Their victims were related or well known to them and had a mean age of 8 years. Other workers found heterosexual as compared with homosexual pedophiles to be more likely to be heavy drinkers, of lower socioeconomic class, to have had little schooling, committed other criminal offenses, and repeated the offense with the same child on many occasions (McConaghy, 1993). Gordon (1989) considered that biological fathers would have greater commitment to the father role than would stepfathers, so that when biological fathers sexually abused daughters it would be in a family environment characterized by relatively high levels of personal, social, and economic stress. Using data from 17 states, drawn from the 1983 National Study on Child Neglect and Reporting, he found, consistent with his expectation, that biological fathers compared with stepfathers showed significantly higher levels of drug or alcohol abuse or both, marital problems, and insufficient income Heterosexual pedophiles who do not show evidence of antisocial behavior, below-average intelligence, or low moral and ethical standards, commonly report total unawareness of any attraction to prepubertal girls prior to their offense. Its initial occurrence was usually impulsive, in response to an unexpected opportunity, such as a female child wrestling with them in their pool, sharing a bath, or cuddling with them. This usually occurred when the subjects were adult and the majority appeared deeply guilty and did not repeat the offense. However, some continued to take advantage of further opportunities and the behavior became compulsive (McConaghy, 1993).

Earlier studies of sexual murderers reported the clinical experience of forensic psychiatrists. Brittain (1970) described the typical sadistic murderer as socially isolated, emotionally flattened, and "weird" in personality or at times psychotic. He may have a record of other paraphilias, such as cross-dressing, peeping, and obscene telephone calls, or a history of extreme cruelty to animals or of firesetting. A surprising number worked as butchers and not infrequently they had an inordinate interest in weapons, guns, or knives, in Nazism, or in black magic. Brittain found that they experienced great excitement during the act of killing, and great relief of tension following its completion. In prison, they were often model prisoners, a fact that he considered could mislead the unwary to believe they had fundamentally changed.

Revitch (1980) also reported a number of these features in male sadistic murderers, as well as a background of maternal overprotection, infantilization, and seduction or rejection. He commented that real or fancied maternal sexual indiscretions were common. In his earlier investigation of men who carried out violent unprovoked sexual assaults or murders of women, Revitch (1965) considered the great majority were overt or latent psychotics, and emphasized their common expression of hatred, and contempt or fear of women. Thirty of the 43 had committed previous offenses, but only three were sex offenses. Twelve of the previous offenses were breaking and entering. Fetishism of female underwear was elicited in 9 cases.

These earlier findings of the characteristics of sexually sadistic criminals contrasted in some respects with those concerning 30 subjects identified by the National Center for the Analysis of Violent Crime (NCAVC) over 5 years (Dietz *et al.,* 1990). The authors agreed the subjects had been sexually aroused in response to images of suffering and humiliation on two or more occasions over at least 6 months. All were male; 73% had murdered their victims, and 56% had murdered at least three, most often by strangulation, and next most often by shooting. Of the 30, 37% collected guns, 33% had military experience, and 30% were police buffs. Thirty percent had an incestuous involvement with their child, and 43% were homosexual. Twenty percent engaged in cross-dressing, and 20% in exposure, peeping, or obscene telephone calling. Forty-three percent had prior arrests for nonsexual or nonsadistic sexual offenses, 50% abused drugs other than alcohol, and all had engaged in an extensive pattern of antisocial behavior in adulthood. Nevertheless, 30% had an established reputation as solid citizens and none were perceived as particularly odd by those who knew them well before their offenses. None were psychotic at the time of onset of the pattern of sexually sadistic behavior; 1 became psychotic later in life. The authors did not report how many cases were referred to NCAVC and if so, how they differed from the 30 selected. It is, therefore, not possible to determine the appropriateness of the authors' restriction of the diagnosis of sexually sadistic criminals to those selected.

Burgess, Prentky, Burgess, Douglas, and Ressler (1994) investigated 36 male sexual murderers, selected for their repetitiveness (i.e., they had an average of three victims). Almost all were White, usually eldest sons, first or second born, and average or above in intelligence; a third were in the superior to very superior range. However, the majority had to repeat elementary grades, did not complete high school, and had poor work histories in unskilled jobs. Only 4 of the 14 who entered the military received honorable discharges. They did not report an extensive peer-related sexual history; their sexual performance was generally limited to self-stimulation. The feature emphasized by the authors was the dominant fantasy life of these men, which was suggested to be a drive mechanism for sexual murder. The highest ranked sexual interest of the subjects was pornography (81%), followed by compulsive masturbation (79%), fetishism (72%), and voyeurism (71%). Their fantasies were often violent and sadistic in nature; 20 had rape fantasies prior to the age of 18, and 7 of these men acted out these fantasies within a year of being aware of them. Burgess and colleagues did not relate the prevalence of the rape fantasies or behaviors to their prevalence in normal males (McConoghy, 1993). They commented that their subjects as adults had pleasant general appearances, and do not suggest that they seemed odd in their presentation. However, 25 of the 36 had histories of early psychiatric difficulties. While their mothers were at home and their fathers were stably employed in unskilled jobs, there was a high degree of family instability.

The relationship of sexual murders and violent rapes to sexual sadism as a paraphilia seems uncertain. The *DSM-IV* account of sexual sadism includes acts of rape, cutting, stabbing, strangulation, torture, mutilation, or killing, and states that usually the severity of sadistic acts increases over time, and that when severe and especially when associated with antisocial personality disorder, individuals with sexual sadism may seriously injure or kill their victims. However, it would seem that the masochistic victims of self-identified sadists rarely require medical attention. Recent U.S. studies (Breslow, Evans, & Langley, 1985; Moser & Levitt, 1987) found that most members of "S & M" clubs were both sadistic and masochistic. Beating, bondage, and fetishistic practices were common, but more extreme or dangerous practices were rare. Subjects were above average in intelligence and social status, and most preferred to continue sadomasochistic activities.

Family Patterns

As stated earlier, marked similarities found by Knight and colleagues (1985) between convicted rapists, child molesters, and the general prison population were their poor and alcoholic families of origin. Child molesters who gave a history of adolescent offenses were likely to have experienced more physical abuse than those without such histories; rapists with adolescent offenses reported more neglect (Knight & Prentky, 1993). Early exposure to family violence, along with childhood sexual abuse and early age of sexual initiation, predicted later sexually aggressive behaviors in the national sample of 2,972 male students investigated by Koss and Dinero (1988). Marshall and Barbaree (1990a) reviewed evidence indicating that poor socialization and, in particular, exposure to parental violence in the sex offender's childhood facilitated his use of aggression as well as cutting him off in adolescence from access to more appropriate sociosexual interactions. They found the family backgrounds of sex offenders were similar to those of people with antisocial personalities. As this personality disorder is partly inherited (Schulsinger, 1972), genetic factors as well as modeling of the disturbed childhood relationships may have contributed to the later aggression of the offender.

In adolescents who sought treatment following rape, the emotional impact was rated by health professionals as more severe on the parents: 71% were assessed as showing a severe response, compared with 37% of victims (Mann, 1981); none showed a mild response as compared with 20% of victims. The major concern reported by 65% of victims was fear for life or bodily harm, a concern shared by only 50% of parents, almost exclusively those whose children had been physically injured. The next concern of victims were feelings of shame, self-blame, and guilt. Forty percent of parents blamed their child directly for the rape, especially if there were preceding intrafamilial problems. Two thirds of parents but only 21% of victims believed the assault would cause future sexual anxieties or problems. Eighty percent of the victims complained about increased communication problems with their parents after the rape. Silverman (1992) reported that "male co-survivors," the term he used for the boyfriends, husbands, brothers, and fathers of raped women, may find it difficult to offer unequivocal support to the victims because of their ambivalent attitudes, misconceptions, and beliefs concerning rape. These included that rape was a sexual experience rather than a violent and life-threatening event with sexual elements; that "women who get raped are asking for it"; that the victim did not take adequate precautions or seek help to prevent the rape; and that she has allowed herself to become "damaged merchandise." Silverman pointed out that powerful fantasies of revenge against the rapist were a response of male cosurvivors; this reaction could protect them from directly experiencing feelings of powerlessness, vulnerability, and impotent rage. Overt expressions of anger by the female survivor were less common.

Silverman (1992) considered that the question of when to resume sexual relations was perhaps the most common and problematic aspect of sexual functioning after rape. Both partners may fear sexual contact will revive painful or frightening memories of the rape. Their capacity for open communication was seen as determining the degree of sexual dysfunction. Fear of the responses discussed could explain why more than two thirds of the adolescent girl victims in Ageton's study (1983) did not inform their parents; more than three quarters told their friends. Twenty years earlier, Kanin (1959) noted that few of the university students who reported sexual aggression from a partner informed their parents.

Cammaert (1988) commented that the literature prior to this decade concerning the family in father–child incest based on clinical impression tended to treat the wife of an incestuous husband as a facilitator if not the primary cause of the incest. She was seen as failing to make sex gratifying for her husband, reversing roles with her daughter by deliberately working outside the home, or collusively providing opportunities for incest to occur and then turning a blind eye. Cammaert pointed out that little research had investigated incestuous families to substantiate these beliefs. The few studies she found indicated these families were experiencing stress caused by larger than average family size, high family discord, wife battering, and mental health problems. Although problems existed in the marital sexual relationship, the father was usually able to command sex from his wife. Cammaert also reviewed a number of studies investigating the personality of the nonoffending mothers that found them to show low self-esteem, passivity, depression, and alcoholism. She felt that these findings provided little support for the strongly pejorative clinical descriptions of the women and that the negative aspects of their personality reported could be the result of living in an atmosphere of male violence.

De Jong (1988) investigated the mothers of 103 children following their evaluation at a sexual assault center for Philadelphia County. He reported that 31% of the mothers were nonsupportive of the child, believing the abuse complaint to be a lie or due to misunderstanding, or that the abuse was primarily the child's fault. Mothers were more likely to be nonsupportive in cases of abuse by fathers or by mothers' paramours, as compared with cases of abuse by other perpetrators. Nonsupportive mothers felt frustrated that the police and protective services were doing too much, whereas supportive mothers complained they were doing too little. Gomes-Schwartz and colleagues (1990) reported similar findings in their study of 156 sexually abused children: 30% of the mothers punished the child when told about the abuse, and 18% failed to take action to protect the child. Mothers were least protective and most angry with the child when the abuser was a stepfather or boyfriend, and least angry when he was the natural father. They suggested that the latter finding might be due to the fact that in 45% of these cases the incest did not occur in an intact family, and, in some, was initially raised in the context of divorce or custody hearings.

The concept of mother–daughter role reversal was supported in a study (Herman, 1981) that found that 45% of 40 women victims of incest had been pressed into service as "little mothers" by the age of 10. In 55% of these families, the mother was ill, disabled, or absent for a period of time, during which the mother did not assume the maternal role, which fell to the oldest daughter. Fifty-eight percent of the victimized daughters never told their mothers of the incest but gave vague and indirect indications of distress and felt betrayed and disappointed at their mothers' failure to recognize the nature of the problem. Most mothers who knew were unable or unwilling to defend their daughters, seeing no option other than submission to their husbands. They conveyed to their daughters the belief that a woman is defenseless against a man, that marriage must be preserved at all costs, and that a wife's duty is to serve and endure. Like other workers (Browne & Finkelhor, 1986), Herman (1981) found that more victims were hostile to their mothers than to the offending fathers. The tendency of incestuous families to accept a pathological exaggeration of the patriarchal norms of society noted by Herman was also emphasized by Asher (1988) in reviewing evidence supporting the conclusion that the typical family in which incest occurred was male dominated and authoritarian. Asher considered that the girls growing up in such families became passive, dependent, and lacking in coping skills. The boys learned to devalue women at an early age and began to experience power over them, so that the dynamics of such families were transmitted intergenerationally.

Markedly disturbed childhood family patterns were reported in sex murderers. Revitch (1980) found a background of maternal overprotection, infantilization and seduction, or rejection in male sadistic murderers. Real or fancied maternal sexual indiscretions were common. Burgess and colleagues (1994) reported that of the family members of the 36 sexual murderers they studied, half had criminal histories, and more than half had psychiatric problems and histories of alcohol abuse and sexual deviance; a third had histories of drug abuse. Most of the 36 subjects said their relationships with their fathers were unsatisfactory and that their relationships with their mothers were highly ambivalent. Biological fathers left home before 17 subjects reached age 12. Only one third reported growing up in one location. And before they reached age 18, more than 40% lived outside the family (e.g., in foster homes, state homes, detention centers, or mental hospitals). The authors commented that although the parents provided little constructive guidance, they offered ample role modeling of deviant behavior. A possible role of genetic factors was not mentioned.

Little attention has been directed to the consequences of disclosure of the deviant behaviors of sex offenders to their families and social and occupational contacts. In the case of the most unacceptable of these behaviors, those against children, rejection of the offenders by many members of their immediate family is common, at least as an initial response. Loss of employment and threats or acts of violence from neighbors sometimes force them to shift residence. In my experience, the reactions of the majority of wives of pedophiles, particularly those whose victims were outside the family, were or soon became supportive. It is possible that parents of the offenders suffer more distress than spouses, perhaps feeling themselves in some way responsible.

Assessment and Diagnosis

Differences in assessment methods and diagnostic criteria contribute to the marked variation in estimates of the prevalence of sexual violence. Studies that used a number of probing questions produced the highest rates. Face-to-face interviews of women by trained women found that 28% of San Francisco women investigated had experienced sexual abuse before the age of 14 (Russell, 1986). Sexual abuse was defined as any sexual contact or attempted contact with a relative 5 years or more older, whether or not the child considered it neutral or positive; with a relative less than 5 years older if unwanted (e.g., initiated by the relative and causing distress or long-term effects, at the time or in retrospect), and unwanted sexual experiences with persons unrelated by blood or marriage, ranging from attempted or successful touching of breasts or genitals to rape.

Using a similar assessment method, Wyatt (1985) found that 62% of a Los Angeles sample of women experienced sexual abuse prior to the age of 18. A. C. Kilpatrick (1992) administered a questionnaire package to her subjects in groups of 3 to 38 participants following discussion of the study and emphasis on confidentiality and anonymity. Fourteen questions concerning who was the initiator, the age discrepancy, and so on, were asked about 13 sexual behaviors possibly experienced from birth through age 17, ranging from kissing and hugging in a sexual way, to intercourse. Fifty-five percent of the 501 women participants from diverse populations in the southern portion of the United States reported at least one childhood (to age 14) sexual experience: 37% experienced sexual kissing and fondling, 35% were shown the genitals of the partner, 23% displayed their own genitals, 15% had their breasts fondled, 5% participated in masturbation, 2% experienced intercourse, and less than 1%, oral sex. In 37% the partner was an unrelated male, in 13.4% an unrelated female, and in 11.9% a male relative. Kilpatrick commented that incidence of incest varied from 0.6% using Webster's 1978 dictionary definition as "sexual intercourse between persons too closely related to marry," to 24% using Finkelhor's 1979 definition of exhibition, fondling, petting, masturbation, oral-genital contact, and intercourse between any family members. More than 50% of the subjects considered their participation voluntary in all activities except oral sex by themselves, and on themselves, when 57% and 50%, respectively, considered it was forced. Kilpatrick, referring to Finkelhor's definition of a sexually abusive experience when the partner was at least 5 years older than the child, stated that 23% of the women reporting sexual experiences as children (13% of the total sample) had partners at least 5 years older. Kilpatrick combined the subjects' reactions of surprise, interest, and enthusiasm to consider that 68% had a positive reaction to the childhood sexual experiences; only those to oral sex and intercourse, which were uncommon, were predominantly negative. Twenty-eight percent of the women who reported childhood sexual experiences considered they were harmful, and 17% (10% of the total sample) reported they were sexually abused. In contrast to the high rates of childhood sexual experiences reported in these studies, in the Los Angeles Epidemiologic Catchment Area Project (Siegel, Sorenson, Golding, Burnam, & Stein, 1987), in which subjects were asked once if anyone had tried to pressure or force them to have sexual contact, 7% of women reported such experiences before the age of 16 years.

Rosenfeld, Bailey, Siegel, and Bailey (1986) indicated a problem with drawing the line between kissing and touching in families applauded for stimulating children's healthy growth, and abusive behavior that may traumatize children. Parents reported in an anonymous questionnaire that more than 30% experienced daughters at all ages until 10 years recently touching the father's genitals and 45% experienced 8–10-year-old sons touching the mother's breasts or genitals. The authors stated they had been consulted by agencies that presumed that a parent, particularly a father, walking around the house naked, taking a bath with a child of the opposite sex, or on a single occasion letting the child touch their genitals, was strong evidence supporting sexual abuse. Thorough clinical evaluation was required to determine whether these activities constituted incestuous activity.

Differences in diagnostic criteria would appear to be a major factor determining some of the striking discrepancies in two recent studies of childhood sexual experiences in representative samples of U.S. populations. One investigation found the sex of child molesters to be male for 98% of girls and 83% of boys (Finkelhor *et al.*, 1990); the other, to be respectively male, female, and both for 91%, 4%, and 4% of girls and 38%, 54%, and 7% of boys (Laumann *et al.*, 1994). Strangers were molesters of 40% and 4% of boys in the two studies. In the Finkelhor and colleagues study, subjects were asked about experiences they would now consider sexual abuse, in the Laumann and colleagues study, if they had been touched sexually by anyone before puberty (cases were restricted to those with molesters over age 14). In the latter study, 45% of men but 70% of women considered the experience had affected their lives, almost all negatively. Hence, it is like that many men would not regard prepubertal sexual experiences with an older woman as sexual abuse; therefore, they would not report them in the study by Finkelhor and colleagues. Laumann and colleagues agreed with this assessment by their subjects, stating that contacts between boys and older women appear to be less likely to be victim–offender situations than the behavior of sexually precocious boys with girls who are only somewhat older than they are. Yet, in their report of the subjects' adult adjustment, both men and women touched sexually in childhood were relatively equally impaired in comparison with those not touched; both groups were less happy and healthy in the previous year and more sexually dysfunctional. As stated earlier, the finding that victims of childhood sexual experiences report greater psychological dysfunction in adulthood has been the major reason advanced for treating these experiences as forms of sexual violence.

Despite the failure of studies in the 1980s to replicate earlier findings that assessment of subjects' penile circumference responses (PCRs) to deviant sexual stimuli could distinguish groups of child molesters or rapists from controls (McConaghy, 1988, 1992), Quinsey and Earls (1990) contended that it remained central to distinguishing individual sex offenders from nonoffenders in most treatment programs in North America. However, some expression of disquiet emerged. Quinsey and Earls pointed out that normal men with no history of child molestation show sizable PCRs to slides of pubescent females; and that uncertainty existed concerning the ratio of subjects' PCRs to descriptions of coercive as opposed to consenting sexual activity that identified individual rapists from nonrapists. Marshall and Barbaree (1990b) reported failure of posttreatment PCR assessments of child molesters to predict outcome. They commented that "if behaviorists are to maintain (their) exaggerated faith in erectile measurements, they must solve the experimental riddle of demonstrating the relevance of changing such indices to the maintenance of offensive behavior and, particularly, to the issue of treatment benefits" (p. 382).

Clinicians continue to assess sex offenders mainly by unstructured interview, relying on their experience to determine the validity of the subjects' statements, supplemented where possible by information from their social contacts and victims and records of past offenses. Researchers use more structured procedures. Knight and Prentky (1993) described the Developmental Interview, which lasted 2 to 3 hours and was based on several interview schedules, to study incarcerated sex offenders. It consisted of 541 questions and statements regarding the subject's family, developmental experiences, school experiences, and peer relations through childhood, and a lengthy section containing self-descriptive statements. It was programmed for computer administration, permitting considerable flexibility in formatting and presenting questions. In addition, subjects completed an inventory administered in two $1-1\frac{1}{2}$ half hour sessions, which was based on self-report inventories and focused especially on areas such as sexual fantasies.

Course, Prognosis, and Recidivism

Sexual offenses commonly begin in adolescence. Six of 45 sex offenders treated in the community were adolescent and 21 of the 39 adults reported their behavior began in adolescence (McConaghy, Blaszczynski, Armstrong, & Kidson, 1989). Six of the 9 homosexual pedophiles but only one of the 5 heterosexual pedophiles reported this. Sixty-one of 277 rapists and 55 of 239 child molesters admitted to the Massachusetts Treatment Center for sexually dangerous offenders had been convicted of a serious sexual crime before their 19th birthday (Knight & Prentky, 1993). In self-report information from computer interview, one third of the adults with no official charges for juvenile sexual offenses stated they had engaged in sexually coercive activity as adolescents. Unfortunately, as with a number of other studies (McConaghy, 1993), data on child molesters in relation to the sex of the victims were not reported. Knight and Prentky (1993) cited a number of studies indicating that recidivism rates of juvenile offenders were substantially lower than those of adult offenders, indicating that the deviant behavior of many adolescents does not persist into adulthood. This would appear to be true of undetected sexual offenders also, in view of the evidence that the majority of male adolescents carry out undetected sexual offenses (McConaghy, 1993). The younger age of rapists compared with child molesters (Bard *et al.*, 1987) suggests that the former are less likely to continue their offenses than the latter.

Furby, Weinrott, and Blackshaw (1989) concluded, from a review of follow-up studies of sex offenders, that the variability was such that it was difficult to make any meaningful statements about recidivism rate. When they examined North American studies only, to reduce the enormous method variability, they found that eight of the nine studies of untreated offenders had recidivism rates below 12%; two thirds of the studies of treated offenders had rates higher than 12%. They suggest that offenders in the latter studies might have been monitored more closely and pointed out many used treatment models now considered obsolete. Marshall and Barbaree (1990b) reported of the recidivism of untreated offenders that incest offenders showed the lowest rates, 4%–10%. Those for rapists were 7%–35%, for nonfamilial molesters of girls, 10%–29%, and for nonfamilial molesters of boys, 13%–40%. Those for exhibitionists were the highest for all sex offenders, 41%–71%. The longer the period of follow-up, the higher was the rate of reoffending. Adolescent compared to adult offenders were found to require more intensive treatment independent of the nature of their offense (McConaghy *et al.*, 1989).

Clinical Management and Treatment

Modification of inappropriate sexual arousal was considered the central aim of current treatment programs of child molesters and rapists in North America (Quinsey & Earls, 1990). This was usually attempted by an aversive procedure in which cues for the deviant arousal were presented followed by an unpleasant or aversive stimulus. The stimulus could be real, such as an electric shock or noxious smell (Maletzky, 1973), or imagined in a state of relaxation (covert sensitization). In general, therapists in North America following the behaviorist tradition preferred physiological measures to subjects' self-report of behavioral change in assessing treatment outcome (McConaghy, 1990). They determined response of paraphiliacs by change in their penile circumference responses (PCRs) to paraphiliac stimuli, despite the failure to demonstrate that these responses validly discriminated individual paraphiliacs from nonparaphiliacs (McConaghy, 1977, 1993), and the failure of such changes to correlate with the treated subjects' behavioral outcome (Marshall & Barbaree, 1990b; Rice, Quinsey, & Harris, 1991). When subjects' penile circumference responses did not change following covert sensitization and electric shock aversive therapy, satiation therapy was added (Marshall, Earls, Segal, & Darke, 1983). The subject was instructed to masturbate continuously for one hour, whether or not he ejaculated during that time, while verbalizing every variation he could imagine concerning his deviant fantasies.

The most commonly employed behavioral techniques to increase paraphiliacs' heterosexual arousability was orgasmic or masturbatory reconditioning or retraining. The subject was asked to masturbate and to report when orgasm was imminent, whereupon he was shown the picture of an attractive, scantily dressed woman until he reported ejaculation. Ten years after its introduction, Conrad and Winzce (1976) pointed out that the evidence of its efficacy had not transcended the case study level. Evidence indicating that orgasmic reconditioning was likely to be ineffective was reported in an investigation of men who sought treatment for compulsive homosexual feelings (McConaghy, 1978). The ratio of their heterosexual to homosexual feelings was assessed by penile volume (not circumference) changes, the validity of which has been consistently replicated (McConaghy, 1992). Men who had repeatedly experienced orgasm in the presence of female cues, namely, female sexual partners, showed no evidence of increased heterosexual arousability compared with men without this experience.

In the past decade, social skills and assertiveness training have also been employed with the aim of improving paraphilic subjects' heterosocial skills. These therapies usually were incorporated in multimodal approaches, which included one or more of the aversive, satiation, or reconditioning therapies reviewed, aimed to reduce deviant preferences, as well as cognitive therapy. The cognitive modifications most commonly advocated for the treatment of sex offenders against women and children are based on the feminist theory of etiology that the offenses are expressions of men's need to dominate women and children. The aim of treatment is to make the offender aware of and then eliminate cognitions supportive of rape and child sexual abuse and to accept total responsibility for his behavior rather than attribute it to the victim. He is also encouraged to develop understanding of the harmful effects of his behavior on his victims and empathy with their experiences by such techniques as being confronted by them, or by writing accounts of the victim's emotional experience of the offense. It has been recently suggested that such cognitive therapies for sex offenders may not require the addition of behavioral approaches, as the variety of behavioral treatments used to modify sexual arousal patterns may act nonspecifically (Quinsey & Earls, 1990).

Other workers who accept the cognitive feminist perspective regard to the initiation of sexual assault have considered that addiction to sexual assault could develop secondarily and require specific treatment, such as painstaking documentation of the offender's sexual fantasy and arousal, his modus operandi for securing access to his victims and evading detection, his preferred sexual activities, and his system of excuses and rationalizations, and that changes in these must be closely monitored (Herman, 1990). These procedures are similar to those used in relapse prevention (George & Marlatt, 1989) and are commonly included in multimodal approaches. Developed to treat addictive disorders, relapse prevention was extended to treat sex offenders, on the basis that the aim of multimodal treatment packages then in common use was to produce an effect so powerful it would not wear off. However, there was little recognition that maintenance might require qualitatively different analyses and interventions. Offenders were encouraged by preparing life autobiographies and monitoring deviant urges, to identify and avoid high-risk situations (HRSs), identified as emotional states rather than situations where they had previously offended. Apparently irrelevant decisions (AIDS) or seemingly unimportant behaviors that lead to errors (SUBTLE) that enable the offender unconsciously to seek out HRSs are corrected. Examples were pedophiles seeking employment involving contact with children, giving benevolent reasons for their choice, such as their commitment to helping children, or rapists leaving home in the early morning to jog. Other avoidance strategies include recognizing and handling the problem of immediate gratification (PIG) that inches the offender closer to relapse.

It has been argued that aversive therapy does not modify sexual arousal to deviant stimuli and that the evidence to the contrary was based on the use of invalid PCR assessment of arousal (McConaghy, 1977, 1993). Rather, aversive therapy gave subjects control over the compulsion to carry out the deviant behavior, while they continued to experience deviant arousal. This finding led to the development of the "behavior completion hypothesis" that compulsive sexuality is driven by activation of the arousal system when the subject is stimulated to complete the deviant behavior by cues previously associated with the behavior (McConaghy, 1980, 1993). The resulting feeling of excitement and tension leads the subject to complete the behavior even when they wish not to do so. The treatment of alternative behavior completion (imaginal desensitization) was introduced to reduce the conditioned arousal. Subjects were briefly trained to relax, and then instructed to visualize being in situations where they have carried out deviant behaviors in the past, but to visualize not completing the behaviors and leaving the situations while remaining relaxed. The treatment was shown to be more effective than electric shock aversive therapy and covert sensitization in giving subjects control over compulsive urges.

The behavior completion hypothesis also led to modification of medroxyprogesterone acetate (MPA) therapy of sex offenders. As introduced, 200 mg was given intramuscularly 2–3 times weekly before being reduced to 100 mg weekly to monthly. Patients generally became impotent for some period of time (Gagne, 1981), justifying the label of chemical castration. In the modified form (McConaghy et al., 1988), patients were given 150 mg fortnightly for four injections and monthly for four injections. The aim was to reduce their serum testosterone levels sufficiently to weaken the deviant urges while allowing their sexual arousal to physical stimulation to remain unimpaired so they could continue acceptable sexual activities As they continued to experience cues for deviant activities without acting in response to them, the behavior completion mechanisms for the deviant acts gradually weakened, so that when the therapy ceased, the subjects no longer experienced deviant urges as compulsive. In a comparison study of alternative behavior completion and MPA, 30 sex offenders were randomly allocated, 10 to one of the two procedures and 10 to both. Differences in response of the three groups was not significant. Twenty-eight ceased deviant behavior a year following treatment, 2 of the 28 having required aversive therapy in addition. Three relapsed in the following 2 to 5 years, but responded to reinstitution of MPA. This response was in the same range as that to more intensive programs (McConaghy, 1993). In the course of interviewing the patients, cognitive correction was attempted where appropriate and referral to community services made if treatment modules, such as anxiety management or assertive or social skills training, seemed indicated. Few patients made use of these resources; however, the dropout from the basic program was very low.

Multimodal programs in use in North America appear to incorporate these additional modules routinely and more intensively, making the programs more demanding of therapy resources. If the behavior completion model of compulsive sexual offenses is valid, subjects treated in jail will not have the opportunity of learning to control their arousal to the cues in their free environment associated with the carrying out of their offenses and they would require treatment for the compulsion after discharge. Currently, many sex offenders do not obtain treatment due to lack of facilities. Studies comparing the treatments currently in use are urgently needed to establish which are the most cost-effective, so that the maximum number of offenders can be treated with the facilities available.

Summary

Rape is not classified as a paraphilia in the *DSM-IV,* and the current discourse considered sexual violence an expression of power rather than physical force. The concepts of blitz and confidence rapes and of anger and power rapes were discussed, and the recent attention given to the rape of males including male prisoners, and of women in the workplace, the handicapped, and the mentally retarded, and to sexual torture was pointed out. As all child–adult sexual activities tend to be regarded as equally harmful, studies rarely report the degree of physical force involved. Those with fatal consequences receive widespread media attention. Sadistic murders of adults may not involve attempted rape.

The role of feminist politics in establishing the current recognition of the importance of sexual violence was discussed and the concept that rape is on a continuum with normal male behavior modified. The prevalence of rape reported in community surveys is markedly higher than that reported to law-enforcement agencies, although a significant proportion of the latter may represent false allegations. Convicted sex offenders resemble the general prison population in socioeconomic status, poor school and work records and deficient social skills. Rapists are younger than child molesters, and the latter are more likely to show organic brain syndromes and to report experiencing sexual victimization in childhood. A strong relationship between being postpubertally sexually coerced by and postpubertally coercing either men or women was found in a community study. Sex offenders were found to use more pornography than nonoffenders in adulthood but not adolescence. Sexually assaultive males are commonly found to be delinquent, to have been more sexually active than nonassaultive males, and to have used drugs or alcohol prior to the assault. Involvement in sports may be associated more strongly with being sexually coerced than coercive. A causal role for the presence of cognitions supportive of rape in sexually assaultive males has not been established. Differences between heterosexual and homosexual male pedophiles were discussed. Studies differ as to whether sexual murderers show obvious aberrant personalities, although many have a history of antisocial behavior. Families of sex offenders commonly expose them to physical or sexual abuse or both; the nature of families in which incest has been reported was discussed.

Investigations using a number of probing questions produce the highest prevalences of victimization by sexual assault; and differences in definitions of adult–child sexuality seem responsible for the marked variation found in the sex of offenders in two recent surveys of representative samples of the U.S. population. Child molesters and rapists can be distinguished from controls as groups, but not as individuals by their penile responses to deviant sexual stimuli, therefore, use of this assessment in legal proceedings or treatment is unjustified. Reports of outcome of treated and untreated sex offenders are too variable to establish recidivism rates. Modification of inappropriate sexual arousal, usually by aversive procedures, remains the central aim of most treatment programs for child molesters and rapists, although the evidence that this can be accomplished is inadequate. Most programs add social skills and assertiveness training, and cognitive restructuring, with emphasis on relapse prevention; some incorporate use of androgen-reducing chemicals. The need for controlled comparison of treatments currently in use was stressed.

References

Ageton, S. S. (1983). *Sexual assault among adolescents.* Lexington, MA: Lexington Books.

Alzenman, M., & Kelley, G. (1988). The incidence of violence and acquaintance rape in dating relationships among college men and women. *Journal of College Student Development, 29,* 305–311.

American Psychiatric Association (1987). *Diagnostic and statistical manual of mental disorders* (3rd ed., rev.). Washington, DC: Author.

American Psychiatric Association. (1994). *Diagnostic and statistical manual of mental disorders* (4th ed.). Washington, DC: Author.

Asher, S. J. (1988). The effects of childhood sexual abuse: A review of the issues and evidence. In L. E. A. Walker (Ed.), *Handbook on sexual abuse of children* (pp. 3–18). New York: Springer.

Bard, L. A., Carter, D. L., Cerce, D. D., Knight, R. A., Rosenberg, R., & Schneider, B. (1987). A descriptive study of rapists and child molesters: Developmental, clinical, and criminal characteristics. *Behavioral Sciences and the Law, 5,* 203–220.

Barry, K. (1979). *Female sexual slavery.* Englewood Cliffs, NJ: Prentice-Hall.

Becker, J. V. (1988). The effects of child sexual abuse on adolescent sexual offenders. In G. E. Wyatt & G. J. Powell (Eds.), *Lasting effects of child sexual abuse* (pp. 193–207). Newbury Park, CA: Sage.

Bem, S. L. (1974). The measurement of psychological androgyny. *Journal of Consulting and Clinical Psychology, 42,* 155–162.

Berlin, F. S., & Meinecke, C. F. (1981). Treatment of sex offenders with antiandrogenic medication: Conceptualization, review of treatment modalities, and preliminary findings. *American Journal of Psychiatry, 138,* 601–607.

Bourget, D., & Bradford, J. M. W. (1990). Homocidal parents. *Canadian Journal of Psychiatry, 35,* 233–238.

Bowie, S. I., Silverman, D.C., Kalick, S. M., & Edbril, S. D. (1990). Blitz rape and confidence rape: Implications for clinical intervention. *American Journal of Psychotherapy, 44,* 180–188.

Bownes, I. T., & O'Gorman, E. C. (1991). Assailants' sexual dysfunction during rape reported by their victims. *Medicine, Science and the Law, 31,* 322–328.

Breslow, N., Evans, L., & Langley, J. (1985). On the prevalence and roles of females in the sadomasochistic subculture: Report of an empirical study. *Archives of Sexual Behavior, 14,* 303–319.

Brittain, R. P. (1970). The sadistic murderer. *Medicine, Science and the Law, 10,* 198–207.

Browne, A., & Finkelhor, D. (1986). Impact of child sexual abuse: A review of the research. *Psychological Bulletin, 99,* 66–77.

Burgess, A. W. (1985). Sexual victimization of adolescents. In A. W. Burgess (Ed.), *Rape and sexual assault* (pp. 199–208). New York: Garland.

Burgess, A. W, & Holmstrom, L. L. (1980). Rape typology and the coping behavior of rape victims. In S. L. McCombie (Ed.), *Rape crisis intervention handbook* (pp. 27–42). New York: Plenum.

Burgess, A. W., Prentky, R. A., Burgess, A. G., Douglas, J. E., & Ressler, R. K. (1994). Serial murder. In M. Hersen, R. T. Ammerman, & L. A. Sisson (Eds.), *Handbook of aggressive and destructive behavior in psychiatric patients* (pp. 509–530). New York: Plenum.

Cammaert, L. P. (1988). Non offending mothers: A new conceptualization. In L. E. A. Walker (Ed.), *Handbook on sexual abuse of children* (pp. 309–325). New York: Springer.

Chasnoff, M. D., Burns, W. J., School, S. H., Burns, K., Chisum, G., & Kyle-Spore, L. (1986). Maternal-neonatal incest. *American Journal of Orthopsychiatry, 56,* 577–580.

Conrad, S. R., & Winzce, J. P. (1976). Orgasmic reconditioning: A controlled study of its effects upon the sexual arousal and behavior of adult male homosexuals. *Behavior Therapy, 7,* 155–166.

Conte, J. R., & Schuerman, J. R. (1988). The effects of sexual abuse on children. In G. E. Wyatt & G. J. Powell (Eds.), *Lasting effects of child sexual abuse* (pp. 157–170). Newbury Park, CA: Sage.

De Jong, A. H. (1988). Maternal responses to the sexual abuse of their children. *Pediatrics, 81,* 14–21.

Dietz, P. E., Hazelwood, R. R., & Warren, J. (1990). The sexually sadistic criminal and his offenses. *Bulletin of the American Academy of Psychiatry and Law,, 18,* 163–176.

Finkelhor, D. (1985). Sexual abuse of boys. In A. W. Burgess (Ed.), *Rape and sexual assault* (pp. 97–103). New York: Garland.

Finkelhor, D., & Yllo, K. (1985). *License to rape: Sexual abuse of wives.* New York: Holt, Rinehart, & Winston.

Finkelhor, D., Hotaling, G., Lewis, I. A., & Smith, C. (1990). Sexual abuse in a national survey of adult men and women: Prevalence, characteristics, and risk factors, *Child Abuse and Neglect, 14,* 19–28.

Freund, K., & Kuban, M. (1994). The basis of the abused abuser theory of pedophilia: A further elaboration on an earlier study. *Archives of Sexual Behavior, 23,* 553–563.

Freund, K., Heasman, G. A., & Roper, V. (1982). Results of the main studies of sexual offenses against children and pubescents (A review). *Canadian Journal of Criminology, 24,* 387–397.

Freund, K., Watson, R., & Dickey, R. (1990). Does sexual abuse in childhood cause pedophilia: An exploratory study. *Archives of Sexual Behavior, 19,* 557–568.

Furby, L., Weinrott, M. R., & Blackshaw, L. (1989). Sex offender recidivism: A review. *Psychological Bulletin, 105,* 3–30.

Gagne, P. (1981). Treatment of sex offenders with medroxyprogesterone acetate. *American Journal of Psychiatry, 138,* 644–646.

George, W. H., & Marlatt, G. A. (1989). Introduction. In D. R. Laws (Ed.), *Relapse prevention with sex offenders* (pp. 1–33). New York: Guilford.

Gomes-Schwartz, B., Horowitz, J. M., & Sauzier, M. (1990). *Child sexual abuse: The initial effects.* Newbury Park, CA: Sage.

Goodchilds, J. D., & Zellman, G. L. (1984). Sexual signaling and sexual aggression in adolescent relationships. In N. M. Malamuth & E. Donnerstein (Eds.), *Pornography and sexual aggression* (pp. 233–246). New York: Academic Press.

Gordon, M. (1989). The family environment of sexual abuse: A comparison of natal and stepfather abuse. *Child Abuse and Neglect, 13,* 121–130.

Groth, A. N., & Birnbaum, H. J. (1978). Adult sexual orientation and attraction to underage persons. *Archives of Sexual Behavior, 7,* 175–181.

Groth, A. N., & Burgess, A. W. (1977). Sexual dysfunction during rape. *New England Journal of Medicine, 297,* 764–766.

Groth, A. N., & Burgess, A. W. (1980). Male rape: Offenders and victims. *American Journal of Psychiatry, 137,* 806–810.

Groth, A. N., Burgess, A. W., & Holmstrom, L. L. (1977). Rape: Power, anger and sexuality. *American Journal of Psychiatry, 134,* 1239–1243.

Harris, A. R. (1991). Race, class, and crime. In J. F. Sheley (Ed.), *Criminology* (pp. 95–119). Belmont, CA: Wadsworth.

Harris, M. B. (1992). Sex, race, and experiences of aggression. *Aggressive Behavior, 18,* 201–217.

Herman, J. L. (1981). *Father–daughter incest.* Boston: Harvard University Press.

Herman, J. L. (1985). Father–daughter incest. In A. W. Burgess (Ed.), *Rape and sexual assault* (pp. 83–96). New York: Garland.

Herman, J. L. (1990). Sex offenders: A feminist perspective. In W. L. Marshall, D. R. Laws, & H. E. Barbaree (Eds.), *Handbook of sexual assault* (pp. 177–193). New York: Plenum.

Hillman, R. J., O'Mara, N., Taylor-Robinson, D., & Harris, J. R. W. (1990). Medical and social aspects of sexual assault of males: A survey of 100 victims. *British Journal of General Practice, 40,* 502–504.

Holmstrom, L. L. (1985). The criminal justice system's response to the rape victim. In A. W. Burgess (Ed.), *Rape and sexual assault* (pp. 189–198). New York: Garland.

Kanin, E. J. (1959). Male aggression in dating-courtship relations. *American Journal of Sociology, 63,* 197–204.

Kanin, E. J. (1969). Selected dyadic aspects of male sex aggression. *Journal of Sex Research, 5,* 12–28.

Kanin, E. J. (1985). Date rapists: Differential sexual socialization and relative deprivation. *Archives of Sexual Behavior, 14,* 219–231.

Kanin, E. J. (1994). False rape allegations. *Archives of Sexual Behavior, 23,* 81–92.

Kanin, E. J., & Parcell, S. R. (1977). Sexual aggression: A second look at the offended female. *Archives of Sexual Behavior, 6,* 67–76.

Karmen, A. A.. (1991). Victims of crime. In J. F. Sheley (Ed.), *Criminology* (pp. 121–138). Belmont, CA: Wadsworth.

Kaufman, A., DiVasto, P., Jackson, R., Voorhees, D., & Christy, J. (1980). Male rape victims: Noninstitutionalized assault. *American Journal of Psychiatry, 137,* 221–223.

Kilpatrick, A. C. (1992). *Long-range effects of child and adolescent sexual experiences.* Hillsdale, NJ: Erlbaum.

Kilpatrick, D. G., Best, C. L., Saunders, B. E., & Veronen, L. J. (1988). Rape in marriage and in dating relationships: How bad is it for mental health? *Annals of the New York Academy of Sciences, 528,* 335–344.

Kincaid, J. R. (1992). *Child-loving: The erotic child and Victorian culture.* New York: Routledge.

King, M. B. (1992a) Male rape in institutional settings. In G. C. Mezey & M. B. King (Eds.), *Male victims of sexual assault* (pp. 67–74). Oxford, England: Oxford University Press.

King, M. B. (1992b). Male sexual assault in the community. In G. C. Mezey & M. B. King (Eds.), *Male victims of sexual assault* (pp. 1–12). Oxford, England: Oxford University Press.

Knight, R. A., & Prentky, R. A. (1990). Classifying sexual offenders. In W. L. Marshall, D. R. Laws, & H. E. Barbaree (Eds.), *Handbook of sexual assault* (pp. 23–52). New York: Plenum.

Knight, R. A., & Prentky, R. A. (1993). Exploring characteristics for classifying juvenile sex offenders. In H. E. Barbaree, W. L. Marshall, & S. M. Hudson (Eds.), *The juvenile sex offender* (pp. 45–83). New York: Guilford.

Knight, R. A., Rosenberg, R., & Schneider, B. A. (1985). Classification of sexual offenders: Perspectives, methods, and validation. In A. W. Burgess (Ed.), *Rape and sexual assault* (pp. 222–293). New York: Garland.

Koss, M. P. (1985). The hidden rape victim: Personality, attitudinal, and situational characteristics. *Psychology of Women Quarterly, 9,* 193–212.

Koss, M. P., & Dinero, T. E. (1988). Predictors of sexual aggression among a national sample of male college students. *Annals of the New York Academy of Sciences, 528,* 133–147.

Koss, M. P., & Gaines, J. A. (1993). The prediction of sexual aggression by alcohol use, athletic participation, and fraternity affiliation. *Journal of Interpersonal Violence, 8,* 94–108.

Koss, M. P., & Oros, C. J. (1982). Sexual experiences survey: A research instrument investigating sexual aggression and victimization. *Journal of Consulting and Clinical Psychology, 50,* 455–457.

Koss, M. P., Leonard, K. F., Beezley, D. A., & Oros, C. J. (1985). Nonstranger sexual aggression: A discriminate analysis of the psychological characteristics of undetected offenders. *Sex Roles, 12,* 981–992.

Laumann, E. O., Gagnon, J. H., Michael, R. T., & Michaels, S. (1994). *The social organization of sexuality.* Chicago: University of Chicago Press.

Lesieur, H. R., & Welch, M. (1991). Vice, public disorder, and social control. In J. F. Sheley (Ed.), *Criminology* (pp. 175–198). Belmont, CA: Wadsworth.

Los, M, (1990). Feminism and rape law reform. In L. Gelsthorpe & A. Morris (Eds.), *Feminist perspectives in criminology* (pp. 160–172). Bristol, PA: Open University Press.

Lunde, I., & Ortmann, J. (1990). Prevalence and sequelae of sexual torture. *Lancet, 336,* 289–29.

Malamuth, N. M. (1989). The attraction to sexual aggression scale: II. *Journal of Sex Research, 26,* 324–354.

Malamuth, N. M., Sockloskie, R. J., Koss, M. P., & Tonaka, J. S. (1991). Characteristics of aggression against women: Testing a model using a national sample of college students. *Journal of Consulting and Clinical Psychology, 59,* 670–681.

Maletzky, B. M. (1973). "Assisted" covert sensitization: A preliminary report. *Behavior Therapy, 4,* 117–119.

Mann, E. M. (1981). Self-reported stresses of adolescent rape victims. *Journal of Adolescent Health Care, 2,* 29–33.

Marshall, W. L., & Barbaree, H. E. (1990a). An integrated theory of the etiology of sexual offending. In W. L. Marshall, D. R. Laws, & H. E. Barbaree (Eds.), *Handbook of sexual assault* (pp. 257–275). New York: Plenum.

Marshall, W. L., & Barbaree, H. E. (1990b). Outcome of comprehensive cognitive-behavioral treatment programs. In W. L. Marshall, D. R. Laws, & H. E. Barbaree (Eds.), *Handbook of sexual assault* (pp. 363–385). New York: Plenum.

Marshall, W. L., Earls, C. M., Segal, Z., & Darke, J. (1983). A behavioral program for the assessment and treatment of sexual aggressors. In K. D. Craig & R. J. McMahon (Eds.), *Advances in clinical behavior therapy* (pp. 148–174). New York: Brunner/Mazel.

McConaghy, N. (1977). Behavioral treatment in homosexuality. In M. Hersen, R. M. Eisler, & P. M. Miller (Eds.), *Progress in behavior modification* (Vol. 5, pp. 309–380). New York: Academic Press.

McConaghy, N. (1978). Heterosexual experience, marital status and orientation of homosexual males. *Archives of Sexual Behavior, 7,* 575–581.

McConaghy, N. (1980). Behavior completion mechanisms rather than primary drives maintain behavioral patterns. *Activitas Nervosa Superior* (Prague), *22,* 138–151.

McConaghy, N. (1988). Sexual dysfunction and deviation. In A. S. Bellack & M. Hersen (Eds.), *Behavioral assessment* (3rd. ed., pp. 490–541). New York: Pergamon.

McConaghy, N. (1990). Sexual deviation. In A. S. Bellack, M. Hersen, & A. E. Kazdin (Eds.), *International handbook of behavior therapy and modification* (2nd ed., pp. 565–580). New York: Plenum.

McConaghy, N. (1992). Validity and ethics of penile circumference measures of sexual arousal: A response to McAnulty and Adams. *Archives of Sexual Behavior, 21,* 187–195.

McConaghy, N. (1993). *Sexual behavior: Problems and management.* New York; Plenum.

McConaghy, N., & Zamir, R. (1995). "Heterosexual and homosexual coercion, sexual orientation, and sexual roles in medical students. *Archives of Sexual Behavior, 24,* 489–502.

McConaghy, N., Blaszczynski, A., & Kidson, W. (1988). Treatment of sex offenders with imaginal desensitization and/or medroxyprogesterone. *Acta Psychiatrica Scandinavica, 77,* 199–206.

McConaghy, N., Blaszczynski, A., Armstrong, M. S., & Kidson, W. (1989). Resistance to treatment of adolescent sexual offenders. *Archives of Sexual Behavior, 18,* 97–107.

McConaghy, N., Zamir, R., & Manicavasagar, V. (1993). Non-sexist sexual experiences survey and scale of attraction to sexual aggression. *Australian and New Zealand Journal of Psychiatry, 27,* 686–693.

McConaghy, N., Manicavasagar, V., & Zamir, R. (1995). Involvement in sport, sexual orientation and sexual coercion.Paper presented at the 1995 Midcontinental Region Annual Conference of the Seciety for the Scientific Study of Sexuality, Minneapolis.

Messerschmidt, J. W. (1993). *Masculinities and crime.* Lanham, MA: Rowman & Littlefield.

Moser, C., & Levitt, E. E. (1987). An exploratory-descriptive study of a sadomasochistically oriented sample. *Journal of Sex Research, 23,* 322–337.

Muehlenhard, C. L., & Cook, S. W. (1988). Men's self-reports of unwanted sexual activity. *Journal of Sex Research, 24,* 58–72.

Muehlenhard, C. L., & Linton, M. A. (1987). Date rape and sexual aggression in dating situations:Incidence and risk factors. *Journal of Counseling Psychology, 34,* 186–196.

Murrin, M. R., & Laws, D. R. (1990). The influence of pornography on sexual crimes. In W. L. Marshall, D. R. Laws, & H. E. Barbaree (Eds.), *Handbook of sexual assault* (pp. 73–91). New York: Plenum.

Myers, M. F. (1989). Men sexually assaulted as adults and sexually abused as boys. *Archives of Sexual Behavior, 18,* 203–215.

Nacci, P. L., & Kane, T. R. (1984). Sex and sexual aggression in federal prisons. *Federal Probation, 48,* 46–53.

Palmer, C. T. (1988). Twelve reasons why rape is not sexually motivated: A skeptical examination. *Journal of Sex Research, 25,* 512–530.

Parker, R. N. (1991). Violent crime. In J. F. Sheley (Ed.), *Criminology* (pp. 143–158). Belmont, CA: Wadsworth.

Pithers, W. D., Kashima, K. M., Cumming, G. F., & Beal, L. S. (1988). Relapse prevention: A method of enhancing maintenance of change in sex offenders. In A. C. Salter (Ed.), *Treating child sex offenders and victims: A practical guide* (pp. 131–170). Beverley Hills, CA: Sage.

Quinsey, V. L. (1986). Men who have sex with children. In D. N. Weisstub (Ed.), *Law and mental health, international perspectives* (Vol. 2, pp. 140–172). New York: Pergamon.

Quinsey, V. L., & Earls, C. M. (1990). The modification of sexual preferences. In W. L. Marshall, D. R. Laws, & H. E. Barbaree (Eds.), *Handbook of sexual assault* (pp. 279–295). New York: Plenum.

Quinsey, V. L., & Upfold, D. (1985). Rape completion and victim injury as a function of female resistance strategy. *Canadian Journal of Behavioral Science, 31,* 40–50.

Revitch, E. (1965). Sex murder and the potential sex murderer. *Diseases of the Nervous System, 26,* 640–648.

Revitch, E. (1980). Gynocide and unprovoked attacks on women. *Correctional and Social Psychiatry, 26,* 6–11.

Rice, M. E., Quinsey, V. L., & Harris, G. T. (1991). Sexual recidivism among child molesters released from a maximum security psychiatric institution. *Journal of Consulting and Clinical Psychology, 59,* 381–386.

Rinear, E. E. (1985). Sexual assault and the handicapped victim. In A. W. Burgess (Ed.), *Rape and sexual assault* (pp. 139–145). New York: Garland.

Risin, L. I., & Koss, M. P. (1987). Sexual abuse of boys: Prevalence and descriptive characteristics of childhood victimization. *Journal of Interpersonal Violence, 2,* 309–319.

Rosenfeld, A., Bailey, R., Siegel, B., & Bailey, G. (1986). Determining incestuous contact between parent and child: Frequency of children touching parents' genitalia in a nonclinical population. *Journal of the American Academy of Child Psychiatry, 25,* 481–484.

Russell, D. E. H. (1982). *Rape in marriages.* New York: Macmillan.

Russell, D. E. H. (1986). *The secret trauma: Incest in the lives of girls and women.* New York: Basic Books.

Sanday, P. R. (1990). *Fraternity gang rape: Sex, brotherhood, and privilege on campus.* New York: New York University Press.

Sarrel, P., & Masters, W. (1982). Sexual molestation of men by women. *Archives of Sexual Behavior, 11,* 117–133.

Schneider, B. E. (1991). Put up and shut up: Workplace sexual assaults. *Gender and Society, 5,* 533–548.

Schulsinger, F. (1972). Psychopathy heredity and environment. *International Journal of Mental Health, 1,* 190–206.

Seghorn, T. K., Prentky, R. A., & Boucher, R. J. (1987). Childhood sexual abuse in the lives of sexually aggressive offenders. *Journal of the American Academy of Child and Adolescent Psychiatry, 26,* 262–267.

Siegel, J. M., Sorenson, S. B., Golding, J. M., Burnam, M. A., & Stein, J. A. (1987). The prevalence of childhood sexual assault. *American Journal of Epidemiology, 126,* 1141–1153.

Silverman, D. C. (1992). Male co-survivors: The shared trauma of rape. In G. C. Mezey & M. B. King (Eds.), *Male victims of sexual assault* (pp. 87–103). Oxford, England: Oxford University Press.

Silverman, D. C., Kalick, S. M., Bowie, S. I., & Edbril, S. D. (1988). Blitz rape and confidence rape: A typology applied to 1,000 consecutive cases. *American Journal of Psychiatry, 145,* 1438–1441.

Sorenson, S. B., Stein, J. A., Siegel, J. M., Golding, J. M. & Burnam, M. A. (1987). The prevalence of adult sexual assault. *American Journal of Epidemiology, 126,* 1154–1164.

Stein, J. A., Golding, J. M., Siegel, J. M., Burnam, M. A., & Sorenson, S. B. (1988). Long-term psychological sequelae of child sexual abuse. In G. E Wyatt & G. J. Powell (Eds.), *Lasting effects of child sexual abuse* (pp. 135–154). Newbury Park, CA: Sage.

Stermac, L. E., Segal, Z. V., & Gillis R. (1990). Social and cultural factors in sexual assault. In W. L. Marshall, D. R. Laws, & H. E. Barbaree (Eds.), *Handbook of sexual assault,* (pp. 143–159). New York: Plenum.

Struckman-Johnson, C. (1988). Forced sex on dates: It happens to men, too. *Journal of Sex Research, 24,* 234–241.

Swigert, V. L., Farrell, R. A., & Yoels, W. C. (1976). Sexual homicidal: Social, psychological and legal aspects. *Archives of Sexual Behavior, 5,* 391–401.

Tharinger, D., Horton, C. B., & Millea, S. (1990). Sexual abuse and exploitation of children and adults with mental retardation. *Child Abuse and Neglect, 14,* 301–312.

Turner, S. (1992). Surviving sexual assault and sexual torture. In G. C. Mezey & M. B. King (Eds.), *Male victims of sexual assault* (pp. 75–86). Oxford, England: Oxford University Press.

Warr, M. (1991). America's perception of crime and punishment. In J. F. Sheley (Ed.), *Criminology* (pp. 5–19). Belmont, CA: Wadsworth.

Watkins, B., & Bentovim, A. (1992). In G. C. Mezey & M. B. King (Eds.), *Male victims of sexual assault* (pp. 27–66). Oxford, England: Oxford University Press.

White, J. W., & Koss, M. P. (1993). Adolescent sexual aggression within heterosexual relationships: Prevalence, characteristics, and causes. In H. E. Barbaree, W. L. Marshall, & S. M. Hudson (Eds.), *The juvenile sex offender* (pp. 182–202). New York: Guilford.

Winfield, I., George, L. K., Swartz, M. & Blazer, D. G. (1990). Sexual assault and psychiatric disorders among a community sample of women. *American Journal of Psychiatry, 147,* 335–341.

Wyatt, G. E. (1985). The sexual abuse of Afro-American and white-American women in childhood. *Child Abuse and Neglect, 9,* 507–519.

Wyatt, G. E., & Mickey, M. R. (1988). In G. E. Wyatt & G. J. Powell (Eds.), *Lasting effects of child sexual abuse* (pp. 211–226). Newbury Park, CA: Sage.

Yllo, K., & Finkelhor, D. (1985). Marital rape. In A. W. Burgess (Ed.), *Rape and sexual assault* (pp. 146–158). New York: Garland.

13

Rape

William L. Marshall, Yolanda M. Fernandez, and Franca Cortoni

Description and History of the Problem

Definitions of rape vary considerably depending on who is doing the defining and on the context in which the definition is provided. Legal definitions have, until recent years, specified rape as the penile penetration by a male of an unwilling female's vagina. This, of course, excluded male victims, identified rape as a strictly sexual act, and required some demonstration that the victim's vagina had indeed been penetrated specifically by the male's penis. These requirements had the unfortunate consequence of making the victim's prior sexual history seem relevant to the proper adjudication of a charge of rape, and this emphasis tended to obscure the nonsexual components of rape and, most importantly, the assaultive aspects of the crime.

Changes made in 1983 to Canadian law attempted to address this problem by eliminating any reference to vaginal penetration and focusing instead on the forceful and assaultive nature of the offense. In Canadian criminal law, sexual assault (the term that has replaced "rape" and various other offense descriptions) refers to the imposition of unwanted direct sexual contacts where there is some degree of forcefulness, coercion, or power imbalance. This change has (1) markedly reduced the opportunities for defense counsel to examine the victim's sexual history, (2) eliminated the need to demonstrate penile penetration, and (3) emphasized the degree of assault as the factor most influential in determining sentence upon conviction. It also eliminates from consideration the genders of the victim and the offender, and also their relationship since no reference is made to the exclusion of spouses. Some states in the United States have similarly attempted to reformulate the legal description of rape but most have retained, within the definition, references to vaginal intercourse that perpetuate some of the unfortunate implications of the earlier legal term.

In this chapter, the term "rape" is used to refer to what Canadian law now considers to be "sexual assault" where the victim is a teenage or adult person. For us, and

William L. Marshall, Yolanda M. Fernandez, and Franca Cortoni • Department of Psychology, Queen's University, Kingston, Ontario, K7L 3N6, Canada.

Handbook of Psychological Approaches with Violent Offenders: Contemporary Strategies and Issues, edited by Van Hasselt and Hersen. Kluwer Academic/Plenum Publishers, New York, 1999.

it seems for most researchers, rape encompasses all direct sexual contacts involving forcefulness or coercion on the part of the assailant, unwillingness on the part of the victim, or both. Excluded from this definition are so-called "hands off" sexual offenses, such as exhibitionism, voyeurism, obscene telephone calling, and sexual harassment. It also excludes, for research purposes at least, sexual assaults of any kind against children, which we refer to as child molestation. Although there is no universally agreed upon definition of the age at which child and adult victims can be distinguished, we use age 14 years as the cutoff. Our earlier research indicated that offenders who sexually assault adults did not differ from those who assaulted teenagers older than 14 years, whereas both of these groups of offenders differed from those who assaulted children under age 14 years (Baxter, Marshall, Barbaree, Davidson, & Malcolm, 1984).

Epidemiology

The rape of adult or teenage females by male assailants appears to have occurred throughout history in all societies, although there is evidence suggesting that the rate at which these sexual assaults occur varies across societies (Sanday, 1981; Schiff, 1971). It is, however, only in recent years that the prevalence of the problem has been highlighted and more carefully collected data have been available.

The National Opinion Research Center conducted a survey of 10,000 U.S. households in 1967 in an attempt to estimate the rate of rape (Ennis, 1967). They found that the number of rapes reported to the interviewers was almost four times higher than the officially reported rates. The official data are derived from the Federal Bureau of Investigation's Uniform Crime Reports which reveal dramatic increases in the rate of rape up to 1980 when 71 of every 100,000 females at risk were assaulted. Thereafter, there appears to have been a steady but slight decrease in the officially reported rate of rape, although by 1989 the rate was back up to 73 per 100,000 females. A problem with these official figures is not only that they represent an underestimate of the actual occurrence of rape; many rapes are not apparent in the official records as they are frequently plea-bargained down to a lesser crime or are obscured by a conviction for another crime (e.g., murder) when in fact a sexual assault also took place.

As an alternative to the official figures, several researchers have followed the example of the National Opinion Research Center and conducted surveys of samples of the general population. Over the years, these surveys have revealed not only alarmingly high rates of sexual assault, but also rather consistent rates. For example, Kanin and Parcell (1977) replicated a 1957 study and found almost the same incidence; approximately half of the females surveyed reported being the victims of some form of sexual coercion during the previous year. Koss, Gidycz and Wisniewski (1987) found that more than half of a national sample of 3,187 female college students reported some form of sexual victimization since age 14 years (over 15% said they had been raped and an additional 12% reported that a male had unsuccessfully attempted to rape them). In this sample, 76 college women out of every 1,000 (i.e., 7,600 per 100,000) reported experiencing rape or attempted rape in the 12 months prior to the survey. D. E. H. Russell (1984) found that 44% of the 930 women she surveyed in the San Francisco area indicated that they either had been raped or subjected to an attempted rape, but only 8% reported the offense to the police. Based on these and other surveys, it has been estimated that at least 25% of American women will be raped sometime during their life (Kilpatrick & Best, 1990), while as many as 75% will be the victims of some form of coerced sexual activity (Koss, 1985).

Data from other countries reveal similar rates. For example, W. L. Marshall and Barrett (1990), basing their estimates on official police data plus the police estimates of the rate of underreporting, concluded that an adult Canadian woman is sexually assaulted every seven minutes. Results of an international crime survey (van Dijk & Mayhew, 1992) revealed the 1-year rates of sexual assault in several European countries and in North America. In all, just over 55,000 people over age 16 years were interviewed. Figure 13.1 describes these data; as can be seen, in the majority of European countries, women report lower rates of sexual assault than do their North American counterparts, although in all cases the rates appear to be lower than has at times been suggested. It is also important to note that van Dijk and Mayhew report that of those respondents who indicated they had been sexually assaulted, 40% considered the incident to be "very serious" and an additional 35% thought the assault was "fairly serious." Poland and Czechoslovakia have relatively high rates which is rather surprising since they have had a focus on research and treatment of sexual offenders for many years both prior to and after the fall of the Iron Curtain (Weiss, 1995).

Adult males are also raped. Kaufman, DiVasto, Jackson, Voorhees, and Christy (1980) reported that the percentage of male victims among the clients presenting at a New Mexico clinic increased from 1975 to 1978 by which time the male victims constituted 10% of the patients. Recently, Stermac, Sheridan, Davidson, and Dunn (1996) analyzed 29 cases where males were the victims of sexual assault. In 86% of the cases,

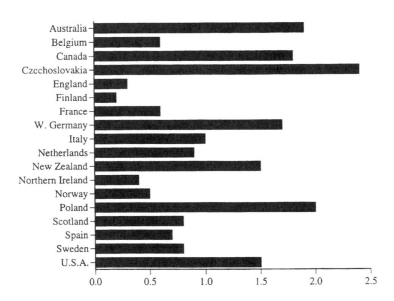

Victimization rates as percentages of the population at risk

FIGURE 13.1. One-year rates of sexual assaults against adult females: A cross-cultural comparison. From *Criminal Victimization in the Industrial World*, by J. J. M. van Dijk and P. Mayhew, 1992, The Hague, Netherlands: Directorate for Crime Prevention. Copyright 1992 by Directorate for Crime Prevention. Adapted with permission.

the victims were assaulted by a male, and in only 3 of the 29 cases was a female perpetrator involved (in 2 of these cases, the females were co-offenders with males). The majority of the victims were young homosexual males who were physically or cognitively disabled, although there was clear evidence in only a minority of the cases that the assaults reflected antigay violence. Various other recent reports also indicate that males are the victims of sexual assault (Groth & Burgess, 1980; Hillman, O'Mara, Taylor-Robinson, & Harris, 1990), but it is important to note that they remain a small proportion of identified rape victims.

Clearly, the incidence of rape and attempted rape is staggeringly high and it is disappointing, if not downright disgraceful, that our society has not made a more concerted effort to deal with the problem. There are a limited number of treatment programs for offenders, even fewer facilities provided for victims, and there has been little effort to develop preventative programs. These glaring deficiencies in society's response to this problem become even more distressing when we consider the effects on victims. There are many articles testifying to the immediate and long-term harmful effects for victims and their families following a sexual assault (Becker, Skinner, Abel, Howell, & Bruce, 1982; Ellis, 1983; Kilpatrick & Amick, 1985; Koss & Harvey, 1991; McCann, Sakheim, & Abrahamson, 1988; Roth & Lebowitz, 1988). These effects include increased anxieties, depression, poor social adjustment, disturbed sexual functioning, increased health problems, frightening memories, guilt, shame, loss of trust, feelings of never being safe, and a loss of self-esteem, to name just some of the more common results of sexual assault. Of course, these effects refer to the distress of the victim, but it is also true that the victim's present and future families also suffer as a result of the trauma of rape. Indeed, the cost to society's health services in dealing with the mental and physical problems of the victims of sexual assault and their families, although presently not well documented, can be expected to be very significant. Obviously, the more we do to assist victims at the time of the sexual assault, the better off they will be and the less burden they will be on our health care systems in the future.

Characteristics of the Offender

Perhaps the most obvious characteristic of identified rapists is that all but a remarkably small number are males. Recent research has certainly begun to reveal a far higher incidence of sexual abuse by females (Knopp & Lackey, 1987; Mathews, Matthews, & Speltz, 1989) than was previously thought to be the case. However, most of these identified female offenders molested children rather than adults, and when they were involved in the sexual assault of an adult, it was often as the accomplice of a male perpetrator.

In terms of intelligence, occupational level and most other socioeconomic features, rapists do not seem to differ from other males, although they tend to have a lower level of educational attainment (Christie, Marshall, & Lanthier, 1979). This latter feature, however, may simply be the result of the fact that those who are studied in research are typically in prison and the processes that lead to incarceration (and those that permit a successful defense at trial) may selectively discriminate for educational qualifications.

Despite popular expectations to the contrary, there is little in the way of convincing evidence that rapists are characterized by psychopathology, other than what may be concluded about their actual deviant acts. Studies have revealed that less than 5% are psychotic (Travin & Protter, 1993). The main characteristics that have received attention in the research literature, however, are those that are the focus of treatment. The following sections, then, consider what we know about those features of rapists that are thought to be the most important to address in treatment.

Deviant Sexual Preferences

Over the years, numerous theorists have suggested that all cases of sexual offending (and, indeed, all eccentric sexual activities) are driven by the desire to fulfill sexual fantasies that originated in the accidental pairing of certain stimuli with sexual arousal (e.g., Abel & Blanchard, 1974; McGuire, Carlisle, & Young, 1965). These theories have been described by Barbaree and Marshall (1991) as variants of the "sexual preference hypothesis." W. L. Marshall (1996c) has pointed out that this hypothesis requires, in the case of rapists, that these men display greater arousal to rape at assessment than would presumptively normal men. Assessments of this kind, where the man's erectile response is measured while he listens to, or watches, depictions of various sexual activities, including rape and consenting sex, are called "phallometry." While there are numerous problems with phallometry (see W. L. Marshall, 1996c, for a review) such assessments, insofar as they are accurate, do permit an evaluation of the sexual preference hypothesis. Unfortunately, currently available data are not clearly supportive of the expectations of this view of rape.

Abel, Barlow, Blanchard, and Guild (1977) reported the first systematic evaluation of the sexual preferences of rapists. Although the rapists appeared more deviant than the comparison group of nonrapist sexual offenders, the rapists were no more aroused to depictions of forced sex than they were to consenting sex. On the other hand, Quinsey, Chaplin, and Upfold (1984) found that rapists were more aroused by rape scenes than by consenting sex, while Barbaree, Marshall, and Lanthier (1979) found less arousal to rape than normative sex in their rapists, although these offenders displayed somewhat greater arousal to rape than did university students. The results of these three early, rather small sample studies are, to say the least, confusing. Subsequent larger sample size studies have not supported the view that rapists differ from other males in terms of their relative arousal to scenes of rape and consenting sex (Baxter et al., 1984; Baxter, Barbaree & Marshall, 1986; Hall, 1989; Hall, Proctor, & Nelson, 1988; Langevin, Paitich & Russon, 1985; W. L. Marshall, Barbaree, Laws, & Baxter, 1986; Murphy, Krisak, Stalgaitis, & Anderson, 1984; Wormith, Bradford, Pawlak, Borzecki, & Zohar, 1988).

It has been suggested that the differences in the findings of these later studies, and the earlier ones just mentioned, may be due to a greater number of sadists (Blader & Marshall, 1989; W. L. Marshall & Eccles, 1991) or a greater number of multivictim offenders in the early investigations (W. L. Marshall, 1996c). Lalumière and Quinsey (1994), in a meta-analysis, produced data that convinced them, however, that the differences in results were due to differences in the stimuli used to elicit arousal rather than to sample differences. While meta-analysis is not without its critics (Eysenck, 1992), Lalumière and Quinsey's findings raise the possibility that stimulus features could be a fruitful area of research. In support of their view, Harris, Rice, Quinsey, Chaplin, and Earls (1992) found that when they made the rape stimuli particularly brutal, rapists were readily distinguished from a community sample of males. Proulx, Aubut, McKibben, and Coté (1994) similarly reported that adding elements depicting the humiliation of the victim to scenes of rape produced distinct differences between rapists and controls that were absent when the elements of humiliation were withdrawn. However, both studies examined rapists held in maximum security psychiatric institutions in Canada, and these facilities accept as residents only those sexual offenders who are insane or whose sanity is in question. In such populations, we might expect a disproportionate number of both sadists and multiple-victim offenders who we might expect would find brutal or humiliating features to be arousing. Consistent with this expectation, Eccles, Marshall, and Barbaree (1994) examined a general prison population of rapists and found that adding elements of brutality and humiliation did not change the fact that the rapists did not differ from matched nonrapists.

Another way to examine the erectile responses of rapists and nonrapists to these stimuli is to look at the individual profiles and determine how many of each group appear deviant. Counting as deviant any response profiles that showed either equal or greater arousal to rape than to consenting sex, W. L. Marshall and Barbaree (1995) found that only 30.8% of 60 rapists could be classified as having a deviant profile. By comparison, 26.8% of 41 nonrapists also showed deviant profiles. These data suggest that examining any individual's responses will not allow us to determine whether he is a rapist or not; that is to say, with rapists, the sensitivity of this test (i.e., the accuracy with which it correctly identifies offenders as deviant) and its specificity (i.e., the accuracy with which it correctly identifies nonoffenders as normal) are both poor.

A consideration of the research findings available to date leads us to conclude that phallometric assessments have not consistently revealed any distinct patterns among rapists. Deviant sexual preferences, then, are either not distinctive features of rapists, or the phallometric test does not constitute an adequate measure of such preferences.

However, we (W. L. Marshall, 1996a; W. L. Marshall & Eccles, 1993) have suggested that it is not so much sexual fantasies, and corresponding sexual motives, that drive sexual offending, but rather fantasies and motives having to do with power, control, aggression, and an intent to humiliate. While it is widely acknowledged that these factors are important in considering the motivational aspects of rape (Amir, 1971; Clark & Lewis, 1977; Groth, 1979; Sanday, 1981), they have not yet been examined in any systematic way in research with rapists, and they have been all but neglected in the assessment and treatment of these offenders.

Social Skills

In their original introduction to the analysis of sexual deviants, social skills were primarily construed as simply conversational skills (Barlow, 1973), although there was at least one early report suggesting that interpersonal and relationship skills should also form part of the assessment and treatment of these men (W. L. Marshall, 1971). Currently, the range of issues subsumed under the rubric "social competence" is quite broad.

Anger problems have frequently been mentioned as an issue with rapists (Groth, 1979), but little systematic research has been conducted on this issue. Using Spielberger's State-Trait Anger measure (Spielberger, 1988), we (Seidman, Marshall, Hudson, & Robertson, 1994) found no differences between rapists and various other sexual offenders, nonsex offenders, and community controls on either trait or state anger.

Lack of self-confidence in social interactions has been proposed as an etiologically significant factor in sexual assault (Groth, 1979; W. L. Marshall & Barbaree, 1990) and, perhaps more importantly, as a factor that maintains the behavior once it is initiated (W. L. Marshall, Anderson, & Champagne, 1996). In a series of studies, Marshall and his colleagues have demonstrated that child molesters suffer from exaggeratedly low social self-esteem (W. L. Marshall, 1995; W. L. Marshall, Champagne, Brown, & Miller, 1995; W. L. Marshall & Mazzucco, 1995; Segal & Marshall, 1986), and two investigations have found similar deficits in rapists (W. L. Marshall, Barbaree, & Fernandez, 1995; Overholser & Beck, 1986). Since these studies were all conducted after the offenders had been reported to the authorities, and most were carried out after the men were incarcerated, it is difficult to interpret the data regarding theories of etiology or maintenance since the iatrogenic effects of identification and imprisonment might be expected to powerfully erode self-esteem. However, the issue seems worth pursuing; in any case, the results suggest that therapists should take these low levels of confidence into account, particularly in the early stages of treatment when we can anticipate that these offenders will be most vulnerable.

Empathy is typically understood as a capacity essential for effective interpersonal relating. We (W. L. Marshall, Hudson, Jones, & Fernandez, 1995) have construed empathy as a four-stage process involving recognition of another's distress, viewing the world from the other's perspective, experiencing some element of the other person's emotional state, and taking some remedial action to reduce the other person's distress. Our research has shown that rapists have trouble recognizing the emotional state of another person and that they particularly confuse surprise, fear, anger, and disgust (Hudson *et al.*, 1993). More recently, we have found that rapists are less empathic toward their own victim than they are toward other sexual assault victims or toward a woman permanently disfigured in an accident (Fernandez & Marshall, 1995).

From a somewhat different perspective, Hanson and Scott (1995) presented subjects with vignettes describing various interactions between males and females, and asked them to identify the distress each participant was experiencing. Rapists tended to underestimate the woman's distress. Deitz, Blackwell, Daley, and Bentley (1982) examined the empathy expressed by nonoffender males toward rapists and their victims Those subjects who demonstrated poor empathy toward the victim, and moderate empathy toward the offender, expressed a desire to actually commit a rape. This finding suggests that a lack of empathy may facilitate rape; this is strengthened by the consistent observation that rapists lack empathy toward women, in general, and toward their own victim, in particular.

This inability to be empathic may arise, as we saw, from deficiencies in recognizing emotional states in others. However, if an offender recognizes the pain he is causing his victim he is likely, if he is not a sadist, to desist. In order to continue to offend, a rapist must therefore either block his feelings of empathy or enjoy his victim's suffering. Since there are, fortunately, few true sadists among rapists (i.e., rapists who are expressively rather than instrumentally aggressive) it appears likely that most rapists are unempathic because they have deliberately initiated processes (presumably cognitive in nature) to suppress or suspend empathy specifically toward an intended victim. Laboratory studies of aggression (Bandura, 1973; Bandura, Underwood, & Fromson, 1975) suggest that the capacity to be cruel (or its converse, the capacity to be empathic) is a function of how similar to himself the aggressor construes the victims to be; the greater the similarity is perceived to be, the less cruel he will be (i.e., the more empathic he will be), while greater perceived dissimilarity will permit greater cruelty and less empathy. Rapists frequently speak of women as though they are radically different from men; even inscrutable. No doubt this construction of women allows rapists to suspend empathy and carry out their assaults.

Several researchers have found rapists to be unassertive (W. L. Marshall, Barbaree, & Fernandez, 1995; Overholser & Beck, 1986; Stermac & Quinsey, 1985) and W. L. Marshall, Barbaree, and Fernandez (1995) reported that rapists held quite different views of what constituted appropriate behavior in an assertive context. For example, rapists thought a verbally aggressive and physically threatening man displayed the most appropriate response to a demanding friend; nonoffender males thought that the polite but firm man displayed the appropriate response. Lipton, McDonel, and McFall (1987) found that rapists consistently misread women's cues in a self-serving way (i.e., they saw negative feedback as positive and encouraging).

Intimacy skills, the experience of loneliness, and attachment styles, have been areas of intense recent research and theoretical focus. W. L. Marshall (1989) suggested that part of the reason men engaged in sexual assault was that they either lacked the skills necessary to establish satisfying intimate relationships, were too afraid to do so, or had learned to dismiss the value of such relationships. Subsequent research has confirmed that both incarcerated rapists (Bumby & Marshall, 1994; Garlick, Marshall, & Thornton, 1996) and rapists attending community clinics (Seidman *et al.*, 1994) have significant deficits in intimacy and are markedly lonely individuals. These problems are not restricted simply to romantic relationships, but also extend to friendships, with rapists being most particularly poor at intimacy with other males (Bumby & Marshall, 1995). Furthermore, rapists blame women for their loneliness and lack of intimacy (Garlick *et al.*, 1996), and these deficiencies in intimacy are strongly related to negative attitudes toward women (Marshall & Hambley, 1996). These findings suggest that rapists may attack women because they desire intimacy and blame women for their inability to establish a meaningful relationship. These attacks may take a sexual form because men characteristically identify sex with intimacy (Perlman & Duck, 1987), and perhaps because they find rape to be the most effective way to strike back at women by humiliating them (Darke, 1990).

Cognitive Distortions

The first and most obvious and problematic distortion is that many rapists, despite overwhelming evidence to the contrary, deny they committed the sexual assault with which they have been charged and convicted (Barbaree, 1991). Some of those who admit the act minimize its importance, deny that they caused the victim any harm, or place responsibility for the act on factors beyond their control (Segal & Stermac, 1990). Although these ideas concerning distortions among rapists enjoy widespread acceptance, there has, in fact, been very little research examining the validity of these notions; most of this research has focused on child molesters (e.g., Abel *et al.*, 1989; W. L. Marshall, 1994; Stermac & Segal, 1987).

Clinicians also characteristically consider rapists to hold an array of attitudes that may be seen as facilitating their offenses. These attitudes include the acceptance of interpersonal violence as a way of resolving problems, particularly problems involving women, a belief in what are called rape myths, and negative views of women suggesting that women should not have political, economic, or social power and that they should be obedient to men's wishes and subservient to men's desires. These attitudes have been examined in the general population of males (Burt, 1980) where they have been related to a self-reported propensity to rape (Koss *et al.*, 1987; Malamuth, 1984; Tieger, 1981). Seidman and colleagues (1994) found that rapists expressed greater hostility toward women than did nonoffender controls, and W. L. Marshall and Hambley (1996) reported that rapists endorsed more rape myths and were more hostile toward women than were matched community males. However, neither Segal and Stermac (1984) nor Overholser and Beck (1986) discerned any differences between rapists and controls in terms of their acceptance of rape myths or in their attitudes about women's roles in society. Perhaps, as Segal and Stermac (1990) suggest, the measures used to assess these attitudes are so transparent that rapists typically (although apparently not always) respond in what they consider to be the socially acceptable manner. While there are measures of dissimulation and of social desirability tendencies, these are not without their own limitations (see, e.g., Holden & Fekken, 1989; Langevin, Wright, & Handy, 1990). The issue concerning rapists' attitudes continues to be of particular clinical and research interest; however, we need to develop better ways of measuring these attributes if we are to make further progress.

Personality

It has for a long time been thought that rapists must have either personality disturbances or a quite different personality profile, since they obviously engage in behaviors that are repugnant to the rest of society. This, however, has been seen by some as an attempt to pathologize rapists and to thereby ignore those sociocultural factors that are said to facilitate or even encourage rape (Brownmiller, 1975). It is interesting that the authors of the *Diagnostic and Statistical Manual of Mental Disorders* of the American Psychiatric Association have steadfastly refused to include rape as a disorder (American Psychiatric Association, 1987, 1994) despite claims by some eminent clinicians that rape meets the criteria for a psychiatric disorder (Abel & Rouleau, 1990b). Of course, when we consider the following facts we might be inclined to think that rapists as a group will appear as normal as other men. For example, a substantial proportion of rapists go unreported, and a significant number of these are men who commit their offenses in the context of a date (Ageton, 1983; Koss *et al.*, 1987). Also, many apparently normal males either admit to having sexually assaulted a woman or say they would if they knew they could get away with it (Malamuth, Heavey, & Linz, 1993). And until recently, men who raped their wives could not be prosecuted; even now, very few are. Evidently, a considerable number of males who we might expect to have normal personalities commit sexual assaults. Unfortunately, the only rapists researchers can assess are those who are reported, prosecuted to conviction, and, in most cases, imprisoned. No doubt these factors select out an unrepresentative group of rapists and this, of course, is relevant to the generalizability of all research findings on sexual offenders. However, what does the available research on the personality of rapists tell us?

Projective tests have been used in some studies (see reviews by Levin & Stava, 1987; Rada, 1978), but recent evaluations of these tests suggest considerable problems with their reliability and validity (Kline, 1993). Laws (1984) concluded that the results revealed by projective tests with sexual offenders should be ignored.

Objective tests, particularly the Minnesota Multiphasic Personality Inventory (MMPI) have enjoyed greater acceptance and there is considerable literature describing the responses of sexual offenders on this test. However, reviewers have concluded that the MMPI has not proved very useful in detecting clear and important differences between sexual offenders of any type and other groups (Hall, 1990; Levin & Stava, 1987; W. L. Marshall & Hall, 1995; Okami & Goldberg, 1992). Several authors (e.g., Armentour & Hauer, 1978; Kalichman, 1991; Panton, 1978) insist that differences between rapists and normal controls are evident on the MMPI with most claiming that there are elevations on Scales 8 and 4 (Schizophrenia and Psychopathic Deviance, respectively). However, when W. L. Marshall and Hall (1995) examined these findings in detail, they observed that while rapists in some studies scored higher on these two scales than controls, their scores were still within normal limits; that is, the rapists were not deviant on these scales. Furthermore, several other studies have found no differences between rapists and other males on the MMPI (Anderson, Kunce, & Rich, 1979; Karacan *et al.*, 1974; Langevin, Ben-Aron, Wright, Marchese, & Handy, 1988; Quinsey, Arnold, & Pruesse, 1980).

Studies using Hare's (1991) Psychopathy Checklist have fared somewhat better in that scores on this measure contribute to the prediction of reoffending among sexual offenders (Quinsey, Rice, & Harris, 1990). Despite this value, very few rapists (12.2%) score within the abnormal range on this measure (Serin, Malcolm, Khanna, & Barbaree, 1994).

Personality measures, then, have not been very productive in research with rapists.

Other Issues

Abel and Rouleau (1990b) reported the presence of multiple paraphilias in rapists. They found that rapists reported on average three or more paraphilias in addition to rape. Freund (1990) found a similar high incidence of multiple paraphilias in rapists. However, Marshall, Barbaree, and Eccles (1991) found that very few of the rapists they studied reported more than one paraphilia. Abel and Rouleau were able to develop excellent procedures to guarantee the confidentiality of their subjects' reports and this may have led to the higher reporting rates they observed, although W. L. Marshall and colleagues also took steps to gain the confidence of their subjects. It is difficult to know how to interpret these discrepant findings, but the issue is quite important, not only for assessment and treatment, but also for theoretical models of rape. A high incidence of paraphilias among rapists would strengthen the notion that this offense is sexually motivated although if rapists are, indeed, characterized by multiple sexual outlets, then the sexual preference hypothesis is in even more serious trouble than the data from phallometric studies would suggest.

Substance abuse of one kind or another is commonly reported among rapists (Amir, 1967; Gebhard, Gagnon, Pomeroy, & Christenson, 1965; Rada, 1975). This is not to say that rapists are typically addicted to alcohol or some other drug, but rather that many of them either use an intoxicant to prime themselves to rape or the use of the intoxicant disinhibits whatever constraints they may have had about forcing an unwilling woman to have sex with them. In a reexamination of some early data collected by Christie and colleagues (1979), W. L. Marshall (1996a) was able to determine that 70% of the rapists in that study were intoxicated by alcohol at the time of their offense and that somewhat more than 60% had a clear drinking problem.

Assessment and Diagnosis

Diagnosis is not an issue with rapists that has received much attention, primarily because the diagnostic manual (American Psychiatric Association, 1994) has no category for rape. Perhaps the only issue of concern is whether or not a particular rapist is a sadist since this is in the diagnostic manual. However, in practice, diagnosticians appear to vary in their use of the term *sadist*. According to *DSM-IV*, a sadist must be sexually excited by the psychological or physical suffering of the victim, where the psychological suffering includes humiliation. Darke (1990; W. L. Marshall & Darke, 1982), in an examination of the motives of rapists, carefully selected only those offense behaviors that were rated by independent judges to be unequivocal signs of intended humiliation. It was found that in 60% of rapes there were clear indications that the offender had attempted to humiliate his victim. Complementing these findings, Darke examined the actual reports of rapists and found that 60% of these men expressed an intent to degrade or humiliate their victims. Presumably this means they enjoyed humiliating their victims, but did it make them sexually excited? If they were sexually excited by humiliating their victims, then as many as 60% of rapists would meet the diagnostic criteria for sadism. This would surprise most clinicians working with these men. Similarly, although Seto and Kubin (1996) classified 7 of their 21 rapists as sadists based on the degree of violence in their offenses, all of these men denied being aroused by violent sexual acts.

Even where it is clear that rapists deliberately cause suffering to their victims, it is not clear that they do this because it makes them sexually aroused. Some rapists (although we presently do not know how many) use violence instrumentally with the intent of frightening their victims into both cooperation and silence so that they will not be reported. Others (again we do not know how many) may use violence expressively because they enjoy making their victims suffer. However, even in the latter cases, this enjoyment may not necessarily be sexualized. In any case, the real diagnostic problem for the clinician in deciding whether or not a rapist is a sadist is to independently determine whether the suffering of the victim is sexually arousing to the offender. The only way this can be done at the moment, other than relying on the clinician's guess as to the man's motivation, is to phallometrically assess him. As we have seen, there are problems with those assessments with rapists, and it appears that very few are aroused by the suffering of the victim although this issue has not yet been examined thoroughly and appropriately. Of course, arousal to victim suffering, on its own, in the absence of clear evidence of excessive and gratuitous force or humiliation, should not be grounds for diagnosing a rapist as sadistic. What difference does a diagnosis of sadism make to decisions about treatment or release from prison? We suggest it should make no difference at all and that the whole issue of diagnosing rapists (or other sexual offenders for that matter) is irrelevant to their proper management (see also W. L. Marshall, 1997, for a consideration of the same issue with child molesters).

The assessment of rapists should be conducted primarily for two reasons (1) to evaluate their risk to re-offend, and (2) to determine their treatment needs. Although some clinicians offer assessments to assist the courts in determining the guilt or innocence of an accused, the data presently available offer no scientific support for such activities (Barbaree & Peacock, 1995; W. L. Marshall, 1996d; Simon & Schouten, 1992).

Quinsey and his colleagues (Quinsey, Lalumière, Rice, & Harris, 1995; Quinsey, Rice, & Harris, 1990, 1995) have completed the best research to date on the prediction of recidivism among sexual offenders. However, it is important to note that their re-search has been based on long-term evaluations of offenders who had either been found to be insane or whose sanity was in serious question. These sexual offenders may not be typical of the more general population of rapists held in prisons or seen at community clinics. Nevertheless, Quinsey's data provide a basis for other researchers to search for factors that predict risk in their own samples.

Quinsey, Lalumière, and colleagues (1995) describe 12 factors that allowed them to sort the offenders into one of six levels of increasing risk based on long-term fol-low-up examinations of recidivism data. All but one of these factors, however, are sta-tic features (e.g., offense history and life history features) that are unchangeable. The only feature identified by these researchers that is open to change is the man's deviant sexual preferences displayed at phallometric evaluation and this, unfortunately, con-tributed a rather small proportion of variance (4.2%) in the prediction of outcome. This is unfortunate because treatment providers hope to reduce recidivism by target-ing those factors that put the offender at risk. Of course, the possible outcomes from the type of research done by Quinsey and colleagues is limited by the variables en-tered into the analyses, and Quinsey (Quinsey, Coleman, Jones, & Altrows, 1996) has recently expanded his evaluations to include potentially modifiable features.

Similarly, assessment conducted to evaluate the need for treatment, and what needs to be targeted in treatment, are limited by the evaluator's belief about what can be treated. The targets addressed in the treatment of rapists are described in the next section, but it is certainly true that these have expanded considerably over the past 25 years. Initially, assessment was restricted to evaluating sexual preferences and some limited aspects of social skills; nowadays the range has been expanded to also include denial and minimization, empathy, relationship skills, psychopathy, cognitive distor-tions, pro-offending attitudes, use of intoxicants, leisure activities, lifestyle features and, indeed, almost an endless list of features depending on the conceptualization of rapists held by the particular clinician. We cannot hope to cover all of these issues; since we have already examined the evidence bearing on most of these problematic aspects of rapists' functioning, we restrict ourselves to an identification of the typical measurement approaches to each area of functioning that most programs evaluate.

Sexual behaviors are assessed by phallometry, but as stated earlier, these proce-dures are of dubious value with rapists. Inventories of sexual practices, sexual inter-ests, and sexual history are necessary. Measures that seem useful for these purposes include the Clarke Sexual History Questionnaire (Langevin, 1983), the Multiphasic Sex Inventory (Nichols & Molinder, 1984), the Derogatis Sexual Functioning Inven-tory (Derogatis, 1980), the Sone Sexual History Form (Maletzky, 1991), and the Sexual Interest Cardsort (Abel & Becker, 1985).

Measures of social functioning encompass a broad range of self-report instru-ments, such as the Social Response Inventory (P. G. Marshall, Keltner, & Marshall, 1981), the Social Self-esteem Inventory (Lawson, Marshall, & McGrath, 1979), the So-cial Avoidance and Distress Scale and its companion, the Fear of Negative Evalua-tions Scale (Watson & Friend, 1969), the Rapist Victim Empathy Measure (Fernandez & Marshall, 1995), the UCLA Revised Loneliness Scale (D. Russell, Peplau, & Cut-rona, 1980), and Miller's Social Intimacy Scale (R. S. Miller & Lefcourt, 1982).

Features of the rapist's life history are also important and available measures that appear useful are the Hassles Scale (Kanner, Coyne, Schafer, & Lazarus, 1981) which assesses life stresses, the Social Network Scale and the Social Buffers Scale (Flannery

& Wieman, 1989) which evaluate social supports, the Multiple Screen Sexual Abuse Questionnaire (Dhawan & Marshall, 1996) which provides a report of childhood sexual abuse, and the Family Environment Scale (Moos & Moos, 1986) which examines the childhood environment of the offender.

As we noted, various cognitive processes produce distortions among rapists. The Hostility Toward Women Scale (Check, 1984), the Rape Myth Acceptance Scale (Burt, 1980), the Attitudes Toward Women Scale (Spence, Helmreich, & Stapp, 1973), and the Attraction to Sexual Aggression Scale (Malamuth, 1989) all assess the complex of pro-rape attitudes. Barbaree, (1991) has used the Multiphasic Sex Inventory to estimate the degree of denial and minimization in rapists, but a more direct measure is needed and awaits development.

Hare's Revised Psychopathy Checklist (Hare, 1991) is particularly useful not only in predicting the likelihood of re-offending but also in assisting the therapist. For example, high scores on this measure may alert the therapist to the propensity among some of these offenders to present themselves in a plausible way that may have little depth and to caution the therapist against a tendency on the part of the offender to manipulate others in ways that may not further the attainment of treatment goals. Finally, the Michigan Alcoholism Screening Test (Selzer, 1971) and the Drug Abuse Screening Test (Skinner, 1982) are satisfactory measures of addictive proclivities.

All of the abovementioned tests are, however, self-report measures and, therefore, rely on the truthfulness of the offender. Rapists clearly have a vested interest in presenting themselves in the best possible light (Stermac, Segal, & Gillis, 1990). Such tendencies are, in any case, a problem with any population when relying on self-reports (Jackson, 1973; Kleinmutz, 1975). In an attempt to circumvent this difficulty, some researchers have employed a measure of social desirability (e.g., Crowne & Marlowe, 1960) in order to partial out this tendency, or, as in the case of the MMPI, they have added "lie" or "faking" scales. However, there are problems with these strategies and it is not clear that they satisfactorily counter these problems (Langevin *et al.*, 1990; W. L. Marshall & Hall, 1995). Furthermore, issues concerning the cultural appropriateness of tests with sexual offenders have been virtually ignored. Yet, there is clear evidence of cultural biases that distort the meaning of the results of self-report tests across different societies and with minority groups within societies (Butcher, Narikiyo, & Vitousek, 1993). All of these issues obfuscate conclusions based on self-report measures; although interviews are definitely valuable supplements to whatever assessment procedures are used, they too have their own problems not the least of which are the biases (many unrecognized) of the interviewer. At the moment, all that can be done with respect to these issues is for assessors to exercise caution in the interpretation of their data until more research is carried out to enhance the value of assessment procedures.

Clinical Management and Treatment

Convicted rapists are typically sent to prison. There are some authors (e.g., J. Miller, 1996; Money, 1986) who consider this to be inappropriate because, it is claimed, these men suffer from a disorder and should not, therefore, be punished for something they cannot control. In addition, it is suggested that doing away with imprisonment would encourage these men to seek treatment before they hurt innocent people. These theorists also suggest that imprisonment, far from reducing the risk to re-offend in rapists, may actually make them worse, presumably meaning that they will, as a result, commit more offenses or commit more severe offenses. Finally, it is thought that treatment cannot be implemented effectively in a prison but can be successfully applied in a community-based facility (Abel & Rouleau, 1990a). There is, however, no evidence in support of any of these propositions, and at least the last suggestion is open to empirical evaluation. No doubt it is theoretically possible to determine whether diversion from imprisonment would have the suggested effects, but it is doubtful anyone will approve of such a strategy. While it is impossible to say with certainty that these rapists do or do not have a disorder of such a nature that they cannot control themselves, the majority of researchers and clinicians working with these offenders reject the contention that rapists have no control over their actions.

While prisons are not ideal places for treatment, most rapists are, in fact, treated in such institutions and in similarly secure psychiatric settings. In many cases, such treatment is followed by careful supervision and further treatment upon release (Marques, Day, Nelson, & Miner, 1989; W. L. Marshall, Eccles, & Barbaree, 1993; Pithers, 1990). Considering the fact that rapists are highly heterogeneous on various factors, including the extent of their treatment needs, we (W. L. Marshall *et al.*, 1993) have structured our prison programs and postrelease treatment accordingly. Those with extensive needs (who are also typically those at greatest risk to re-offend) are involved in more comprehensive and more protracted treatment in prison, and receive the most careful and extended supervision and treatment upon release.

Although some valuable work was done with sexual offenders prior to 1970 (e.g., Frisbie & Dondis, 1965; Pacht, Halleck, & Ehrman, 1962; Peters & Roether, 1971), it was during the early 1970s that more systematic approaches began developing. The two main strategies of treatment that have become established in North America focus on either the physical substrates of the behavior or on the psychological factors. The psychological approach to treatment has led to the development of the cognitive-behavioral approach, which in recent years has incorporated relapse prevention strategies. The physical approach has led to the use of medications that alter hormonal functioning or modify the action of the serotonin system in the brain. Those clinicians who are at the forefront in the use of medications with sexual offenders also typically have their clients participate in psychological treatment programs (e.g., Berlin & Meinecke, 1981; Bradford, 1983). Since there are many clear descriptions in the literature of antiandrogen and hormonal treatments (e.g., Bradford, 1990, 1993), we note here only that the serotonergic drugs seem to have considerable promise (Fedoroff & Fedoroff, 1992). Whichever of these two approaches proves to be the most valuable, it remains very likely that medications will not, on their own, provide a complete treatment for sexual offenders. They are valuable, and for some clients essential, to the best management of these offenders. However, they should be viewed as adjuncts to those psychological treatments that teach rapists the skills and attitudes necessary to build a crime-free future life. Our focus is, therefore, primarily on cognitive-behavioral programs.

We (W. L. Marshall, 1996b; W. L. Marshall & Eccles, 1995; W. L. Marshall & Fernandez, 1998) have distinguished between "offense-specific" and "offense-related" treatment targets. The offense-specific targets are those that need to be addressed for all rapists whereas the offense-related targets are those that may or may not need to be included in treatment.

The following list describes the offense-specific targets and the appropriate references outlining the relevant procedures and their effectiveness: self-esteem enhancement (W. L. Marshall, Champagne, Sturgeon, & Bryce, 1996), reduction of denial and minimization (Barbaree, 1991; W. L. Marshall, 1994), development of victim empathy (W. L. Marshall, O'Sullivan, & Fernandez, 1996; Pithers, 1994), alteration of pro-offending attitudes and correcting cognitive distortions (Murphy, 1990), training intimacy skills and reducing loneliness (W. L. Marshall, Bryce, Hudson, Ward, & Moth, 1996), modifying sexual fantasies (Laws & Marshall, 1991), and generating relapse prevention plans (Laws, 1989; Pithers, 1990).

Offense-related targets include substance abuse, anger management, stress management, assertiveness, sex education, childhood sexual abuse issues, problem solving, and any other problematic issue that appears to be functionally related to the particular individual's offending. We provide treatment for each of these possible offense-related targets by either referring the individual client to an appropriate established program, or where one is not available, we develop procedures specific to the individual.

The overall effectiveness of cognitive-behavioral treatment programs for rapists has been reviewed (W. L. Marshall & Anderson, 1996; W. L. Marshall & Pithers, 1994; W. L. Marshall, Jones, Ward, Johnston, & Barbaree, 1991; Steele, 1993) and not only have these programs been found to reduce subsequent recidivism, analyses have revealed that their benefits (in terms of reduced human suffering and financial savings) far outweigh their costs (W. L. Marshall, 1992; Prentky & Burgess, 1991).

However, there are some suggestions that these treatments, while effective for rapists, are not so markedly effective with these clients as they are with child molesters (W. L. Marshall, Jones, et al., 1991). In response to this, suggestions have been made to alter programs for rapists by shifting the emphases more toward attitude change, by addressing their more characteristically criminal lifestyle and psychopathic tendencies, and by focusing on motives other than the strictly sexual ones (W. L. Marshall, 1993; Pithers, 1993). Whether or not these changes will produce better results remains to be seen. However, it is important to keep in mind that even the earlier programs appear to have produced lower recidivism rates than leaving rapists untreated.

Conclusions

The sexual assault of adult and teenage females by male assailants is a social problem of considerable significance. Definitions of rape have varied over the years and recent changes in the criminal codes have attempted to de-emphasize penile penetration of the woman's vagina so that the assaultive aspects have become more salient. Rapists are characterized by an array of problems, including deviant fantasies (nonsexual fantasies are likely to be more primary than sexual fantasies), social skill deficits (e.g., anger problems, empathy deficits, low self-esteem, relationship difficulties), cognitive distortions and inappropriate attitudes, and various additional, sometimes idiosyncratic problems (e.g., substance abuse). These issues are typically addressed in both the assessment and treatment of rapists. While treatment appears to be effective with rapists, more research is needed to further enhance the efficacy of treatment with these men, and suggestions have been made about how these programs might be valuably expanded.

References

Abel, G. G., & Becker, J. V. (1985). *Sexual Interest Cardsort*. Atlanta, GA: Emory University, Behavioral Medicine Laboratory.

Abel, G. G., & Blanchard, E. B. (1974). The role of fantasy in the treatment of sexual deviation. *Archives of General Psychiatry, 30,* 467–475.

Abel, G. G., & Rouleau, J. L. (1990a). Male sex offenders. In M. E. Thase, B. A. Edelstein, & M. Hersen (Eds.), *Handbook of outpatient treatment of adults* (pp. 271–290). New York: Plenum.

Abel, G. G., & Rouleau, J. L. (1990b). The nature and extent of sexual assault. In W. L. Marshall, D. R. Laws, & H. E. Barbaree (Eds.), *Handbook of sexual assault: Issues, theories and treatment of the offender* (pp. 9–21). New York: Plenum.

Abel, G. G., Barlow, D. H., Blanchard, E. B., & Guild, D. (1977). The components of rapists' sexual arousal. *Archives of General Psychiatry, 34,* 894–903.

Abel, G. G., Gore, D. K., Holland, C. L., Camp, N., Becker, J. V., & Rathner, J. (1989). The measurement of the cognitive distortions of child molesters. *Annals of Sex Research, 2,* 1351–152.

Ageton, S. (1983). *Sexual assault among adolescents*. Lexington, MA: Lexington Books.

American Psychiatric Association. (1987). *Diagnostic and statistical manual of mental disorders* (3rd ed., rev.). Washington, DC: Author.

American Psychiatric Association. (1994). *Diagnostic and statistical manual of mental disorders* (4th ed.). Washington, DC: Author.

Amir, M. (1967). Alcohol and forcible rape. *British Journal of Addictions, 62,* 219–232.

Amir, M. (1971). *Patterns of forcible rape*. Chicago: University of Chicago Press.

Anderson, W. P., Kunce, J. T., & Rich, B. (1979). Sex offenders: Three personality types. *Journal of Clinical Psychology, 35,* 671–676.

Armentour, J. A., & Hauer, A. L. (1978). MMPIs of rapists of adults, rapists of children, and nonrapist sex offenders. *Journal of Clinical Psychology, 34,* 330–332.

Bandura, A. (1973). *Aggression: A social learning analysis*. Englewood Cliffs, NJ: Prentice-Hall.

Bandura, A., Underwood, B., & Fromson, M. E. (1975). Disinhibition of aggression through diffusion of responsibility and dehumanization of victims. *Journal of Research in Personality, 9,* 253–269.

Barbaree, H. E. (1991). Denial and minimization among sex offenders: Assessment and treatment outcome. *Forum on Corrections Research, 3,* 300–333.

Barbaree, H. E., & Marshall, W. L. (1991). The role of male sexual arousal in rape: Six models. *Journal of Consulting and Clinical Psychology, 59,* 621–630.

Barbaree, H. E., & Peacock, E. J. (1995). Phallometric assessment of sexual preferences as an investigative tool in cases of alleged child sexual abuse. In T. Ney (Ed.), *Allegations in child sexual abuse: Assessment and case management* (pp. 242–259). New York: Brunner/Mazel.

Barbaree, H. E., Marshall, W. L., & Lanthier, R. D. (1979). Deviant sexual arousal in rapists. *Behaviour Research and Therapy, 14,* 215–222.

Barlow, D. H. (1973). Increasing heterosexual responsiveness in the treatment of sexual deviation: A review of the clinical and experimental evidence. *Behavior Therapy, 4,* 655–671.

Baxter, D. J., Marshall, W. L., Barbaree, H. E., Davidson, P. R., & Malcolm, P. S. (1984). Deviant sexual behavior: Differentiating sex offenders by criminal and personal history, psychometric measures, and sexual responses. *Criminal Justice and Behaviors, 11,* 477–501.

Baxter, D. J., Barbaree, H. E., & Marshall, W. L. (1986). Sexual responses to consenting and forced sex in a large sample of rapists and nonrapists. *Behaviour Research and Therapy, 24,* 513–520.

Becker, J. V., Skinner, L., Abel, G. G., Howell, J., & Bruce, K. (1982). The effects of sexual assault on rape and attempted rape victims. *Victimology: An International Journal, 7,* 106–113.

Berkin, F. S., & Meinecke, C. F. (1981). Treatment of sex offenders with antiandrogen medication: Conceptualization, review of treatment modalities and preliminary findings. *American Journal of Psychiatry, 138,* 601–607.

Blader, J. C., & Marshall, W. L. (1989). Is assessment of sexual arousal in rapists worthwhile? A critique of current methods and the development of a response compatibility approach. *Clinical Psychology Review, 9,* 569–587.

Bradford, J. M. W. (1983). Research in sex offenders. In R. L. Sadoff (Ed.), *The psychiatric clinics of North America* (pp. 715–733). Philadelphia: Saunders.

Bradford, J. M. W. (1990). The antiandrogen and hormonal treatment of sex offenders. In W. L. Marshall, D. R. Laws, & H. E. Barbaree (Eds.), *Handbook of sexual assault: Issues. theories, and treatment of the offender* (pp. 297–310). New York: Plenum.

Bradford, J. M. W. (1993). The pharmacological treatment of the adolescent sex offender. In H. E. Barbaree, W. L. Marshall, & S. M. Hudson (Eds.), *The juvenile sex offender* (pp. 278–288). New York: Guilford.

Brownmiller, S. (1975). *Against our will: Men, women, and rape.* New York: Bantam Books.

Bumby, K., & Marshall, W. L. (1994, November). *Loneliness and intimacy dysfunction among incarcerated rapists and child molesters.* Paper presented at the 13th annual Research and Treatment Conference of the Association for the Treatment of Sexual Abusers, San Francisco.

Bumby, K. M., & Marshall, W. L. (1995, October). *Intimacy deficits, fears of intimacy and emotional loneliness: Evidence of avoidant adult attachments of sexual offenders.* Paper presented at the 14th annual Research and Treatment Conference of the Association for the Treatment of Sexual Abusers, New Orleans, LA.

Burt, M. (1980). Cultural myths and supports for rape. *Journal of Personality and Social Psychology, 38,* 217–230.

Butcher, J. N., Narikiyo, T., & Vitousek, K. B. (1993). Understanding abnormal behavior in cultural context. In P. B. Sutker & H. E. Adams (Eds.), *Comprehensive handbook of psychopathology* (pp. 83–105). New York: Plenum.

Check, J. V. (1984). *The Hostility Towards Women Scale.* Unpublished doctoral dissertation, University of Manitoba, Winnipeg, Manitoba, Canada.

Christie, M. M., Marshall, W. L., & Lanthier, R. D. (1979). *A descriptive study of incarcerated racists and pedophiles.* Report to the Solicitor General of Canada, Ottawa.

Clark, L., & Lewis, D. (1977). *Rape: The price of coercive sexuality.* Toronto, Ontario, Canada: Women's Educational Press.

Crowne, D. P., & Marlow, D. (1960). A new scale of social desirability independent of psychopathology. *Journal of Consulting Psychology, 24,* 349–354.

Darke, J. L. (1990). Sexual aggression: Achieving power through humiliation. In W. L. Marshall, D. R. Laws, & H. E. Barbaree (Eds.), *Handbook of sexual assault: Issues, theories, and treatment of the offender* (pp. 55–72). New York: Plenum.

Deitz, S. R., Blackwell, K. T., Daley, P.C., & Bentley, B. J. (1982). Measurement of empathy toward rape victims and rapists. *Journal of Personality and Social Psychology, 43,* 372–384.

Derogatis, L. R. (1980). Psychological assessment of psychosexual functioning, *Psychiatric Clinics of North America, 3,* 113–131.

Dhawan, S., & Marshall, W. L. (1996). Sexual abuse histories of sexual offenders. *Sexual Abuse: A Journal of Research and Treatment, 8,* 7–15.

Eccles, A., Marshall, W. L., & Barbaree, H. E. (1994). Differentiating rapists and non-offenders using the Rape Index. *Behaviour Research and Therapy, 32,* 539–546.

Ellis, E. M. (1983). A review of empirical rape research: Victims' reactions and response to treatment. *Clinical Psychology Review, 3,* 473–490.

Ennis, P. H. (1967). *Criminal victimization in the United States: A report of a national survey* (National Opinion Research Center (NORC), University of Chicago). Washington, DC: U.S. Government Printing Office.

Eysenek, H. J. (1992). Meta-analysis, sense or non-sense? *Pharmaceutical Medicine, 6,* 113–119.

Fedoroff, J. P., & Fedoroff, I. C. (1992). Buspirone and paraphilic sexual behavior. In E. Coleman, S. M. Dwyer, & N. J. Pallone (Eds.), *Sex offender treatment: Psychological and medical approaches* (pp. 89–108). New York: Haworth.

Fernandez, Y. M., & Marshall, W. L. (1995, October). *Victim empathy in rapists.* Paper presented at the 14th annual Research and Treatment Conference of the Association for the Treatment of Sexual Abusers, New Orleans, LA.

Flanery, R. B., & Wieman, D. (1989). Social support, life stress, and psychological distress: An empirical assessment. *Journal of Clinical Psychology, 45,* 867–872.

Freund, K. (1990). Courtship disorder. In W. L. Marshall, D. R. Laws, & H. E. Barbaree (Eds.), *Handbook of sexual assault: Issues, theories, and treatment of the offender* (pp. 195–207). New York: Plenum.

Frisbie, L. V., & Dondis, E. H. (1965). *Recidivism among treated sex offenders.* Sacramento: California Department of Mental Hygiene.

Garlick, Y., Marshall, W. L., & Thornton, D. (1996). Intimacy deficits and attribution of blame among sexual offenders. *Legal and Criminological Psychology, 1,* 251–258.

Gebhard, P. H., Gagnon, J. H., Pomperoy, W. H., & Christenson, C. V. (1965). *Sex offenders.* New York: Harper & Row.

Groth, A. N. (1979). *Men who rape: The psychology of the offender.* New York: Plenum.

Groth, A. N, & Burgess, A. W. (1980). Male rape: Offenders and victims. *American Journal of Psychiatry, 137,* 806–810.

Hall, G. C. N. (1989). Sexual arousal and arousability in a sexual offender population. *Journal of Abnormal Psychology, 98,* 145–149.

Hall, G. C. N. (1990). Prediction of sexual aggression. *Clinical Psychology Review, 10,* 229–245.

Hall, G. C. N., Proctor, W. C., & Nelson, G. M. (1988). Validity of physiological measures of pedophilic sexual arousal in a sexual offender population. *Journal of Consulting and Clinical Psychology, 56,* 118–122.

Hanson, K., & Scott, H. (1995). Assessing perspective taking among sexual offenders, nonsexual criminals and nonoffenders. *Sexual Abuse: A Journal of Research and Treatment, 7,* 259–277.

Hare, R. D. (1991). *Manual for the Revised Psychopathy Checklist.* Toronto, Ontario, Canada: Multi-Health Systems.

Harris, G. T., Rice, M. E., Quinsey, V. L., Chaplin, T. C., & Earls, C. M. (1992). Maximizing the discriminant validity of phallometric assessment data. *Psychological Assessment: A Journal of Consulting and Clinical Psychology, 4,* 502–511.

Hillman, R. J., O'Mara, N., Taylor-Robinson, D., & Harris, J. R. W. (1990). Medical and social aspects of sexual assault of males: A survey of 100 victims. *British Journal of General Practice, 40,* 502–504.

Holden, R. R., & Fekken, G. C. (1989). Three common social desirability scales: Friends, acquaintances, or strangers? *Journal of Research in Personality, 23,* 180–191.

Hudson, S. M., Marshall, W. L., Wales, D., McDonald, E., Bakker, L. W., & McLean, A. (1993). Emotional recognition skills of sex offenders. *Annals of Sex Research, 6,* 199–211.

Jackson, D. N. (1973). Structural personality assessment. In B. B. Wolman (Ed.), *Handbook of general psychology* (pp. 44–68). Englewood Cliffs, NJ: Prentice-Hall.

Kalichman, S. C. (1991). Psychopathology and personality characteristics of criminal sexual offenders as a function of victim age. *Archives of Sexual Behavior, 20,* 187–197.

Kanin, E. J., & Parcell, S. R. (1977). Sexual aggression: A second look at the offended female. *Archives of Sexual Behavior, 6,* 67–76.

Kanner, A. D., Coyne, J. C., Schafer, C., & Lazarus, R. S. (1981). Comparison of two modes of stress management: Daily hassles and uplifts versus major life events. *Journal of Behavioral Medicine, 4,* 1–39.

Karacan, I., Williams, R. L., Guerrero, M. W., Scales, P. J., Thornby, J. L., & Hursch, C. J. (1974). Nocturnal penile tumescence and sleep of convicted rapists and other prisoners. *Archives of Sexual Behavior, 3,* 19–26.

Kaufman, A., DiVasto, P., Jackson, R., Voorhees, D., & Christy, J. (1980). Male rape victims: Noninstitutionalized assault. *American Journal of Psychiatry, 137,* 221–223.

Kilpatrick, D. G., & Amick, A. E. (1985). Rape trauma. In M. Hersen & C. G. Last (Eds.), *Behavior therapy casebook* (pp. 86–103). New York: Springer.

Kilpatrick, D. G., & Best, C. L. (1990, April). *Sexual assault victims: Data from a random national probability study.* Paper presented at the annual Convention of the Southeastern Psychological Association, Atlanta, GA.

Kleinmutz, B. (1975). *Personality measurement: An introduction.* Huntington, NY: Krieger.

Kline, P. (1993). *The handbook of psychological testing.* New York: Routledge.

Knopp, F. H., & Lackey, L. B. (1987). *Female sexual abusers: A summary of data from 44 treatment providers.* Orwell, VT: Safer Society Press.

Koss, M. P. (1985). The hidden rape victim: Personality, attitudinal, and situational characteristics. *Psychology of Women Quarterly, 9,* 193–212.

Koss, M. P., & Harvey, M. R. (1991). *The rape victim: Clinical and community interventions* (2nd ed.). Newbury Park, CA: Sage.

Koss, M. P., Gidycz, C. A., & Wisniewski, N. (1987). The scope of rape: Incidence and prevalence of sexual aggression and victimization in a national sample of higher education students. *Journal of Consulting and Clinical Psychology, 55,* 162–170.

Lalumière, M. L., & Quinsey, V. L. (1994). The discriminability of rapists from non-sex offenders using phallometric measures: A meta-analysis. *Criminal Justice and Behavior, 21,* 150–175.

Langevin, R. (1983). *Sexual stands: Understanding and treating sexual anomalies in men.* Hillsdale, NJ: Erlbaum.

Langevin, R., Paitich, D., & Russon, A. E. (1985). Are rapists sexually anomalous, aggressive, or both? In R. Langevin (Ed.), *Erotic preference, gender identity, and aggression in men: New research studies* (pp. 130–38). Hillsdale, NJ: Erlbaum.

Langevin, R., Ben-Aron, M. H., Wright, P., Marchese, V., & Handy, L. (1988). The sex killer. *Annals of Sex Research, 1,* 263–301.

Langevin, R., Wright, P., & Handy, L. (1990). Use of the MMPI and its derived scales with sex offenders: 1. Reliability and validity studies. *Annals of Sex Research, 3,* 245–291.

Laws, D. R. (1984). The assessment of dangerous sexual behavior in males. *Medicine and Law, 3,* 127–140.

Laws, D. R. (Ed.). (1989). *Relapse prevention with sex offenders.* New York: Guilford.

Laws, D. R., & Marshall, W. L. (1991). Masturbatory reconditioning: An evaluative review. *Advances in Behaviour Research and Therapy, 13*, 13–25.

Lawson, J. S., Marshall, W. L., & McGrath, P. (1979). The Social Self-Esteem Inventory. *Educational and Psychological Measurement, 39*, 803–811.

Levin, S. M., & Stava, L. (1987). Personality characteristics of sex offenders: A review. *Archives of Sexual Behavior, 16*, 57–79.

Lipton, D. N., McDonel, E. C., & McFall, R. M. (1987). Heterosocial perception in rapists. *Journal of Consulting and Clinical Psychology, 55*, 17–21.

Malamuth, N. M. (1984). Aggression against women: Cultural and individual causes. In N. M. Malamuth & E. Donnerstein (Eds.), *Pornography and sexual aggression* (pp. 19–52). Orlando, FL: Academic Press.

Malamuth, N. M. (1989). The Attraction to Sexual Aggression Scale: Part One. *Journal of Sex Research, 26*, 26–49.

Malamuth, N. M., Heavey, C. L., & Linz, D. (1993). Predicting men's antisocial behavior against women: The interaction model of sexual aggression. In G. C. N. Hall, R. Hirschman, J. R. Graham, & M. S. Zaragoza (Eds.), *Sexual Aggression: Issues in etiology, assessment and treatment* (pp. 63–97). Washington, DC: Taylor & Francis.

Maletzky, B. M. (1991). *Treating the sexual offender*. Newbury Park, CA: Sage.

Marques, J. K., Day, D. M. , Nelson, C., & Miner, M. H. (1989). The Sex Offender Treatment and Evaluation Project: California's relapse prevention program. In D. R. Laws (Ed.), *Relapse prevention with sex offenders* (pp. 96–104). New York: Guilford.

Marshall, P. G., Keltner, A., & Marshall, W. L. (1981). Anxiety reduction, assertive training, and enactment of consequences: A comparative study in the modification of nonassertion and social fear. *Behavior Modification, 5*, 85–102.

Marshall, W. L. (1971). A combined treatment method for certain sexual deviations. *Behaviour Research and Therapy, 9*, 292–294.

Marshall, W. L. (1989). Intimacy, loneliness and sexual offenders. *Behaviour Research and Therapy, 27*, 491–503.

Marshall; W. L. (1992). The social value of treatment for sexual offenders. *Canadian Journal of Human Sexuality, 1*, 109–114.

Marshall, W. L. (1993). A revised approach to the treatment of men who sexually assault adult females. In G. C. Nagayama Hall, R. Hirschman, J. R. Graham, & M. S. Zaragoza (Eds.), *Sexual aggression: Issues in etiology, assessment and treatment* (pp. 143–165). Bristol, PA: Taylor & Francis.

Marshall, W. L. (1994). Treatment effects on denial and minimization in incarcerated sex offenders. *Behaviour Research and Therapy, 32*, 559–564.

Marshall, W. L. (1995). *The relationship between self-esteem and deviant sexual arousal in nonfamilial child molesters*. Submitted for publication.

Marshall, W. L. (1996a). Assessment, treatment, and theorizing about sex offenders: Development over the past 20 years and future directions. *Criminal Justice and Behavior, 23*, 162–199.

Marshall, W. L. (1996b). Current status of North American assessment and treatment programs for sexual offenders. In W. L. Marshall & J. Frenken (Eds.), *North American and European approaches to assessment, treatment, and research with sexual offenders*. Manuscript submitted for publication.

Marshall, W. L. (1996c). *Phallometric testing with sexual offenders: Scientifically sound or a matter of faith?* Manuscript submitted for publication.

Marshall, W. L. (1998). Pedophilia: Psychopathology and theory. In D. R. Laws & W. O'Donohue (Eds.), *Handbook of sexual deviance: Theory and applications* (pp. 162–174). New York: Guilford.

Marshall, W. L. (1996d). Psychological evaluations in sexual offense cases. *Queen's Law Journal, 21*, 499–514.

Marshall, W. L., & Anderson, D. (1996). An evaluation of the benefits of relapse prevention programs with sexual offenders. *Sexual Abuse: A Journal of Research and Treatment, 8*, 209–221.

Marshall, W. L., & Barbaree, H. E. (1990). An integrated theory of sexual offending. In W. L. Marshall, D. R. Laws, & H. E. Barbaree (Eds.), *Handbook of sexual assault: Issues, theories, and treatment of the offender* (pp. 257–275). New York: Plenum.

Marshall, W. L., & Barbaree, H. E. (1995). *Heterogeneity in the erectile response patterns of rapists and nonoffenders*. Unpublished manuscript, Queen's University, Kingston, Ontario, Canada.

Marshall, W. L., & Barrett, S. (1990). *Criminal neglect: Why sex offenders go free*. Toronto, Ontario, Canada: Doubleday.

Marshall, W. L., & Darke, J. (1982). Inferring humiliation as motivation in sexual offenses. *Treatment for Sexual Aggressives, 5*, 1–3.

Marshall, W. L., & Eccles, A. (1991). Issues in clinical practice with sex offenders. *Journal of Interpersonal Violence, 6,* 68–93.

Marshall, W. L., & Eccles, A. (1993). Pavlovian conditioning processes in adolescent sex offenders. In H. E. Barbaree, W. L. Marshall, & S. M Hudson (Eds.), *The juvenile sex offender* (pp. 118–142). New York: Guilford.

Marshall, W. L., & Eccles, A. (1995). Cognitive-behavioral treatment of sex offenders. In V. M. B. Hasselt & M. Hersen (Eds.), *Sourcebook of psychological treatment manuals for adult* (pp. 295–332). New York: Plenum.

Marshall, W. L., & Fernandez, Y. M. (1998). Cognitive/behavioral approaches to the treatment of the paraphilias. In V. E. Caballo (Ed.)., *International handbook of cognitive/behavioral treatment disorders for psychological disorders.* (pp. 1–32). Shannon, Ireland: Elsevier Science.

Marshall, W. L., & Hall, G. C. N. (1995). The value of the MMPI in deciding forensic issues in accused sexual offenders. *Sexual Abuse: A Journal of Research and Treatment, 7,* 203–217.

Marshall, W. L., & Hambley, L. S. (1996) Intimacy and loneliness, and their relationship to rape myth acceptance and hostility toward women among rapists. *Journal of Interpersonal Violence, 11,* 586–592.

Marshall, W. L., & Mazzucco, A. (1995). Self-esteem and parental attachments in child molesters. *Sexual Abuse: A Journal of Research and Treatment, 7,* 279–285.

Marshall, W. L., & Pithers, W. D. (1994). A reconsideration of treatment outcome with sex offenders. *Criminal Justice and Behavior, 21,* 10–27.

Marshall, W. L., Barbaree, H. E., Laws, D. R., & Baxter, D. J. (1986, September). *Rapists do not have deviant sexual preferences: Large scale studies from Canada and California.* Paper presented at the 12th annual Meeting of the International Academy of Sex Research, Amsterdam.

Marshall, W. L., Barbaree, H. E., & Eccles, A. (1991). Early onset and deviant sexuality in child molesters. *Journal of Interpersonal Violence, 6,* 323–336.

Marshall, W. L., Jones, R. L., Ward, T., Johnston, P., & Barbaree, H. E. (1991). Treatment outcome with sex offenders. *Clinical Psychology Review, 11,* 465–485.

Marshall, W. L., Eccles, A., & Barbaree, H. E. (1993). A three-tiered approach to the rehabilitation of incarcerated sex offenders. *Behavioral Sciences and the Law, 11,* 441–445.

Marshall, W. L., Anderson, D., & Champagne, F. (1996). Self-esteem and its relationship to sexual offending. *Psychology, Crime & Law, 3,* 81–106.

Marshall, W. L., Barbaree, H. E., & Fernandez, Y. M. (1995). Some aspects of social competence in sex offenders. *Sexual Abuse: A Journal of Research and Treatment, 7,* 113–127.

Marshall, W. L., Hudson, S. M., Jones, R. L., & Fernandez, Y. M. (1995). Empathy in sex offenders. *Clinical Psychology Review, 15,* 99–113.

Marshall, W. L., Champagne, F., Sturgeon, C., & Bryce, P. (1996). *Increasing the self-esteem of child molesters.* Sexual Abuse: A Journal of Research and Treatment, 9, 321–333.

Marshall, W. L., O'Sullivan, C., & Fernandez, Y. M. (1996). The enhancement of victim empathy among incarcerated child molesters. *Legal and Criminological Psychology, 1,* 95–102.

Marshall, W. L., Bryce, P., Hudson, S. M., Ward, T., & Moth, B. (1996). The enhancement of intimacy and the reduction of loneliness among child molesters. *Journal of Family Violence, 11,* 219–235.

Marshall, W. L., Champagne, F., Brown, C., & Miller, S. (1997). Empathy, intimacy, loneliness and self-esteem in nonfamilial child molesters. *Journal of Child Sexual Abuse, 6,* 87–97.

Mathews, R., Matthews, J., & Speltz, K. (1989). *Female sex offenders.* Orwell, VT: Safer Society Press.

McCann, I. L., Sakheim, D. K., & Abrahamson, D. J. (1988). Trauma and victimization: A model of psychological adaptation. *The Counselling Psychologist, 6,* 531–594.

McConaghy, N. (1993). *Sexual behavior: Problems and management.* New York: Plenum.

McGuire, R. J., Carlisle, J. M., & Young, B. G. (1965). Sexual deviations as conditioned behavior: A hypothesis. *Behaviour Research and Therapy, 2,* 185–190.

Miller, J. (1996, January). *Treatment of sex offenders.* Paper presented at the Hennepin County Sexual Offending Conference, Minneapolis, MN.

Miller, R. S., & Lefcourt, H. M. (1982). The assessment of social intimacy. *Journal of Personality Assessment, 46,* 514–518.

Money, J. (1986). *Love maps: Clinical concepts of sexual/erotic health and pathology, paraphilias and gender transposition, childhood, adolescence and maturity.* New York: Irving.

Moos, R., & Moos, B. S. (1986). *Family Environment Scale manual.* Palo Alto, CA: Consulting Psychologists.

Murphy, W. D. (1990). Assessment and modification of cognitive distortions in sex offenders. In W. L. Marshall, D. R. Laws, & H. E. Barbaree (Eds.), *Handbook of sexual assault: Issues, theories, and treatment of the offender* (pp. 331–342). New York: Plenum.

Murphy, W. D., Krisak, J., Stalgaitis, S. J., & Anderson, K. (1984). The use of penile tumescence measures with incarcerated rapists: Further validity issues. *Archives of Sexual Behavior, 13,* 545–554.

Nichols, H.R., & Molinder, I. (1984). *Multiphasic Sex Inventory manual.* Tacoma, WA: Authors.

Okami, P., & Goldberg, A. (1992). Personality correlates of pedophiles: Are they reliable indicators? *Journal of Sex Research, 39,* 297–328.

Overholser, J. C., & Beck, S. (1986). Multimethod assessment of rapists, child molesters, and three control groups on behavioral and psychological measures. *Journal of Consulting and Clinical Psychology, 54,* 682–687.

Pacht, A. R., Halleck, S. L., & Ehrman, J. C. (1962). Diagnosis and treatment of the sexual offender: A nine-year study. *American Journal of Psychiatry, 118,* 802–808.

Panton, J. H. (1978). Personality differences appearing between rapists of adults, rapists of children, and non-violent sexual molesters of female children. *Research Communications in Psychology, Psychiatry and Behavior, 3,* 385–393.

Perlman, D., & Duck, S. (1987). *Intimate relationships: Development, dynamics, and deterioration.* Beverly Hills, CA: Sage.

Peters, J. J., & Roether, H. A. (1971). *Success and failure of sex offenders.* Philadelphia: American Association for the Advancement of Science.

Pithers, W. D. (1990). Relapse prevention with sexual aggressors: A method for maintaining therapeutic gain and enhancing external supervision. In W. L. Marshall, D. R. Laws, & H. E. Barbaree (Eds.), *Handbook of sexual assault: Issues, theories and treatment of the offender* (pp. 343–361). New York: Plenum.

Pithers, W. D. (1993).Treatment of rapists: Reinterpretation of early outcome data and explanatory constructs to enhance therapeutic efficacy. In G. C. N. Hall, R. Hirschman, J. R. Graham, & M. S. Zaragoza (Eds.), *Sexual aggression: Issues in etiology, assessment, and treatment* (pp. 167–196). Washington, DC: Taylor & Francis.

Pithers, W. D. (1994). Process evaluation of a group therapy component designed to enhance sex offenders' empathy for sexual abuse survivors. *Behaviour Research and Therapy, 32,* 565–570.

Prentky, R., & Burgess, A. W. (1991). Rehabilitation of child molesters: A cost-benefit analysis. *American Journal of Orthopsychiatry, 60,* 108–117.

Proulx, J., Aubut, J., McKibben, A., & Coté, M. (1994). Penile responses of rapists and nonrapists to rape stimuli involving physical violence or humiliation. *Archives of Sexual Behavior, 23,* 295–310.

Quinsey, V. L., Arnold, L. S., & Pruesse, M. G. (1980). MMPI profiles of men referred for pretrial psychiatric assessment as a function of offense type. *Journal of Clinical Psychology, 36,* 410–417.

Quinsey, V. L., Chaplin, T. C., & Upfold, D. (1984). Sexual arousal to nonsexual violence and sadomasochistic themes among rapists and non-sex-offenders. *Journal of Consulting and Clinical Psychology, 52,* 651–657.

Quinsey, V. L., Rice, M. E., & Harris, G. T. (1990). *Psychopathy, sexual deviance, and recidivism among sex offenders released from a maximum security institution* (Penetanguishene Research Report, Vol. 7, No. 1). Penetanguishene, Ontario: Oak Ridge, Mental Health Center.

Quinsey, V. L., Lalumière, M. L., Rice, M. E., & Harris, G. T. (1995). Predicting sexual offenses. In J. C. Campbell (Ed.), *Assessing dangerousness: Violence by sexual offenders, batterers, and child abusers* (pp. 116–137). Thousand Oaks, CA: Sage.

Quinsey, V. L., Coleman, G., Jones, B., & Altrows, I. (1996). *Proximal antecedents of absconding and reoffending among supervised mentally disordered offenders.* Manuscript submitted for publication.

Quinsey, V. L., Rice, M. E., & Harris, G. T. (1995). Actuarial prediction of sexual recidivism. *Journal of Interpersonal Violence, 10,* 85–105.

Rada, R. T. (1975). Alcohol and rape. *Medical Aspects of Human Sexuality, 9,* 48–65.

Rada, R. T. (1978). *Clinical aspects of the rapist.* New York: Grune & Stratton.

Roth, S., & Lebowitz, L. (1988). The experience of sexual trauma. *Journal of Traumatic Stress, 1,* 79–107.

Russell, D., Peplau, L. A., & Cutrona, C. A. (1980). The Revised UCLA Loneliness Scale. *Journal of Personality and Social Psychology, 39,* 472–480.

Russell, D. E. H. (1984). *Sexual exploitation: Race, child sexual abuse, and workplace harassment.* Newbury Park, CA: Sage.

Sanday, P. R. (1981). The socio-cultural context of rape: A cross-cultural study. *Journal of Social Issues, 37,* 5–27.

Schiff, A. F. (1971). Rape in other countries. *Medicine, Science and the Law, 11,* 139–143.

Segal, Z. V., & Marshall, W. L. (1986). Discrepancies between self efficacy predictions and actual performance in a population of rapists and child molesters. *Cognitive Therapy and Research, 10,* 363–376.

Segal, Z. V., & Stermac, L. E. (1984). A measure of rapists' attitudes towards women. *International Journal of Law and Psychiatry, 7,* 437–440.

Segal, Z. V., & Stermac, L. E. (1990). The role of cognition in sexual assault. In W. L. Marshall, D. R. Laws, & H. E. Barbaree (Eds.), *Handbook of sexual assault: Issues, theories, and treatment of the offender* (pp. 161–174). New York: Plenum.

Seidman, B. T., Marshall, W. L., Hudson, S. M., & Robertson, P. J. (1994). An examination of intimacy and loneliness in sex offenders. *Journal of Interpersonal Violence, 9,* 518–534.

Selzer, M. L. (1971). The Michigan Alcoholism Screening Test (MAST): The quest for a new diagnostic instrument. *American Journal of Psychiatry, 127,* 1653–1658.

Serin, R. C., Malcolm, P. B., Khanna, A., & Barbaree, H. E. (1994). Psychopathy and deviant sexual arousal in incarcerated sexual offenders. *Journal of Interpersonal Violence, 9,* 3–11.

Seto, M. C., & Kubin, M. (1996). Criterion-related validity of a phallometric test for paraphilic rape and sadism. *Behaviour Research and Therapy, 34,* 175–183.

Simon, W. T., & Schouten, P. G. W. (1992). Problems in sexual preferences testing in child sexual abuse cases: A legal and community perspective. *Journal of Interpersonal Violence, 7,* 503–506.

Skinner, H. A. (1982). The Drug Abuse Screening Test. *Addictive Behaviors, 7,* 363–371.

Spence, J. T., Helmreich, R., & Stapp, J. (1973). A short version of the Attitudes Towards Women Scale (ATW). *Bulletin of the Psychonomic Society, 2,* 219–220.

Spielberger, C.D. (1988). *State-trait Anger Expression Inventory: Professional manual research edition.* Odessa, FL: Psychological Assessment Resources.

Steele, N. (1995). Cost effectiveness of treatment. In B. K. Schwartz & H.R. Cellini (Eds.), *The sex offender: Corrections, treatment and legal practice* (pp. 4.1–4.19). Kingston, NJ: Civic Research Institute.

Stermac, L. E., & Quinsey, V. L. (1985). Social competence among rapists. *Behavioral Assessment, 8,* 171–185.

Stermac, L. E., & Segal, Z. V. (1987, November). *Cognitive assessment of child molesters.* Paper presented at the annual meeting of the Association for the Advancement of Behavior Therapy, Boston.

Stermac, L. E., Segal, Z. V., & Gillis, R. (1990). Social and cultural factors in sexual assault. In W. L. Marshall, D. R. Laws, & H. E. Barbaree (Eds.), *Handbook of sexual assault: Issues, theories, and treatment of the offender* (pp. 143–159). New York: Plenum.

Stermac, L. E., Sheridan, P. M., Davidson, A., & Dunn, S. (1996). Sexual assault of adult males. *Journal of Interpersonal Violence, 11,* 52–64.

Tieger, T. (1981). Self-rated likelihood of raping and the social perception of rape. *Journal of Research in Personality, 15,* 147–158.

Travin, S., & Protter, B. (1993). *Sexual perversion: Integrative treatment approaches for the clinician.* New York: Plenum.

van Dijk, J. J. M., & Mayhew, P. (1992). *Criminal victimization in the industrial world.* The Hague, Netherlands: Directorate for Crime Prevention.

Watson, D., & Friend, R. (1969). Measurement of social evaluation anxiety. *Journal of Consulting and Clinical Psychology, 33,* 448–457.

Weiss, P. (1995). Sexology in the Czech Republic. In W. L. Marshall & J. Frenken (Eds.), *North American and European approaches to assessment, treatment, and research with sexual offenders.* Manuscript submitted for publication.

Wormith, J. S., Bradford, J. M. W., Pawlak, A., Borzecki, M., & Zohar, A. (1988). The assessment of deviant sexual arousal as a function of intelligence, instructional set and alcohol ingestion. *Canadian Journal of Psychiatry, 33,* 800–808.

$$14$$

Child Sexual Molestation

Robert A. Prentky

Description of the Problem

Over the past several decades, our awareness of the magnitude and the impact of sexual victimization has increased considerably. Sexual abuse has become an acute problem, manifested in ever increasing costs to society as well as to its victims. The costs incurred by society include medical and psychological services to aid victim recovery, the apprehension and disposition of offenders, and the invisible climate of fear that makes safety a paramount consideration in scheduling normal daily activities. In addition to the monetary costs associated with sexual abuse (Prentky & Burgess, 1990), the impact of such abuse on its victims has been well documented. Indeed, there is a large and growing literature on the proximal (short-term) and distal (long-term) effects of child sexual abuse (see Table 14.1).

Most of these studies have focused on *adult* outcomes (i.e., samples of adults who were sexually abused as children and who are now the subject of an outcome study to determine the long-term effects of the abuse). A recent meta-analytic study of the long-term effects of child sexual abuse aggregated 2,774 women who reported a victimization history and 8,388 women who reported no such history (Neumann, Houskamp, Pollock, & Briere, 1996). Neumann and colleagues found that depression, suicidality, anger, anxiety, revictimization, self-mutilation, sexual problems, abuse of substances, impaired self-concept, interpersonal problems, obsessive-compulsive symptoms, somatization, dissociation, and symptoms of posttraumatic stress were all significantly associated with sexual abuse.

Relatively few studies have focused on the short-term sequelae of sexual abuse in samples of children, and those that have, usually focus on the children who have been identified as victims through contact with a social service agency or through the court system. Although family histories often are collected, the empirical spotlight focuses almost exclusively on the index child. The literature on short-term outcomes of identified victims clearly suggests a wide range of responses to the abuse, from no apparent symptoms to *mild symptomatology* (situation-specific anxiety or phobic

Robert A. Prentky • Justice Resource Institute at the Massachusetts Treatment Center, Bridgewater, Massachusetts 02324.

Handbook of Psychological Approaches with Violent Offenders: Contemporary Strategies and Issues, edited by Van Hasselt and Hersen. Kluwer Academic/Plenum Publishers, New York, 1999.

TABLE 14.1
Empirical Support for the Primary Effects of Chilhood Sexual Abuse

Primary Short-Term Effects

(A) Anxiety/Phobic Reactions & *Posttraumatic Stress Disorder* (PTSD)
(Kendall-Tackett, Williams, & Finkelhor, 1993; Kiser, Ackerman, Brown, Edwards, McColgan, Pugh, & Pruitt, 1988; McLeer, Deblinger, Atkins, Foa, & Ralphe, 1988; Porter, Blick, & Sgroi, 1982)
(B) *Dissociation/Multiple Personality Disorder* (MPD)
(Braun & Sachs, 1985; Kluft, 1985)
(C) *Depression/Poor Self-Esteem*
(Cavaiola & Shiff, 1988; Dubowitz, Black, Harrington, & Verschoore, 1993); Friedrich, Urquiza, & Beilke, 1986; Kendall-Tackett, *et al.*, 1993; Livingston, 1987; Mennen & Meadow, 1995; Sansonnet-Hayden, Haley, Marriage, & Fine, 1987; Sgroi, 1982)
(D) *Sexually Inappropriate & Promiscuous Behavior*
(Dubowitz *et al.*, 1993; Friedrich, 1988; Friedrich & Reams, 1987; Goodwin, 1985; Kendall-Tackett, *et al.*, 1993; Sgroi, 1982; Yates, 1982).

Primary Long-Term Effects

(A) *Dissociation/MPD & PTSD*
(Anderson, Yasenik, & Ross, 1993; Bagley, 1991; Briere & Runtz, 1990b; Briere & Runtz, 1993; Chu & Dill, 1990; Coons, 1986; Lindberg & Distad, 1985; Nash, Hulsey, Sexton, Harralson, & Lambert, 1993; Ross, Norton, & Wozney, 1989; Ross , Anderson, Heber, & Norton, 1990; Ross, Miller, Reagor, Bjoinson, Fraser & Anderson, 1991; Rowan, Foy, Rodriguez, & Ryan, 1994; Schultz, Braun, & Kluft, 1989; Swett & Halpert, 1993; Winfield, George, Swartz, & Blazer, 1990; Wolfe, Sas, & Wekerle, 1994)
(B) *Serious Psychopathology* (e.g., Borderline Personality Disorder)
(Alexander, 1993; Anderson *et al.*, 1993; Briere & Zaidi, 1989; Brown & Anderson, 1991; Bryer, Nelson, Miller, & Krol, 1987; Gold, 1986; Gross, Doerr, Caldirola, Guzinski, & Ripley, 1980–1981; Herman, Perry, & van der Kolk, 1989; Nash *et al.*, 1993; Ogata *et al.*, 1990; Stone, 1990; Swett & Halpert, 1993; Westen, Ludolph, Misle, Ruffins, & Block, 1990; Winfield *et al.*, 1990)
(C) *Eating Disorders*
(Bulik, Sullivan, & Rorty, 1989; Coons, Bowman, Pellow, & Schneider, 1989; Goldfarb, 1987; Hall, Tice, Beresford, Wolley, & Hall, 1989; Moeller, Bachmann, & Moeller, 1993; Palmer, Oppenheimer, Dignon, Chaloner, & Howells, 1990; Schecter, Schwartz, & Greenfield, 1987)
(D) *Alcohol and Drug Abuse*
(Anderson *et al.*, 1993; Briere & Zaidi, 1989; Brown & Anderson, 1991; Moeller *et al.*, 1993; Peters, 1988; Pribor & Dinwiddie, 1992; Stein, Golding, Siegel, Burnam, & Sorenson, 1988; Winfield *et al.*, 1990)
(E) *Depression and Suicidality*
(Anderson *et al.*, 1993; Bagley, 1991; Briere & Zaidi, 1989; Brown & Anderson, 1991; Elliott & Briere, 1992; Gold, 1986; Moeller *et al.*, 1993; Pribor & Dinwiddie, 1992; Stein *et al.*, 1988; Winfield *et al.*, 1990)
(F) *Revictimization*
(Briere & Runtz, 1988; Jackson, Calhoun, Amick, Madderer, & Habif, 1990; Kendall-Tackett & Simon, 1988; Moeller *et al.*, 1993; Wyatt, Guthrie, & Notgrass, 1992)
(G) *Prostitution/Promiscuous Behavior*
(Bagley, 1991; Burgess, Hartman, & McCormack, 1987; James & Meyerding, 1977; Silbert & Pines, 1981; Widom & Ames, 1994)
(H) *Victimization of Others*
(Garland & Dougher, 1990; Groth, 1979; Hanson & Slater, 1988; Rivera & Widom, 1990; Seghorn, Prentky, & Boucher, 1987; Widom, 1989; Widom & Ames, 1994).

reactions, depression, delays in acquisition of normal developmental skills, especially social and interpersonal skills), *moderate symptomatology* (anxiety or phobic reactions and possibly some signs of posttraumatic stress disorder [PTSD], sexually inappropriate acting out and sexualized aggression, depression, impaired self-esteem), and *severe symptomatology* (in addition to the preceeding symptoms, clear signs and symptoms of PTSD and Dissociative Disorder, and, in the most extreme cases, Dissociative Identity Disorder, or Multiple Personality Disorder [MPD]). The multiplicity and complexity of outcomes of childhood sexual abuse is attributable not only to the nature of the abuse, but to a host of other concurrent experiences, both positive and negative, to which the victim is exposed.

Although the task of examining the short-term impact of sexual abuse in the context of the family environment (taking into account the numerous factors that potentially influence outcome) is an extraordinarily difficult one, this is the essential "next step" in research on childhood abuse. The need for an integrative, developmental perspective, one that embraces not only the index child but *all* children within the family unit, has been articulated in several recent reviews.

Cole and Putnam (1992) stated, for example, that, "one major difficulty in this research is the lack of a developmentally sensitive model for conceptualizing short and long term effects and continuity and discontinuity of effects over time" (p. 174). Finkelhor and Dziuba-Leatherman (1994b) concluded in their excellent review that "the field needs a more developmental perspective on child victimization. This would start with an understanding of the mix of victimization threats that face children of different ages" (p. 182). In addition to a more sophisticated approach to investigating the complex interplay of risk factors at different developmental stages, Finkelhor and Dziuba-Leatherman (1994b) also underscored the need for "research that cuts across and integrates the various forms of child victimization" (p. 182). This latter point is especially important, since it is relatively rare that abuse is isolated to only one "form" (e.g., sexual abuse in the absence of any form of psychological or emotional abuse, physical abuse, and neglect).

When sexual abuse is an isolated incident, noninvasive (e.g., caressing or fondling), without physical violence, and perpetrated by a stranger, the child often can recover without major disruption to normal development. Quite often, however, the abuse that children suffer is protracted and is perpetrated by a member of the nuclear, extended, step or foster family. Moreover, these children often are subjected to other forms of pathology within the family, such as physical abuse, emotional or psychological abuse, domestic violence, alcohol and drug abuse, promiscuity, and inappropriate or blurred sexual boundaries, and neglect of emotional and physical needs. In these instances, the sexual abuse invariably is associated with psychiatric sequelae that are manifested in a variety of maladaptive outcomes, including many forms of self-destructive or other-destructive behavior. Although these destructive behaviors often emerge in adolescence, they begin to take a significant toll in adulthood. Indeed, it is quite clear at this point that childhood sexual abuse has the potential to cast a long shadow into adulthood, effectively undermining normal adult adaptation in a wide variety of domains.

Because the adult manifestations of childhood sexual abuse are so varied, we rarely think of them as falling under one umbrella with common roots. This heterogeneous group of maladaptive and destructive behaviors imposes an enormous burden on many facets of the system, from outpatient medical clinics, emergency rooms and hospitalization to child protective services, the police, the court system, the prison system, and public assistance–welfare services. Table 14.2 provides an overview of the unwieldy burden imposed by sexual abuse. Effective treatment of child victims of sexual abuse *can* reduce the long-term maladaptive consequences of

TABLE 14.2
Maladaptive Adult Outcomes of Sexual Abuse and Their Impact on the System

Maladaptive outcomes	System impact
Deficits in educational and vocational skills	Unstable employment Underemployment (below potential) Public assistance/welfare
Depression & suicidality	Outpatient Treatment Possible hospitalization
Severe mental illness (e.g., Borderline P.D., Dissociation/MPD, and P.T.S.D.)	Unstable employment Underemployment Dysfunctional and abusive relationships Outpatient treatment Periodic hospitalization Neglect and abuse of children leading to placement
Alcohol and drug abuse	Unstable employment Neglect and abuse of offspring (D.H.S. response) Outpatient treatment Possible hospitalization Possible criminal justice system response
Eating disorders	Outpatient treatment Possible hospitalization
Prostitution and promiscuous behavior	Medical treatment for STD's Criminal justice system response Possible imprisonment Unplanned/unwanted pregnancies Border babies (abandoned)
Revictimization (e.g., wife abuse)	Substance abuse Neglect and abuse of offspring Unstable employment Use of community shelters Use of restraining orders Emergency medical response Death
Victimization of others	Outpatient treatment Criminal justice system response Possible imprisonment Treatment of victims Continuation of the cycle of abuse

the abuse, and thus the burdens imposed on our already beleaguered medical, social service, and criminal justice systems.

Historical Background

Although it obviously is impossible to identify the earliest instances in recorded history when children were sexually exploited, there is ample evidence of such activity in Greek literature about 2,500 years ago. Pederasty (or "love of boys") was so widespread in Greece during the 4th century B.C. that "many of the outstanding men of the time" participated and the literature of the time proclaimed "this love as the highest form of wisdom" (Fisher, 1965). In early European cities, particularly Rome and Athens, marriages between boys and adult men were permitted and "rent-a-boy" sexual services were common (Schultz, 1980). Although the sexual interest was focused on boys, rather than girls, the onset of menses was considered the time when girls were marriage eligible (L. G. Schultz, 1980) and thus were available as sexual "partners."

In 1440, Baron de Rais, the Protector of Joan of Arc, was executed for the rape-murder of 800 children (Ruggiero, 1975). Apparently, the need for criminal sanctions against child sexual abuse was noted in England and one of the first of such laws was passed in 1548, protecting boys from sodomy (Radzinowicz, 1948). A second law was passed in 1576, protecting girls under the age of 10 from forcible rape. Both of these offenses carried the death penalty. A post–French Revolution wave of reform eliminated the death penalty for sexual offenses against children and liberalized most sexual activity. Although the continental European countries followed the French Napoleonic lead, England and America did not. As L. G. Schultz (1980) noted, in 18th-century England "in sex crimes against children, both victim and offender were equally guilty and both were to be punished, a condition not likely to result in complaints to the police" (p. 6).

It is well beyond the scope of this chapter to cover the long, sinuous and often grim history of child sexual abuse. Over the past two millennia, sexual activity with children has been tolerated, criminalized, and pathologized at different times, in different societies, and in different ways. Cushing (1950), in his discussion of the psychopathology of sexual delinquency, noted that the only difference between the cave man living in 8000 B.C. and Americans in 1948 is the evolution of "culture, social philosophies and religious philosophies" (p. 49). We may infer from available sources, primarily literary and historical, that sexual contact between adults and children has been an ever present part of the human experience and that its expression has been modified, shaped, and controlled over the generations, depending on prevailing social customs, governing law, and religious canons.

The current, arguably more enlightened, era of social and political sensitivity to child sexual abuse is the outgrowth of a coalescence of forces, particularly the women's movement and the children's protection movement (Finkelhor, 1984). A groundswell of support for legislative response to the problem of child sexual abuse led to the formation of a large network of private, state, and federal agencies, as well as organizations composed of clinicians and other practitioners, social activists, and researchers. Most of this response has been within the past 25 years, with the federal Child Abuse Prevention and Treatment Act of 1978, the Protection of Children Against Sexual Exploitation Act of 1977 (amended in 1990 by the Anti–Child Pornography Act), and the founding of the National Committee to Prevent Child Abuse in 1972, the International Society for Prevention of Child Abuse and Neglect in 1977, the Association for the Treatment of Sexual Abusers in 1984, and the American Professional Society on the Abuse of Children in 1987. In addition, the past several decades have witnessed a veritable explosion of clinical and empirical articles and books addressing every aspect of child sexual abuse. Extrapolating from the winds of change, it does not appear that we are likely to see major faltering or retrenching in support and resources as long as it remains politically expedient to oppose child sexual abuse.

Epidemiology

An epidemiological analysis, in the broader sense, refers to the full ecology of a disease. Recent reviews of the epidemiology of child sexual abuse, however, have focused on the frequency of occurrence (e.g., Cappelleri, Eckenrode, & Powers, 1993; Finkelhor, 1994). This section undertakes the simpler task of addressing frequency and leaves topics such as causes and control for subsequent sections.

Perhaps one of the murkiest and most debated areas of sexual violence concerns its frequency of occurrence. More than any other type of criminal conduct, a great number of sexual offenses, in their extraordinary diversity, are likely to fade into the unfathomable abyss of human experience, never to be known by the criminal justice system. The innumerable problems that plague investigators who have estimated the frequency (or incidence) of rape and child molestation have been discussed in detail elsewhere (V. L. Quinsey, 1986) and will be only briefly mentioned here. It is helpful to begin by at least defining relevant terms, particularly since they are often confused. Incidence refers to the number of behaviors of a particular type and may, at least at the present time, be more reliable than prevalence, which refers to the proportion of people who engage in the behavior. Incidence should provide a larger predictive target and be less sensitive to underreporting. Other problems include the lack of precision in the specification of the domain of criminal behaviors being estimated, sampling biases, definitional ambiguities, and the variety of sources used for data acquisition. Although these methodological problems plague incidence estimates in most areas of criminal conduct, sexual crimes seem to be especially affected. Sexual offenses, for example, are not as behaviorally "clean" as nonsexual crimes such as robbery, burglary, auto theft, or armed robbery. That is, a sexual assault often includes nonsexual offenses (e.g., kidnap, breaking and entering, robbery, simple assault) and a variety of different sexual offenses. The charges resulting from such a string of criminal acts differ from one district attorney's office to another, and the resulting conviction may be for a "lesser" offense that is nonsexual (e.g., "pleading out" to simple assault). Given all of these constraints imposed by the vagaries of the legal system, it is not surprising that incidence and prevalence estimates are remarkably "soft" (i.e., wide variations between estimates and wide ranges within estimates).

The assumption that sexual crimes against children and teenagers are drastically underreported is now accepted as a virtual truism. One of the strongest sources of evidence for this assumption comes from offenders themselves, who report vastly more victims than they have been convicted of.

Perhaps the most dramatic self-report data on victimization rates *from offenders* comes from the research of Abel and his colleagues (Abel & Rouleau, 1990; Abel *et al.,* 1987). Abel and colleagues (1987) recruited 561 subjects through a variety of different sources (e.g., health care workers, media advertising, presentations at meetings). Subjects were given a lengthy structured clinical interview covering standard demographic information and a history of deviant sexual behavior. The 561 subjects reported a total of 291,737 "paraphilic acts" committed against 195,407 victims. The five most frequently reported paraphilic acts all involved criminal conduct: (1) nonincestuous child molestation with a female victim (224 of the 561 subjects reported 5,197 acts against 4,435 victims); (2) nonincestuous child molestation with a male victim (153 of the 561 subjects reported 43,100 acts against 22,981 victims); (3) incest with a female victim (159 of the 561 subjects reported 12,927 acts against 286 victims); (4) incest with a male victim (44 of the 561 subjects reported 2,741 acts against 75 victims); and (5) rape (126 of the 561 subjects reported 907 acts against 882 victims). The remaining 16 categories included a wide range of paraphilias, which may or may not have involved coercion. The first 5 categories included a total of 64,872 acts. The total number of subjects and victims involved cannot be determined since the categories are overlapping (i.e., many subjects reported multiple paraphilias and hence were recorded in multiple categories). As Chappell (1989) pointed out, it is impossible to determine how representative these offenders are compared with all of the nonincarcerated or unidentified sex offenders in the population.

Fromuth, Burkhart, and Jones (1991) examined the "hidden child molestation" of adolescents by asking 582 college men to fill out a questionnaire. Only 3% of the sample acknowledged that they had sexually abused a child, prompting the authors to offer a host of possible reasons for this presumed underestimate. J. Briere and Runtz (1989) found that 21% of their college students reported some degree of sexual attraction to children and 7% revealed some inclination to have sex with a child if they could be assured immunity from prosecution. The 7% figure might have come very close to the 3% figure reported by Fromuth and colleagues if Briere and Runtz had asked whether the subjects had in fact molested a child. Based on data averaged from two telephone surveys, Finkelhor and Lewis (1988) estimated that 10% of the adult men admitted to sexually abusing a child.

Rather than relying on the veridicality of adults' reports of highly socially disapproved behavior, Finkelhor and Dziuba-Leatherman (1994a) conducted a national telephone survey of 2,000 children between the ages of 10 and 16. Sexual abuse involving physical contact was reported by 3.2% of the girls and 0.6% of the boys, revealing "levels of child victimization that far exceed those reported in official government victimization statistics" (Finkelhor & Dziuba-Leatherman, 1994a, p. 415). The rape rate, for example, was about five times higher than the estimate of 0.1% reported in the National Crime Survey. Finkelhor and Dziuba-Leatherman (1994b) concluded: "One reality, not widely recognized, is that children are more prone to victimization than adults are" (p. 173). One example offered is the rape rate, which is 1.60 per 1,000 for adolescents (ages 12 to 19) and 0.50 per 1,000 for adults. The overall rate for sexual abuse among children and teenagers (ages 0 to 17) in 1991 was 6.3 per 1,000, a threefold increase since 1986 when the equivalent rate was determined to be 2.1 (Finkelhor & Dziuba-Leatherman, 1994b).

Finkelhor (1994) surveyed the estimates of child sexual abuse in 21 countries, including the United States and Canada. All studies reported rates of abuse that were quite comparable to the rates in North America, ranging from 7% to 36% for women and 3% to 29% for men. In general, females are abused $1\frac{1}{2}$ to 3 times more frequently than males. Given the aforementioned methodological problems that undermine the accuracy of frequency estimates of child sexual abuse, the ranges provided in these recent studies, particularly the studies employing national probability samples, are our "best guesses" at this time.

Characteristics of the Offender

Given the manifest heterogeneity of child molesters, it is impossible to identify any single factor or even group of factors that can be said to "characterize" all such offenders. Indeed, there is probably only one dimension that may be applied to *all* child molesters: degree of sexual preoccupation with children. Although all child molesters, by definition, fall somewhere along this dimension, as a group, child molesters vary considerably even on this seemingly obvious dimension. The core distinction is the extent to which the offender is child focused. As noted, many terms (e.g., fixated, exclusive, pedophile, and preferential) have been used to identify a group of child molesters who appear to have an exclusive, or almost exclusive, sexual and social preference for children. Many child molesters, however, are *not* exclusively child focused (e.g., most incest offenders) or have lesser degrees of preoccupation with children (e.g., low fixated or nonpreferential extrafamilial offenders).

It is logical to conclude that a behavioral dimension of sexual interest in children should be accompanied by physiological arousal to children. There is indeed a very sizable literature on the discriminant and predictive validity of plethysmographically assessed sexual arousal in child molesters and various comparison groups (e.g., Abel, Becker, Murphy, & Flanagan, 1981; Avery-Clark & Laws, 1984; Barbaree & Marshall, 1988; Freund, 1967a, 1967b; Freund & Blanchard, 1989; Freund & Langevin, 1976; G. C. N. Hall, Proctor, & Nelson, 1988; Malcolm, Andrews, & Quinsey, 1993; Marshall & Christie, 1981; V. L. Quinsey & Chaplin, 1988). Although inevitably there are negative or mixed findings, the results, by and large, demonstrate the ability to discriminate between child molesters and nonmolesting comparison groups, as well as between subgroups of child molesters defined by victim gender preference (e.g., same-sex vs. opposite-sex) and by relationship to victim (e.g., incest vs. nonincest). Exclusive incest offenders, for example, evidence far less inappropriate arousal to children than extrafamilial child molesters. Thus, we can support the general hypothesis that men who prefer children as sexual companions evidence greater sexual arousal to stimuli depicting children. Evidence for the predictive validity of phallometric assessment has been, not surprisingly, more equivocal. That is, the relation between deviant sexual arousal and the likelihood of reoffending (acting on the arousal) is not linear or direct. As we see in the section "Course, Prognosis, and Recidivism," prediction of recidivism is a complex, multivariate problem and reliance on any single factor, such as inappropriate sexual arousal, is unlikely to yield optimum results.

An often cited precursor of child molestation is childhood sexual abuse. Although sexual abuse is commonly reported in the early lives of adult child molesters (Abel, 1982; Brant & Tisza, 1977; Groth, 1979; Groth, Hobson, & Gary, 1982; Hanson & Slater, 1988; Langevin, Day, Handy, & Russon, 1985; Langevin, Wright, & Handy, 1989; Marshall & Mazzucco, 1995; Seghorn, Prentky, & Boucher, 1987), as well as child and juvenile sex offenders (Becker, Kaplan, Cunningham-Rathner, & Kavoussi, 1986; Fehrenbach, Smith, Monastersky, & Deisher, 1986; Friedrich & Luecke, 1988; Johnson, 1988; Longo, 1982; Vizard, Monck, & Misch, 1995; Worling, 1995), the estimates vary enormously. Vizard and colleagues (1995) pointed out, for instance, that the reported rates of sexual abuse in the histories of young sexual offenders range from 30% to 70%. In their review of the literature, Hanson and Slater (1988) found an even wider range of reported sexual victimization among sex offenders (0% to 67%). Although a higher proportion of child molesters than rapists appear to have been sexually victimized (Seghorn *et al.*, 1987), the rates among child molesters also vary considerably. Thus, although as many as 40% to 50% of all child molesters may have been sexually abused, at least half, by definition, were not.

There has been considerable speculation about whether child molestation may be related to the offender's recapitulation of his own sexual victimization (Finkelhor *et al.*, 1986; Garland & Dougher, 1990; Kempe & Kempe, 1984; Lanyon, 1986; Rogers &

Terry, 1984). We tested the recapitulation theory on a sample of 131 rapists and child molesters, hypothesizing that the earlier and the more serious or protracted the sexual abuse, the more likely the sexual victimization of others (Prentky & Knight, 1993). We found no evidence of recapitulation of sexual abuse among the rapists (i.e., there were no differences among our three groups of rapists, classified by the age at which they first committed a sexual assault, on the age of onset of their own sexual abuse or the nature of the sexual abuse). We did find support for this notion among child molesters. Those child molesters who committed their first assault when they were 14 or younger had been sexually victimized at a younger age than those offenders who committed their first assault in adulthood. Similarly, that same group of offenders who committed their first sexual assault early also had experienced more severe sexual abuse than the offenders with an adult onset of sexual aggression. We should hasten to emphasize, however, that *all* men in our study went on to commit sexual offenses, irrespective of whether they were sexually abused and, if they were, their age at first incident.

Taken alone, sexual victimization is an overly parsimonious explanation of child molestation. Most victims of childhood sexual abuse do *not*, as Finkelhor (1984) pointed out, become perpetrators of sexual abuse. We must conclude that childhood sexual abuse, like other forms of abuse, becomes critical in the presence of a variety of other factors (Kaufman & Zigler, 1987), such as the age of onset, the duration of abuse, the child's relationship to the perpetrator, the invasiveness, and/or violence, in the abuse, the co-occurrence of other types of abuse, the availability of supportive caregivers, the ego strength of the child at the time of the abuse, and treatment. All of these variables may be moderators of outcome. The complexity of the role of sexual abuse in the lives of child molesters illustrates the multiplicity of etiologic paths that lead to different types of outcomes.

Another commonly reported characteristic of child molesters, social skills deficits, appears in many guises. Although there seems to be an implicit assumption that child molesters are, by definition, socially deficient, and a variety of studies have documented the deficient social and interpersonal skills, underassertiveness, and poor self-esteem of child molesters (Araji & Finkelhor, 1985; Finkelhor & Araji, 1986; Glueck, 1956; Marshall & Mazzucco, 1995; Marshall, Christie, & Lanthier, 1979; Marshall, Barbaree, & Fernandez, 1995; Quinsey 1977; Segal & Marshall, 1985, 1986; Whitman & Quinsey, 1981), there seems to be an equally accepted corollary that these offenders are highly variable with respect to social skills.

Marshall and colleagues (1995) compared 36 nonfamilial child molesters with college students and nonstudent male volunteers on self-reported social confidence, social anxiety, and assertiveness. The child molesters did not differ from the matched community control group. Both groups reported more social anxiety, lower self-esteem, and less assertiveness than the college students. The importance of this study is not that it provides further evidence for the social and self-esteem deficits of child molesters, but that these deficits were equally observed among the matched nonoffending controls. Thus, low social competence does not, in and of itself, forecast an outcome of child molestation.

Social competence deficits, nevertheless, are pervasive among child molesters and must be considered to be of etiologic importance. Pithers, Beal, Armstrong, and Petty (1989) reported, for example, that low self-esteem was an immediate precursor to offending in 61% of their child molesters. As with the role of sexual abuse, we must conclude that these deficits, in their remarkable diversity and variability among child molesters, occupy an important, though not exclusive, link in the chain of contributory events.

The last characteristic that should be mentioned is impulsive, antisocial personality. As noted in the section "Assessment," many typologies have described an impulsive, exploitative type of child molester whose sexual offenses are part of an extensive criminal history and antisocial lifestyle. Recent empirical studies support the predictive utility of antisocial behavior (e.g., Prentky, Knight, & Lee, 1996; V. L. Quinsey, Rice, & Harris, 1995). V. L. Quinsey and colleagues (1995) reported that psychopathy ratings were one of three factors that predicted sexual recidivism in their mixed sample of 178 sex offenders (124 of whom were child molesters). Prentky, Knight, and Lee (1997) reported that antisocial behavior predicted nonsexual, victim-involved recidivism *and* violent recidivism (any battery offense classified as very high in physical injury to the victim) in their sample of 111 child molesters. Prentky and Knight (1993) had previously reported on age of onset of sexual assault among 53 child molesters, finding that those offenders who committed their first offense in childhood or adolescence evidenced more disruptiveness in school (verbal or physical assaults on peers and teachers), were higher in juvenile antisocial behavior, and, as adults, manifested a higher degree of nonsexual aggression.

Family Patterns

Although there has been relatively little empirical research on familial antecedents of child molestation, there have been many reports on familial abuse, particularly sexual abuse. Recently, recognition of the multidetermined nature of child molestation has led clinicians and investigators to examine the antecedent and concurrent experiences that place sexual abuse in a developmental context and provide a much richer developmental picture. Borrowing from the language of forensic science, there are innumerable aggravating and mitigating factors that determine the impact of sexual abuse, as well as all other forms of child trauma.

The most interesting and promising developments have come from the literature on attachment. Alexander (1992, 1993) proposed the use of attachment theory to help understand the family antecedents and distal effects of sexual abuse, and B. James (1994) eloquently documented the role of abuse-related trauma in undermining the development of healthy attachments in children. Attachment theory has been adopted, moreover, as the centerpiece of an etiologic model of sexual aggression (Marshall, 1989; Marshall, Hudson, & Hodkinson, 1993; Ward, Hudson, Marshall, & Siegert, 1995). This important theoretical contribution proposes a number of aberrant attachment styles, deriving from the work of Bartholomew and Horowitz (1991), that characterize different child molesters. Each maladaptive attachment style emerges from a hypothesized pattern of early life experiences, is associated with presumptive interpersonal deficits, and leads to a different pattern of sexually deviant behavior. The anxious-ambivalent style, for example, is characterized by a desire for intimacy that is undermined by anxiety in adult relationships. When the anxiety becomes too crippling to develop and sustain relationships with adults, the individual turns to children to gratify needs for emotional intimacy. As noted, each of these attachment styles is presumed to be a developmental byproduct, a "proximal effect," of, as Ward,

Hudson, Marshall, and Siegert (1995) noted, problematic parent-child relationships. Ward, Hudson, Marshall, and Siegert speculated, for instance, that the child molester with an anxious-ambivalent style experienced marked inconsistency in parental affection. Thus, specifiable early childhood experiences lead to interpersonal deficits and low self-esteem that severely undermine the development of secure adult attachments (Bumby & Marshall, 1994; Marshall & Mazzucco, 1995).

We found, in early studies on the developmental antecedents of sexual aggression, that a dimension of "caregiver inconstancy" was a powerful predictor of subsequent sexual violence (Cerce, Day, Prentky, & Knight, 1984; Prentky, Knight, Sims-Knight, et al., 1989). Caregiver inconstancy, which measured the frequency of changes in primary caregivers and the longest time spent with any single caregiver, reflected the permanence and consistency of the child's interpersonal relationships with significant adults. Prentky, Knight, Sims-Knight and colleagues (1989) noted: "Whereas stable contact with a caregiver over a long duration provides the opportunity for the establishment of secure relationships with adults, frequent changes in caregivers would most likely disrupt such relationships. The fact that repeated interruptions in relationships with caregivers, independent of other factors such as abuse and nonintactness, predicted greater sexual violence, suggests that early caregiver relationships may be important in modulating aggression in potentially intimate relationships" (p. 164). In a subsequent study, caregiver inconstancy was treated as both a dependent and independent variable (Prentky, Holland, & Lee, 1996). The most powerful predictor of caregiver inconstancy was maternal violence, accounting for 36% of the variance. This finding seems to be consistent with Marshall and Mazzucco (1995), who reported that maternal rejection was the best predictor of low self-esteem in their child molesters. In the study by Prentky and colleagues (1996), sexual abuse was *unrelated* to caregiver inconstancy, accounting for only 2% of the variance. Caregiver inconstancy was then treated as an independent variable in an attempt to predict the proximal effects of such instability. Six proximal outcome variables were significantly related to caregiver inconstancy: health, depression, anxiety, school problems, aggression, and juvenile antisocial behavior.

Other studies have supported and elaborated on the potential importance of early childhood attachments. Kobayashi, Sales, Becker, Figueredo, and Kaplan (1995) found in their study of 117 juvenile sex offenders that the child's bonding to his mother decreased the level of sexual aggression. In a review of the relevant attachment literature, Marshall, Hudson, and Hodkinson (1993) examined the role of mal-attachment (insecurity, rejection, lack of warmth, inconsistency, disruptions in continuity, abuse) on the development of an avoidant or anxious-ambivalent interpersonal style. Marshall and colleagues (1993) observed that sex offenders "seem to have experienced a disproportionate degree of problems or disruptions in the development of appropriate attachment bonds with their parents," (pp. 173–174). Marshall and colleagues (1993) proposed an integrative, developmental theory in which failure to develop secure attachments in infancy and childhood impairs one's ability to form and sustain intimate relationships. Such an individual is fearful of intimacy and lacks the skills and self-confidence necessary to establish and maintain close relationships. Thus, childhood trauma disrupts or prevents the development of normal attachments, leading to an incapacity for intimacy and emotional loneliness (see B. James, 1994). Seidman, Marshall, Hudson, and Robertson (1994) found, in fact, that sex offenders had acute deficits in their capacity for intimacy. We may thus hypothesize that chronic failure to gratify social, sexual, and affiliative needs may result in, depending on the interpersonal style of the offender, a passive refocusing onto less intimidating sources of gratification (i.e., children) or an aggressive exploitation of children that satisfies sexual needs and discharges anger. It would be reasonable to hypothesize, moreover, that the age range of the children that an offender seeks reflects the severity of the deficits that obviate the establishment of adult relationships (i.e., those who seek 6–8-year-old children have more severe deficits than those who seek 13–15-year-old adolescents).

Assessment and Diagnosis

One of the few indisputable conclusions about child molesters is that they constitute a markedly heterogeneous group (Knight, Rosenberg, & Schneider, 1985). Their childhood and developmental experiences, adult competencies, and criminal histories differ considerably. Moreover, the motives that underlie their sexual abuse of children and the patterns of behavior that characterize their offenses differ considerably. Therefore, it is virtually impossible to make informed decisions about these offenders without some understanding of the hypothetically important dimensions that discriminate among them.

The fundamental purpose of diagnosing an offender is to reduce this heterogeneity by assigning the offender to a class or group of individuals with similar relevant characteristics. Identifying and measuring these relevant characteristics is the task of assessment. Proper diagnosis or classification can be of enormous assistance in improving decision making with sex offenders, particularly child molesters. A reliable, valid classification system can improve accuracy of decisions: (a) in the criminal justice system, where decisions about dangerousness and reoffense risk are routinely made and influence discretionary allocation of resources, (b) in the clinical setting, where the development of treatment plans can be optimized by a more informed understanding of what is most effective with that class of offenders, and (c) in designing more effective primary prevention strategies. In addition, a classification model may also be helpful in deciphering the critical antecedent factors that lead to different types of outcome (i.e., different "types" of child molesters). In this section, I briefly examine some of the attempts to classify child molesters.

The Utility of the DSM

The *Diagnostic and Statistical Manual of Mental Disorders* of the American Psychiatric Association (1952, 1968, 1980, 1987, 1994) has consistently included a category for pedophilia. In the original *DSM*, published in 1952, pedophilia was included under Sexual Deviation. Sexual Deviation was one of four Sociopathic Personality Disturbances (along with Antisocial Reaction, Dyssocial Reaction, and Addiction) included within the broader category of Personality Disorders. In this version of the *DSM*, an assignment to the category of Sexual Deviation was guided by the following statement: "This diagnosis is reserved for deviant sexuality which is not symptomatic of more extensive syndromes, such as schizophrenic and obsessional reactions. The term includes most of the cases formerly classified as 'psychopathic personality with pathologic sexuality.' The diagnosis will specify the type of the pathologic behavior, such as homosexuality, transvestism, pedophilia, fetishism and sexual sadism (including rape, sexual assault, mutilation)" (pp. 38–39). No specific criteria for classifying pedophilia, or any of the other Sexual Deviations, were provided.

In the second version of *DSM*, published in 1968, pedophilia was again included under Sexual Deviation and again no classification criteria were provided. In the *DSM-III*, published in 1980, pedophilia was classified under Psychosexual Disorders. The age of onset was identified as "frequently middle age" and the course was stated to be "unknown." Two criteria were provided: (1) the act or fantasy of engaging in sexual activity with prepubertal (age not specified) children is a repeatedly preferred or exclusive method of achieving sexual excitement and (2) if the subject is an adult, the victim is at least 10 years younger; if the subject is a late adolescent, no age difference is required.

The revision of the third edition of the *DSM* (*DSM-III-R*), published in 1987, reflected the first attempt to provide operational criteria that were consistent with current thinking. Pedophilia was included under Sexual Disorders. The age of onset was revised to "usually begins in adolescence" and the course was now identified as "usually chronic." The *DSM-III-R* provided more specific, behavioral criteria for pedophilia, including (1) recurrent intense sexual urges or fantasies involving sexual activity with a prepubescent child (generally age 13 or younger) for at least 6 months, (2) the subject has acted on these urges *or* is markedly distressed by them, (3) the subject is at least 16 years old and at least 5 years older than the victim, (4) late adolescent subjects who are involved in ongoing relationships with 12- or 13-year-olds are *excluded*. The *DSM-III-R* also required that the clinician specify (1) whether the client's victims were all males, all females, or both, (2) whether the offenses were limited to incest, and (3) whether the client is an "exclusive type" (i.e., attracted only to children) or a nonexclusive type.

The *DSM-IV*, published in 1994, included pedophilia under Sexual and Gender Identity Disorders. The age of onset, course and criteria were the same as in the *DSM-III-R*. The only technical difference is that the first criterion in the *DSM-IV* added the word "behaviors" to urges and fantasies.

Although the *DSM-III-R* and *DSM-IV* provide greater specificity and clarity when it comes to classifying someone as a "pedophile," the clinician who uses the *DSM* is still left with a single categorical diagnosis for all those who engage in sexual activity with children. From a taxonomic standpoint, the critical question is whether the classification system does an adequate job of capturing as many individuals as possible (i.e., "coverage") and sorting them accurately into theoretically meaningful groups. If the intent is to classify the larger world of child molesters, the *DSM* fails to provide adequate coverage. One may reasonably argue, of course, that the intent of the *DSM* was not to classify all child molesters but rather to define and capture a subset of individuals with a distinct paraphilic attraction to children. The *DSM-III-R* and *DSM-IV* certainly accomplish that narrow goal more effectively than any preceding version of the *DSM*. In general, however, the *DSM* is not a useful taxonomic system for classifying child molesters.

Unidimensional Classification: Sex of Victim

One of the earliest classificatory variables to receive empirical scrutiny was the proposed subdivision of child molesters on the basis of the sex of their victims (Fitch,

1962; Gebhard, Gagnon, Pomeroy, & Christenson, 1965; Mohr, Turner, & Jerry, 1964). Trichotomization of child molesters into same-sex, opposite-sex, and mixed groups has been shown to have some cross-temporal stability (Fitch, 1962; Langevin, Hucker, *et al.*, 1985) and predictive validity (Fitch, 1962; Frisbie, 1969; Frisbie & Dondis, 1965; Radzinowicz, 1957). In addition, sexual preference among child molesters appears to have some concurrent validity. It has been shown to covary in a systematic way with penile plethysmographic responsiveness to stimuli depicting specific ages and sexes (e.g., Freund, 1965, 1967a, 1967b; Laws & Osborn, 1983, V. L. Quinsey & Chaplin, 1988).

The most frequent use of sex of victim has been in the area of recidivism. Early reports suggested that reoffense rates among same-sex child molesters were higher than rates for opposite-sex child molesters (e.g., Fitch, 1962; Frisbie & Dondis, 1965; Radzinowicz, 1957). More recent support came from a study by Hanson, Steffy, and Gauthier (1993), who found that offenders against boys were at higher risk for recidivism than offenders against girls, and the mixed group was nonsignificantly different from the other two groups.

The sex of victim distinction has not, however, received consistent support. Langevin, Hucker, and colleagues (1985), for example, found that the same-sex offenders evidenced the fewest number of criminal charges (8%, compared with 22% for the opposite-sex group), and Abel and colleagues (1981) found that their opposite-sex child molesters reported more than twice as many victims as their same-sex child molesters (62.4% and 30.6%, respectively). Abel, Mittelman, Becker, Rathner, and Rouleau (1988) subsequently reported that mixed-sex preference "was exceedingly effective on its own at predicting recidivism" (p. 230), correctly classifying 83.7% of their subjects.

Marques (1995) reported sex of victim differences in reoffense rates among 110 treated child molesters. The opposite-sex child molesters had a slightly higher rate of recidivism than the same-sex child molesters (13.9% and 12.1%, respectively). The treated mixed-sex group of offenders had the highest reoffense rate (16.7%), a finding that would support Abel and colleagues (1988). Among volunteer controls, Marques found that the same-sex offenders had a 5.5% higher recidivism rate than the opposite-sex offenders (13.9% and 8.4%, respectively).

In another recent study, we found no evidence for the utility of sex of victim as a predictor of reoffense (Prentky, Knight, & Lee, 1997). We examined recidivism data on 111 child molesters who had been discharged from the Massachusetts Treatment Center over a 25-year period. The sexual recidivism rates for opposite-sex, mixed-sex, and same-sex offenders were .33, .35, and .38, respectively. In a series of discriminant function analyses, using different domains of criminal behavior as the criterion, the univariate F values for victim sex in all three analyses were < 0.50, and the correlations between victim sex and the criterion were .07 (opposite), .12 (mixed), and −.03 (same).

Although the reasons for these inconsistent findings remain unclear, there are two obvious potential sources of methodological variability. The first problem concerns the adequacy with which sexual preference has been operationally defined. The most frequent definition has focused on the sex of victims in reported crimes (V. Quinsey, 1977). The large number of unreported sexual assaults on children (Abel, 1982; Finkelhor, 1984), possible biases against reporting homosexual encounters, situational factors that might lead to assaults on the less preferred sex, and incarceration after a single assault might all contribute to unreliability in the assignment of offenders to victim-sex categories.

The second problem involves confounding variables that may artifactually contribute to victim-sex subtype differences. Many studies, for example, have not distinguished between incest and nonincest offenders. Incest cases differ from nonincest cases in several important ways. Most important, incest offenders are almost exclusively heterosexual in their choice of victims (Dixon, Arnold, & Calestro, 1978; Langsley, Schwartz & Fairbairn, 1968). Assuming that "true" (i.e., exclusive) incest offenders constitute a clinically and theoretically meaningful group of child offenders, the proportion of such cases in any particular sample might artifactually effect the differences between same- and opposite-sex offenders.

Clinically Derived Multidimensional Systems

Table 14.3 presents most of the prominent classification systems for child molesters in the extant literature and the subtypes that comprise those systems, partitioning by subtype comparability. That is, all of the subtypes in the first row (Common Type 1) are roughly comparable. The same is true for each of the successive rows. Although the most recent version of the classification system for child molesters developed at the Massachusetts Treatment Center (MTC:CM3) is included in Table 14.3, identifying comparable types in extant systems is complicated by the fact that MTC:CM3 includes two independent axes and Axis I separates social competence and intensity of pedophilic interest (i.e., fixation). Although space does not permit discussion of these historical systems, they are discussed in detail elsewhere (R. Knight *et al.*, 1985).

As one may note from Table 14.3, there are three subtypes that appear in most prior systems. Every child molester classification system has included a subtype with an exclusive and long-standing sexual and social preference for children (Common Type 1) and most systems have contrasted this type with a second whose offenses were seen as a shift or a "regression" from a higher, adult level of psychosexual adaptation, typically in response to stress (Common Type 2). Most systems have also posited a third type comprising psychopaths or sociopaths with very poor social skills who turned to children largely because they are easy to exploit, not because they are preferred or even desired partners (Common Type 3).

Fixation–Regression and Social Competence

Although the three aforementioned subtypes certainly possess clinical salience, it is only recently that these subtypes have been the subject of empirical scrutiny. The most important of these hypothetical subtypes are the "fixated" and the "regressed." As noted, these two types have had counterparts in virtually every classification system. The primary intent of this distinction is to differentiate offenders with longstanding, exclusive preferences for children as sexual and social companions from child molesters whose offenses are seen as a departure under stress from a more age-appropriate social and psychosexual adaptation. These two types, therefore, appear to present clinically meaningful and distinct profiles.

Despite this legacy, the validity of the fixation–regression dichotomy is questionable (Conte, 1985). Conte pointed out that this dichotomy evolved solely out of clinical experience, had never been subjected to any form of empirical validation, and that the two groups were not, in fact, homogeneous. Finkelhor and Araji (Araji & Finkelhor, 1985; Finkelhor & Araji, 1986) raised an important theoretical problem. In their four-factor model, they distinguished between "emotional congruence" (which

TABLE 14.3

Comparable Types on Child Molester Classification Systems

Fitch (1962)	Kopp (1962)	Gebhard et al. (1965)	McCaghy (1967)	Swanson (1971)	Groth (1981)	Dietz (1983) Lanning (1986)	Knight et al. (1989) [MTC:CM3]
				Common Type 1			
Immature	Type	Socio-sexually underdeveloped	High interaction molester	Classic pedophiliac	Molestation fixated	Preferential: seduction or Preferential: introverted	Axis I: Fixated/low social competence [#0] and Axis II: Interpersonal [#1] or Narcissistic [#2]
				Common Type 2			
Frustrated	Type II	Situational		Situational Violator	Molestation regressed	Situational: regressed	Axis I: Low fixated/hi social competence [#3] and Axis II: Interpersonal [#1] or Narcissistic [#2] or Exploitative [#3]
				Common Type 3			
Sociopathic		Amoral delinquent	Asocial molester	Inadequate sociopathic violator	Rape: power	Situational: morally indiscriminate	Axis I: any type Axis II: Exploitative [#3] or Muted Sadistic [#4]

Types Characterized by Expressive Aggression

Spontaneous/aggressive[a]	Rape: anger type Rape: sadistic type	Preferential: sadistic type	Axis I: Low social competence types [0 & 2] Axis II: Aggressive [#5] Sadistic [#6]

Types Characterized by Psychosis, Mental Defect or Organicity

Pathological	Mentally defective Senile deteriorate Psychotic	Incestuous molester Senile molester	Brain damaged

Additional Unrelated Types

Miscel-laneous	Drunken	Career molester[a]	Situational: sexually indiscriminate Situational: inadequate

[a]Comparability for these types is unclear

involves arrested development and low self-esteem) and "blockage" (which involves fear of adult females, poor social skills, and marital disturbance). Finkelhor and Araji's conceptual and theoretical contribution suggested that social and interpersonal competence may have to be considered independently of fixation. Implicit or explicit in the various systems that have described fixated and regressed types is an assessment of achieved level of social competence. Fixated offenders have typically been differentiated from regressed offenders by marital status, number and quality of age-appropriate heterosexual relationships, acquired level of education, and achieved skill level. The fixated child molester is hypothesized to have a negligible history of dating or peer interaction in adolescence or adulthood and, if married, the quality of his relationship is considered to be poor. Regressed offenders, on the other hand, are more likely to have been married and to have developed age-appropriate heterosexual relationships prior to their "regressive" sexual offense or offenses. Thus, the construct of social competence is clearly evident in this distinction.

Our own work on the development of taxonomic models for child molesters (see R. A. Knight, 1992; R. A. Knight & Prentky, 1990) clearly pointed to the need for a reconceptualization of the fixation–regression dichotomy. The fixation and regression groups in our second generation model (MTC:CM2) had unacceptably low interrater reliabilities and some of the subgroups (e.g., the Exploitative-Fixated type) were clearly *not* homogeneous (R. A. Knight & Prentky, 1990). In addition, there were those offenders that fell between the two groups (e.g., that were fixated but had high social competence). In our most recent model (MTC:CM3), intensity of pedophilic interest (i.e., fixation) and social competence were partitioned into two independent factors. The unconfounding of these two dimensions improved reliability substantially (R. A. Knight, Carter, & Prentky, 1989). In addition, the two dimensions were completely independent (Knight, 1989) and each evidenced distinct developmental antecedents and adult adaptations (Prentky, Knight, Rosenberg, & Lee, 1989).

Development of MTC:CM3

The classification system reported by Cohen and Seghorn (Cohen, Seghorn, & Calmas, 1969; Cohen, Boucher, Seghorn, & Mehegan, 1979) served as the point of departure for our programmatic efforts to develop taxonomic models for the classification of child molesters (see R. A. Knight, 1992; R. A. Knight & Prentky, 1990). In this first model (MTC:CM1), Cohen and Seghorn described four types of child molesters: (1) the Pedophile-Fixated type, (2) the Pedophile-Regressed type, (3) Pedophile-Aggressive type, and (4) the Exploitative type. An attempt to operationalize these four types and assign them to cases resulted in poor reliability, and led to the first major revision of the model (MCT:CM2). The revised model was applied to a sample of 68 child molesters and a series of interrater discrepancy analyses, cluster analyses, and target analyses on specific questions (R. A. Knight, 1988, 1992) resulted in three major structural changes in the model: (1) the concept of regression was dropped and a newly defined fixation dimension (operationalized as intensity of pedophilic interest) was crossed with a dimension of social competence, yielding four independent types, (2) a new behavioral dimension (Amount of Contact with Children) became the prepotent discriminator on a separate axis, and (3) the degree of violence was differentiated into physical injury (high-low) and sadism (present-absent) dimensions (R. A. Knight, Carter, & Prentky, 1989). This model is depicted in Figure 14.1.

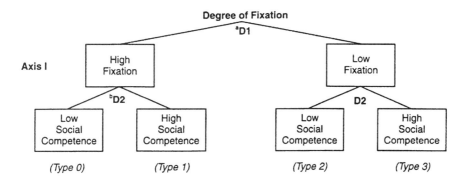

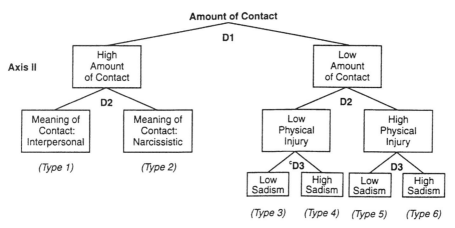

ᵃ**D1** Decision 1
ᵇ**D2** Decision 2
ᶜ**D3** Decision 3

FIGURE 14.1 Flow design of the decision process forclassifying child molesters on Axis I and Axis II of MTC: CM3

The following profiles include hypothetical characteristics of the six Axis II subtypes:

1. *Type 1: Interpersonal*
   - high contact with children
   - nongenital, nonorgasmic sexual acts (e.g., fondling, caressing, frottage)
   - offender knew victim prior to sexual assault
   - offender often has long-term relationship or multiple contacts with the same victim
   - offenses reflect a high degree of planning
2. *Type 2: Narcissistic*
   - high contact with children
   - primary motive is sexual gratification; interests are self-centered
   - phallic sexual acts (i.e., primary aim is achieving orgasm; victim is used as a masturbatory object

TABLE 14.4
Hypothetical Profiles of MTC: CM3 Axis II Types

Characteristic	Interpersonal (Type 1)	Narcissistic (Type 2)	Muted Exploitative (Type 3)	Nonsadistic sadistic (Type 4)	Aggressive (Type 5)	Sadistic (Type6)
Amount of contact with children	High	High	Low	Low	Low	Low
Sexual acts	Nongenital Foundling, caressing Frottage	—	—	Sodomy "Sham" sadism[a]	-	Sadism
Relationship of offender to victim	Known	Stranger	Stranger	—	Stranger	Stranger
Amount of physical injury to victim	Low	Instrumental[b]	Instrumental	Instrumental	High	High
Amount of planning in offenses	High	Low	Low	Moderate	Low	High

— implies no hypothesized characteristic; Types 2, 3, and 5, for example, may evidence any sexual acts
[a]Sham sadism implies behaviors or reported fantasies that reflect sadism without the high victim injury present in Type 6
[b]Instrumental aggression implies only enough force to gain victim compliance

- victims are typically strangers
- offenses are usually single encounters with each victim
- offenders tend to be promiscuous (i.e., with many victims)
- offenders are likely to be spontaneous with little planning

3. *Type 3: Exploitative*
   - low contact with children
   - relatively little physical injury to victims (i.e., only enough aggression to gain victim compliance)
   - there is no evidence that the aggression is eroticized
   - sexual acts are likely to be phallic
   - victims are typically strangers
   - offenses will have very little evidence of planning

4. *Type 4: Muted Sadistic*
   - low contact with children
   - relatively little physical injury to victims
   - evidence that aggression was eroticized (e.g., sexual acts included bondage, spanking, urination, use of feces, bizarre, peculiar or ritualized acts; insertion of nondamaging foreign objects; or offender reports presence of sadistic fantasies)
   - victims are typically strangers
   - offenses reflect a moderate degree of planning

5. *Type 5: Aggressive*
   - low contact with children
   - high degree of physical injury to victims (injury may be accidental, resulting from offender's climsiness or ineptitude, or from aggression rooted in anger at the victim
   - there is no evidence that the aggression is eroticized
   - sexual acts are likely to be phallic
   - victims are typically strangers
   - offenses will have very little evidence of planning
6. *Type 6: Overt Sadistic*
   - low contact with children
   - high degree of physical injury to victims
   - offender is highly aroused or derives pleasure from putting victim in fear or subjecting victim to pain
   - presence of violence appears to increase sexual arousal
   - presence of bizarre, ritualized, or peculiar sexual acts
   - victims are typically strangers
   - offenses reflect a high degree of planning

Although further revision of this model, including the integration of the two axes, is necessary, the validity studies accomplished thus far (R. A. Knight, 1988, 1989, 1992; Prentky *et al.*, 1989; Prentky, Knight, & Lee, 1997) clearly support the primary structural changes in MTC:CM3. As may be apparent, MTC:CM3 was not designed to include exclusive incest offenders. Including such offenders in this system will require considerable reconceptualization and revision.

Course, Prognosis, and Recidivism

Course typically refers to the progression of symptoms associated with a disease, and prognosis is a forecast of the probable course and the likelihood of recovery. It is difficult to offer guidelines as to course and prognosis with child molesters. The course varies, in some cases significantly, among child molesters, with onset ranging from early adolescence to middle adulthood (as in the case of some exclusive incest offenders). Prognosis too may vary markedly, from cases of lifelong, intractable pedophilic interest that is refractory to treatment, to isolated instances of incest in adults with a sexual preference for peers, ample remorse and victim empathy, and a high likelihood of complete recovery. In summary, the best that we can say is that course and prognosis are highly variable among child molesters as a group.

In one of the largest recidivism studies with sex offenders, Christiansen, Elers-Nielsen, Le Maire, and Strup (1965) followed up a heterogeneous sample of 2,934 rapists, child molesters, and exhibitionists for a period ranging from 12 to 24 years. Of the entire sample, 714 offenders (24.3%) received a sentence for some type of reoffense. Less than half (43.4%) of the 714 recidivists were sentenced for a sexual offense (10.6% of the entire sample). The highest subgroup reoffense rate was for exhibitionists, followed by rapists, opposite-sex child molesters, and same-sex child molesters.

Soothill, Jack, and Gibbens (1976) reported on a 22-year follow-up of 119 offenders who had been charged with some form of sexual offense in 1951. Of the 119 men,

95 had been charged with rape or attempted rape, and of this group, 86 were convicted. Of that cohort of 86 convicted offenders, 13 were reconvicted of some type of sexual offense. Soothill and Gibbens (1978) appears to have been the first study of its kind to adopt "life-table methodology." Using their life table, Soothill and Gibbens recalculated recidivism rates at the end of the observation period, noting an increase from 18.4% to 23% for sexual offenses, and an increase from 38.5% to 48% for any reconviction by the end of the study period.

Romero and Williams (1985) divided 231 sex offenders into three groups (21% exhibitionists, 17% child molesters with victims ages 10 or younger, and 62% sexual assaulters with female victims ages 13 or older). Their 10-year follow-up revealed an 11.3% rearrest rate for a sexual offense. Of that group, the sexual recidivism rate for pedophiles was 6.2%. G. C. N. Hall and Proctor (1987) studied a sample of 342 nonpsychotic sex offenders who had been committed to a state hospital. Most of the sex offenders in their sample (about 85%) were child molesters. Of the 342 subjects, 139 were rearrested, 90 (26.3%) for a sexual offense. Of that group, 67 (19.6% of original sample) committed a sexual offense against a child.

Rice, Quinsey, and Harris (1991) followed up 136 extrafamilial child molesters for an average period of 6.3 years. About one third of the sample (50 men) received behavior therapy. Of the entire sample, 31% were convicted of a new sexual offense and 43% were convicted of a new violent or sexual offense. Therapy did not affect recidivism. Hanson and colleagues (1993) followed up 197 child molesters for a period ranging from 15 to 31 years. This sample included 125 men who participated in a nonbehavioral treatment program. Of that group, 82 (42%) were reconvicted for a new sexual offense, violent offense, or both during the study period. There were no differences in recidivism between the treated and nontreated offenders. A subsequent study by Hanson, Scott, and Steffy (1995) compared 191 child molesters with 137 nonsexual offenders. Hanson and colleagues (1995) reported that 83.2% of the nonsexual offenders and 61.8% of the child molesters were reconvicted of any offense during the study period (same as Hanson *et al.*, 1993). The sexual recidivism rate was 35.1% for the child molesters and 1.5% for the nonsexual offenders.

We completed a 25-year follow-up of 251 sex offenders (115 child molesters and 136 rapists) discharged from the Massachusetts Treatment Center (Prentky, Lee, Knight & Cerce, 1997). As in the Hanson and colleagues (1993) study, these men participated in a nonbehavioral treatment program. By the end of the study period, 52% of the child molesters had been charged with a new sexual offense and 42% had been convicted.

The following treatment studies examined what would generally be regarded as state-of-the-art programs. Marques, Day, Nelson, and West (1993) reported on an outcome study of treated sex offenders in California. By the end of 1991, 95 sex offenders (19 rapists and 76 child molesters) completed treatment and had been discharged. Of that group, 4.6% were arrested for a new sexual offense during the follow-up (average 34 months). Pithers and Cumming (1989) reported a 3% sexual recidivism rate during a 6-year follow-up period for 147 pedophiles that had been treated in their Vermont program. Maletzky (1987) completed a 14-year follow-up of 2,232 pedophiles treated at his Oregon clinic. Of that group, 12.7% of the opposite-sex pedophiles and 13.6% of the same-sex pedophiles committed a new sex offense. Marshall and Barbaree (1988) followed up 126 child molesters who were treated at their Sexual Behavior Clinic in Kingston, Ontario, Canada. The length of follow-up ranged from 12 months to 117 months. Of that group, 17.9% of the opposite-sex pedophiles, 13.3% of the same-sex pedophiles, and 8% of the incest offenders committed a new sex offense. In their matched sample of untreated child molesters, 42.9% reoffended.

As may be apparent, recidivism rates are highly variable, making it impossible to draw any reliable conclusions about recidivism among child molesters as a group. Most recent recidivism studies have been done in the context of evaluating treatment efficacy. Consequently, we know relatively little about recidivism independent of some treatment intervention. Moreover, variations in recidivism rates associated with different treatment programs are very difficult to interpret. Differences in recidivism rates across studies are confounded with legal jurisdiction, duration of exposure time (i.e., time in the community), characteristics of the offender, differential attrition rates, differences in program integrity and amount of treatment, amount and quality of posttreatment supervision, and a host of other variables. In addition, recidivism measures tend to be subject to error and to result in comparisons of low statistical power. Even without attempting to attribute variations in recidivism to treatment program characteristics, the variation in recidivism rates in the published literature is truly remarkable.

Clinical Management

Since the primary purpose of offender treatment is to decrease victimization rates, thereby increasing community safety, it has become clear that an indispensable part of any rehabilitation program is community-based maintenance. Pithers (1990) developed the External Supervisory Dimension of the relapse prevention model specifically to increase community safety. This supervisory dimension includes a network of informed "collateral contacts" or monitors (e.g., spouse or girlfriend, family members, employer, coworkers, friends) along with probation or parole officers. All such individuals are trained to observe and detect high-risk situations, offense precursors, and lapses. Marques and colleagues (1993) included an aftercare component in their treatment model to achieve the same end. The aftercare phase of treatment requires, as a condition of parole, that all men attend two sessions a week for the first year after release. These sessions were intended to be "boosters" (i.e., to refresh and enhance relapse prevention techniques).

We have offered a number of recommendations for instituting a potentially effective, community-based maintenance program for child molesters (Prentky, 1996). First, the program should be coordinated by highly trained and well-supervised parole agents and probation officers who carry small caseloads. Caseloads should not exceed about 15 offenders to ensure intensive surveillance and supervision. Offenders should be mandated for treatment by therapists who are trained and supervised in cognitive-behavior therapy with sex offenders. Effective treatment in the community is particularly critical for adjustment and maintenance. Treatment should, however, be considered only one aspect of an overall maintenance program for the offender. The second component of maintenance must be the proper monitoring and supervision around vocational, social, recreational, and leisure activities. Finally, the third component of maintenance is the confidential notification of local police departments and the district attorney's office. Registration with the criminal justice system provides an important part of the triad of community maintenance for sex offenders. Registration helps to keep the "price of failure" in conscious awareness. Registration *alone*, however, is unlikely to deter most sex offenders who have reached a point where they are at high risk to reoffend. Once they have entered their offense cycle, they have started down a slippery slope toward reoffense and the mere awareness that they are registered is unlikely to interrupt the cycle.

The essential principle in management of many child molesters, certainly most extrafamilial child molesters, is continuity of care. As Pithers, Kashima, Cumming, Beal, and Buell (1988) concluded, "No final therapy session is conducted under the RP [relapse prevention] model. RP is not an activity that a sex offender completes. Offenders who believe that their treatment ends with the termination of formal therapy have failed to learn the crucial lesson that maintenance is forever" (p. 258). Since the vast majority of child molesters eventually return to the community, the clinical management of these offenders must extend beyond incarceration or inpatient care and into the community. Commmunity-based clinical management must be supportive, vigilant, and informed by current wisdom about maximally effective strategies for maintaining child molesters. Community-based social and legal responses that are inflamed by sentiment and driven by punitive motives are likely to increase, rather than decrease, the probability of reoffense.

Treatment

The past decade has witnessed considerable progress in the refinement and specification of treatment interventions for sex offenders. Service provision has increased over the past decade in response to the seeming epidemic of sexual violence. The most recent survey by the Safer Society Program (Longo, Bird, Stevenson, & Fiske, 1995), completed in 1994, reported on 710 treatment programs for adult sex offenders and 684 treatment programs for juvenile sex offenders. Since the last Safer Society survey in 1985 (Knopp, Rosenberg, and Stevenson, 1986), there has been more than a 100% increase in treatment programs for adults (297 programs as of 1985) and almost a 100% increase in programs for juveniles (346 programs as of 1985).

Broadly speaking, sex offender treatment programs employ four approaches: (a) *evocative therapy*, which focuses on understanding the causes and motivations leading to sexually deviant and coercive behavior, as well as increasing empathy for the victims of sexual assault; (b) *cognitive behavior therapy*, which focuses on sexual assault cycles and techniques that interrupt those cycles, altering cognitions that justify and perpetuate sexually aggressive behavior, and controlling and managing anger; (c) *psychoeducation* groups or classes that use a more didactic approach to remedy deficits in social and interpersonal skills, teach techniques for managing anger, teach principles of relapse prevention, and teach a range of topics having to do with human sexuality, dating and communication skills, myths about sexuality and relationships, and so on; and (d) *pharmacological treatment*, which focuses on reducing sexual arousability and the frequency of deviant sexual fantasies through the use of antiandrogens and antidepressants. These approaches are not mutually exclusive and the ideal treatment program would employ combinations of these approaches.

Evocative therapy may include individual therapy, group therapy, couples and marital therapy, and family therapy. Group therapy may be eclectic or issue-focused. In the latter case, specialty groups may include substance abuse (AA or NA), Adult

Children of Alcoholics, victim empathy, victim survivors, social skills and assertiveness training, A Way of Life, Black Awareness, Gay Identity, Vietnam Veterans, and so on.

The most commonly employed cognitive-behavioral model in sex offender treatment programs is relapse prevention (RP) (Pithers, 1990; Pithers, Marques, Gibat, & Marlatt, 1983). In the RP model, sexually aggressive behavior is conceptualized as an ingrained response set to engage in maladaptive behavior that is sparked by a series of antecedent (or signal) events. This chain of events often takes the form of a series of "seemingly unimportant decisions" that lead to the maladaptive behavior (i.e., relapse). The task of therapy in the RP model is to provide the offender with the cognitive and behavioral skills necessary to short-circuit the chain of events that leads to reoffense. Although the chain (or cycle) is unique for each individual, the most common class of events anteceding relapse among sex offenders was thought to be a negative emotional state (Pithers *et al.*, 1983). Pithers and his colleagues (Pithers, 1990; Pithers, Martin, & Cumming, 1989) subsequently reported, however, that for child molesters, the most frequently identified experience prior to the offense was not an emotional state (as was the case with rapists) but planning the offense (73% of sample) and low victim empathy (71% of sample).

The relapse prevention model targets three areas of assessment: (1) those situations that place an individual at risk for relapse, (2) the adequacy of the individual's skills for coping with high-risk situations, and (3) the identification of those antecedent events that permit hypotheses about why the maladaptive coping response is to aggress sexually. Once this information is elicited, two interventions are employed: (1) strategies that help the individual avoid high risk situations, and (2) strategies that minimize the likelihood that high-risk situations, once encountered, will lead to relapse.

Perhaps the best-known residential treatment and evaluation program for sex offenders was in California under the direction of Marques (e.g., Marques *et al.*, 1993). The centerpiece of the program was relapse prevention. In addition, it included an aftercare component in which, as a condition of parole, offenders were required to attend two treatment sessions a week for the first year. Marques and colleagues (1993) reported that of 108 treated sex offenders, roughly three quarters of whom were child molesters, 4.6% were rearrested for a sexual offense, 6.5% were rearrested for a nonsexual violent offense, and 5.6% violated some other condition of parole. The average exposure time for this group was 34 months.

Another equally well-known treatment program is the one directed by Pithers (e.g., Pithers, Martin, & Cumming, 1989) in Vermont. The Vermont program is a combination of community-based outpatient and residential inpatient therapy groups. As with Marques's program, the treatment model is cognitive-behavioral with a focus on relapse prevention. Pithers and Cumming (1989) reported that 3% of a sample of 147 treated child molesters committed a new sexual offense during a 6-year follow-up period.

Maletzky (1987) conducted a 1- to 14-year follow-up of child molesters treated at his clinic in Oregon. Maletzky reported that 12.7% of 1,719 opposite-sex child molesters (girl victims) and 13.6% of 513 same-sex child molesters (boy victims) committed another sexual offense. In another cognitive-behavioral treatment program at the Kingston Sexual Behaviour Clinic (Ontario, Canada), Marshall and Barbaree (1988) reported similar findings. Of the opposite-sex child molesters, 17.9% reoffended, compared with 42.9% of the matched untreated child molesters. Of the same-sex child molesters, 13.3% reoffended, compared with 42.9% of the matched untreated offenders. Of the incest offenders, 8% of the treated and 21.7% of the untreated men reoffended.

Although we still are in the early stages of identifying optimal treatment interventions and reliably documenting treatment effects, it seems reasonable to conclude at this point that "state-of-the-art" intervention (cognitive-behavioral therapy and medication when appropriate) can effectively reduce reoffense rates. A more problematic question, and one that is central to the determination of treatment effects, is the probability of reoffense among untreated offenders. In our 25-year follow-up of 115 child molesters who did not receive cognitive-behavioral treatment, the cumulative failure rate for sexual offenses by the end of the 25-year study period was 52% charged and 42% convicted (Prentky, Lee, Knight & Cerce, 1997). These figures are comparable to what Marshall and Barbaree (1988) reported for untreated child molesters. In a recent meta-analysis on 12 sex offender treatment studies ($N = 1,313$), G. C. N. Hall (1995) found that the overall recidivism rate for untreated sex offenders was only .27, compared with .19 for treated offenders. Thus, based on Hall's meta-analysis, the treatment effect is 8%. If the recidivism rate for untreated offenders approached what Marshall and Barbaree (1988) and Prentky, Knight, and Lee (1996) reported (i.e., 40% to 50%), the treatment effect would be considerably larger than 8%. In reality, of course, the likelihood of reoffense among untreated child molesters is highly variable.

As noted at the beginning of this section, the most compelling motive for treating child molesters is the presumptive reduction in victimization rates. As a society, however, we resist treating sexual offenders, because it is perceived to be a "humane" response to egregious behavior (Prentky & Burgess, 1990). If the overriding goal is, in fact, reduction in the number of victims, and if treatment can be demonstrated to reduce the probability of reoffense, then it is essential that we overcome our resistance to treatment and work toward the optimization of treatment interventions and treatment conditions that most effectively reduce risk.

References

Abel, G. G. (1982, July). Viewpoint: Who is going to protect our children? *Sexual Medicine Today, 32,* p. 32.

Abel, G. G., & Rouleau, J. L. (1990). The nature and extent of sexual assault. In W. L. Marshall, D. R. Laws, & H. E. Barbaree (Eds.), *Handbook of sexual assault: Issues, theories and treatment of the offender* (pp. 9–21). New York: Plenum.

Abel, G. G., Becker, J. V., Murphy, W. D., & Flanagan, B. (1981). Identifying dangerous child molesters. In R. B. Stewart (Ed.), *Violent behavior: Social learning approaches to prediction, management and treatment* (pp. 116–137). New York: Brunner-Mazel.

Abel, G. G., Becker, J. V., Mittelman, M. S., Cunningham-Rathner, J., Rouleau, J. L., & Murphy, W. D. (1987). Self-reported sex crimes of nonincarcerated paraphilics. *Journal of Interpersonal Violence, 2,* 3–25.

Abel, G. G., Mittelman, M., Becker, J. V., Rathner, J., & Rouleau, J. L. (1988). Predicting child molesters response to treatment. In R. A. Prentky & V. L. Quinsey (Eds.), *Human sexual aggression: Current perspectives* (pp. 223–234). New York: New York Acadey of Sciences.

Abel, G. G., Lawry, S. S., Karlstrom, E., Osborn, C. A., & Gillespie, C. F. (1994). Screening tests for pedophilia. *Criminal Justice and Behavior, 21,* 115–131.

Alexander, P. C. (1992). Application of attachment theory to the study of sexual abuse. *Journal of Counsulting and Clinical Psychology, 2,* 185–195.

Alexander, P. C.. (1993). The differential effect of abuse characteristics and attachment in the prediction of long-term effects of sexual abuse. *Journal of Interpersonal Violence, 3,* 346–362.

American Psychiatric Association. (1952). *Diagnostic and statistical manual of mental disorders*. Washington, DC: Author.

American Psychiatric Association. (1968). *Diagnostic and statistical manual of mental disorders* (2nd ed). Washington, DC: Author.

American Psychiatric Association. (1980 *Diagnostic and statistical manual of mental disorders* (3rd ed.). Washington, DC: Author.

American Psychiatric Association. (1987). *Diagnostic and statistical manual of mental disorders* (3rd ed., rev.). Washington, DC: Author.

American Psychiatric Association. (1994). *Diagnostic and statistical manual of mental disorders* (4th ed.). Washington, DC: Author.

Anderson, G., & Yasenik, L., & Ross, C. A. (1993). Dissociative experiences and disorders among women who identify themselves as sexual abuse survivors. *Child Abuse & Neglect, 17,* 677–686.

Araji, S., & Finkelhor, D. (1985). Explanations of pedophilia: Review of empirical research. *Bulletin of the American Academy of Psychiatry and the Law, 13,* 17–37.

Avery-Clark, C. A., & Laws, D. R. (1984). Differential erection response patterns of sexual child abusers to stimuli describing activities with children. *Behavior Therapy, 15,* 71–83.

Bagley, C. (1991). The long-term psychological effects of child sexual abuse: A review of some British and Canadian studies of victims and their families. *Annals of Sex Research, 4,* 23–48.

Barbaree, H. E., & Marshall, W. L. (1988). Deviant sexual arousal, offense history, and demographic variables as predictors of reoffense among child molesters. *Behavioral Sciences and the Law, 6,* 267–280.

Barbaree, H. E., Seto, M. C., & Serin, R. C. (1994). *Comparisons between low- and high-fixated child molesters: Psychopathy, criminal history, and sexual arousal to children.* Manuscript submitted for publication.

Bartholomew, K., & Horowitz, L. M. (1991). Attachment styles among young adults: A test of a four-category model. *Journal of Personality and Social Psychology, 2,* 226–244.

Becker, J. V., Abel, G. G., Blanchard, E. B., Murphy, W. D., & Coleman, E. (1978). Evaluating social skills of sexual aggressives. *Criminal Justice and Behavior, 5,* 357–367.

Becker, J. V., Kaplan, M. S., Cunningham-Rathner, J., & Kavoussi, R. (1986). Characteristics of adolescent incest sexual perpetrators: Preliminary findings. *Journal of Family Violence, 1,* 85–97.

Brant, R. S. T., & Tisza, V. B. (1977). The sexually misused child. *American Journal of Orthopsychiatry, 47,* 80–90.

Braun, B. G., Sachs, R. G. (1985). The development of multiple personality disorder: Predisposing, precipitating, and perpetuating factors. In R. P. Kluft (Ed.), *Childhood antecedents of multiple personality* (pp. 38–64). Washington, DC: Psychiatric Press.

Briere, J. (1992). Methodological issues in the study of sexual abuse effects. *Journal of Consulting and Clinical Psychology, 60,* 196–203.

Briere, J., & Elliot, M. D., (1993). Sexual abuse, family environment, and psychological systems. *Journal of Consulting and Clinical Psychology, 61,* 216–288.

Briere, J., & Runtz, M. (1988). Symptomatology associated with childhood sexual victimization in a nonclinical adult sample. *Child Abuse & Neglect, 12,* 51–59.

Briere, J., & Runtz, M. (1989). University males' sexual interest in children: Predicting potential indices of "pedophilia" in a nonforensic sample. *Child Abuse & Neglect, 13,* 65–75.

Briere, J., & Runtz, M. (1990a). Augmenting Hopkins SCL scales to measure dissociative systems: Data from two nonclinical samples. *Journal of Personality Assessment, 55,* 376–379.

Briere, J., & Runtz, M. (1990b). Differential adult symptomatology associated with three types of child abuse histories. *Child Abuse & Neglect, 14,* 357–364.

Briere, J., & Runtz, M. (1993). Childhood sexual abuse: Long-term sequelae and implications of psychological assessment. *Journal of Interpersonal Violence, 8,* 312–330.

Briere, J., & Zaidi, L. Y. (1989). Sexual abuse histories and sequelae in female psychiatric emergency room patients. *American Journal of Psychiatry, 146,* 1602–1606.

Briere, J. N. (1992). *Child abuse trauma: Theory and treatment of the lasting effects.* Newbury Park, CA: Sage.

Brown, G. R., & Anderson, B. (1991). Psychiatric morbidity in adult inpatients with childhood histories of sexual and physical abuse. *American Journal of Psychiatry, 148,* 55–61.

Bryer, J. B., Nelson, B. A., Miller, J. B., & Krol, P. A. (1987). Childhood sexual and physical abuse as factors in adult psychiatric illness. *American Journal of Psychiatry, 144,* 1426–1430.

Bulik, C. M., Sullivan, P. E., & Rorty, M. (1989). Childhood sexual abuse in women with bulimia. *Journal of Clinical Psychiatry, 50,* 446–464.

Bumby, K., & Marshall, W. L. (1994, November). *Loneliness and intimacy dysfunction among incarcerated rapists and child molesters.* Paper presented at the annual meeting of the Association for the Treatment of Sexual Abusers, San Francisco.

Burgess, A., Hartman, C., & McCormack, A. (1987). Abused to abuser: Antecedents of socially deviant behaviors. *American Journal of Orthopsychiatry, 144,* 1431–1436.

Cappelleri, J. C., Eckenrode, J., & Powers, J. L. (1993). The epidemiology of child abuse: Findings from the Second National Incidence and Prevalence Study of Child Abuse and Neglect. American Journal of *Public Health, 83,* 1622–1624.

Carlson, V., Cicchetti, D., Barnett, D., & Braunwald, K. (1989). Disorganized/disoriented attachment relationships in maltreated infants. *Development and Psychopathology, 25,* 525–531.

Cavaiola, A., & Schiff, M. (1988). Behavioral sequelae of physical and/or sexual abuse in adolescents. *Child Abuse & Neglect, 12,* 181–188.

Cerce, D., Day, S. R., Prentky, R. A., & Knight, R. A. (1984, August). *The correlative relationship between family instability in childhood and sexually aggressive behavior in adulthood.* Paper presented at the second National Family Violence Research Conference, University of New Hampshire, Durham.

Cernkovich, S. A., & Giordano, P. C. (1987). Family relationships and delinquency. *Criminology, 2,* 295–321.

Cernkovich, S. A., & Giordano, P. C. (1992). School bonding, race, and delinquency. *Criminology, 2,* 261–291.

Chappell, D. (1989). Sexual criminal violence. In N. A. Weiner and M. E. Wolfgang (Eds.), *Pathways to criminal violence* (pp. 68–108). Newbury Park, CA: Sage.

Christiansen, K. O., Elers-Nielsen, M., Le Maire, L., & Strup, G. K. (1965). Recidivism among sexual offenders. In K. O. Christiansen (Ed.)., *Scandinavian studies in criminology,* (pp. 55–85). London, England: Tavistock.

Chu, J. A., & Dill, D. L. (1990). Dissociative symptoms in relation to childhood physical and sexual abuse. *American Journal of Psychiatry, 147,* 887–892.

Cohen, M. L., Seghorn, T., & Calmas, W. (1969). Sociometric study of sex offenders. *Journal of Abnormal Psychology, 74,* 249–255.

Cohen, M. L., Boucher, R. J., Seghorn, T. K., & Mehegan, J. (1979, March). *The sexual offender against children.* Paper presented at a meeting of the Association for Professional Treatment of Offenders, Boston.

Cole, P. M., & Putman, F. W. (1992). Effect of incest on self and social functioning: A developmental psychopathology perspective. *Journal of Consulting and Clinical Psychology, 60,* 174–184.

Conte, J. R. (1985). Clinical dimensions of adult sexual abuse of children. *Behavioral Sciences and the Law, 3,* 341–354.

Coons, P. M. (1986). Psychiatric problems associated with child abuse: A review. In J. J. Jacobson (Ed.), Psychiatric sequelae of child abuse and incest. *Psychiatric Clinics of North America, 12,* 325–335.

Coons, P. M., Bowman, E. S., Pellow, T. A., & Schneider, P. (1989). Posttraumatic aspects of the treatment of victims of sexual abuse and incest. *Psychiatric Clinics of North America, 12,* 325–335.

Cushing, J. G. N. (1950). Psychopathology of sexual delinquency. *Journal of Clinical Psychopathology, 11,* 49–56.

Dhawan, S., & Marshall, W. L. (1996). Sexual abuse histories of sexual offenders. *Sexual Abuse: A Journal of Research and Treatment, 8,* 7–15.

Dietz, P. E. (1983). Sex offenses: Behavioral aspects. In S. H. Kadish *et al.* (Eds.), *Encyclopedia of crime and justice.* New York: Free Press.

Dixon, K. N., Arnold, E., & Calestro, K. (1978). Father–son incest: Underreported psychiatric problem? *American Journal of Psychiatry, 135,* 835–838.

Dubowitz, H., Black, M., Harrington, D., & Verschoore, A. (1993). A follow-up study of behavior problems associated with child sexual abuse. *Child Abuse & Neglect, 17,* 743–754.

Egeland, B., & Sroufe, L. A. (1981). Attachment and early maltreatment. *Child Development, 52,* 44–52.

Elliott, D. M., & Briere, J. (1992). The sexually abused boy: Problems in manhood. *Medical Aspects of Human Sexuality, 26,* 68–71.

Fehrenbach, P. A., Smith, W., Monastersky, C., & Deisher, R. W. (1986). Adolescent sexual offenders: Offender and offense characteristics. *American Journal of Orthopsychiatry, 56,* 225–233.

Finkelhor, D. (1984). *Child sexual abuse: New theory and research.* New York: Free Press.

Finkelhor, D. (1994). The international epidemiology of child sexual abuse. *Child Abuse & Neglect, 18,* 409–417.

Finkelhor, D., & Araji, S. (1986). Explanations of pedophilia: A four factor model. *Journal of Sex Research, 22,* 145–161.

Finkelhor, D., & Dziuba-Leatherman, J. (1994a). Children as victims of violence: A national survey. *Pediatrics, 94,* 413–420.

Finkelhor, D., & Dziuba-Leatherman, J. (1994b). Victimization of children. *American Psychologist, 49,* 173–183.

Finkelhor, D., & Lewis, I. S. (1988). An epidemiologic approach to the study of child molestation. In R. A. Prentky & V. L. Quinsey (Eds.), *Human sexual aggression: Current perspectives* (Vol. 528, pp. 64–78). New York: New York Academy of Sciences.

Finkelhor, D., Araji, S., Baron, L., Browne, A., Peters, S. D., & Wyatt, G. E. (1986). *A sourcebook on child sexual abuse*. Beverly Hills, CA: Sage.

Fisher, S. H. (1965). A note on male homosexuality and the role of women in Ancient Greece. In J. Marmor (Ed.), *Sexual inversion* (pp. 165–172). New York: Basic Books.

Fitch, J. H. (1962). Men convicted of sexual offenses against children: A descriptive follow-up study. British *Journal of Criminology, 3,* 18–37.

Freund, K. (1965). Diagnosing heterosexual pedophilia by means of a test for sexual interest. *Behavior Research and Therapy, 3,* 229–234.

Freund, K. (1967a). Diagnosing homo- and heterosexuality and erotic age preference by means of a psychophysiological test. *Behaviour Research and Therapy, 5,* 209–228.

Freund, K. (1967b). Erotic preference in pedophilia. *Behavior Research and Therapy, 5,* 339–348.

Freund, K., & Blanchard, R. (1989). Phallometric diagnosis of pedophilia. *Journal of Consulting and Clinical Psychology, 57,* 100–105.

Freund, K., & Langevin, R. (1976). Bisexuality in homosexual pedophilia. *Archives of Sexual Behavior, 5,* 415–423.

Friedrich, W. N. (1988). Behavior problems in sexually abused children: An adaptational perspective. In G. E. Wyatt & G. J. Powell (Eds.), *Lasting effects of child sexual abuse* (pp. 171–191). Beverly Hills, CA: Sage.

Friedrich, W. N., & Luecke, W. (1988). Young school age sexually aggressive children. *Professional Psychology: Research and Practice, 19,* 155–164.

Friedrich, W. N., & Reams, R. A. (1987). Course of psychological symptoms in sexually abused young children. *Psychotherapy, 24,* 160–170.

Friedrich, W. N., Urquiza, A. J., & Beilke, R. (1986). Behavioral problems in sexually abused young children. *Journal of Pediatric Psychology, 11,* 47–57.

Frisbie, L. V. (1969). *Another look at sex offenders in California* (California Mental Health Research Monograph, No. 12), Sacramento, State of California Department of Mental Hygiene.

Frisbie, L. V., & Dondis, E. H. (1965). *Recidivism among treated sex offenders* (California Mental Health Research Monograph No. 5). Sacramento: State of California Department of Mental Hygiene.

Fromuth, M. E., Burkhart, B. R., & Jones, C. W. (1991). Hidden child molestation. An investigation of adolescent perpetrators in a nonclinical sample. *Journal of Interpersonal Violence, 6,* 376–384.

Garland, R. J., & Dougher, M. J. (1990). The abused-abuser hypothesis of child sexual abuse: A critical review of theory and research. In J. R. Feierman (Ed.), *Pedophilia: Biosocial dimensions* (pp. 488–509). New York: Springer-Verlag.

Gebhard, P. H., Gagnon, J. H., Pomeroy, W. B., & Christenson, C. V. (1965). *Sex offenders: An analysis of types.* New York: Harper & Row.

Glueck, B. C. (1956). *Research Project for the study and treatment of persons convicted of crimes involving sexual aberrations* (Final Report: June 1952–June 1955). New York: State Department of Hygiene.

Gold, E. R. (1986). Long-term effects of sexual victimization in childhood an attributional approach. *Journal of Consulting and Clinical Psychology, 4,* 471–475.

Goldfarb, L. A. (1987). Sexual abuse antecedent to anorexia nervosa, bulimia, and compulsive eating: Three case reports. *International Journal of Eating Disorders, 6,* 665–680.

Goodwin, J. M. (1985). Post-traumatic symptoms in incest victims. In S. Eth & R. Pynoos (Eds.), *Post-traumatic stress disorder in children.* (pp. 157–168). Washington, DC: American Psychiatric Press.

Gross, R. J., Doerr, H., Caldirola, D., Guzinski, G. M.,& Ripley, H. S. (1980–1981). Borderline syndrome and incest in chronic pelvic pain patients. *International Journal of Psychiatry in Medicine, 10,* 79–96.

Groth, A. N. (1978). Patterns of sexual assault against children and adolescents. In A. W. Burgess, A. N. Groth, L. L. Holmstrom, & S. M. Sgroi (Eds.), *Sexual assault of children and adolescents* (pp. 3–24). Lexington, MA: Heath.

Groth, A. N. (1979). Sexual trauma in the life histories of rapists and child molesters. *Victimology: An International Journal, 4,* 10–16.

Groth, A. N. (1981). *Sexual offenders against children.* Distributed by Forensic Mental Health Associates, Webster, MA 01570.

Groth, A. N., Hobson, W. F., Gary, T. S. (1982). The child molester: Clinical observations. *Social Work and Human Sexuality, 1,* 129–144.

Hall, G. C. N. (1995). Sexual offender recidivism revisited: A meta-analysis of recent treatment studies. *Journal of Consulting and Clinical Psychology, 63,* 802–809.

Hall, G. C. N., & Proctor, W. C. (1987). Criminological predictors of recidivism in a sexual offender population. *Journal of Consulting and Clinical Psychology, 55,* 111–112.

Hall, G. C. N., Proctor, W. C., & Nelson, G. M. (1988). Validity of physiological measures of pedophilic sexual arousal in a sexual offender population. *Journal of Consulting and Clinical Psychology, 56,* 118–122.

Hall, R. C., Tice, L., Beresford, T. P., Wolley, B., & Hall, A. K. (1989). Sexual abuse in patients with anorexia nervosa and bulimia. *Psychosomatics, 30,* 73–79.

Hanson, R. K., & Slater, S. (1988). Sexual victimization in the history of sexual abusers: A review. *Annals of Sex Research, 1,* 485–500.

Hanson, R. K., Steffy, R. A., & Gauthier R. (1993). Long-term recidivism of child molesters. *Journal of Consulting and Clinical Psychology, 61,* 646–652.

Hanson, R. K., Scott, H., & Steffy, R. A. (1995). A comparison of child molesters and nonsexual criminals: Risk predictors and long-term recidivism. *Journal of Research in Crime and Delinquency, 32,* 325–337.

Herman, J. L., Perry, J. C., & van der Kolk, B. A. (1989). Childhood trauma in borderline personality disorder. *American Journal of Psychiatry, 146,* 405–490.

Jackson, J. L., Calhoun, K. S., Amick, A. E., Madderer, H. M., & Habif, V. L. (1990). Young adult women who report childhood intrafamilial sexual abuse: Subsequent adjustment. *Archives of Sexual Behavior, 19,* 211–221.

James, B. (1994). *Handbook for treatment of attachment-trauma problems in children.* New York: Lexington Books.

James J., & Meyerding, J. (1977). Early sexual experience and prostitution. *American Journal of Psychiatry, 134,* 1381–1386.

Johnson, T. C. (1988). Child perpetrators—children who molest other children: Preliminary findings. *Child Abuse & Neglect, 12,* 219–229.

Kaufman, J., & Zigler, E. (1987). Do abused children become abusive parents? *American Journal of Orthopsychiatry, 57,* 186–192.

Kempe, R. S., & Kempe, C. H. (1984). *The common secret: Sexual abuse of children and perpetrators.* New York: Freeman.

Kendall-Tackett, K., & Simon, A. (1988). Molestation and the onset of puberty: Data from 365 adults molested as children. *Child Abuse & Neglect, 12,* 73–81.

Kendall-Tackett, K., Williams, L. M., & Finkelhor, D. (1993). Impact of sexual abuse on children: A review and synthesis of recent empirical studies. *Psychological Bulletin, 113,* 164–180.

Kiser, L. J., Ackerman, B. J., Brown, E. Edwards, N. B., McColgan, E., Pugh, R., & Pruiff, D. B. (1988). Posttraumatic stress disorder in young children: A reaction to purported sexual abuse. *Journal of the American Academy of Child and Adolescent Psychiatry, 27,* 645–649.

Kluft, R. (1985). *Childhood antecedents of multiple personality.* Washington, DC: American Psychiatric Press.

Knight, R., Rosenberg, R., & Schneider, B. (1985). Classification of sexual offenders: Perspectives, methods and validation. In A. Burgess (Ed.), *Rape and sexual assault: A research handbook* (pp. 222–293). New York: Garland.

Knight, R. A. (1988). A taxonomic analysis of child molesters. In R. A. Prentky & V. Quinsey (Eds.), *Human sexual aggression: Current perspectives* (Vol. 528, pp. 2–20). New York: Annals of the New York Academy of Sciences.

Knight, R. A. (1989). An assessment of the concurrent validity of a child molester typology. *Journal of Interpersonal Violence, 4,* 131–150.

Knight, R. A. (1992). The generation and corroboration of a taxonomic model for child molesters. In W. O'Donohue & J. H. Geer (Eds.), *The sexual abuse of children: Theory, research, and therapy* (pp. 24–70). Hillsdale, NJ: Erlbaum.

Knight, R. A., & Prentky, R. A. (1990). Classifying sexual offenders: The development and corroboration of taxonomic models. In W. L. Marshall, D. R. Laws, & H. E. Barbaree (Eds.), *The handbook of sexual assault: Issues, theories, and treatment of the offender* (pp. 23–52). New York: Plenum.

Knight, R. A., Carter, D. L., & Prentky, R. A. (1989). A system for the classification of child molesters: Reliability and application. *Journal of Interpersonal Violence, 4,* 3–23.

Knopp, F. H., Rosenberg, J., & Stevenson, W. (1986). *Report on nationwide survey of juvenile and adult sex-offender treatment programs and providers.* Syracuse, NY: Safer Society Press.

Kobayashi, J., Sales, B. D., Becker, J. V., Figueredo, A. J., & Kaplan, M. S. (1995). Perceived parental deviance, parent–child bonding, child abuse, and child sexual aggression. *Sexual Abuse: A Journal of Research and Treatment, 7,* 25–44.

Kopp, S. B. (1962). The character structure of sex offenders. *American Journal of Psychotherapy, 16,* 64–70.

Langevin, R., Day, D., Handy, L., & Russon, A. (1985). Are incestuous fathers pedophilic, aggressive, and alcoholic? In R. Langevin (Ed.), *Erotic preference, gender identity, and aggression in men: New research studies* (pp. 161–179). Hillsdale, NJ: Erlbaum.

Langevin, R., Hucker, S. J., Handy, L., Hook, H. J., and Purins, J. E., & Russon, A. E. (1985). Erotic preference and aggression in pedophelia: A comparison of heterosexual, homosexual, and bisexual types. In R. Langevin (Ed.), *Erotic preference, gender identity, and aggression in men: New research studies* (pp. 137–160). Hillsdale, NJ: Erlbaum.

Langevin, R., Wright, P., & Handy, L. (1989). Characteristics of sex offenders who were sexually victimized as children. *Annals of Sex Research, 2,* 227–253.

Langsley, D. G., Schwartz, M. N., & Fairbairn, R. H. (1968). Father–son incest. *Comprehensive psychiatry, 9,* 218–226.

Lanning, K. V. (1986). *Child molesters: A behavioral analysis for law-enforcement officers investigating cases of child exploitation.* Washington, DC: National Center for Missing and Exploited Children.

Lanyon, R. I. (1986). Theory and treatment in child molestation. *Journal of Consulting and Clinical Psychology, 54,* 176–182.

Laws, D. R., & Osborn, C. A. (1983). How to build and operate a behavioral laboratory to evaluate and treat sexual deviance. In J. G. Greer & I. R. Stuart (Eds.), *The sexual aggressor* (pp. 293–335). New York: Van Nostrand Reinhold.

Lindberg, F. H., & Distad, L. J. (1985). Post-traumatic stress disorders in women who experienced childhood incest. *Child Abuse & Neglect, 9,* 329–334.

Lipovsky, J. A., Saunders, B. E., & Murphy, S. M. (1989). Depression, anxiety, and behavior problems among victims of father–child sexual assault and nonabused siblings. *Journal of Interpersonal Violence, 4,* 452–468.

Livingston, R. (1987). Sexually and physically abused children. *Journal of the American Academy of Child and Adolescent Psychiatry, 26,* 413–415.

Longo, R. F. (1982). Sexual learning and experience among adolescent sexual offenders. *International Journal of Offender Therapy and Comparative Criminology, 26,* 235–241.

Longo, R. F., Bird, S., Stevenson, W. F., & Fiske, J. A. (1995). *1994 nationwide survey of treatment programs and models.* Brandon, VT: Safer Society Program & Press.

Malcolm, P. B., Andrews, D. A., & Quinsey, V. L. (1993). Discriminant and predictive validity of phallometrically measured sexual age and gender preference. *Journal of Interpersonal Violence, 8,* 486–501.

Maletzky, B. (1987 May). *Data generated by an outpatient sexual abuse clinic.* Paper presented at the third annual conference of the Association for the Treatment of Sexual Abusers, Newport, OR.

Marques, J. K. (1995, September). *How to answer the question: Does sex offender treatment work?* Paper presented at the International Expert Conference on Sex Offenders: Issues, Research and Treatment, Utrecht, The Netherlands.

Marques, J. K., Day, D. M., Nelson, C., & West, M. A. (1993). Findings and recommendations from California's experimental treatment program. In G. C. Nagayama Hall, R. Hirschman, J. R. Graham, & M. S. Zaragoza (Eds.), *Sexual aggression: Issues in etiology, assessment, and treatment* (pp. 197–214). Washington, DC: Taylor & Francis.

Marshall, W. L. (1989). Invited essay: Intimacy, loneliness and sexual offenders. *Behavior Research and Therapy, 27,* 491–503.

Marshall, W. L., & Barbaree, H. E. (1988). The long-term evaluation of a behavioral treatment program for child molesters. *Behaviour Research and Therapy, 26,* 499–511.

Marshall, W. L., and Mazzucco, A. (1995). Self-esteem and parental attachments in child molesters. *Sexual Abuse: A Journal of Research and Treatment, 7,* 279–285.

Marshall, W. L., Christie, M. M., & Lanthier, R. D. (1979). *Social competence, sexual experience and attitudes to sex in incarcerated rapists and pedophiles.* Report to the Solicitor General of Canada. Ottawa.

Marshall, W. L., & Christie, M. M. (1981). Pedophilia and aggression. *Criminal Justice and Behavior, 8,* 14–158.

Marshall, W. L., Earls, C. M., Segal, Z., & Darke, J. (1983). A behavioral program for the assessment and treatment of sexual aggressors. In K. Craig & R. McMahon (Eds.), *Advances in clinical behavior therapy* (pp. 148–174). New York: Brunner/ Mazel.

Marshall, W. L., Hudson, S. M., & Hodkinson, S. (1993). The importance of attachment bonds in the development of juvenile sex offending. In H. E. Barbaree, W. L. Marshall, & S. M. Hudson (Eds.), *The juvenile sex offender* (pp. 164–181). New York: Guilford.

Marshall, W. L., Barbaree, H. E., & Fernandez, M. (1995). Some aspects of social competence in sexual offenders. *Sexual Abuse: A Journal of Research and Treatment, 7,* 113–127.

McCaghy, C. H. (1967). *Child molesters: A study of their careers as deviants.* New York: Holt, Rinehart, and Winston.

McLeer, S. V., Deblinger, E., Atkins, M. S., Foa, E. B., & Ralphe, D. L. (1988). Post-traumatic stress disorder in sexually abused children. *Journal of the American Academy of Child and Adolescent Psychiatry, 27,* 650–654.

Mennen, F., & Meadow, D. (1995). The relationship of abuse characteristics to symptoms in sexually abused girls. *Journal of Interpersonal Violence, 10,* 259–274.

Moeller, T. P., Bachmann, G. A., & Moeller, J. R. (1993). The combined effects of physical, sexual and emotional abuse during childhood: Long-term health consequences for women. *Child Abuse & Neglect, 17,* 623–640.

Mohr, J. W., Turner, R. E., & Jerry, M. B. (1964). *Pedophilia and exhibitionism.* Toronto, Ontario, Canada: University of Toronto Press.

Nash, M. R., Hulsey, T. L., Sexton, M. C., Harralson, T. L., & Lambert, W. (1993). Long-term sequelae of childhood sexual abuse: Perceived family environment, psychology, and dissociation. *Journal of Consulting and Clinical Psychology, 61,* 276–283.

Neumann, D. A., Houskamp, B. H., Pollock, V. E., & Briere, J. (1996). The long-term sequelae of childhood sexual abuse in woman: A meta-analytic review. *Child Maltreatment, 1,* 6–16.

Ogata, S. N., Silk, K. R., Goodrich, S., Lohr, N. E., Westen, D., & Hill, E. M. (1990). Childhood sexual and physical abuse in adult patients with borderline personality disorder. *American Journal of Psychiatry, 147,* 1008–1013.

Palmer, R. L., Oppenheimer, R., Dignon, A., Chaloner, D. A., & Howells, K. (1990). Childhood sexual experiences with adults reported by women with eating disorders: An extended series. *British Journal of Psychiatry, 156,* 699–703.

Parker, G., Tupling, H., & Brown, L. B. (1979). A parental bonding instructment. *British Journal of Medical Psychology, 52,* 1–10.

Peters, S. D. (1988). Child sexual abuse and later psychological problems. In G. E. Wyatt & G. J. Powell (Eds.), *Lasting effects of child sexual abuse* (pp. 101–117). Newbury Park, CA: Sage.

Pithers, W. D. (1990). Relapse prevention with sexual aggressors. A method for maintaining therapeutic gain and enhancing external supervision. In W. L. Marshall, D. R. Laws, & H. E. Barbaree (Eds.), *Handbook of sexual assault. Issues, theories, and treatment of the offender* (pp. 343–361). New York: Plenum.

Pithers, W. D., & Cumming, G. F. (1989). Can relapses be prevented? Initial outcome data from the Vermont Treatment Program for Sexual Aggressors. In D. R. Laws (Ed.), *Relapse prevention with sex offenders* (pp. 313–325). New York: Guilford.

Pithers, W. D., Marques, J. K., Gibat, C. C., & Marlatt, G. A. (1983). Relapse prevention with sexual aggressives: A self-control model of treatment and maintenance of change. In J. G. Greer & I. R. Stuart (Eds.), *The sexual aggressor: Current perspectives on treatment* (pp. 214–239). New York: Van Nostrand Reinhold.

Pithers, W. D., Kashima, K. M., Cumming, G. F., Beal, L. S., & Buell M. M. (1988). Relapse prevention of sexual aggression. In R. A. Prentky & V. L. Quinsey (Eds.), *Human sexual aggression: Current perspectives* (pp. 244–260). New York: Annals of the New York Academy of Sciences, Vol. 528.

Pithers, W. D., Beal, L. S., Armstrong, J., & Petty, J. (1989). Identification of risk factors through clinical interviews and analysis of records. In D. R. Laws (Ed.), *Relapse prevention with sexual offenders* (pp. 77–87). New York: Guilford.

Pithers, W. D., Martin, G. R., & Cumming, G. F. (1989). Vermont treatment program for sexual aggressors. In D. R. Laws (Ed.), *Relapse prevention with sex offenders* (pp. 292–311). New York: Guilford.

Porter, F. S., Blick, L. C., & Sgroi, S. M. (1982). Treatment of the sexually abused child. In S. M. Sgroi (Ed.), *Handbook of clinical intervention in child sexual abuse* (pp. 109–145). Lexington, MA: Lexington Books.

Prentky, R. A. (1996). Community notification and constructive risk reduction. *Journal of Interpersonal Violence, 11,* 295–298.

Prentky, R. A., & Burgess, A. W. (1990). Rehabilitation of child molesters: A cost-benefit analysis. *American Journal of Orthopsychiatry, 60,* 108–117.

Prentky, R. A., & Knight, R. A. (1993). Age of onset of sexual assault: Criminal and life history correlates. In G. C. N. Hall, R. Hirschman, J. R. Graham, & M. S. Zaragoza (Eds.), *Sexual aggression: Issues in etiology, assessment, and treatment* (pp. 43–62). Washington, DC: Taylor & Francis.

Prentky, R. A., Knight, R. A., Rosenberg, R., & Lee, A. (1989). A path analytic approach to the validation of a taxonomic system for classifying child molesters. *Journal of Quantitative Criminology, 5,* 231–257.

Prentky, R. A., Knight, R. A., Sims-Knight, J., Straus, H., Rokous, F., & Cerce, D. (1989). Development antecedents of sexual aggression. *Development and Psychopathology, 1,* 153–169.

Prentky, R. A., Holland, A., & Lee, A. F. (1996). *Caregiver instability in the life histories of adult sex offenders.* Manuscript in preparation.

Prentky, R. A., Knight, R. A., & Lee, A. F. S. (1997). Risk factors associated with recidivism among extra-familial child molesters. *Journal of Consulting and Clinical Psychology, 65,* 141–149.

Prentky, R. A., Lee, A. F. S., Knight, R. A., & Cerce, D. (1997). Recidivism rates among child molesters and rapists: A methodological analysis. *Law and Human Behavior, 21,* 635–659.

Pribor, E. F., & Dinwiddie, S. H. (1992). Psychiatric correlates of incest in childhood. *American Journal Psychiatry, 1,* 52–56.

Quinsey, V. (1977). The assessment and treatment of child molesters: A review. *Canadian Psychological Review, 18,* 204–220.

Quinsey, V. L. (1986). Men who have sex with children. In D. Weisstub (Ed.)., *Law and mental health: International perspectives* (Vol. 2, pp. 140–172). New York: Pergamon.

Quinsey, V. L., & Chaplin, T. C. (l988). Penile responses of child molesters and normals to descriptions of encounters with children involving sex and violence. *Journal of Interpersonal Violence, 3,* 259–274.

Quinsey, V. L., Rice, M. E., & Harris, G. T. (1995). Actuarial prediction of sexual recidivism. *Journal of Interpersonal Violence, 10,* 85–105.

Radzinowicz, L. (1948). *History of English criminal law* (Vol. 1). New York: Macmillan.

Radzinowlcz, L. (1957). *Sexual offenses.* London: Macmillan.

Rice, M. E., Quinsey, V. L., & Harris, G. T. (1991). Sexual recidivism among child molesters released from a maximum security psychiatric institution. *Journal of Consulting and Clinical Psychology, 59,* 381–386.

Rivera, B., & Widom, C. S. (1990). Childhood victimization and violent offending. *Violence and Victims, 5,* 19–35.

Rogers, C. M., & Terry, T. (1984). Clinical interventions with boy victims of sexual abuse. In I. Stuart & J. Greer (Eds.), *Victims of sexual aggression* (pp. 91–104). City: Publisher.

Romero, J. J., & Williams, L. M. (1985). Recidivism among convicted sex offenders: A 10-year follow-up study. *Federal Probation, 49,* 58–64.

Ross, C. A., Norton, G. R., & Wozney, K. (1989). Multiple personality disorder: An analysis of 236 cases. *Canadian Journal of Psychiatry, 34,* 413–418.

Ross, C. A., Anderson, G., Heber, S., & Norton, G. R. (1990). Dissociation and abuse among multiple personality patients, prostitutes, and exotic dancers. *Hospital and Community Psychiatry, 41,* 328–330.

Ross, C. A., Miller, S. D., Reagor, P., Bjornson, L., Fraser, G. A., & Anderson, G. (1991). Abuse histories in 102 cases of multiple personality disorder. *Canadian Journal of Psychiatry, 36,* 97–101.

Rowan, A. B., Foy D. W., Rodriguez N., & Ryan, S. (1994). Posttraumatic stress disorder in a clinical sample of adults sexually abused as children. *Child Abuse & Neglect, 18,* 51–61.

Ruggiero, C. (1975). Sexual criminality in early Renaissance. *Journal of Social History, 8,* 18–37.

Sansonnet-Hayden, H., Haley G., Marriage, K., & Fine, S. (1987). Sexual abuse and psychopathology in hospitalized adolescents. *Journal of the American Academy of Child and Adolescent Psychiatry, 26,* 753–757.

Schecter, J. O., Schwartz, H. P., & Greenfield, D. G., (1987). Sexual assault and anorexia nervosa. *International Journal of Eating Disorder, 5,* 313–316.

Schultz, L. G. (1980). The sexual abuse of children and minors: A short history of legal control efforts. In L. G. Schultz (Ed.), *The sexual victimology of youth* (pp. 3–17). Springfield, IL: Thomas.

Schultz, R., Braun, B. G., & Kluft, R. P. (198′9). Multiple personality disorder: Phenomenology of selected variables in comparison to major depression. *Dissociation, 2,* 45–51.

Segal, Z. V., & Marshall, W. L. (1985). Heterosexual social skills in a population of rapists and child molesters. *Journal of Consulting and Clinical Psychology, 53,* 55–63.

Segal, Z. V., & Marshall, W. L. (1986). Discrepancies between self-efficacy predictions and actual performance in a population of rapists and child molesters. *Cognitive Therapy and Research, 10,* 363–376.

Seghorn, T. K., Prentky, R. A., & Boucher, R. J. (1987). Childhood sexual abuse in the lives of sexually aggressive offenders. *Journal of the American Academy of Child and Adolescent Psychiatry, 26,* 262–267.

Seidman, B., Marshall, W. L., Hudson, S., & Robertson, P. J. (1994). An examination of intimacy and loneliness in sex offenders. *Journal of Interpersonal Violence, 9,* 518–534.

Sgroi, S. (1982). Handbook of clinical intervention in child sexual abuse. Lexington, MA: Lexington Books.

Silbert, M. H., & Pines, A. M. (1981). Sexual child abuse as an antecedent to prostitution. *Child Abuse & Neglect, 5,* 407–411.

Simon, L. M. J., Sales, B., Kaszniak, A., & Kahn, M. (1992). Characteristics of child molesters. Implications for the fixated–regressed dichotomy. *Journal of Interpersonal Violence, 7,* 211–225.

Soothill, K. L., & Gibbens, T. C. N. (1978). Recidivism of sexual offenders: A re-appraisal. *British Journal of Criminology, 18,* 267–276.

Soothill, K. L., Jack, A., & Gibbens, T. C. N. (1976). Rape: A 22-year cohort study. *Medicine, Science and Law, 16,* 62–69.

Stein J. A., Golding, J. M., Siegel, J. M., Burnam, A. M., & Sorenson, S. B. (1988). Long-term psychological sequelae of child sexual abuse. In G. E. Wyatt & G. J. Powell (Eds.), *Lasting effects of child sexual abuse* (pp. 135–154), Newbury Park, CA: Sage.

Stone, M. H. (1990). Incest in the borderline patient. In R. P. Kluft (Ed.), *Incest-related syndromes in adult psychopathology* (pp. 183–204). Washington, DC: American Psychiatric Press.

Swanson, D. W. (1971). Who violates children sexually? *Medical Aspects of Human Sexuality, 5,* 184–197.

Swett, C., & Halpert, M. (1993). Reported history of physical and sexual abuse in relation to dissociation and other symptomatology in women psychiatric inpatients. *Journal of Interpersonal Violence, 8,* 545–555.

Vizard, E., Monck, E., & Misch, P. (1995). Child and adolescent sex abuse perpetrators: A review of the research literature. *Journal of Child Psychology & Psychiatry, 36,* 731–756.

Ward, T., Hudson, S. M., & Marshall, W. L. (1995). Cognitive distortions and affective deficits in sex offenders: A cognitive deconstructionist interpretation. *Sexual Abuse: A Journal of Research and Treatment, 7,* 67–83.

Ward, T., Hudson, S. M., Marshall, W. L., & Siegert, R. (1995). Attachment style and intimacy deficits in sexual offenders: A theoretical framework. *Sexual Abuse: A Journal of Research and Treatment, 7,* 317–335.

Westen, D., Ludolph, P., Misle, B., Ruffins, S., & Block, J. (1990). Physical and sexual abuse in adolescent girls with borderline personality disorder. *American Journal of Orthopsychiatry, 60,* 55–66.

Whitman, W. P., & Quinsey, V. L. (1981). Heterosexual skill training for institutionalized rapists and child molesters. *Canadian Journal of Behavioral Science, 13,* 105–114.

Widom, C. S. (1989). The cycle of violence. *Science, 244,* 160–166.

Widom, C. S., & Ames, A. (1994). Criminal consequences of childhood sexual victimization. *Child Abuse & Neglect, 18,* 303–318.

Winfield, I., George, L. K., Swartz, M., & Blazer, D. G. (1990). Sexual assault and psychiatric disorders among a community sample of women. *American Journal of Psychiatry, 147,* 335–341.

Wolfe, D. A., Sas, L., & Wekerle, C. (1994). Factors associated with the development of posttraumatic stress disorder among child victims of sexual abuse. *Child Abuse & Neglect, 18,* 37–50.

Wolfe, V. V., Gentile, C., Michienzi, T., Sas, L., & Wolfe, D. A. (1991). The Children's Impact of Traumatic Events Scale: A measure of post-sexual-abuse PTSD symptoms. *Behavioral Assessment, 13,* 359–383.

Worling, J. R. (1995). Sexual abuse histories of adolescent male sex offenders: Differences on the basis of the age and gender of their victims. *Journal of Abnormal Psychology, 104,* 610–613.

Wyatt, G. E., & Guthrie, D., & Notgrass, C. M., (1992). Differential effects of women's child sexual abuse and subsequent sexual revictimization. *Journal of Consulting and Clinical Psychology, 60,* 167–173.

Yates, A. (1982). Children eroticized by incest. *American Journal of Psychiatry, 139,* 482–485.

V

FAMILY VIOLENCE

Adolescent Victims and Intergenerational Issues in Sexual Abuse

Debra B. Hecht and David J. Hansen

Introduction

The transitional period of adolescence is characterized by a number of changes and challenges that occur both within and outside the individual. Many developmental events occur during adolescence that have a significant impact on an adolescent's functioning, including a variety of physical, cognitive, emotional, behavioral, and social changes. In addition, adolescents may experience a variety of other important events, such as peer group changes, school moves, changes in family structure or functioning, and alterations in societal and community expectations (Hansen, Giacoletti, & Nangle, 1995; Peterson & Hamburg, 1986). Unfortunately, many adolescents are further challenged by being a victim of sexual abuse.

The widespread prevalence of sexual abuse and the numerous problems and consequences associated with it have been increasingly recognized in recent decades (e.g., Browne & Finkelhor, 1986; Faller, 1993; V. V. Wolfe & Wolfe, 1988). In addition, much has been learned about the treatment of sexually abused children and adolescents during that time (e.g., Hansen, Hecht, & Futa, 1998; O'Donohue & Elliot, 1992). Given that victims of sexual abuse are at risk to develop sexualized behaviors, and that adolescents, for a variety of reasons (e.g., puberty, peer influences) are likely to begin engaging in sexual acts, this population needs special attention to help prevent the intergenerational transmission of abuse.

This chapter addresses sexual abuse of adolescent victims and intergenerational issues in sexual abuse. The problem of sexual abuse is described, including historical background and epidemiological information. The potential impact and correlates of sexual abuse are discussed, including characteristics of adolescent victims and their

Debra B. Hecht and David J. Hansen • Department of Psychology, University of Nebraska–Lincoln, Lincoln, Nebraska 68588-0308.

Handbook of Psychological Approaches with Violent Offenders: Contemporary Strategies and Issues, edited by Van Hasselt and Hersen. Kluwer Academic/Plenum Publishers, New York, 1999.

families. The assessment and treatment of sexually abused adolescents is described, with attention to issues of prognosis and clinical management.

Description of the Problem

Child sexual abuse is a growing problem in today's society, and surprisingly, no definitional criteria have been universally accepted (Hansen *et al.*,1998; V. V. Wolfe & Wolfe, 1988). Most definitions of sexual abuse consist of two main components: the specific sexual behaviors involved and the ages of the victim and the perpetrator (Browne & Finkelhor, 1986; V. V. Wolfe & Wolfe, 1988). Definitions usually emphasize that the sexual activity has occurred between children (e.g., under the age of 16) and older persons (generally defined as more than 5 years older than the child). This often creates some ambiguity when deciding whether sexual abuse has occurred with an adolescent, either as a victim or a perpetrator, because often the age difference is not as great as 5 years, but nonconsensual sex has occurred.

Sexual abuse tends to refer to a broad range of behaviors from noncontact to contact offenses. Noncontact activities include behaviors such as genital exposure, voyeurism, and pornography. Contact offenses refer to genital manipulation, digital or object penetration, penile penetration, and oral sex. In addition to the age and sexual behavior components, the relationship between the child and perpetrator is usually considered in the definition of sexual abuse. If the perpetrator is a family member, including distant relations, in-laws, and step-relatives, the abuse is considered intrafamilial sexual abuse or incest. If the perpetrator is an individual not related by marriage or blood, the abuse is considered extrafamilial. Most cases of abuse involve someone known to the family, however, whether or not an official family member (V. V. Wolfe & Wolfe, 1988).

Lourie (1977) outlined a typology describing the onset of adolescent maltreatment. Type I refers to abuse that began in childhood and has continued into adolescence. Type II describes those cases in which the nature and amount of abuse increases in severity during the adolescent years, and is seen to be a result of the parents' inability or unwillingness to accept the adolescent's attempts at separation and individuation (Lourie, 1977; Williamson, Borduin, & Howe, 1991). Type III abuse includes those instances when the abuse begins in adolescence, and again it is hypothesized that issues surrounding autonomy are a major contributing factor.

The effects and incidence of adolescent abuse may be overlooked for various reasons (Blythe, Hodges, & Guterman, 1990; Lourie, 1977). Adolescent victims often are not brought to the attention of the authorities. Abuse in adolescence is thought to be harder to identify; there often is confusion between some of the telltale acting-out behaviors that are present in child victims and the normal developmental changes that are present in many adolescents (Blythe *et al.*, 1990). This may be especially true with respect to sexual behaviors. It can be quite difficult at times to draw the line between normal experimentation and deviant behaviors. More details about the incidence and effects of abuse are described in later sections.

Historical Background

Adolescence covers the period typically beginning at puberty and extending to a socially defined period of "adulthood" which is not marked by any physical change.

The end of adolescence tends to be defined more by legal statutes (e.g., voting and military age, ability to get married without parental consent or purchase alcohol). Although adolescents are now considered a distinct category of people in our society, this was not always true. Throughout much of history, adolescents were considered to be adults; with puberty came the rights and responsibilities of adulthood (Gonsiorek, 1994b). In our society, the concept of adolescence was largely initiated during the social and political changes of the industrial revolution, with larger cities, immigration of many youth, more property subject to delinquency, and changes in social policies and laws (e.g., compulsory education, child labor laws, special legal procedures for juveniles) (Gonsiorek, 1994b). With the concept of adolescence came changes in societal expectations regarding education, work, sexual activity, and marriage. Now with so many young people attending college, there appears to be a trend to prolong adolescence past the age of majority (Gonsiorek, 1994a).

Children and adolescents throughout much of history often have been treated with cruelty and received little protection from such treatment. Unfortunately, widespread societal concern over any form of child abuse as a significant problem dates back only to the 1950s and 1960s. Some of the original professional and public attention was focused more on the impact of physical abuse, following the description of the "battered child syndrome" (Kempe, Silverman, Steele, Droegenmueller, & Silver, 1962). In recent decades, protection efforts for sexually abused children and adolescents have steadily increased, perhaps because of frequent and intense attention from diverse sectors of society—the media, the general public, the professional community, and legislators. The study of sexual abuse is also a relatively recent development, with a surge of attention in the 1970s as victims came forward and talked about their experiences.

Historically, the involvement of adolescents in committing sexual offenses also received little attention and youth involved in committing sexual assaults were not held responsible for their acts. They were explained as "experimentation," "adolescent adjustment reactions," or as a symptom of a greater emotional disturbance (National Adolescent Perpetrator Network [NAPN], 1993). Cases that were brought to court usually were not prosecuted, or the charges were reduced to a nonsexual offense before being filed (NAPN, 1993). It was not until the late 1970s to early 1980s that the issue of adolescent perpetrators was seriously addressed and interventions were considered and developed (NAPN, 1993). This was partly due to the discovery that adult perpetrators report beginning their offending behaviors while in their teens (Groth, Longo, & McFadin, 1982). The increased attention to adolescent perpetrators logically followed the increased attention to victims, especially when some studies show that more than 50% of male victims were molested by an adolescent (Rogers & Terry, 1984; Showers, Farber, Joseph, Oshino, & Johnson, 1983).

Epidemiology

The National Center on Child Abuse and Neglect (NCCAN, 1996) recently reported the results of the Third National Incidence Study of Child Abuse and Neglect (NIS-3). The NIS-3 is the most comprehensive study of the incidence of child abuse and neglect in the United States. The data were collected in 1993 from a nationally representative sample of more than 5,600 professionals from 842 agencies in 42 counties. The NIS-3 used two types of definitions of abuse and neglect. Children were considered maltreated under the harm standard only if they had already experienced harm (i.e., physical, emotional, or behavioral injury) from maltreatment. Children were considered maltreated under the more inclusive endangerment standard if they experienced maltreatment that put them at risk of harm or if they had already experienced harm. The endangerment standard enlarges the set of those to be considered perpetrators of sexual abuse by permitting children to count in the estimates if they are abused by teenage (i.e., nonadult) caretakers. Overall, there were substantial increases in the incidence of abuse and neglect since the earlier National Incidence Studies (NCCAN, 1996).

Based on the harm standard, it was estimated that 3.2 children per 1,000 (for a total of 217,700 nationwide) were known to be sexually abused in the United States. This is a significant increase over estimates from the earlier NIS Studies (NIS-2 was 1.9 per 1,000; NIS-1 was .7 per 1,000). Based on the endangerment standard, it was estimated that 4.5 children per 1,000 (for a total of 300,200 nationwide) were sexually abused. This is also a significant increase over the 1986 NIS-2 estimates of 2.1 per 1,000. (Endangerment definitions were not used in NIS-1.)

A variety of possible demographic correlates of maltreatment were examined in the NIS-3. The rates of sexual abuse (based on the harm standard) for males was 1.6 per 1,000 while the rate for females was over three times higher at 4.9 per 1,000. The rates according to the endangerment standard were 2.3 per 1,000 for males and 6.8 per 1,000 for females. Children from birth to 2 years were least likely to be sexually abused, and the rates of abuse were relatively constant across the ages from 3 years on. There were no significant race differences in the incidence of maltreatment or maltreatment-related injuries.

Rates of sexual abuse (harm standard) by family income were 7.0 per 1,000 for incomes less than $15,000 per year, 2.8 per 1,000 for incomes between $15,000 and $29,000, and .4 per 1,000 for incomes of $30,000 and greater. The rates according to the endangerment standard for these income groups were 9.2., 4.2, and 0.5 per 1,000, respectively. No differences in rates of sexual abuse were found for families of different sizes (i.e., number of children) or structure (i.e., single or two-parent family). No differences were found for metropolitan status of the community (i.e., very large urban, moderate urban, suburban, and rural).

Of the children who were sexually abused, 34% were reported to have serious or even fatal injury, 12% were reported to have moderate injury, and the remainder were determined to have inferred injury (i.e., it was assumed that some emotional, physical, or behavioral consequences of various levels of severity would have occurred). Across forms of abuse, males were 24% more likely than females to suffer serious injury. Children from the lowest income families (less than $15,000) were over 22 times more likely to be seriously injured from maltreatment than children from the higher income families.

These incidence figures probably underestimate the extent of the problem because these are only cases known to relevant agencies. Because of changes in child abuse definitions and the identification and handling of cases, estimates of the number of children abused in the United States have increased greatly over the past several years. It is unclear whether the figures reflect an actual increase in incidence or an increase in reporting due to growing public awareness, or both. Sexual abuse of adolescents is believed to be more underreported than sexual abuse of children because the public does not perceive adolescents at as much risk and adolescents are seen as better able to fight back or remove themselves from the situation.

Incidence figures reflect only cases that occurred and were identified during the year investigated (e.g., 1993 for the NIS-3). Estimates of the prevalence of sexual abuse, which addresses the total number of persons sexually abused during childhood, are much larger and rather speculative. Professionals estimate that between1 in 3 and 1 in 4 females are sexually abused in some way during childhood (Faller, 1993). Rates for males are believed to be approximately 1 in 10, with some suggesting that it may be as many as 1 in 6 (Faller, 1993).

It may be that male victims are less likely to be reported or identified compared with female victims. It is often suggested that sexual abuse of males is more underreported than that of females, due to societal tendencies not to view the behavior as abusive (e.g., sexual acts with an older female may be viewed by many, including the victim, as "experience" rather than abuse) (Faller, 1993). In addition, boys tend to be more reluctant to talk about their own victimization (Watkins & Bentovim, 1992). This may be partially due to fears of homosexuality, or their socialization taught them that boys are supposed to be "tough" and the abuse was a failure on their part because they were unable to protect themselves.

Characteristics of the abuse experience also appear to be different between boys and girls. Boys tend to be victimized at younger ages especially when abused within the family (although reports vary on this account), are less likely to present as adolescents, are more likely to have been also physically abused, to have been sexually abused with force, or both, and tend to experience more severe and repeated abuse (Faller, 1989; Watkins & Bentovim, 1992). As mentioned earlier, boys are more likely to be victims of extrafamilial abuse, and tend not to be solo victims (Faller, 1989).

The NIS-3 also collected information about the perpetrators of maltreatment. The perpetrators of sexual abuse (according to the harm standard) were 29% birth parents, 25% other parents and parent substitutes (e.g., adoptive parents, stepparents, foster parents), and 46% others (e.g., other family members or other individuals) (NCCAN, 1996). Approximately 89% of perpetrators were male.

As many as 60% to 80% of adult offenders reported the onset of their sexual offenses as occurring in adolescence (Groth *et al.*, 1982). Some studies have shown that about 20% of sexual assaults on children were committed by adolescents (Bagley & Shewchuk-Dann, 1991; Johnson, 1988), accounting for about 8% of male victims and 15% to 25% of female victims (Ryan, 1988).

Although not all victims of sexual abuse engage in sexually exploitive acts, a large proportion of adult and juvenile offenders report a history of victimization (Johnson, 1988; Watkins & Bentovim, 1992; Worling, 1995). Adolescent offenders against children were significantly more likely to have been abused than those who assaulted peers or adults (20% vs. 4%; Worling, 1995). In addition, those offenders who had male victims had a higher chance of having a history of sexual abuse (Worling, 1995).

Characteristics of the Victim

Developmental Context

Adolescence is a time of individuation and experimentation, marked by the onset of puberty and the emergence of sexual activity. During adolescence, social interactions and relationships become increasingly complicated and adult-like. The peer group becomes larger and more complex, more time is spent with peers, and interactions with opposite-sex peers increase (Hansen *et al.*, 1995). The desire for close friends increases, as adolescents turn to their peers for support formerly provided by the family, and the primarily same-sex interests and playmates of childhood give way to opposite-sex interests and friendships (Hansen, Christopher, & Nangle, 1992; Hansen *et al.*, 1995). The more advanced cognitive and verbal abilities and the physical and emotional changes associated with puberty alter the adolescent's interactions with both same-sex and opposite-sex peers (Hansen *et al.*, 1992). In addition, adolescents experience a variety of other changes within their family, peer group, school, and community (Peterson & Hamburg, 1986).

Kirsh (1984) suggests that adolescence can be divided into three stages. Early adolescence characterizes males ages 12–14 and females ages 11–13. These youth are primarily concerned with adjusting to the changes that their bodies are going through, new sexual feelings, and the fear that they will no longer be cared for as a child. Middle adolescence covers the period 14–16 for males and 13–15 for females. These adolescents tend to focus on becoming emotionally independent of their parents, the attractiveness of their bodies, and their sexual adequacy. Finally, late adolescence describes males and females ages 16–19. These youth are preoccupied with concerns about their adequacies as men and women, their ability to form permanent relationships and to integrate sex and intimacy. As so many of these issues focus around sexuality, adolescents are particularly vulnerable to the impact of sexual abuse and the development of deviant behavior as a result of such abuse.

These developmental considerations are often overlooked in the understanding of the dynamics of abuse, specifically the vulnerability or risk of being abused and the impact that an occurrence of abuse will have on the individual. A recent conceptualization by Finkelhor (1995), developmental victimology, addresses these issues. Throughout childhood, individuals gain and lose characteristics that may make them more or less vulnerable for various types of victimization. For example, sexual maturation may make children, especially girls, at increased risk for sexual abuse (Finkelhor, 1995). As children grow older, they may be more able to run away, fight back, and utilize their social networks to gain support, and therefore are better able to protect themselves and prevent the recurrence of abuse. There also has been a tendency to believe that adolescents, due to their increased control over their environment, are largely responsible for their own victimization (Finkelhor, 1995). In fact, adolescents may give in to social pressures and engage in behaviors (e.g., using drugs and alcohol) that do not facilitate self-protection (Finkelhor, 1995).

The impact of abuse also appears to be related to developmental level. For example, there is some evidence suggesting that prepubescent abuse affects endocrine secretions, possibly resulting in the early onset of puberty (Finkelhor, 1995; Gil, 1996). Puberty brings about many uncomfortable feelings and issues related to body image, and an abusive experience during this time can have wide-ranging impact on an adolescent (Gil, 1996). Cognitively, an important dimension appears to be how children understand the concept of victimization and the perception of responsibility for the event (Finkelhor, 1995). Older children may be more at risk in this respect, as they are more able to understand the stigma associated with victimization. Also, the victim's sense of morality may be impacted, which would affect the way they view their own abuse and would have possible consequences on their future behaviors (Finkelhor, 1995). Their perception of power, right and wrong, and fairness may be shaped by abusive incidents, thus limiting their moral development and creating or encouraging a tendency to commit an abusive act.

Correlates and Possible Consequences

There is no single profile of a sexually abused child, and the extent of the impact of abuse varies from individual to individual. Much of the research has been conducted with children. However, the dynamics and the consequences involved also apply to adolescents, especially since abuse often starts in childhood. Unfortunately, the research evidence is inconclusive as many practical and methodological issues make it difficult to identify the consequences of sexual abuse (Browne & Finkelhor, 1986; Faller, 1993; Finkelhor, 1990; V. V. Wolfe & Wolfe, 1988). The research is primarily correlational; therefore, causal relationships cannot be identified. The research evidence is further limited by the fact that it is unclear whether symptoms in abused children are directly a result of the abuse or more globally a by-product of family pathology and problems (Berliner, 1991; Hansen *et al.*, 1998). As mentioned earlier, normal developmental changes also play a role. Research designs are extremely difficult to implement under these circumstances (e.g., heterogeneous population, developmental considerations, inability to randomly assign subjects or manipulate variables of interest, multiple possible variables to assess, multiple etiological and maintaining factors). The fact that abusive acts are illegal, private, and sometimes of relatively low frequency, also complicates research efforts because of the difficulty of assessment. The secrecy and shame associated with the abuse may cause many people never to disclose their experiences. Typically the most severe cases are the most likely to come to the authorities' attention, thus creating a biased sample. Despite the complexity of the issue, the available research in the field provides some insights regarding the varied possible consequences of child sexual abuse.

A number of studies and reviews have addressed the consequences of child sexual abuse (see reviews by Browne & Finkelhor, 1986; Faller, 1993; Finkelhor, 1990; V. V. Wolfe & Wolfe, 1988). The possible psychological consequences of sexual abuse are numerous and variable and no symptom or syndrome is found universally in all victims. It has been estimated that as many as 50% of abuse victims may be asymptomatic (Beutler *et al.*, 1994). Many variables may affect whether and how abuse has an impact, including factors such as the gender of the victim and perpetrator, the type and severity of abuse, and the duration of and time since the abuse, and family reaction following disclosure (Browne & Finkelhor, 1986; Faller, 1993). It may be that some victims are not strongly affected by abuse due to "protective" factors that prevent the negative effects of maltreatment (e.g., good family and social support, positive school experiences, therapy) (Falshaw, Browne, & Hollin, 1996).

Research has found sexual abuse to be associated with a number of internalizing behaviors, including anxiety (e.g., McClellan, Adams, Douglas, McCurry, & Storck, 1995), depression (e.g., Livingston, 1987; Wozencraft, Wagner, & Pelligrin, 1991), problems with self-esteem (e.g., Tong, Oates, & McDowell, 1987), suicidal ideation and attempts (e.g., Bayatpour, Wells, & Holford, 1992; McClellan *et al.*, 1995; Wozencraft *et al.*, 1991), sleep disturbances (e.g., McClellan *et al.*, 1995; Wells, McCann, Adams, Voris, & Ensign, 1995), somatic complaints (e.g., Livingston, 1987), and fear of males (e.g., Wells *et al.*, 1995). A number of studies have also noted the presence of externalizing behavior problems, including self-abusive behaviors (e.g., McClellan *et* al., 1995), delinquency (e.g., Einbender & Friedrich, 1989), and cruelty (e.g., Einbender & Friedrich, 1989; McClellan et al., 1995). In addition, problems with school performance (e.g., Einbender & Friedrich, 1989; Wells et al., 1995) and concentration (e.g., Wells et al., 1995), as well as problems with relationships and social competence (e.g., Einbender & Friedrich, 1989) have been identified as correlates of child sexual abuse.

Adolescent victims of sexual abuse may also exhibit substance abuse problems (Harrison, Hoffman, & Edwall, 1989; McClellan et al., 1995; Singer, Song, & Ochberg, 1994).). It has been suggested that the antecedents of alcoholism are similar to the consequences of sexual abuse, especially the factors of social isolation and emotional disturbances (B. A. Miller, Downs, Gondoli, & Keil, 1987) Further, youth with a history of victimization saw greater perceived benefits (e.g., tension reduction, escape from family problems) in using substances, which led to increased levels of intoxication and drug use (Harrison et al., 1989; Singer et al., 1994).

Sexual behavior is another possible area of impact. Sexually abused children appear to know more about sex and are more interested and curious about sexual matters or genital regions (e.g., Friedrich & Reams, 1987; Wells et al., 1995). Heightened sexual activity, such as compulsive masturbation, precocious sexual play, and overt sexual acting out toward adults and peers have been found among abused youth (e.g., McClellan et al., 1995). Another possible consequence of sexual abuse is self-consciousness about the youth's own body (Wells et al., 1995).

Reviews of teen pregnancies show that 50%–66% of adolescents who become mothers have a history of sexual abuse (Lanz, 1995; Rainey, Stevens-Simon, & Kaplan, 1995). These rates greatly exceed the incidence of reported rape and child sexual abuse found in the general population (Lanz, 1995; Rainey et al., 1995). There is some evidence that sexually abused youth who become pregnant are likely to have multiple behavior problems, such as prepregnancy and perinatal substance abuse and suicide attempts (Bayatpour et al., 1992; Lanz, 1995). Pregnant teens with a history of sexual abuse also report higher levels of depression, anxiety, family dysfunction, and lower self-esteem than those without a history of victimization (Lanz, 1995; Rainey et al., 1995).

It commonly is believed that males tend to respond to abuse, as well as other stressors, with externalizing behaviors while females typically exhibit internalizing problems. Research to date with victims of sexual abuse does not support this general proposition (Watkins & Bentovim, 1992). Initially, boys, like girls, may respond with sexualized behavior (Watkins & Bentovim, 1992). Sexually abused boys are seen to have greater sexual identity confusion, lower self-esteem, and greater sexual dysfunction (Watkins & Bentovim, 1992). Although sexually abused males report less psychological harm than sexually abused females, abused males exhibit more depression, anxiety, and interpersonal problems than nonabused males, and also have a greater preponderance of suicidal feelings and behaviors (Watkins & Bentovim, 1992).

For males, an additional consideration may be their sexual self-concept (Richardson, Meredith, & Abbot, 1993). Sexual self-concept is defined as the sex-typed role that a person identifies with and uses to describe oneself. This type of self-concept is typically categorized as masculine, feminine, androgynous, or undifferentiated (Bem, 1974). Sexually abused adolescent males are more likely than nonabused males to report undifferentiated sexual self-concepts, suggesting a poorly developed sense of sexual identity (Richardson et al., 1993). Correlates of this undifferentiated concept include poor adjustment, poor social relations, and lower self-esteem.

Many scholars have tried to characterize the effects that abuse has on children and adolescents (e.g., Conte, 1985; Finkelhor, 1984; Friedrich, 1995). A conceptualization offered by Friedrich (1995), for example, categorizes the impact of trauma according to three dimensions: attachment, self-regulation, and self-perspective. Attachment problems refer to the detachment and interpersonal problems that are often present in abuse victims. This includes difficulties in trusting others and hypervigilance. Difficulties in self-regulation include behavioral problems such as impulsivity, aggression, and sexual acting out. Finally, self-perspective refers to the adolescent's integration of the abuse into his or her own sense of self, often leading to a negative self-image and identity problems.

Conceptualizations About the Impact of Sex Abuse

A variety of conceptualizations have also been offered to explain how sexual abuse has an impact. Understanding the possible mechanisms for the impact of abuse may be useful for assessment and treatment, as well as prevention of further problems, including offending behavior. Finkelhor (Browne & Finkelhor, 1985, 1986; Finkelhor & Browne, 1985) proposed one of the best-known conceptualizations of the psychological impact of sexual abuse. In this model, sexual abuse is analyzed in terms of four trauma causing factors or "traumagenic dynamics": traumatic sexualization, betrayal, powerlessness, and stigmatization. Traumatic sexualization is the process by which the child's sexuality is affected in a way that is developmentally inappropriate and interpersonally dysfunctional. Betrayal refers to the dynamic wherein a person upon whom the child once depended has caused harm. The child's trust and vulnerability are manipulated, expectations that others will provide protection are violated, and there is a lack of support and protection from caregivers. Powerlessness or disempowerment refers to the dynamic in which the victim's will, desires, and sense of efficacy are compromised. The dynamic includes the invasion of bodily territory, the use of force or trickery to involve the child, the child's inability to believe the abuse occurred, and feelings of vulnerability, fear, and the inability to protect oneself. The final traumagenic dynamic is stigmatization, which refers to the negative feelings of guilt, shame, lowered self-esteem, and a sense of differentness from others. This traumagenic conceptualization of the impact of sexual abuse is one of the most parsimonious and comprehensive models to date; yet, the model is subject to criticism. For example, these dynamics have not been demonstrated to be consequences of abuse, the extent or presence of these dynamics varies considerably, and not all victims experience all dynamics (Conte, 1990).

Conte (1985, 1990) suggested that sexual abuse has first- and second-order sources of trauma or impact. First-order factors are the direct result of sexual abuse, such as the sexual behavior itself and actions by perpetrators to gain sexual access to the child and maintain silence (e.g., threat, force, bribes). Second-order factors result from processing first-order events. For example, threats or force may create fear, which may result in the development of abuse-specific fears (e.g., fear of the perpetrator or the location where the abuse occurred) or more general fear (e.g., men).

Newberger and DeVos (1988) offered a transactional model that identifies the process of interaction among three dimensions in the impact and recovery from sexual abuse: social cognition, environmental sensitivity, and emotional-behavioral functioning. The social cognition domain consists of the youth's cognitive appraisal of the event. Beliefs about control and personal efficacy potentially influence the outcome of abuse. For example, the belief that the victimization is one's own fault may contribute to poorer outcomes. The second domain, environmental sensitivity, suggests that the environmental context influences the youth's psychological processes and functioning. Interactions with parents, relatives, friends, adults, community institutions (i.e., school, sports teams), legal and law enforcement institutions, and therapists may lessen or exacerbate the impact of abuse. The final domain consists of the youth's emotional (e.g., distress, anxiety, depression) and behavioral functioning (e.g., aggression, somatization, sexualized behavior, achievement). The domains are believed to be active and mutually influence one another, so that alterations in one domain change functioning in other domains (Newberger & DeVos, 1988).

Risk of Becoming an Offender

Victims of sexual abuse are at increased risk of becoming offenders (e.g., Bagley & Shewchuk-Dann, 1991; Rasmussen, Burton, & Christopherson, 1992). In fact, many of the correlates of sexual abuse also are correlates of offending; such correlates are marital tension in the family, maternal psychopathology, paternal psychopathology (particularly alcoholism), and harsh discipline (Bagley & Shewchuk-Dann, 1991). Other factors associated with sexual offending include depression, anxiety, social inadequacy and self-concept problems, lack of intimacy, and lack of accountability for one's actions (Bagley & Shewchuk-Dann, 1991; Rasmussen *et al.*, 1992). Additional common precursors to offending behavior include hyperactivity, impulsiveness, and learning disorders (Bagley & Shewchuk-Dann, 1991; Watkins & Bentovim, 1992). Since the majority of known sex offenders are male, special consideration needs to be paid to the circumstances surrounding male victims (Faller, 1989).

Based on the available research, Watkins and Bentovim (1992) have proposed a model of perpetrator risk following sexual abuse. They proposed that being male is a risk, and that being molested by a male or having had multiple perpetrators places one at greater risk. If the perpetrator is a close relative, risk is also increased. In addition, more severe abuse, repeated over time increases the chances that the victim will later offend. When the victim is young (e.g., under 8 years of age), the chances are increased that he will eventually offend. Other risk factors include the diagnoses of Conduct Disorder, Posttraumatic Stress Disorder, Attention Deficit Disorder, and Learning Disabilities. In addition, children exhibiting anxious sexualization (e.g., a dysphoric aspect associated with the sexualized behavior), externalized coping strategies, sexual identity confusion, or who identify with the aggressor are at greater risk. Those who are isolated and do not get treatment for their own abuse also may be at increased risk to offend.

Finkelhor (1984) has developed the Four Preconditions Model of Sexual Abuse; a potential offender must meet these preconditions before committing an assault. First, the potential offender must be motivated to abuse. This suggests that the offender feels that relating to the child will fulfill an emotional need, and that other sources of sexual release are not perceived to be available, or are not as satisfying. This motivation may also be connected to a need for power and control, or it may be a reenactment of the potential offender's own personal trauma. This "cycle of abuse," or reenactment, may be an attempt to achieve mastery over the conflicts of past history, and may condition the potential offender to become sexually aroused by assaultive fantasies (Worling, 1995). Second, Finkelhor (1984) discussed the importance of overcoming internal inhibitors. The use of alcohol or the presence of psychosis or an impulse disorder may enable the potential offender to overcome these inhibitions. Family dynamics that support incestuous relationships also may contribute, and may help to explain the intergenerational transmission of abuse. The third precondition involves predispositions to overcoming external inhibitors. These consist of having an absent, ill or emotionally distant mother in the child's family, a patriarchical father, or social isolation of the family. Poor supervision of the child and the potential offender helps to remove some of these external constraints. Finally, the potential offender must overcome the child's resistance. In many cases, this means that the child trusts the offender due to their prior relationship, or the child is insecure, deprived, or both, or merely lacks knowledge of sexual abuse.

Lane (1991) has proposed a Sex Abuse Cycle, which details the thoughts and characteristics of potential offenders that may contribute to their behavioral choices. Lane focused on the power-based thinking and cognitive errors in which these individuals engage. Specifically, these adolescents feel that they are unable to control the environment (perhaps due to their own victimization), and think that gaining power and domination resolves problems. This identification with their own offender is not uncommon, and often can lead to the reduction of anxiety surrounding their own abuse (Watkins & Bentovim, 1992). These youth also tend to exhibit some conduct disordered beliefs, such as that having an urge or impulse, acting on it, and "getting away" with it is a sign of competence, and that it is acceptable to manipulate others (Lane, 1991). Acts of delinquency might actually give these youth a sense of control, and they might learn that intimidation and coercion are reliable ways of meeting their goals. Lane (1991) further described these potential offenders as having no empathy. They typically have unrealistic expectations and a sense of ownership and entitlement. They refuse to accept responsibility for their acts, and often do not think ahead to the consequences of their actions. Ryan (1991a) suggested that the anxiety that occurs after the first offense is commonly overcome by feelings of entitlement.

Family Patterns

The response to adolescence often depends on the type of family structure that is present and the family response can affect the likelihood of maltreatment and its impact (Garbarino, 1989; Lourie, 1977; Ryan, 1991b). In authoritarian families, there usually is not much freedom afforded to the adolescent, which may lead the adolescent to either rebel or become overly dependent (Garbarino, 1989). If the parental discipline has been unduly harsh, there is a chance that the youth will become overtly aggressive and hostile (Garbarino, 1989). Parents in these authoritarian families typically use considerable denial and minimizing, and their marriages are characterized by a lack of intimacy and availability (Pelcovitz, Kaplan, Samit, Krieger, & Cornelius, 1984). The parents are then united when dealing with the acting-out behaviors of their child. Permissive or overindulgent parents may create resentment in adolescents if they are viewed as overprotective, overly indulgent, or enmeshed (Garbarino, 1989). The parents often have a hard time dealing with the potential threat of separation, and due to the overindulgent patterns throughout the youth's childhood, the adolescent may not be prepared for the responsibilities of growing up (Pelcovitz *et al.*,

1984). These adolescents may feel "smothered," especially in intimate and sexual relationships (Garbarino, 1989). Poor supervision in these families may also be a risk related to victimization as well as offending behavior.

Lourie (1977) hypothesized that, for some adolescents, abuse can be a result of the failure of the family to readjust to the structural changes that are created by the youth's movement toward autonomy. In this stage the youth and the family need to accept that the child is moving out of the role of a "controlled and dependent" family member and is separating from the family (Lourie, 1977). The family and adolescent also must adapt to physical changes and sexual maturity.

As some adolescent victims become sexual offenders, it is important to look at family patterns of offenders. Family characteristics that are common among juvenile sex offenders include distant or unstable relationships and unhealthy sexual activities of the adults (e.g., sexually deviant acts or open behavior in front of the child) (Becker, Harris, & Sales, 1993). Coercive patterns may exist, and these manipulative behaviors may be reinforced in the family environment, teaching the youth that coercion is a means of controlling others. These families also tend to be emotionally impoverished, utilizing inappropriate affect and often "scapegoating" the offender with the negative feelings of the family (Ryan, 1991b).

Ryan (1989) went farther to explain three types of family systems associated with juvenile sex offending. The "exploitive family" is characterized by a lack of unconditional positive regard and the child is typically used by the parent or parents to meet their own needs. These parents tend to have very high expectations for their children. The "rigid/enmeshed family" typically has many secrets and is isolated from the external community. Family members are dependent on each other and are afraid of abandonment. "Chaotic/disengaged family" members cannot provide support for one another. They tend to interact in immature ways and concentrate on their own individual crises.

Clinical lore has supported the belief that the intergenerational transmission of maltreatment is a common occurrence. Given the relative lack of empirical evidence to support this link, however, the best that can be said is that a history of abuse is a risk factor to offending behavior (Falshaw et al., 1996; Kaufman & Zigler, 1989; Widom, 1989). Research provides some evidence for the intergenerational transmission of sexual abuse; however, these studies generally suffer from methodological flaws, such as small, nonrepresentative samples and retrospective designs (Kaufman & Zigler, 1989; Watkins & Bentovim, 1992; Widom, 1989). Specific estimates regarding rates of intergenerational transmission of sexual abuse are described later.

Special considerations may be in place for the intergenerational transmission of abuse with adolescent parents. As noted earlier, sexual abuse increases the likelihood of adolescent pregnancy (Lanz, 1995; Rainey et al., 1995). In addition, these mothers may be more likely to have children who are abused. A prospective study by Boyer and Fine (1992) indicated that adolescent mothers who were sexually abused were three times more likely to have children who were maltreated than nonabused adolescent mothers. Another recent investigation showed that a history of chronic sexual abuse increased the chances that an adolescent mother would be involved with Child Protective Services (Spieker, Bensley, McMahon, Fung, & Ossiander, 1996). The majority of cases were reported for neglect, not sexual abuse, however. The mothers who reported histories of abuse also reported less supportive relationships with their families and more prepregnancy drug use (Spieker et al., 1996), suggesting that assessment of additional contextual variables (e.g., family support, substance abuse) is also important in examining possible intergenerational links.

Several theories have attempted to address the mechanisms of transmission. For example, a sociological view suggests that when parents and children share an environment and culture with norms that support abusive behavior, the continuance of abuse is likely (Kaufman & Zigler, 1989). Social learning theory suggests that by witnessing and experiencing the behavior, children are experiencing conditioned patterns of arousal, learning that it is appropriate, and are forming rules and cognitive distortions around these beliefs (Kaufman & Zigler, 1989; Widom, 1989). Psychodynamic approaches suggest that the victim is attempting to overcome the trauma of abuse by identifying with the aggressor (Bagley, Wood, & Young, 1994). Similarly, attachment theory states that internalized representations of past relationships serve as templates that dictate future relationships, and abusive patterns are integrated into these models (Kaufman & Zigler, 1989).

Assessment and Diagnosis

There are two core parts to assessment in cases of adolescent abuse: (1) defining the symptoms that are consequences of the abuse that the adolescent experienced, and (2) identifying the risk factors that may lead the youth to later offend. Of course, there are some unique problems associated with getting information from adolescents, and these are compounded for sexually abused adolescents who for a variety of reasons are often untrusting of others (Azima & Dies, 1989). In cases where perpetration is an issue, the youth may be even less willing to comply, especially given that they are likely to have committed offenses that have not yet been discovered. Adolescents may be unwilling to fill out the "school-like forms" that characterize many assessment measures (Azima & Dies, 1989). These youth also may be afraid of exposing secrets and admitting feelings related to inferiority, sexual inadequacy, and their drug and alcohol use (Azima & Dies, 1989) and will minimize these behaviors. It is important, therefore, to be very straightforward and honest with the adolescent, explaining the constraints of confidentiality, and stressing that honesty in the assessment process will help ensure better treatment. It is helpful to start with some of the more general, less threatening topics in the assessment process, such as measures of global adjustment, mood, or personality, before addressing some of the more intimate topics, such as substance use, sexual history, victimization, and perpetration.

Building rapport is very important, as the clinical interview will often provide some of the most critical information. Given the wide range of possible consequences of sexual abuse, it is necessary to gather information about the youth's functioning across domains (e.g., school, home, peers), as well as a thorough description of family dynamics and their current complaints, symptoms, and level of functioning. Conducting collateral interviews with parents and other significant people (e.g., teachers) is also recommended. Special attention should be paid to those issues that are identified with the risk to sexually offend. These include social isolation, impulsivity, conduct disordered behaviors, and limited cognitive abilities (Watkins & Bentovim, 1992). Questions about any prior involvement with the legal system are also important (Perry & Orchard, 1992), and any deviant activities of the peer group should also be explored (Watkins & Bentovim, 1992). Family characteristics, such as parental behavior and attitudes about sex, as well as parent–child and marital relationships, should be discussed (Watkins & Bentovim, 1992).

Given the range of possible psychological consequences associated with sexual abuse, assessments should address a variety of internalizing and externalizing symptoms. Measures such as the Child Behavior Checklist, Youth and Parent Report (Achenbach, 1991) for younger adolescents and the Symptom Checklist–90-R (Derogatis, 1994) for older adolescents are good measures of global functioning and symptomatology. More specific measures of anxiety and depression may also be helpful. Such measures as the Children's Depression Inventory (Kovacs, 1992), the Reynolds Adolescent Depression Scale (W. M. Reynolds & Coats, 1985), and the Revised Children's Manifest Anxiety Scale (C. R. Reynolds & Richmond, 1978) all contain norms for adolescents. Because higher rates of suicidal ideation and behavior are found among this population of adolescents, special attention should be paid to this issue, and the youth should be asked about suicidal thoughts directly, even if they do not endorse the specific items on the measures. The Inventory of Suicidal Orientation–30 (ISO-30; King & Kowalchuk, 1994) is a useful tool for measuring the magnitude of suicidal thoughts and orientation in adolescents.

Personality measures can also provide useful information about current psychopathology and patterns of functioning that may be maladaptive. The Minnesota Multiphasic Personality Inventory–Adolescent (MMPI-A; Butcher *et al.*, 1992) is a widely used measure of adolescent pathology and functioning, including dimensions such as treatment compliance, attitudes towards therapeutic change, drug and alcohol use, and adolescent-specific areas (e.g., family relationships, school behavior, peer-group influences). This measure also contains validity scales that help indicate whether the respondent is being open or defensive in his or her report. Another measure is the Millon Adolescent Clinical Interview (MACI; Millon, Millon, & Davis, 1993). This self-report inventory was designed specifically to assess adolescent personality characteristics (e.g., submissive, dramatizing, unruly, oppositional) and adolescent concerns (e.g., sexual discomfort, peer insecurity, identity diffusion). It also measures clinical syndromes such as eating dysfunctions, delinquent predisposition, impulsive propensity, and others.

As mentioned earlier, youth who have a history of sexual abuse are well represented among those with substance abuse problems. In addition to the subscales of the MMPI-A and the MACI that address these concerns and the propensity to develop addiction problems, direct measurement and questioning should be used surrounding this issue. The Substance Abuse Subtle Screening Inventory (SASSI), Adolescent Version (G. A. Miller, 1985) differentiates substance abusers from social users, regardless of deliberate deception attempts on the part of the respondent.

In order to assess the risk of an adolescent's turning to sexually aggressive behavior, the clinician has to consider several dimensions. The clinical interview should address accountability, cognitive distortions, self-esteem, and conduct disordered behaviors, since these are all precursors or correlates of offending behavior. Issues of power, entitlement, and poor empathy skills also are important in determining an individual's risk to offend. Even though sexually assaultive behavior may not be present, some of the attitudes and thinking errors that are expressed may be associated with offending behaviors. The assessment should also address attitudes toward sex and dating. Many rape prevention programs work under the assumption that the development of empathy will increase prosocial behavior and decrease aggression

(Schewe & O'Donohue, 1993). Measures such as the Attitudes Towards Rape scale (Feild, 1978) and the Rape Empathy Scale (Deitz, Blackwell, Daley, & Bentley, 1982) can give some indication of an adolescent's beliefs. In addition, knowledge about their fantasies and their initiation into sexual experiences should be obtained. It also might be helpful to ask about family attitudes toward sex and how the youth learned about sex.

If it is known that the youth has sexually offended, additional information should be obtained. Details about the assaults, including the sexual acts performed, the duration and frequency of the offending behavior, the use of force, and the age of the victim or victims are all important. Questions pertaining to victim empathy (e.g., "How did she respond?" "What do you think she was feeling?") should be asked to assess the offender's level of empathy and the extent of distorted thinking that may be present. Other information about the selection and "grooming" of victims, fantasies, and feelings of the offender before and after the assault are important as well, to identify problems and guide treatment.

Course and Prognosis

As noted earlier, research has identified a variety of possible short-term consequences of sexual abuse (Browne & Finkelhor, 1986; Faller, 1993; Finkelhor, 1990; V. V. Wolfe & Wolfe, 1988). Somewhat less is known about the long term consequences of sexual abuse. The research on long-term effects is also complicated by even more obstacles (e.g., the need for longitudinal design) that make it more difficult to identify the correlates and possible consequences of sexual abuse. Commonly identified long-term effects include anxiety, depression, self-destructive behavior, poor self-esteem, feelings of isolation, difficulty trusting others, substance abuse, patterns of revictimization, sexual dysfunction, and sexual deviance (Browne & Finkelhor, 1986; Falshaw et al., 1996; V. V. Wolfe & Wolfe, 1988).

It was also noted earlier that one of the most critical possible consequences of sexual abuse is sexual offending (Bagley & Shewchuk-Dann, 1991; Lane, 1991; Rasmussen et al., 1992). Like all of the research on sexual abuse, however, research in the area of intergenerational effects of sexual abuse on sexual offending is also difficult to conduct and inherently contains some serious methodological problems. For example, longitudinal designs are most informative but few researchers have the resources available for that type of undertaking. In addition, legal records as sources of data on sexual offending do not reflect the cases in which a sexual offense or other deviant act was perpetrated but not reported. The sample sizes are often small and good comparison groups are hard to find.

Although such limitations prevent drawing firm conclusions from the literature, there is some useful information available. For example, research with small samples of male adolescents has found rates of sexual offending subsequent to sexual abuse in 13% (Friedrich, Beilke, & Urquiza, 1988) to 50% (Sansonnett-Hayden, Hayley, Marriage, & Fine, 1987). In a review of the pooled prevalence rate across available research, Watkins and Bentovim (1992) found that 22% of the sexually abused male youth in the various samples exhibited offending behavior. Looking prospectively or retrospectively may affect the results of the studies. Watkins and Bentovim (1992) referred to a study that claimed that a retrospective analysis indicated a 90% rate of intergenerational transmission of physical abuse, while a prospective analysis indicated a rate of only 18%. In a review of related studies involving adolescent male offenders, Worling (1995) found that 31% (range = 19%–55%) reported some form of sexual abuse, which is triple the rate of men in the general population who have experienced sexual abuse.

As we know very little about sexual offending by adolescent females, an unanswered question is why so few females, as compared with males, become abusers as a consequence of their own abuse, especially since higher numbers of female victimization are reported. It has been suggested that women are socialized to be more sexually submissive than men, as well as more nurturing; this socialization pattern decreases the chances that they will act out by creating more internal inhibitions that they must overcome before offending (Watkins & Bentovim, 1992). In addition, boys may have more childhood sexual experiences than girls, and may actually become physiologically aroused and sexually conditioned more quickly than girls (Watkins & Bentovim, 1992).

Some authors have suggested that a specific form of abuse is most likely to lead to the same type of violence (e.g., sexual abuse leads to sexual violence, physical abuse leads to physical violence) (e.g., Bagley *et al.;* Falshaw *et al.,* 1996; Rasmussen *et al.,* 1992; Ryan, 1989). In contrast, some authors have suggested that specific maltreatment type does not lead to the same type of offending and that any type of victimization may lead to any category of crime (Benoit & Kennedy, 1992; Widom & Ames, 1994). There is, however, no clear or inevitable progression from victim to offender (Falshaw *et al.,* 1996). The majority of maltreated children do not become aggressive or delinquent (Falshaw *et al.,* 1996; Widom, 1989).

Clinical Management

Clinical assessment and treatment with adolescents are commonly believed to pose special clinical challenges. In the case of adolescent victims, clinical management is further challenged by the complex picture of sexual abuse. For example, the adolescent can be removed from the home for several reasons. The family may have difficulties that interfere with their ability to take care of the teen. The teen may be in immediate danger from another family member, or the youth's own behavior may be endangering another family member. In addition, there is a need to determine whether the youth can be treated on an outpatient basis. Psychosis, poor impulse control, severe conduct problems, prior treatment failures, and, in the cases of offenders, the amount and severity of the assaults may suggest a more restrictive setting (Di-Giorgio-Miller, 1994). Given the complexities associated with treatment of adolescent sexual abuse, systematic consideration of treatment adherence, generalization, and social validity are needed to facilitate effective assessment, treatment, and research.

The full involvement of the adolescent and family in treatment is essential for treatment success. Three types of treatment adherence are needed: attending sessions regularly, participating within sessions, and completing out-of-session assignments or tasks (e.g., using skills learned) (Lundquist & Hansen, 1998). A variety of possible contextual factors may increase or decrease the likelihood of treatment adherence, including stress factors or setting events, such as conflict within the family, social isolation, low parental education, low socioeconomic status, and so forth. A variety of specific problems can arise, such as transportation problems, illness, forgetting, and parent or family concerns about obtaining mental health services. In addition, the adolescents often do not come to treatment of their own accord. Their parents or other authority figures usually have identified a problem and have required the adolescent to enter treatment. In some cases, the court might be involved and therapy may be mandated.

Given the growing importance of autonomy during adolescence, and the lack of control and power that often goes along with being a victim of abuse, a certain amount of resistance should be expected with this population. Resistance can be seen at micro or macro levels (Sutton & Dixon, 1986). At the micro level, clients can challenge, disagree, and otherwise negate the therapist's suggestions within the session. At the macro level, resistance is evidenced by clients not completing homework assignments, missing appointments, or dropping out of the session. Newman (1994) suggested that the therapist consider the following questions when dealing with client resistance: (a) "What is the function of the client's resistant behaviors?" (b) "How does the client's current resistance fit into his or her developmental/historical pattern of resistance?" (c) "What might be some of the client's idiosyncratic beliefs that are feeding into his or her resistance?" (d) "What might the client fear will happen if he or she complies?" (e) "What skills does the client lack that might make it practically difficult or impossible at this point for him or her to actively collaborate with treatment?" and (f) "What factors in the client's natural environment may be punishing the client's attempts to change?" (pp. 51–55).

In addition to completion of a specific functional analysis of each client's adherence, the clinician should note the general antecedent and consequent strategies that may facilitate treatment adherence. Antecedent strategies include addressing client cognitions that precede or accompany negative reactions to therapy, having an empathic or skilled therapist, involving the client in goal and procedure selection, providing additional stimuli such as reminder cards, beginning with small homework requests and gradually increasing assignments, ensuring that assignments contain specific details relevant to the desired behavior, and providing specific training for the tasks to be implemented (Lundquist & Hansen, 1998). Consequent strategies that may promote adherence include use of praise or tangible reward, and feedback and shaping procedures. In addition, approaches that use both antecedent and consequent strategies are valuable; these approaches include working with referral sources (e.g., schools, courts, Child Protective Services), advocating for the client, using cognitive rehearsal strategies (e.g., self-management, self-reinforcement), and using contingency management and behavioral contracting. Proactive problem solving for potential obstacles to adherence may increase the likelihood of adherence.

As noted earlier, there are some unique problems associated with getting information from adolescents, as they are often untrusting of others and reluctant to comply and participate (Azima & Dies, 1989). In addition, sexual abuse is typically surrounded by secrecy and shame, and is difficult to talk about. The client must be informed that some things cannot be kept confidential (e.g., disclosures of assaults). If the assessment is court-ordered, the information will go to the courts. If new victims or perpetrators are discussed, these must also be reported through the appropriate channels. It is helpful to start with some of the more general, less threatening topics. Building rapport is very important, and could be especially challenging in cases where assessment or treatment is court-ordered. Many times adolescent victims of abuse prefer a female therapist (DiGiorgio-Miller, 1994).

Three types of generalization treatment effects are usually needed: (a) stimulus generalization, including demonstration of behavior gains in other settings or with new people, or both; (b) response generalization, including changes in behaviors that have not been specific targets of intervention; and (c) temporal generalization or maintenance of treatment effects over time. To achieve generalization it is important to program for it actively (Stokes & Osnes, 1989). A wide variety of strategies are possible, including contacting and recruiting natural consequences (e.g., appropriate peer and family reinforcers), training diversely (e.g., using sufficient stimulus and response exemplars), incorporating functional mediators (e.g., common salient physical and social stimuli, self-mediated physical and verbal stimuli), and targeting contextual factors (e.g., social isolation, family stressors) that interfere with skill acquisition or limit use of newly acquired skills (Lundquist & Hansen, 1998; Stokes & Osnes, 1989). Teaching general strategies for problem solving and coping can enhance generalization and maintenance (Stokes & Osnes, 1989). Use of relevant and effective treatment strategies is, of course, the most critical part of achieving lasting, generalized impact.

Group treatment is believed to be useful for enhancing the generalization of treatment (Damon & Waterman, 1986; Hansen *et al.*, 1998). Group treatment provides increased exposure to the problems, strategies, and solutions of others; additional opportunity for modeling of appropriate behaviors and responses; opportunities to rehearse skills with more individuals; and extensive opportunity for feedback, support, and reinforcement from group members and the therapist.

The involvement of the parents in treatment is probably the most important strategy for enhancing maintenance and generalization. Parents are the persons who are responsible for the health, well-being, and safety of the child, and are generally with the child more than any other adult. They are going to be most able to identify and address problems that may arise, both during and long after treatment. The family, as well as the victim, might have faulty attributions about the abuse and the adolescent that need to be addressed (Berliner, 1991). For example, it can be very helpful to deal with the parents' expectations and anxiety about the impact of the abuse on their child (Hansen *et al.*, 1998).

Because of the often intergenerational nature of sex abuse, it is frequently found that the mothers have been sexually abused and they need to work through their own trauma again so that they can be helpful to their children (Damon & Waterman, 1986). There is often an impaired relationship between victims and their mothers, especially in incest cases, and it is often unclear whether symptoms in these youth are directly a result of the abuse or more globally a by-product of family pathology (Berliner, 1991). Involvement of parents in treatment facilitates the identification and remediation of these issues; this should lead to more lasting and generalized effects.

Ensuring that the goals, procedures, and outcomes of therapy are socially or functionally valid is also valuable (Kazdin, 1977). Therapists need to consider whether the treatment goals are what the adolescent, family, and society want and whether achieving the goals would actually improve the adjustment and effectiveness of the individual. Therapists also need to consider whether the adolescent victim and family members consider the assessment and treatment procedures acceptable. Finally, therapists need to consider whether clients and relevant others (e.g., family, teachers, judges, other legal authorities) are satisfied with all of the effects of treatment (i.e., whether behavior changes of individual, social, or applied importance have been achieved).

Treatment adherence, generalization, and social validity have generally been discussed as separate concepts, but it is important to note that there is significant overlap among the concepts (Lundquist & Hansen, 1998). For example, the more socially valid the goals and the procedures, the more likely the client is to adhere to treatment; the more likely the client is to participate in treatment, the more likely the effects will generalize and maintain; the more the effects generalize and maintain, the more socially valid and functional the effects.

Treatment

Given the well-documented problems of sexual abuse, the lack of empirically validated treatments is surprising. Although we have learned much over the years, treatments have typically lacked a theoretical basis and evaluation has been minimal and poorly conducted (Conte, 1990; Hansen et al., 1998; O'Donohue & Elliot, 1992). The treatment literatures relevant for sexually abused adolescents have, for the most part, been developed and evaluated separately; some research addresses the needs of victims (e.g., internalizing and externalizing behaviors, sexual education) and some addresses prevention of sexual offending.

Many of the treatments for adolescents with a history of sexual abuse are described in the literature that focuses on females (e.g., Blick & Porter, 1982; Furniss, Bingley-Miller, & Van Elburg, 1988). The goals of therapy generally deal with helping the adolescents communicate about the abuse experiences, enhance self-esteem, learn and discuss issues surrounding normal sexuality, talk about appropriate family roles and boundaries, overcome isolation, and develop healthy peer relationships (Blick & Porter, 1982; Furniss et al., 1988). Special considerations have been suggested for boys. Specifically, boys need help opening up, especially in asking for help (Watkins & Bentovim, 1992). They also need to discuss their fears and issues surrounding homosexuality and their attitudes toward women, especially family members (Watkins & Bentovim, 1992).

As noted previously, group treatment has advantages for facilitating generalization. Azima and Dies (1989) suggested that a group modality with adolescents has advantages because the format reflects the shift in importance that adolescents typically place on their peers and away from their parents. Group therapy allows them to see themselves in relation to others within a safe environment. It also lets them work through some of their feelings of rebelliousness and hostility toward authority. Mainly, group therapy allows the youth to see that they are not alone, that their problems are not unique, and that there are other people who understand what they are going through, thus reducing their feelings of isolation. The emotional support provided by the group has immediate effects that may ultimately facilitate continued involvement in therapy. Of course, not every youth is a candidate for group therapy, and many adolescents may also require individual and family therapy in addition to the group.

The importance of parental involvement in treatment for enhancing generalization and maintenance has also been discussed. Research indicates that parental support after disclosure may be a key factor in reducing the impact of sexual abuse, including maintaining school performance and peer relations and protection against serious mental health symptoms (Hansen et al., 1998). Poor family support, as evidenced by conflict and poor cohesion, is related to increased likelihood of internalizing and externalizing problems (Friedrich et al., 1988). Support may protect the victims by assisting them in processing what happened to them in a less negative way and ensuring that they obtain needed services (Wozencraft et al., 1991).

Although parental support is important for reducing the effects of sexual abuse, it is important to remember that the family may be experiencing its own emotional distress in reaction to the youth's victimization. When a youth is victimized, it affects not only the abuse victim but the entire family system, and family members may need support for the feelings and stressors that they are experiencing. Davies (1995) examined parental distress and ability to cope following disclosure of extrafamilial sexual abuse. Most parents felt that they needed assistance dealing with the abuse, especially during the early postdisclosure stage. Problems experienced by parents following disclosure included increased strain for both parent–child and spousal relationships, depression, posttraumatic stress, and unresolved anger. Families may not only need assistance in dealing with the aftermath of child sexual abuse, but parents may also need assistance in adjusting to their own preexisting mental health issues. For example, maternal history of sexual abuse or maternal psychiatric symptoms may interact with the youth's response to the sexual abuse (Friedrich & Reams, 1987). Family variables may interact with abuse related variables in a manner that exacerbates or modifies the possible maladjustment noted in sexually abused youth, and thus family therapy may be needed.

A limited number of treatment programs are available for sexual abuse victims and the research evidence supporting them is limited (Hansen et al., 1998; O'Donohue & Elliot, 1992). The majority of available research and treatment programs have addressed younger child victims (e.g., Berliner, 1991; Damon & Waterman, 1986), though clinicians have begun to address the treatment needs of adolescent victims (e.g., Blythe et al., 1990; Gil, 1996; Prendergast, 1994). Unfortunately, even when research or clinical experience suggests that a procedure is effective, other sites may not be able to replicate the process because of the lack of standardized treatment protocols (Hansen et al., 1998).

A newly developed treatment protocol for child and adolescent sexual abuse victims and their nonoffending parents, referred to as Project SAFE (or Sexual Abuse Family Education), was developed from a systematic analysis of the literature (Hecht, Futa, & Hansen, 1995) and based on a three-factor model of the target areas impacted by sexual abuse: the individual or "self" (e.g., self-esteem, guilt, fears); relationships (peer, family); and sex (sexual knowledge, sexual abuse–specific knowledge) (Hansen et al., 1998). This treatment protocol utilizes a parallel group format, with separate groups running simultaneously for the youth and their nonoffending parents. Treatment procedures include education, skill building, problem solving, and support. Treatment modules cover topics such as understanding and recognizing feelings, sharing what happened, addressing family and social support issues, relaxation and coping with feelings, basic education about sex and sexual abuse, and empowerment and self-assertion. Although such standardized treatment programs are valuable and provide guidance for clinicians and researchers alike, more evaluation is needed to firmly establish their impact (Hansen et al., 1998; O'Donohue & Elliot, 1992). The treatment literature in this area is plagued by the methodological problems commonly found in sexual abuse research (e.g., small and heterogenous samples, inability to randomly assign subjects, multiple possible variables to assess and treat) as well as all of the difficulties found in the conduct of treatment research (e.g., difficulty of demonstration of experimental control, lack of adequate comparison groups).

Addressing the current psychological needs of the victims of abuse can also impact the conditions that are associated with the likelihood of future offending. Victims and offenders share many similar characteristics, such as low self-esteem, peer problems, social isolation, feelings of powerlessness, and behavior problems (Watkins & Bentovim, 1992). Certain principles are suggested in the treatment of victims that also pertain to the prevention of future offending. Control is an important factor in abuse, and victims often perceive a lack of control that generalizes from the abuse experience to other aspects of their life. Returning control to the victim is a powerful intervention strategy, and can be accomplished through assisting the victim to make appropriate decisions (Prendergast, 1994). Ambivalent feelings toward the perpetrator also need to be addressed. In many cases, such ambivalence might result in identification with the abuser, leading the victim to then become a perpetrator (Pescosolido, 1993). It is important to teach these adolescents the distinction between caring about a person and liking their behaviors (Prendergast, 1994). Dealing with identity confusion is another critical component of treatment (Pescosolido, 1993; Prendergast, 1994). As discussed earlier, traumatic events can have a considerable impact on the development of a sense of self. This disruption may lead the victim to identify with the abuser, or may create a negative self-image that affects many other aspects of the adolescent's life. Thus, reforming self-image can be an important part of therapy.

Schacht, Kerlinsky, and Carlson (1990) discussed a coed group run with inpatient psychiatric patients who were both victims and offenders. In addition to histories of abuse, these youth also exhibited behaviors such as poor impulse control, poor problem solving, limited insight, and problems with regulation of emotions. The goals of this therapy included ending abusive relationships and developing victim empathy, increased self-respect, willingness to take responsibility for own behaviors, increased impulse control, improved problem-solving skills, decreased anger and depression, improved trust and peer relations, and a positive, open attitude toward sexuality. The therapists reported several special issues that needed to be addressed during treatment. They found that some of the boys felt that they had to be the "abuser" within the group in order to deal with their discomfort. This led to a broader discussion of abuse, including emotional abuse, intimidation, humiliation, and invasion of personal space.

In order to interrupt the cycle of intergenerational abuse, efforts at primary and secondary prevention with high-risk groups are necessary. Primary prevention of perpetration involves social, cultural, and familial change in order to help change the early socialization experiences of the children in the family and community (Ryan, 1991c). Secondary prevention efforts involve intervention with children who have been abused and neglected, physically or sexually or both, institutionalized, or undersocialized (Ryan, 1991c). The approach with adolescents in these preventive efforts should focus on the fostering of empathy in order to prevent exploitive behavior (Hagan, King, & Patros, 1994; Ryan, 1991c). Issues such as helplessness, powerlessness, and perceived lack of control have been identified as triggers that start the assault cycle (Ryan, 1991c). Specifically, youth who are trying to regain a sense of control and well-being often harbor negative and unrealistic expectations about interpersonal relationships, and think that an external source of gratification may compensate for negative experiences.

D. A. Wolfe and his colleagues (1996) have developed an impressive program targeting adolescents at-risk to become offenders. Adolescents with a history of victimization are involved in groups designed to help them understand the abuse of power and control on their own relationships and how this may impact their future behaviors. Specifically, goals for males include being able to identify and express their feelings assertively, recognizing and respecting the personal rights of others, especially in dating situations, and learning to take responsibility for their behavior. For females, the goals are understanding their own personal rights, learning how to take care of their own personal safety, and developing assertive communication skills. This program teaches adolescents the skills to help them build healthy relationships and to recognize and respond to abuse in their own relationships as well as those of peers. It focuses on power dynamics, interpersonal violence, and ways of breaking out of the cycle. Specifically, positive and assertive communication and problem-solving skills are emphasized. In addition to instruction about the skills, the youth are asked to actively use these skills during role-plays. Gender stereotypes are addressed and corrected as well. This treatment protocol has been empirically validated, and is one of the few available programs aimed specifically at the prevention of offending by targeting potential offenders.

Other treatment approaches focus specifically on the problems of an identified adolescent perpetrator, which is tertiary prevention. These programs must address issues such as accountability, the abuse cycle, arousal and fantasy, power and control, the consequences of sexual abuse and victim empathy, cognitive distortions (e.g., denial, minimization), positive and healthy sexuality, impulse control, and skills deficits (NAPN, 1993). Treatment of adolescent sex offenders also involves relapse prevention, or teaching the youth to recognize the precursors to offending behaviors and teaching the skills to interrupt the assault cycle. A variety of literature (e.g., Becker *et al.*, 1993; Perry & Orchard, 1992; Ryan, 1989), including several workbooks and treatment materials (e.g., Kahn, 1990; Steen, 1993), is available that addresses these issues. Detailed elaboration of these approaches is beyond the scope of this chapter but more information can be found in Becker and colleagues (1993) on adolescent sexual offenders.

Conclusion

Adolescence is a transitional developmental period that is characterized by physical, cognitive, social, and emotional changes. Many adolescents are further stressed by being a victim of sexual abuse. Sexual abuse is a widespread problem with serious and varied consequences for adolescent victims. Adolescents, for a variety of reasons (e.g., puberty, peer influences), are likely to begin engaging in sexual acts and victims of sexual abuse are particularly at risk to develop sexualized behaviors. Research evidence suggests that adolescent victims need special attention to help prevent the intergenerational transmission of abuse. Despite the increased attention to the problem of adolescent sexual abuse in recent decades, there is still much to learn about providing effective treatment. Future research must further develop and evaluate effective intervention strategies for adolescent sexual abuse victims, including treatment for the varied consequences of abuse and prevention of offending behavior.

References

Achenbach, T. M. (1991). *Manual for the Child Behavior Checklist/4–18 and 1991 Profile*. Burlington: University of Vermont Press.

Azima, F. J. C., & Dies, K. R. (1989). Clinical research in adolescent group psychotherapy: Status, guidelines, and directions. In F. J. C. Azima & L. H. Richmond (Eds.), *Adolescent group psychotherapy* (pp. 193–223). Madison, CT: International Universities Press.

Bagley, C., & Shewchuk-Dann, D. (1991). Characteristics of 60 children and adolescents who have a history of sexual assault against others: Evidence from a controlled study. *Journal of Child and Youth Care* [Special issue], 43–52.

Bagley, C., Wood, M., & Young, L. (1994). Victim to abuser: Mental health and behavioral sequelae of child sexual abuse in a community survey of young adult males. *Child Abuse & Neglect, 18,* 683–697.

Bayatpour, M., Wells, R. D., & Holford, S. (1992). Physical and sexual abuse as predictors of substance use and suicide among pregnant teenagers. *Journal of Adolescent Health, 13,* 128–132.

Becker, J. V., Harris, C. D., & Sales, B. D. (1993). Juveniles who commit sexual offenses: A critical review of research. In G. C. N. Hall, R. Hirschman, J. R. Grahm, & M. S. Zaragoza (Eds.), *Sexual aggression: Issues in etiology, assessment, and treatment* (pp. 215–228). Washington, DC: Taylor & Francis.

Bem, S. L. (1974). The measurement of psychological androgeny. *Journal of Consulting and Clinical Psychology, 42,* 155–162.

Benoit, J. L., & Kennedy, W. A. (1993). The abuse history of male adolescent sex offenders. *Journal of Interpersonal Violence, 7,* 543–548.

Berliner, L. (1991). Therapy with victimized children and their families. *New Directions for Mental Health Services, 51,* 29–46.

Beutler, L. E., Williams, R. E., & Zetzer, H. A. (1994) Efficacy of treatment for victims of child sexual abuse. *The Future of Children, 4,* 156–175.

Blick, L. C., & Porter, F. S. (1982). Group therapy with female adolescent incest victims. In S. M. Sgroi (Ed.), *Handbook of clinical intervention in child sexual abuse* (pp. 147–176). Lexington, MA: Lexington Books.

Blythe, B., Hodges, V., & Guterman, N. (1990). Intervention for maltreated adolescents. In M. Rothery & G. Cameron (Eds.), *Child maltreatment: Expanding our concept of helping* (pp. 33–47). Hillsdale, NJ: Erlbaum.

Boyer, D., & Fine, D. (1992). Sexual abuse as a factor in adolescent pregnancy and child maltreatment. *Family Planning Perspectives, 24,* 4–12.

Browne, A., & Finkelhor, D. (1985). The traumatic impact of child sexual abuse: A conceptualization. *American Journal of Orthopsychiatry, 55,* 530–541.

Browne, A., & Finkelhor, D. (1986). Impact of child sexual abuse: A review of the research. *Psychological Bulletin, 99,* 66–77.

Butcher, J. N., Williams, C. L., Graham, J. R., Archer, R. P., Tellegen, A., Ben-Porath, Y. S., & Kaemmer, B. (1992). *MMPI-A: Minnesota Multiphasic Personality Inventory–Adolescent*. Minneapolis: University of Minnesota Press.

Conte, J. R. (1985). The effects of sexual abuse on children. A critique and suggestions for future research. *Victimology, 10,* 110–130.

Conte, J. R. (1990). Victims of child sexual abuse. In R. T. Ammerman & M. Hersen (Eds.), *Treatment of family violence: A sourcebook* (pp. 50–76). New York: Wiley.

Damon, L., & Waterman, J. (1986). Parallel group treatment of children and their mothers. In K. MacFarlane & J. Waterman (Eds.), *Sexual abuse of young children* (pp. 244–298). New York: Guilford.

Davies, M. G. (1995). Parental distress and ability to cope following disclosure of extrafamilial sexual abuse. *Child Abuse & Neglect, 19,* 399–408.

Deitz, S., Blackwell, K., Daley, P., & Bentley, B. (1982). Measurement of empathy toward rape victims and rapists. *Journal of Personality and Social Psychology, 43,* 372–383.

Derogatis, L. R. (1994). *SCL-90-R: Administration, scoring, and procedures manual* (3rd ed.). Towson, MD: Clinical Psychometric Research.

DiGiorgio-Miller, J. (1994). Clinical techniques in the treatment of juvenile sex offenders. *Journal of Offender Rehabilitation, 21,* 117–126.

Einbender, A. J., & Friedrich, W. N. (1989). Psychological functioning and behavior of sexually abused girls. *Journal of Consulting and Clinical Psychology, 57,* 155–157.

Faller, K. C. (1989). Characteristics of a clinical sample of sexually abused children: How boy and girl victims differ. *Child Abuse & Neglect, 13,* 281–291.

Faller, K. C. (1993). *Child sexual abuse: Intervention and treatment issues.* Washington, DC: U.S. Department of Health and Human Services.

Falshaw, L., Browne, K. D., & Hollin, C. R. (1996). Victim to offender: A review. *Aggression and Violent Behavior, 4,* 389–404.

Feild, H. S. (1978). Attitudes towards rape: A comparative analysis of police, rapists, crisis counselors and citizens. *Journal of Personality and Social Psychology, 36,* 156–179.

Finkelhor, D. (1984). *Child sexual abuse: New theories and research.* New York: Free Press.

Finkelhor, D. (1990). Early and long-term effects of child sexual abuse: An update. *Professional Psychology: Research and Practice, 21,* 325–330.

Finkelhor, D. (1995). The victimization of children: A developmental perspective. *American Journal of Orthopsychiatry, 65,* 177–193.

Finkelhor, D., & Browne, A. (1985). The traumatic impact of sexual abuse: An update. *Professional Psychology: Research and Practice, 21,* 325–330.

Friedrich, W. N. (1995). Managing disorders of self-regulation in sexually abused boys. In M. Hunter (Ed.), *Child survivors and perpetrators of sexual abuse: Treatment innovations* (pp. 3–23). Newbury Park, CA: Sage.

Friedrich, W. N., & Reams, R. A. (1987). Course of psychological symptoms in sexually abused young children. *Psychotherapy, 24,* 160–170.

Friedrich, W. N., Beilke, R. L., & Urquiza, A. J. (1988). Behaviour problems in young sexually abused boys. *Journal of Interpersonal Violence, 3,* 21–28.

Furniss, T. , Bingley-Miller, L. , & Van Elburg, A. (1988). Goal-oriented group treatment for sexually abused adolescent girls. *British Journal of Psychiatry, 152,* 97–106.

Garbarino, J. (1989). Troubled youth, troubled families: the dynamics of adolescent maltreatment. In D. Cicchetti & V. Carlson (Eds.), *Child maltreatment: Theory and research on the causes and consequences of child abuse and neglect* (pp. 685–706). New York: Cambridge University Press.

Gil, E. (1996). *Treating abused adolescents.* New York: Guilford.

Gonsiorek, J. C. (1994a). Diagnosis and treatment of young adult and adolescent male victims: An individual psychotherapy model. In J. C. Gonsiorek, W. H. Bera, & D. LeTourneau (Eds.), *Male sexual abuse: A trilogy of intervention strategies* (pp. 56–110). Thousand Oaks, CA: Sage.

Gonsiorek, J. C. (1994b). Historical and background perspectives on adolescent and male sexual abuse. In J. C. Gonsiorek, W. H. Bera, & D. LeTourneau (Eds.), *Male sexual abuse: A trilogy of intervention strategies* (pp. 3–20). Thousand Oaks, CA: Sage.

Groth, A. N., Longo, R. E., & McFadin, J. B. (1982). Undetected recidivism among rapists and child molesters. *Crime & Delinquency, 28,* 450–458.

Hagan, M. P., King, R. P., & Patros, R. L. (1994). Recidivism among adolescent perpetrators of sexual assault against children. *Journal of Offender Rehabilitation, 21,* 127–137.

Hansen, D. J., Christopher, J. S., & Nangle, D. W. (1992). Adolescent heterosocial interactions and dating. In V. B. Van Hasselt & M. Hersen (Eds.), *Handbook of social development: A lifespan perspective* (pp. 371–394). New York: Plenum.

Hansen, D. J., Giacoletti, A. M., & Nangle, D. W. (1995). Social interactions and adjustment. In V. B. Van Hasselt & M. Hersen (Eds.), *Handbook of adolescent psychopathology: A guide to diagnosis and treatment* (pp. 102–129). New York: Macmillan.

Hansen, D. J., Hecht, D. B., & Futa, K. T. (1998). In V. B. Van Hasselt & M. Hersen (Eds.), *Handbook of psychological treatment protocols for children and adolescents* (pp. 153–178). New York: Erlbaum.

Harrison, P. A., Hoffman, N. G., & Edwall, G. E. (1989). Sexual abuse correlates: Similarities between male and female adolescents in chemical dependency treatment. *Journal of Adolescent Research, 4,* 382–399.

Hecht, D. B., Futa, K. T., & Hansen, D. J. (1995, November). *A qualitative analysis of group therapy for sexually abused children and adolescents: How prior treatments can guide future interventions.* Paper presented at the Convention of the Association for the Advancement of Behavior Therapy, Washington, DC.

Johnson, T. C. (1988). Child perpetrators—Children who molest other children: Preliminary findings. *Child Abuse & Neglect, 12,* 219–229.

Kahn, T. J. (1990). *Pathways: A guided workbook for youth beginning treatment.* Brandon, VT: Safer Society Press.

Kaufman, J., & Zigler, E. (1989). The intergenerational transmission of child abuse. In D. Cicchetti & V. Carlson (Eds.), *Child maltreatment: Theory and research on the causes and consequences of child abuse and neglect* (pp. 129–150). New York: Cambridge University Press.

Kazdin, A. E. (1977). Assessing the clinical or applied importance of behavior change through social validation. *Behavior Modification, 1,* 427–452.

Kempe, C. H., Silverman, F., Steele, B., Droegenmueller, W., & Silver, H. (1962). The battered child syndrome. *Journal of the American Medical Association, 181,* 17–24.

King, J. D., & Kowalchuk, B. (1994). *ISO-30-Adolescent: Inventory of Suicide Orientation-30.* Minneapolis, MN: National Computer Systems.

Kirsh, S. (1984). Adolescent problems and related practices. In F. Maidman (Ed.), *Child welfare: A source book of knowledge and practice* (pp. 289–323). New York: Child Welfare League of America.

Kovacs, M. (1992). *Children's Depression Inventory.* North Tonowonda, NY: Multi-Health Systems.

Lane, S. (1991). The sexual abuse cycle. In G. D. Ryan & S. L. Lane (Eds.), *Juvenile sexual offending: Causes, consequences, and correction* (pp. 103–141). Lexington, MA: Lexington Books.

Lanz, J. B. (1995). Psychological, behavioral, and social characteristics associated with early forced sexual intercourse among pregnant adolescents. *Journal of Interpersonal Violence, 10,* 188–200.

Livingston, R. (1987). Sexually and physically abused children. *Journal of the American Academy of Child and Adolescent Psychiatry, 26,* 413–415.

Lourie, I. S. (1977). The phenomenon of the abused adolescent: A clinical study. *Victimology: An International Journal, 2,* 268–276.

Lundquist, L. M., & Hansen, D. J. (1998). Enhancing treatment adherence, social validity, and generalization of parent-training interventions with physically abusive and neglectful families. In J. R. Lutzker (Ed.), *Handbook of child abuse research and treatment* (pp. 449–471). New York: Pergamon.

McClellan, J., Adams, J., Douglas, D., McCurry, C., & Storck, M. (1995). Clinical characteristics related to severity of sexual abuse: A study of seriously mentally ill youth. *Child Abuse & Neglect, 19,* 1245–1254.

Miller, B. A., Downs, W. R., Gondoli, D. M., & Keil, A. (1987). The role of childhood sexual abuse in the development of alcoholism in women. *Violence and Victims, 2*(3), 157–172.

Miller, G. A. (1985). *The Substance Abuse Subtle Screening Inventory (SASSI) manual.* Spencer, IN: Spencer Evening World.

Millon, T., Millon, C., & Davis, R. (1993). *MACI manual: Millon Adolescent Clinical Inventory.* Minneapolis. MN: National Computer Systems.

National Adolescent Perpetrator Network. (1993). The revised report from the national task force on juvenile sexual offending. *Juvenile and Family Court Journal, 44*(4), 5–121.

National Center on Child Abuse and Neglect. (1996). *Third national incidence study of child abuse and neglect.* Washington, DC: U.S. Department of Health and Human Services.

Newberger, C. M., & DeVos, E. (1988). Abuse and victimization: A life-span developmental perspective. *American Journal of Orthopsychiatry, 58,* 505–511.

Newman, C. (1994). Understanding client resistance: Methods for enhancing motivation to change. *Cognitive and Behavioral Practice, 1,* 47–69.

O'Donohue, W. T., & Elliot, A. N. (1992). Treatment of the sexually abused child: A review. *Journal of Clinical Child Psychology, 21,* 218–228.

Pelcovitz, D., Kaplan, S., Samit, C., Krieger, R., & Cornelius, D. (1984). Adolescent abuse: Family structure and implications for treatment. *Journal of the American Academy of Child Psychiatry, 23,* 85–90.

Perry, G. P., & Orchard, J. (1992). *Assessment and treatment of adolescent sex offenders.* Sarasota, FL: Professional Resource Press.

Pescosolido, F. J. (1993). Clinical considerations related to victimization dynamics and post-traumatic stress in the group treatment of sexually abused boys. *Journal of Child and Adolescent Group Therapy, 3,* 49–73.

Petersen, A. C., & Hamburg, B. A. (1986). Adolescence: A developmental approach to problems and psychopathology. *Behavior Therapy, 17,* 480–499.

Prendergast, W. E. (1994). Initial steps in treating child and adolescent survivors of sexual abuse. *Journal of Offender Rehabilitation, 21,* 89–115.

Rainey, D. Y., Stevens-Simon, C., & Kaplan, D. W. (1995). Are adolescents who report prior sexual abuse at higher risk for pregnancy. *Child Abuse & Neglect, 10,* 1283–1288.

Rasmussen, L. A., Burton, J. E., & Christopherson, B. J. (1992). Precursors to offending and the trauma outcome process in sexually reactive children. *Journal of Child Sexual Abuse, 1,* 33–48.

Reynolds, C. R., & Richmond, B. O. (1978). What I think and feel: A revised measure of children's manifest anxiety. *Journal of Abnormal Child Psychology, 6,* 271–280.

Reynolds, W. M., & Coats, K. I. (1985). A comparison of cognitive-behavioral therapy and relaxation training for the treatment of depression in adolescents. *Journal of Consulting and Clinical Psychology, 54,* 653–660.

Richardson, M. F., Meredith, W., & Abbot, D. A. (1993). Sex-typed role in male adolescent sexual abuse survivors. *Journal of Family Violence, 8,* 89–100.

Rogers, C. M., & Terry, T. (1984). Clinical intervention with boy victims of sexual abuse. In I. R. Stuart & J. G. Greer (Eds.), *Victims of sexual aggression: Treatment of children, women, and men* (pp. 91–104). New York: Van Nostrand Reinhold.

Ryan, G. (1988, April). *The juvenile sexual offender: A question of diagnosis.* Paper presented at the National Symposium on Child Victimization, Anaheim, CA.

Ryan, G. (1989). Victim to victimizer: Re-thinking victim treatment. *Journal of Interpersonal Violence, 4,* 325–341.

Ryan, G. (1991a). Consequences for the juvenile sex offender. In G. D. Ryan & S. L. Lane (Eds.), *Juvenile sexual offending: Causes, consequences, and correction* (pp. 175–181). Lexington, MA: Lexington Books.

Ryan, G. (1991b). The juvenile sex offender's family. In G. D. Ryan & S. L. Lane (Eds.), *Juvenile sexual offending: Causes, consequences, and correction* (pp. 143–160). Lexington, MA: Lexington Books.

Ryan, G. (1991c). Perpetration prevention: Primary and secondary. In G. D. Ryan & S. L. Lane (Eds.), *Juvenile sexual offending: Causes, consequences, and correction* (pp. 393–408). Lexington, MA: Lexington Books.

Sansonnett-Hayden, H., Hayley, G., Marriage, C., & Fine, S. (1987). Sexual abuse and psychopathology in hospitalized adolescents. *Journal of the American Academy of Child and Adolescent Psychiatry, 26,* 753–757.

Schacht, A. J., Kerlinsky, D., & Carlson, C. (1990). Group therapy with sexually abused boys: Leadership, projective identification, and countertransference issues. *International Journal of Group Psychotherapy, 40,* 401–417.

Schewe, P. A., & O'Donohue, W. (1993). Sexual abuse prevention with high-risk males: The roles of victim empathy and rape myths. *Violence and Victims, 8,* 339–351.

Showers, J., Farber, E. D., Joseph, J. A., Oshino, L., & Johnson, C. F. (1983). The sexual victimization of boys: A three year study. *Health Values: Achieving High Level Wellness, 7,* 15–18.

Singer, M. I., Song, L., & Ochberg, B. (1994). Sexual victimization and substance abuse in psychiatrically hospitalized adolescents. *Social Work Research, 18,* 97–103.

Spieker, S. J., Bensley, L., McMahon, R. J., Fung, H., & Ossiander, E. (1996). Sexual abuse as a factor in child maltreatment by adolescent mothers of preschool aged children. *Development and Psychopathology, 8,* 497–509.

Steen, C. (1993). *The relapse prevention workbook for youth in treatment.* Brandon, VT: Safer Society Press.

Stokes, T. F., & Osnes, P. G. (1989). An operant pursuit of generalization. *Behavior Therapy, 20,* 337–355.

Sutton, C. S., & Dixon, D. (1986). Resistance in parent training: A study of social influence. *Journal of Social and Clinical Psychology, 4,* 133–144.

Tong, L., Oates, K., & McDowell, M. (1987). Personality development following sexual abuse. *Child Abuse & Neglect, 11,* 371–383.

Watkins, B. , & Bentovim, A. (1992). The sexual abuse of male children and adolescents: A review of current research. *Journal of Child Psychology and Psychiatry, 33,* 197–248.

Wells, R. D., McCann, J., Adams, J., Voris, J., & Ensign, J. (1995). Emotional, behavioral, and physical symptoms reported by parents of sexually abused, nonabused, and allegedly abused prepubescent females. *Child Abuse & Neglect, 19,* 155–163.

Widom, C. S. (1989). Does violence beget violence? A critical examination of the literature. *Psychological Bulletin, 106,* 3–28.

Widom, C. S., & Ames, M. A. (1994). Criminal consequences of childhood sexual victimization. *Child Abuse & Neglect, 18,* 308–318.

Williamson, J. M., Borduin, C. M., & Howe, B. A. (1991). The ecology of adolescent maltreatment: A multilevel examination of adolescent physical abuse, sexual abuse, and neglect. *Journal of Consulting and Clinical Psychology, 59,* 449–457.

Wolfe, D. A., Wekerle, C., Gough, R., Reitzel-Jaffe, D., Grasley, C., Pittman, A., Lefebvre, L., & Stumpf, J. (1996). *The youth relationships manual: A group approach with adolescents for the prevention of woman abuse and the promotion of healthy relationships.* Thousand Oaks, CA: Sage.

Wolfe, V. V., & Wolfe, D. A. (1988). The sexually abused child. In E. J. Mash & L. G. Terdal (Eds.), *Behavioral assessment of childhood disorders* (2nd ed., pp. 670–714). New York: Guilford.

Worling, J. R. (1995). Sexual abuse history of adolescent male sex offenders: Differences on the basis of the age and gender of their victims. *Journal of Abnormal Psychology, 104,* 610–613.

Wozencraft, T., Wagner, W., & Pelligrin, A. (1991). Depression and suicidal ideation in sexually abused children. *Child Abuse & Neglect, 15,* 505–511.

Child Physical Abuse and Neglect

Jody E. Warner-Rogers, David J. Hansen, and Debra B. Hecht

Introduction

Children ideally develop and learn about their world from the safe and stimulating environment of their home. Therefore, it is quite disturbing when violence occurs within the supposedly protective domains of the home and the parent–child relationship, although such acts have been committed throughout history (Zigler & Hall, 1989). Even though acts of child maltreatment have a long history, the concept that society should be responsible for the protection of children, including identification, reporting, and treatment of both the victims and perpetrators of maltreatment, is a relatively recent development.

This chapter addresses the physical abuse and neglect of children by their parents. The problems of child physical abuse and neglect are described, including historical and epidemiological information and the characteristics of maltreating parents and families. A discussion of assessment methods as they apply to case conceptualization and treatment is provided. The basis for any well-planned treatment lies in a thorough assessment, and this is particularly true for the complex problem of child maltreatment. Interventions to address the needs of abusive and neglectful parents and prevent the recurrence of maltreatment are also described. In addition, issues in the clinical management of the problems and treatment of these challenging families are discussed.

Description of the Problem

Physical abuse can be defined as an act of "commission," in which physically aggressive behavior on the part of a caretaker is directed toward a child and results in injury or harm to that child (Kelly, 1983b; National Center on Child Abuse and Neglect [NCCAN], 1988). Neglect can take many forms, but has been defined globally as an act of "omission," in which caretakers fail to provide for a child's basic physical,

Jody E. Warner-Rogers • MRC Child Psychiatry Unit, de Crespigny Park, Denmark Hill, London SE5 8AF United Kingdom. *David J. Hansen and Debra B. Hecht* • Department of Psychology, University of Nebraska–Lincoln, Lincoln, Nebraska 68588-0308.

Handbook of Psychological Approaches with Violent Offenders: Contemporary Strategies and Issues, edited by Van Hasselt and Hersen. Kluwer Academic/Plenum Publishers, New York, 1999.

medical, educational, or emotional needs (Kelly, 1983b; NCCAN, 1988). Physical abuse involves discrete incidents of violence directed toward a child. In contrast, neglect is characterized by more chronic patterns of substandard care in which a parent fails to meet the child's basic needs (Kelly, 1983b; Wolfe, 1988). Direct observation of physically abusive or neglectful behavior is uncommon, since it occurs in the relative privacy of the home environment. As a result, identification of both physical abuse and neglect is often based on the consequences of maltreatment rather than observation of actual maltreating behavior (Hansen & Warner, 1994). The immediate consequences of physical abuse (i.e., physical trauma) may be more easily identified compared with the consequences of neglect, which may have neither an immediate nor obvious effect on children's health and development. Although neglect does not involve violent behavior, and the causes of neglect may differ from those involved in physical abuse, the two forms of maltreatment often co-occur (Hansen, Warner-Rogers, & Hecht, 1998).

Throughout their early years, children must learn to negotiate certain central and specific developmental tasks, such as acquiring communication and social skills and learning to regulate their behavior and affect in response to the environment. Maltreatment has been conceptualized as a failure of the environment to provide a child with opportunities for normal development and the acquisition of such knowledge and skills (Cicchetti & Lynch, 1995). Maltreatment undoubtedly presents a serious impediment to a child's behavioral, social, and academic development. In addition to the possibility of physical injury or health problems as a result of maltreatment, physically abused and neglected children have been shown to have delays in language acquisition, deficits in intellectual and academic functioning, aggression and peer problems, and emotional problems such as hopelessness, depression, and low self-worth (see Ammerman, Cassisi, Hersen, & Van Hasselt, 1986; Azar & Wolfe, 1989; Hansen, Conaway, & Christopher, 1990; Malinosky-Rummell & Hansen, 1993). In the most severe cases, the consequences of maltreatment can be fatal—more than 1,000 children die from physical abuse and neglect each year (NCCAN, 1988, 1996).

Abusive and neglectful families tend not to report themselves for treatment; less than 1% of reports to statewide protection agencies are made by the perpetrators (NCCAN, 1994). This has important implications for treatment, as abusive families may not view themselves as having any problems or difficulties in need of intervention. Thus, identification and reporting of physically abusive and neglectful families by professionals is often the first step in the treatment process (Warner & Hansen, 1994). In fact, all states have mandated reporting laws through which physicians, psychologists, teachers, and other professionals are required to report suspected instances of child maltreatment. Despite such laws, research suggests that as many as one third of possible child physical abuse cases remain unidentified or unreported (e.g., NCCAN, 1988, 1996).

Historical Background

Throughout history, children have often been treated with incredible cruelty, including abandonment, domination, beatings, murder, forced labor, and imprisonment (Zigler & Hall, 1989). The historical context of child abuse can be useful for understanding its senselessness and brutality. For example, infanticide during some points of history in some cultures occurred as a population control measure to help the community survive (Zigler & Hall, 1989). Other abuse events have no such contextual factors and appear only senseless and extreme. Although there is evidence in recent decades that child abuse is increasing, Zigler and Hall point out that if one takes a historical view, there has been much improvement in how children have been treated over the ages. Evidence of the abuse of children is as old as recorded history, but the study of child abuse has relatively recent beginnings. Widespread societal concern over child abuse as a significant problem dates back only to the 1950s and 1960s (Hansen *et al.*, 1990; Wolfe, 1988).

"Why does a parent physically abuse his or her child?" is a question professionals have been trying to answer for well over 30 years (Spinetta & Rigler, 1972, p. 296). The medical community was among the first group of professionals to question how and why certain types of childhood injuries could be obtained "accidentally." This line of questioning culminated in the seminal paper by Kempe, Silverman, Steele, Droegemuller, and Silver (1962), which described the "battered child syndrome" and formed the foundations on which theories of assessment and intervention for physically abusive parents were based for many subsequent years.

Initially, a categorical approach was used to conceptualize physically abusive behavior, in part because the initial focus was on very severe maltreatment. Such aggressive and hostile behavior directed toward a child was viewed as a distinct deviation from "normal" parenting behavior and, as such, was thought to be due to severe psychopathology in the parent (Kempe *et al.*, 1962; Steele & Pollack, 1974). The cause of maltreatment was considered unidimensional and direct: psychiatrically disturbed parents abused children.

However, within a few years of the identification of the "battered child syndrome," research showed that the majority of abusive parents were not psychotic and the majority of maltreatment did not result in severe, life-threatening injuries but rather moderate or mild injuries (Kempe & Helfer, 1972; Spinetta & Rigler, 1972). The field broadened from the narrow focus on psychiatric illness of offenders to the more general aspects of parental functioning and the context in which parenting occurs (Belsky & Vondra, 1989). Efforts were made to determine the characteristics of those most at risk for maltreating their children and to identify the situations in which abuse was most likely to occur.

A dimensional approach, which places abusive behavior on a general continuum of parenting practices, evolved to replace the categorical model (Azar & Wolfe, 1989; Hansen *et al.*, 1990; Wolfe, 1988). Those parenting practices considered most unsuitable and harmful to a child are at the negative end of the continuum, while those actions that facilitate social, emotional, and cognitive development comprise the positive end (Azar & Wolfe, 1989). Similarly, disciplinary strategies such as attending to and rewarding prosocial behavior fall at the positive end while harsh, aggressive physical discipline is found at the negative end.

Epidemiology

The Third National Incidence Study of Child Abuse and Neglect (NIS-3), the most comprehensive study of the incidence of child abuse and neglect in the United States, was recently reported by the National Center on Child Abuse and Neglect

(NCCAN, 1996). The NIS-3 data were collected during 1993 from a nationally representative sample of more than 5,600 professionals from 842 agencies in 42 counties. Abuse and neglect were defined according to two standards: (a) the harm standard, in which children were considered maltreated if they had already experienced harm (i.e., physical, emotional, or behavioral injury); and (b) the endangerment standard, a more inclusive standard in which children were considered maltreated if they experienced maltreatment that put them at risk of harm or if they had already experienced harm.

Overall, there were significant increases in the incidence of physical abuse and neglect since the previous National Incidence Studies (NCCAN, 1988, 1996). Based on the harm standard, it was estimated that 5.7 children per 1,000 were physically abused, with an estimated total of 381,700 children nationwide. This is a substantial increase from the earlier studies; the NIS-2 in 1986 was 4.3 children per 1,000 and the NIS-1 in 1980 was 3.1 children per 1,000. Based on the endangerment standard, it was estimated that 9.1 children per 1,000 were physically abused, with an estimated total of 614,100 nationwide. This is also a significant increase over the NIS-2 estimates of 4.9 per 1,000. (Endangerment definitions were not used in NIS-1.)

The incidence of neglect is substantially higher than physical abuse. Based on the harm standard, it was estimated that 13.1 children per 1,000 were neglected, with an estimated total of 879,000 children nationwide. This is a significant increase from the earlier studies; the NIS-2 was 7.5 children per 1,000 and the NIS-1 was 4.9 children per 1,000. Harm standard rates across types of neglect were as follows: physical neglect, 5.0 per 1,000; emotional neglect, 3.2 per 1,000; and educational neglect, 5.9 per 1,000. Based on the endangerment standard, it was estimated that 29.2 children per 1,000 were neglected, with an estimated total of 1,961,300 nationwide. This is also a significant increase over the NIS-2 estimates of 14.6 per 1,000. Endangerment standard rates across types of neglect were as follows: physical neglect, 19.9 per 1,000; emotional neglect, 8.7 per 1,000; and educational neglect, 5.9 per 1,000.

A variety of possible demographic correlates of physical abuse and neglect were examined in the NIS-3. Rates of physical abuse and neglect did not differ for male and female children. The only significant difference found in age for physical abuse was that the incidence of abuse among 12- to 14-year-old youth was more than double the incidence for those 0 to 2 years of age. For neglect the only age difference found was for emotional neglect, where the incidence for children ages 6 and older was six times higher than the incidence for children ages 5 and younger. There were no significant race differences for physical abuse or neglect.

The incidence of physical abuse in low-income families (less than $15,000 family income per year) was more than twice the rate in middle-income families ($15,000 to $29,999 per year) and sixteen times the rate for children in high-income families (more than $30,000 per year). Patterns of neglect showed similar differences. In addition, the abuse experienced by children of lower income families tends to be more severe than that experienced by children from higher income families. These families may be more likely to reside in impoverished communities where resources are scarce.

Physical abuse was significantly more common in father-only households than with two-parent families, whereas rates for single-mother households were not different from two-parent families. Neglect was significantly higher among children with a single parent, father or mother, than two-parent families. Physical abuse rates did not differ across family size, whereas neglect was most likely in larger families (i.e., with four or more children). Metropolitan status of the community (i.e., very large urban, moderate urban, suburban, and rural) was not related to the incidence of physical abuse or neglect.

The NIS-3 estimated that approximately 1,500 children a year died from maltreatment, with 80% of those deaths being caused by natural parents. Approximately 78% of fatalities were due to a female parent or parent substitute. Serious injury (i.e., involving a life-threatening condition, representing a long-term impact, or requiring professional treatment to prevent long-term impairment) occurred in approximately 565,000 children nationwide, with 87% caused by natural parents.

Most physical abuse (71%) was committed by natural parents, with 21% being other parents (e.g., step or foster) or parent substitutes, and the remainder being committed by others (e.g., other family members or unrelated adults). Most neglect was by natural parents (91%), with other parents or parent substitutes responsible for 9%.

Characteristics of the Offender

A host of factors can impact parenting and these factors can be associated with the parents themselves, their child, the relationships in the family, and the broader context in which parenting occurs. Physical abuse is most likely to occur when parents are attempting to discipline their child or otherwise manage the behavior of their child (Wolfe, 1988). Certain situational factors may have a direct, immediate influence on maltreatment by escalating the intensity of these parent–child interactions. Other factors may contribute to maltreatment more indirectly by compromising the overall quality of parenting or the home environment. Poor child management skills, stress, knowledge deficits, motivational and anger control problems have all been identified as factors that can compromise parenting (Hansen et al., 1990; Hansen & Warner, 1992). Parental psychopathology, such as depression, can strain parental resources and thus interfere with the ability to provide an optimal home environment (Quamma & Greenberg, 1994). Furthermore, marital discord has been shown to have a negative impact on parenting skills and the availability of the parents (Kerig, 1995).

Certain models of maltreatment focus on the etiology and maintenance of abusive behavior by attempting to account for how and why parents move along the continuum from milder to more harmful interactions with their child. For example, Wolfe (Azar & Wolfe, 1989; Wolfe, 1987) described a three-stage transitional model. Stage 1 is characterized by a reduced tolerance to stress and disinhibition of aggression in the parent. Stage 2 is associated with poor handling of acute crises, precipitated by the parent's early, failed attempts at controlling stress and misbehavior that lead to more power-assertive, punitive methods. Stage 3 consists of the habitual, coercive patterns of aggression and arousal in which excessive punishment functions to decrease child misbehavior. At each stage, compensatory factors (e.g., supportive spouse, social support) may decrease negative interactions, whereas destabilizing factors (e.g., stressful life event, increase in child behavior problems) may increase negative interactions and thus heighten the risk for abuse.

An interactive model of child abuse views parenting as occurring in the context of other behavioral, biological, affective, cognitive, and societal variables. This provides a useful and contemporary conceptualization of physically abusive behavior. One such model, provided by Walker, Bonner, and Kaufman (1988), involves the fol-

lowing four tenets: (a) certain parental factors (e.g., personality characteristics) predispose individuals toward abusive behavior, (b) these factors can lead parents to
have a disturbed relationship with their child (e.g., unrealistic expectations, inconsistent child management strategies), (c) certain factors associated with the child may
render their behavior more difficult to manage (e.g., high rates of challenging behaviors), and (d) sociological issues (e.g., low income) can contribute to a negative environment in which abuse is more likely to occur. In summary, physical abuse and
neglect can be viewed as a multifaceted problem that results from complex maladaptive interactions between parents and children, combined with a lack of essential
caregiving behaviors.

Appropriate parenting that is characterized by predictability, responsiveness,
and sensitivity, and is provided within a structured and organized home environment, has long been recognized as crucial for optimal child development (Maccoby &
Martin, 1983). The ability to provide such parenting is multidetermined (Belsky &
Vondra, 1989); the inability to provide such parenting is also multidetermined. It is
not surprising, therefore, that there is no adequately validated "typical perpetrator
profile" of a maltreating parent (Milner & Chilamkurti, 1991). Rather, it is more useful to view maltreatment in the context of a continuum of parenting and to examine
the factors that compromise the quality of parenting and thus increase the risk of
abuse and neglect.

Research suggests areas of parenting behaviors that may differentiate abusive
from nonabusive parents, including child-management techniques, anger and impulse control, and parent–child interactions (Azar & Wolfe, 1989; Walker *et al.*, 1988;
Wolfe, 1988). For example, when observed in play or other interactive situations with
their children, abusive mothers tend to interact less often with their children than
do nonabusive mothers (e.g., Schindler & Arkowitz, 1986). The interactions that
do occur tend to be more negative and less supportive (e.g., Bousha & Twentyman, 1984). Abusive mothers have been found to engage in less positive nonverbal
and verbal behavior and more verbal and nonverbal aggression (e.g., Reid, Kavanagh, & Baldwin, 1987). Abusive mothers also tend to use more power-assertive
child-management strategies (e.g., disapproval, humiliation, threat) and less positive
techniques (e.g., approval, cooperation, reasoning), and to issue more commands
compared with nonabusive counterparts (e.g., Oldershaw, Walters, & Hall, 1989).
Overall, abusive mothers have been noted to view their children less favorably than
nonabusive mothers view their children (e.g., Oldershaw *et al.*, 1989). Like many issues in maltreatment, the majority of research has been on abusive mothers. Much
less is known about the qualitative aspects of interactions between abusive fathers
and their children.

Parents need to be sensitive to their child's changing needs at different stages of
development. They also need to be attentive to and perceptive of the cues provided
by their child's behavior and learn to respond to those cues appropriately. Abusive
parents tend to lack accurate knowledge about child rearing and have unrealistic expectations for their children's behavior (e.g., Azar, Robinson, Hekimian, & Twentyman, 1984; Spinetta & Rigler, 1972). They may have a tendency to view their child's
behavior in a negative manner, and describe their children as purposefully disruptive, noncompliant, and annoying (e.g., Bauer & Twentyman, 1985). Abusive parents
may also view misbehavior differently from nonabusive parents and therefore may
not be reliable reporters of their own child's behavior. For example, though they may

describe their child as exhibiting more behavioral difficulties than other children, independent observation may fail to detect such differences (Reid *et al.*, 1987).

General life stressors appear more pronounced in maltreating families. Chaotic lifestyles, characterized by problems such as marital discord and frequent moves are often evident (Azar & Wolfe, 1989; Lundquist & Hansen, 1998). Physical health issues may be present, as abusive parents tend to report more health problems than would be expected in the general population (Milner, 1986). Overall psychological health can impact coping and parenting. High rates of depression have been linked to maltreatment, with physically abusive mothers in particular reporting more physical symptoms (Lahey, Conger, Atkeson, & Treiber, 1984). The higher number and increased intensity of stressors faced by parents may place an unrealistic demand on coping skills already compromised by a weak preparation for the parenting role, increasing the likelihood that a parent will react to situations with aggressive behavior (Milner & Chilamkurti, 1991).

Coping with stressors requires identifying the cause of the stress, generating and implementing a plan to reduce the stress, and attempting to prevent the stress from occurring or increasing in the future. All of these skills require some degree of insight, planning, and organization. Inability to solve problems related to parenting and other aspects of daily living is hypothesized to result in frustration or inability to cope and lead to problematic parental behavior such as physical abuse or neglect (Hansen, Pallotta, Christopher, Conaway, & Lundquist, 1995). General coping and problem-solving skills are widely acknowledged to be underdeveloped in abusive parents and this observation has received some empirical support (e.g., Azar *et al.*, 1984; Hansen *et al.*, 1995; Hansen, Pallotta, Tishelman, Conaway, & MacMillan, 1989). Limited problem-solving skills for child-management situations may result in a tendency to use verbal and physical aggression as conflict-resolution techniques. As noted earlier, compared with nonabusive mothers, abusive mothers tend to rely on more power-assertive, negative child-management strategies, such as hitting and pushing (Lahey *et al.*, 1984; Oldershaw *et al.*, 1989), and verbal reprimands and response cost punishment (Trickett & Susman, 1988) when attempting to manage child behavior.

Although low intelligence has been identified in the literature as a possible risk factor for abuse (Kaufman & Zigler, 1989; Schilling, Schinke, Blythe, & Barth, 1982), support for this conclusion is debatable (Dowdney & Skuse, 1993). Rather than focus on general intellectual ability, research suggests that the emphasis should be placed on specific problem-solving skills, including abstract reasoning and the ability to generate appropriate child-management strategies (Azar *et al.*, 1984; Hansen *et al.*, 1989; Hansen *et al.*, 1995).

Anger can be seen as a natural occurrence of parenting. All children become difficult and oppositional at times, especially during certain developmental periods, and parental anger can be a natural and expected response to some child behavior (Hecht, Hansen, & Chandler, 1996). In certain cases, however, anger may be an inherent part of a parent's style or can arise as a result of the incongruence between their expectations and the reality of parenting (Hecht *et al.*, 1996). Abusive parents may have increased sensitivity to anger- or stress-inducing cues. For example, research has found abusive mothers to be more physiologically aroused by and averse to infant cries (Frodi & Lamb, 1980) and to have greater and longer arousal to stressful stimuli (Wolfe, Fairbank, Kelly, & Bradlyn, 1983). Maltreating parents may not recognize the physiological and cognitive cues of anger arousal or they may be less able to reduce their arousal level. Poor coping strategies and a lack of anger-management techniques may increase the likelihood that abusive parents will react in a hostile or angry manner. Poor impulse control may exacerbate the problems even further.

Social cognition is an important component in the conceptualization of parental anger. Milner (1993) proposed that maltreating parents have preexisting cognitive schemas, which include beliefs and values that impact the way they perceive, evaluate, integrate, and act on child-specific information. In the first stage of Milner's Social Information Processing Model, misperceptions of child behavior occur when parents focus on only part of the situation. This selective attention may be a result of predispositions or existing schemas, or could be due to the increased arousal and distress that maltreating parents report with respect to child behavior. The next stage involves the parents' interpretations and evaluations of the child's behavior. In particular, parental attributions of hostile intent by the child may contribute to aggression. Third, parents use the information they have obtained to choose a response, and parents may be poor observers and interpreters of anger cues. Alternatively, they may ignore the cues in order to maintain their preferred power-assertive behaviors.

Substance abuse may contribute to the problems of maltreatment. Estimates of the association between alcohol use and child maltreatment vary, probably due to the various definitions and samples used. Several studies in the 1970s found that approximately 50% of all child-abusing parents drank heavily or were intoxicated at the time abuse occurred (Orme & Rimmer, 1981). Other reviews of the literature suggest that alcohol use was involved in 40%–95% of marital violence cases and in 32%–62% of child abuse cases (Coleman & Straus, 1983). Studies have shown similar environmental and personality characteristics in alcohol abusers and child abusers (Milner & Chilamkurti, 1991; Vaillant, 1995), including low levels of social support and self-esteem, high levels of stress and marital discord, and poor impulse control (e.g., Bavolek & Henderson, 1990; Muller, Fitzgerald, Sullivan, & Zucker, 1994).

Although child maltreatment and alcoholism may share similar etiologies and co-occur frequently, there is little convincing evidence that one phenomenon leads to the other (Orme & Rimmer, 1981). Milner and Chilamkurti (1991) are hesitant to establish a causal link between alcohol use and maltreatment, especially given the lack of adequate controls and clear definitions in the literature. Rather, they suggest that alcohol may mediate cognition, and maltreating parents who drink might have their attention narrowed so that they concentrate only on the most immediate stimuli. Furthermore, abusers tend to make faulty attributions about child behavior. This processing style taken together with a diminished cognitive ability might lead to a violent response. Alternative hypotheses suggest that if maltreating parents are more easily aroused, they may drink to decrease this arousal (Stasiewicz & Lisman, 1989).

The nature and quality of social contacts and social support also have important implications for child maltreatment. There is a link between elevated scores on the Child Abuse Potential Inventory on social isolation and the parent's perception of lack of support (Milner, 1994). The marital relationship, extended family, neighborhood network, and community outreach services can all be potential sources of support. These sources can have many positive functions such as educating parents about child rearing, modeling appropriate child-management techniques, giving or loaning money when necessary, or providing respite childcare. Supportive relationships can also provide outlets for talking through stressful situations or validating one's feelings about an issue. However, not all social networks support optimal parenting. Social networks can serve a negative function if maltreating parents select a peer group with similar problems who also exhibit maladaptive child-rearing strategies. Wahler (1980) was one of the first researchers to draw empirical attention to the issue that abusive mothers tend to have fewer social contacts than nonabusive mothers. Furthermore, the contacts they do have tend to be negative, rather than positive, and to involve professionals or relatives rather than friends.

Factors associated with the child, including gender, age, ordinal position, temperament, and behavioral characteristics, can influence parenting (Belsky & Vondra, 1989; Maccoby & Martin, 1983) and therefore can be possible risk factors for abuse. For example, with regard to physical abuse, there is some evidence that a gender effect emerges in later childhood with males under the age of 12 years and females over the age of 13 at most risk (NCCAN, 1994). In addition, children with developmental disabilities, especially those with oppositional or disruptive behaviors, are at increased risk for maltreatment (Ammerman, Hersen, Van Hasselt, Lubetsky, & Sieck, 1994).

Abusive parents report more behavior problems in their children, focusing on negative, noncompliant behavior and ignoring the more positive, prosocial behaviors (Bousha & Twentyman, 1984). When high levels of behavioral difficulties are paired with parenting skills already compromised by the presence of other risk factors, the potential for maltreatment may increase. Furthermore, because abusive parents may engage in less effective child-management strategies overall, they may actually exacerbate existing behavioral difficulties in their children by selectively attending to inappropriate or aggressive behavior, thus increasing the likelihood that these behaviors will occur more frequently. Although occurrence of abuse and neglect can co-vary with child behavior problems, it is important not to place any responsibility on the child for the occurrence of maltreatment (Hansen et al., 1990).

Family Patterns

Many family characteristics may not necessarily be targets for intervention, yet they are relevant for treatment planning through their association with increased risk for maltreatment or potential impact on treatment adherence (e.g., low socioeconomic status, marital or relationship problems). These factors may interact in a complex manner. For example, limited financial resources may place additional stress on a fragile marital relationship. Friction between caregivers may, in turn, exacerbate an already low tolerance for child misbehavior and trigger an angry, aggressive response to a rather minor incident of child noncompliance. Residing in a rural community may impact access to resources in general and increase likelihood of social isolation. In some communities, external supports may be available, but families most in need may not be able to access the support or may choose not to utilize it.

There is a long-standing belief that a childhood history of abuse significantly increases the likelihood of being an abusive parent and there is considerable evidence to support this link (Falshaw, Browne, & Hollin, 1996; Kaufman & Zigler, 1989; Widom, 1989). However, there are also problems with the research in the area, such as correlational and retrospective designs, and small, nonrepresentative samples (Falshaw et al., 1996; Spinetta & Rigler, 1972; Widom, 1989). Despite the research difficulties and limitations, there appears to be a relationship between the seriousness and chronicity of childhood abuse and measures of adult child abuse, as well as associations between the observation of abuse in childhood and the potential to engage in abusive behaviors in adulthood (e.g., Milner, Robertson, & Rogers, 1990). Even those adults who experienced less severe corporal punishment may be at increased risk for physically abusing their children (e.g., Straus & Kantor, 1994).

The exact processes through which experiencing childhood maltreatment exerts its influence across generations are not known. There has been debate about the specificity of the effects of abuse—whether a specific form of abuse (e.g., physical abuse) is most likely to result in the intergenerational transmission of the same form of abuse (Falshaw *et al.*, 1996). At the minimum, one can conclude that a history of abuse is a risk factor for offending behavior and that a childhood characterized by maltreatment provides weak preparation and poor modeling for the role of parenting in adulthood. A sociological view suggests that if parents and children share an environment and culture in which abusive behavior is frequent and acceptable, then the continuance of abuse is likely (Kaufman & Zigler, 1989). Similarly, social-learning theory suggests that by witnessing and experiencing maltreatment, children are experiencing conditioned patterns of arousal, learning that it is appropriate, and forming rules and cognitive distortions around these beliefs (Kaufman & Zigler, 1989; Widom, 1989). Attachment theory would suggest that internalized representations of past relationships serve as templates that dictate future relationships and that abusive patterns of interaction are integrated into these models (Kaufman & Zigler, 1989).

Maltreatment in the home may not be the only violence children experience. Children who live in violent communities may be exposed to unpredictable violence directly (as victims of violence) or indirectly (as witnesses of violent acts). In such communities, the use of violence may be modeled repeatedly and even accepted as a solution to difficult situations. Exposure to increased crime and violence in the day-to-day community life may add yet more stress to parenting skills already taxed by limited personal resources. Cicchetti and Lynch (1995) present an ecological-transactional view to conceptualize the manner in which the effects of violence in the community interact with violence in the home to exert a negative influence on child development. The manner in which parents cope specifically with violence in their community may be influenced by levels of education, financial resources, and involvement with a support network such as church groups (Hill, Hawkins, Raposo, & Carr, 1995).

Assessment and Diagnosis

If maltreatment is viewed in the context of parenting, then the focus of assessment must be based on the variables, such as those just discussed, that are known to impact parenting. In some cases, the most urgent and immediate goal of assessment may be to determine dangerousness and risk to the child; in other cases, the goal of assessment may be to determine whether abuse has occurred (Wolfe, 1988). However, if the family has been referred from social services or a child protection agency, the immediate decision about whether abuse occurred or whether to remove the child from the environment already may be resolved.

If that is the case, then the purpose of the assessment is more likely to involve the recognition of needs, the conceptualization of the problems, and the identification of targets for intervention. Thus, the initial step in the assessment process is to examine the basic skills and background that parents bring with them to the parenting role and to evaluate the context in which parenting occurs. The skills and background of parents includes their own childhood history of discipline, their knowledge of child development, problems with anger or impulse control, characteristics of the parent–child relationship, level of behavior problems exhibited by the child, and investigation of the child-management strategies currently used. Assessment should identify areas of strength and weakness in parenting and highlight possible risk factors. Evaluation of the parenting context involves consideration of the home environment, social support, and community resources. The assessment process also requires an in-depth, functional analysis of discrete episodes of maltreatment or times in which the parent found his or her skills particularly challenged. Antecedents that precipitate abuse should be identified (e.g., child misbehavior, spousal conflict, parental anger over a nonrelated issue), and consequences of abuse should be explored (e.g., child stops misbehaving, parent experiences release of stress).

Ideally, assessment is highly individualized, as every family will differ in terms of their strengths and vulnerabilities. A multimethod, multi-informant approach to assessment will yield the most valid and useful data and clinicians should view the information gathered via each separate method in conjunction with data from the other sources. Some techniques are most useful for the initial assessment to aid in problem identification and conceptualization. Other techniques can be incorporated into an ongoing assessment that is integral for documenting behavior change and monitoring progress throughout treatment. More extensive reviews of assessment measures and issues are available for interested readers (e.g., Hansen & Warner, 1992; Milner, 1991).

Clinical Interview

Interviewing is an essential tool for gathering background information, assessing risk, and identifying antecedents and consequences of maltreatment. Data on parental knowledge regarding general child development and behavior can be collected via interview as well. Specific information on how parents view their own child and how they respond to problematic behavior is also easily gathered in this manner. Anger control issues can be raised in the neutral context of the interview. Similarly, topics such as quality of relationships and possibility of substance abuse can be addressed. Details as to availability and use of social supports can be gathered. Such support may include guidance and advising, emotional support, tangible assistance, self-disclosure, and support related to management of child problems. Wolfe (1988) has developed a useful outline, entitled the Parent Interview and Assessment Guide, that can be a valuable resource. The Child Abuse and Neglect Interview Schedule, a detailed semistructured interview, is also available (Ammerman, Hersen, & Van Hasselt, 1988).

It is not uncommon for people within a family to view the same child or set of problems quite differently. Therefore, it is ideal if all caregivers are interviewed, even if only one has been identified as "the client," or if only one will be participating in treatment. Furthermore, there are few data on the actual correspondence between parental report and actions. Maltreating parents may underreport the frequency of their own negative responses or inappropriate behaviors. As mentioned earlier, their reports regarding the level of their child's misbehavior may not match the reports of others, nor match actual rates of misbehavior, thus highlighting the need for interviewing multiple informants.

Self-Report Measures

Several well-validated self-report measures are available that target a wide range of potentially important factors. In many cases, the paper-and-pencil measures can be given to the client to complete at home, thereby allowing the clinician to spend more actual assessment time in interview or direct observation of parent–child interaction. Clearly, it is not necessary to include all of the measures here in a comprehensive battery. Those devices that best match the referral concerns and client needs are needed.

Commonly used measures available for assessing general psychological functioning are the Minnesota Multiphasic Personality Inventory–2 (MMPI-2; Butcher, Dahlstrom, Graham, Tellegen, & Kaemmer, 1989) or the Symptom-Checklist–90–Revised (SCL-90-R; Derogatis, 1983). The validity scales of the MMPI-2 are valuable for screening for deviant test-taking attitudes (e.g., attempts to present oneself in an overly positive fashion). The SCL-90-R is particularly useful in that it is brief, yet covers a variety of symptoms (global indices of functioning as well as Somatization, Obsessive-Compulsive, Interpersonal Sensitivity, Depression, Anxiety, Hostility, Phobic Anxiety, Paranoid Ideation, Psychoticism).

Specific assessment of parental knowledge about and expectations of child development is more complicated, as normative levels and timing of developmental milestones are relatively variable. The Parent Opinion Questionnaire (Azar & Rohrbeck, 1986) is useful to assess the appropriateness of a range of child behaviors. A total score is obtained and six subscales are scored: Self-Care, Family Responsibility and Care of Siblings, Help and Affection to Parents, Leaving Children Alone, Proper Behavior and Feelings, and Punishment. A second device, useful when older children are involved, is the Family Beliefs Inventory (Roehling & Robin, 1986), which provides a measure of adherence to unreasonable beliefs particular to parent–adolescent conflict situations. On the parent side, the beliefs measured include ruination, perfectionism, approval, obedience, self-blame, and malicious intent. On the adolescent side, the beliefs are ruination, unfairness, autonomy, and approval.

Many devices are available to assess child behavior problems and child-management and parent–child interaction skills. The informants for the devices can be parents, teachers, or other adults familiar with the child. Two of the most commonly used devices are the Child Behavior Checklist (CBCL; Achenbach, 1991) and the Eyberg Child Behavior Inventory (ECBI; Eyberg & Ross, 1978). The CBCL consists of two main scales: Social Competence and Behavior Problems. The Social Competence scales include Activities, Social, and School subscales. The Behavior Problems scale is composed of 118 items. The actual subscales vary according to the gender and age of the child, but may include Anxious, Depressed, Uncommunicative, Obsessive-Compulsive, Somatic Complaints, Social Withdrawal, Ineffective, Aggressive, and Delinquent. The ECBI is shorter than the CBCL and can be used more easily as a repeated measure to assess behavior change during and after treatment. The ECBI is composed of 36 behavior problems that are rated on a 7-point scale for frequency. Respondents are also asked to indicate which behaviors they consider a problem.

Knowledge about behavioral principles as they apply to child management is an area of particular relevance to skills-based interventions for maltreatment. A measure designed to assess parental knowledge about child management is the Knowledge of Behavioral Principles as Applied to Children, which is composed of 50 multiple-choice items (KBPAC; O'Dell, Tarler-Benlolo, & Flynn, 1979). Although the KBPAC can be a useful clinical tool, the length and relatively advanced reading level may make it difficult for many maltreating parents to complete independently (Hansen *et al.*, 1998).

Stress can arise from many different sources, some of which may be particular to the role of parenting (e.g., child misbehavior) and some of which may not (e.g., poor physical health). General measures of stress may be valuable to identify the impact of recent stressful experiences of maltreating parents. The Life Experiences Survey (Sarason, Johnson, & Siegel, 1978) assesses the occurrence and impact of major life events and the Hassles Scale (Kanner, Coyne, Schaefer, & Lazarus, 1981) assesses occurrence of more minor, commonly occurring stressors. Both of these measures provide data on stressors outside the parent–child relationship that can impact the quality of parenting. The Parenting Stress Index (PSI; Abidin, 1986) was developed for evaluating stress associated specifically with parenting and the parent–child relationship. The PSI is composed of two domains. The Child Domain has scales of Adaptability, Acceptability, Demandingness, Mood Distractibility/Hyperactivity, and Reinforces Parent. The Parent Domain scales include Parent Health, Depression, Attachment, Restrictions of Role, Sense of Competence, Social Isolation, and Relationship with Spouse. There is an optional Life Stress scale.

Often parents must cope with stressors, solve problems, and manage anger simultaneously. The Parental Problem-Solving Measure (PPSM; Hansen *et al.*, 1989; Hansen *et al.*, 1995) measures problem-solving skills for child-related and non-child-related areas. Problem situations for the PPSM are classified into one of five problem areas: (a) child behavior and child management, (b) anger and stress control, (c) finances, (d) child care resources, and (e) interpersonal problems. Responses are rated for the number of solutions generated and the effectiveness of the chosen solution. Other self-report problem-solving measures that have shown promise with other populations may also be helpful. For example, the Social Problem-Solving Inventory (D'Zurilla & Nezu, 1988) is a measure of multiple components of problem-solving ability.

Because parental anger responses may follow or be intensified by child behavior problems, anger specifically related to child behavior should be an assessment priority. The Parental Anger Inventory (PAI; DeRoma & Hansen, 1994; V. M. MacMillan, Olson, & Hansen, 1988) was developed to assess anger experienced by maltreating parents in response to child misbehavior and other child-related situations. Parents rate 50 child-related situations (e.g., child refuses to go to bed, child throws food) as problematic or nonproblematic and rate the degree of anger evoked by each situation. Other paper-and-pencil measures of adult anger may also be useful, such as the State-Trait Anger Scale (STAS; Spielberger, Jacobs, Russel, & Crane, 1983) or the Multdimensional Anger Inventory (Siegel, 1986).

Presence of positive relationships and social supports within the community can decrease the risk of maltreatment. Wahler's (1980) Community Interaction Checklist is useful for evaluating the frequency and tone of social contacts. The marital relationship is a potentially powerful source of support as well as problems. The quality of the caregiver's relationship can be assessed using the Dyadic Adjustment Scale (DAS; Spanier, 1976), a brief measure that uses mostly Likert-type rating scales to assess the quality of the relationship. The DAS provides a standard score that corresponds to the degree of dissatisfaction in the relationship and the score can be compared with normative data from distressed and nondistressed couples.

Given the likelihood of aggression between adults within the home, the brief Conflict Tactics Scales (CTS; Straus, 1979) or the more thorough Revised Conflict Tactics Scales (CTS2; Straus, Hamby, Boney-McCoy, & Sugarman, 1996) are valuable for assessing the extent to which partners engage in physical or psychological attacks when in conflict and their use of negotiation or reasoning. The CTS2 has added scales to address sexual coercion and injury. Items assess a wide range of tactics, from items such as "I agreed to try a solution to a disagreement my partner suggested" to "I used a gun or a knife on my partner." Respondents are asked to report on their own and their significant other's behavior.

For the specific assessment of the risk of maltreatment, the Child Abuse Potential Inventory (CAPI; Milner, 1986) can be used. This device provides an Abuse Potential Scale, which is divided into six factor scales: Distress, Rigidity, Unhappiness, Problems with Child and Self, Problems with Family, and Problems with Others. Three validity scales, Lie, Random Response, and Inconsistency, allow for examination of deviant response styles, including Fake-Good, Fake-Bad, and Random Responding. Elevated abuse scores indicate that the respondent exhibits an assortment of personal and interpersonal features that are similar to characteristics found in known child physical abusers (Milner, 1994). As highlighted by the test's author, it is inappropriate to use any one test, such as the CAPI, as a "diagnostic criterion" (Milner, 1991). Therefore, although the CAPI can identify risk, it is not to be used for the identification or substantiation of actual maltreatment.

Direct Observation

Direct observations of parent–child interactions and parenting behavior are essential for a complete assessment. Given that physical abuse is composed of discrete episodes of aggression perpetrated by a caretaker, and given that these episodes generally occur in the relative privacy of the home environment, it is unlikely that professionals will actually observe abuse as it occurs. The initial identification of maltreatment is generally made based on the consequences of abuse, rather than direct observation of abusive behavior (Warner & Hansen, 1994). Direct observation of any behavior can be a time-consuming, costly method of assessment. Yet, direct observation of parent–child interactions, in both the clinic and the home, can yield extremely useful data, which would definitely not be available through other methods (Hansen *et al.*, 1998). Initial observations can serve as baseline data against which behavior change during and after treatment can be evaluated. Videotaping can be an informative, integral part of assessment, especially given the availability and portability of videorecording equipment.

Parent–child interactions can be observed in unstructured play situations, such as the commonly used Child's Game procedure (Forehand & McMahon, 1981). In this procedure, parents are told to play with their child but to allow the child to structure the activity. The interactions are observed for approximately 10 min, after which the parents ask the child to put away the toys. The Behavioral Coding System (Forehand & McMahon, 1981) is straightforward and particularly useful for observing such parent–child interactions in the context of parent training. The appropriateness of child behavior is recorded, as well as the parental antecedents (command, warning, question, attend, reward), child responses (compliance, noncompliance), and parental consequences (attend, reward).

More complex observational codes are available for scoring quality and content of parent–child interactions; examples are the Dyadic Parent–Child Interaction Coding System (DPICS; Eyberg & Robinson, 1981) and the Family Interaction Coding System (Reid, 1978). The DPICS, for example, assesses a variety of positive and negative behaviors. Frequency of 14 parent behaviors (e.g., direct or indirect commands, descriptive or reflective statements, physical positive or negative) and 10 child behaviors (e.g., cry, yell, destructive, compliance, noncompliance) are coded.

Assessment of abusive parents in high-demand child-management situations is particularly important, given the connection between parental discipline efforts and physically abusive behavior (V. M. MacMillan, Olson, & Hansen, 1991). Parenting skills may be mastered only during low-demand clinic assessments, but not rehearsed in high-arousal situations that are more representative of the parent's natural environment. Because directly observing actual discipline is often difficult, assessments utilizing adult actors (e.g., therapists, research assistants) to present deviant child behavior can be useful. For example, the Home Simulation Assessment (HSA; V. M. MacMillan *et al.*, 1991) measures parent ability to apply child-management skills in realistic problem situations that may occur in the home. Parents are provided with instructions about tasks (e.g., dry the dishes) and asked to do their best at prompting the actors to complete the tasks. "Deviant" scripted behaviors are exhibited by the actors. Parent self-report ratings of stress, anger, and anxiousness are also collected.

Direct observation of the home environment is a necessary component in the assessment of neglect. Lutzker and colleagues developed two very helpful observational rating systems designed to identify and monitor problems in the home. The Checklist for Living Environments to Assess Neglect (CLEAN; Watson-Perczel, Lutzker, Greene, & McGimpsey, 1988) is a measure of home cleanliness. Item areas in targeted places (e.g., sink, counter) are rated for cleanliness on three dimensions: presence of dirt or organic matter, number of clothes or linens in contact with the item area, and number of nonclothing items or other nonorganic matter in contact with the area.

The actual physical safety of the home environment may be another issue for assessment. The Home Accident Prevention Inventory (HAPI; Tertinger, Greene, & Lutzker, 1984) was devised to evaluate the safety of home environments of physically abusive and neglectful families. Five categories of potential hazards in the home are evaluated: fire and electrical hazards, suffocation by ingested objects; suffocation by mechanical objects, firearms, and solid and liquid poisons. The type and number of categories under which these hazards are organized can be identified and a summary score of total number of hazardous items can be obtained. In addition to their role in the initial assessment, both the CLEAN and the HAPI can be quite useful throughout treatment to monitor specific changes in the home environment.

Self-Monitoring

A complete functional analysis of the factors that operate to initiate or maintain abusive interactions often requires asking the parents to record the occurrence of specific behaviors, such as child tantrums or use of current child-management techniques (e.g., spanking). It is possible that the very act of having to record the frequency of punitive or aggressive management techniques may decrease the likelihood that parents will use them. Of course, as with any self-report measure, it is equally possible that parents may continue to use such techniques, but underreport the frequency with which they do so. Self-monitoring has been useful with maltreatment parents in assessing responses triggered by arousing events (Hansen *et al.*, 1998). Parents can be asked to note a description of each incident that triggered angry feelings, including frustration or tension, and the way in which they dealt with the incident and their feelings (Hansen & Warner, 1992). Presence and function of potentially positive factors, such as the frequency and quality of social contacts, can also be measured using self-monitoring.

Self-monitoring techniques are particularly adaptable to individualized assessment, as therapists can operationalize a host of different factors or behaviors and devise unique and personalized assessment forms. Alternative arrangements can be provided for clients who have reading or writing difficulties (e.g., tape-recording their data). For example, V. M. MacMillan, Guevremont, and Hansen (1988) developed a self-report measure of stress and anxiety that was completed two to three times a week by a client during audiotaped telephone interviews. Individual items were created based on her own descriptions of her experience in stressful situations (e.g., "light-headed," "headachy") and read to her over the telephone because she was unable to read.

Information from Others Outside the Family

Information from professionals outside the family is an integral part of a multi-method, multi-informant approach to assessment. Interagency collaboration is important throughout assessment and treatment. Professionals from schools, medical facilities, and social services may all have various types of contact with the families in different settings and provide data not obtainable from other methods. Interviews and monitoring can all be utilized with professionals in the community, both in the initial assessment and in the monitoring of treatment progress. In cases of neglect, for example, teachers may be in the best position to provide daily, independent ratings of children's hygiene or appropriateness of dress (Hansen *et al.*, 1998).

Maltreating families may be involved with the legal system. In such cases, particularly if the family has been court-mandated for assessment or treatment, it is important that the therapist clarify his or her role and the issue of confidentiality (or the possible lack thereof) at the onset of the assessment process. Milner (1991) and Melton and Limber (1989) provide useful discussions of assessment and testimony issues that may arise when the judicial system is involved.

Issues in Clinical Management

As noted throughout this chapter, maltreating families are well recognized for their heterogeneity and complexity. Typically, maltreatment is only one of a host of difficulties experienced by the family at any given time. Practical problems may arise, such as lack of transportation to clinics, limited financial resources, and lack of motivation for change (Hansen *et al.*, 1998; Lundquist & Hansen, 1998). The multiproblem nature of these families presents several issues in terms of their clinical management and a hierarchy of needs and target areas must be developed very early in the treatment. Naturally, decisions about what treatments or combinations of treatments to use will depend heavily on the assessment results. Several other pragmatic issues must be addressed, including the selection of (a) the "client" targeted (e.g., parent, child, family unit), (b) the type of intervention (e.g., group versus individual treatment), and (c) the context of treatment (e.g., home versus clinic). Poor adherence to treatment recommendations and coordination of interagency collaboration present additional challenges to clinical management. Finally, the client may not necessarily be a willing participant in treatment and may not agree with the need for professional involvement.

Because of the complexities associated with treatment of maltreating families, careful consideration of treatment adherence, generalization, and social validity are needed. The full involvement of the parent in treatment is essential and three types of treatment adherence are needed: attending sessions regularly, participating in sessions, and completing out-of-session assignments or tasks (Lundquist & Hansen, 1998). Completion of a specific functional analysis of adherence and nonadherence responses is important. A variety of factors may contribute to nonadherence, including inadequate instructions and rationale, lack of skills or motivation, and competing contingencies that reinforce noncompliance or punish compliance (Lundquist & Hansen, in press). Professionals report using a wide variety of strategies for increasing adherence with maltreating families, including antecedent prompting strategies (e.g., telephone reminders, providing training in tasks to be implemented) and consequent strategies (e.g., praise and rewards, feedback), though the effectiveness of such strategies has not been demonstrated empirically (Hansen & Warner, 1992). In addition, addressing contextual factors that may interfere with compliance (e.g., family conflict, financial problems) can be valuable. Coordination with other agencies (e.g., Child Protective Services, schools) is essential to maximize service provision and minimize service overlap or "splintering of allegiances" (Hansen et al., 1998).

Professionals who work with maltreating parents will, at some time, become involved in the legal system. Melton and Limber (1989) provided a good discussion of the issues involved and suggested that practitioners confine their role in the legal process to investigator, evaluator, or therapist. Abusive and neglectful parents who are court-ordered for assessment or treatment present unique issues for treatment. If the family is involved with the legal system, a certain level of severity or chronicity of maltreatment probably existed that prompted legal involvement. Therefore, patterns of behavior and interacting may be more entrenched and resistant to modification than those present in high-risk families. Despite court mandates, some parents remain noncompliant in terms of attending sessions. These parents tend to be younger and more disadvantaged then those who are more compliant (Butler, Radia, & Magnatta, 1994). Adherence becomes very critical when the courts are involved. Atkinson and Butler (1996), in a study of mothers court-ordered for assessment, found that mothers who are noncompliant were more likely eventually to lose custody of their children

Generalization is needed across stimuli, responses, and time, and it is important to program actively for it (Stokes & Osnes, 1989). A number of strategies may be useful for facilitating generalization, including contacting and recruiting natural consequences (e.g., reinforcers within the family), training diversely (e.g., using sufficient stimulus and response exemplars), and incorporating functional mediators (e.g., common salient physical and social stimuli as well as self-mediated physical and verbal stimuli) (Stokes & Osnes, 1989). It is also useful to target contextual factors (e.g., family stressors) that interfere with assessment or treatment (Lundquist & Hansen, 1998).

Extended home visitation is a critical element of successful programs designed to prevent the occurrence of child maltreatment among high-risk (e.g., single parent, teenage parent, low socioeconomic status) families (H. L. MacMillan, MacMillan, Offord, Griffith, & MacMillan, 1994). Home visitation may be the best technique to promote treatment adherence in families in which abuse has already occurred (Hansen & Warner, 1992; Hansen *et al.,* 1998; Wekerle & Wolfe, 1993). It is not yet known which exact aspect or aspects of a home visit increase compliance.

It is also important to ensure that the goals, procedures, and outcomes of therapy are socially or functionally valid (Lundquist & Hansen, 1998). This includes consideration of whether the goals are what the family and society wants and whether achieving the goals would lead to real, functional improvements. Establishing the acceptability of the assessment and treatment procedures and satisfaction with the effects of treatment is also important.

One evaluation of the social validity of behaviorally based interventions suggests that physically abusive and neglectful families find the format of individualized behavioral intervention to be useful (Warner, Ujcich, Ellis, Malinosky-Rummell, & Hansen, 1992). In particular, maltreating parents found practicing new skills with the therapist and receiving written information most useful. In contrast, practicing a new skill with their child was rated as the least useful aspect of treatment. Thus, professionals working with physically abusive and neglectful parents should be aware that not all aspects of behavioral treatment programs will be equally well accepted or adhered to (Kelley, Grace, & Elliot, 1990).

Treatment adherence, generalization, and social validity are usually considered separate concepts, but it is important to note that there is significant overlap among the concepts. The more socially valid the goals and the procedures, the more likely the client is to participate in treatment; the more likely the client is to participate in treatment, the more likely the effects will generalize and maintain; the more the effects generalize and maintain, the more socially valid and functional the effects (Lundquist & Hansen, 1998).

Treatment

The basic goals of treatment should be to terminate ongoing maltreatment and to prevent future occurrences of maltreatment. These goals are addressed by targeting stressors that compromise parenting, increasing knowledge about child development and behavior, and teaching new skills. It is not enough only to target the acquisition of new skills. Parents who are knowledgeable about child development and have adequate parenting skills may still maltreat their children. Factors that impact utilization of skills must also be targeted.

The literature suggests that if a thorough assessment can identify the probable variables that are contributing to maltreatment, then cognitive-behavioral intervention programs can be very effective in treating physically abusive and neglectful families (Azar & Wolfe, 1989; Kelly, 1983b; Wolfe & Wekerle, 1993). Competency-based programs are a good fit with abusive and neglectful families in that the programs can be concrete, educational, and problem-focused (Azar & Wolfe, 1989; Hansen *et al.,*

1998; Wolfe & Wekerle, 1993). Interventions can be tailor-made to suit individual family needs and therefore are very face valid and perhaps less threatening, which may enhance family cooperation with treatment.

Intervention can occur at different levels. The parent, the family situation, resources in the community, or some combination may be targeted. At the level of the maltreating parent, Wolfe and Wekerle (1993) suggest five areas of intervention: (a) symptoms of emotional distress, cognitive impairments, and psychological problems that limit coping; (b) emotional arousal and reactivity to child behavior, anger control, and hostility; (c) poor child management (teaching, discipline, and stimulation); (d) inflexible and limited beliefs and expectations regarding child behavior and development; and (e) negative lifestyle habits (drugs, alcohol). Family issues may need to be addressed, including marital discord or domestic violence, chronic poverty, and social isolation. At the community level, contact with support services (e.g., housing, financial advice, church groups, respite day care) can be initiated or facilitated.

Overall, a variety of factors contribute to difficulties in treating these families: (a) the presence of multiple stressors and limited financial, personal, and social resources within the family for coping with stressors; (b) the often coercive nature of the referral and the possibility that participation in services may be involuntary or under duress; (c) the difficulty of observing abusive behavior; and (d) the need for multiple interventions to treat multiple target areas and family members (Azar & Wolfe, 1989; Hansen *et al.*, 1998; Wolfe, 1988). Description of approaches for specific treatment of the child, beyond intervention for child management or parent– child interactions, is beyond the offender focus of this chapter; reviews of the treatment of child victims of physical abuse and neglect are available (e.g., Hansen *et al.*, 1990; Walker *et al.*, 1988).

Intervention for Parenting and Related Behaviors

Research with individual parents or small groups of maltreating parents has suggested that parent training may be effective for improving family functioning and reducing the recurrence of maltreatment (e.g., V. M. MacMillan *et al.*, 1991; Wolfe, Edwards, Manion, & Koverola, 1988). However, the multiplicity of problems characteristic of maltreating families, in combination with the need for individualized and comprehensive intervention has made the evaluation of such treatment procedures very difficult (Hansen *et al.*, 1998; Wolfe & Wekerle, 1993).

When general parenting skills are targeted, the goals of intervention typically include (a) increasing knowledge of child development; (b) helping parents establish realistic expectations for child behavior; (c) teaching parents to identify, define, and record common classes of behavior; (d) educating parents on the role of the environment (e.g., antecedents, consequences) in eliciting and maintaining problem behaviors or interactions; and (e) teaching parents nonphysical, nonaggressive techniques of interaction, child management, and problem solving (Walker *et al.*, 1988).

Teaching parents about child development and helping them adopt realistic expectations for child behavior can be achieved by discussing these issues in session and providing parents with reading materials to review outside of session. Evaluations of maltreating parents' perceptions of treatment indicates that they consider interventions such as talking with therapists about new skills, practicing skills with a therapist and receiving written materials to be very useful (Hansen *et al.*, 1998).

At the time of intervention, parents may need information specific to the needs of their own children, but must develop an appreciation that the needs of children change throughout development. Work with parents of infants should stress the developmental tasks of physiological regulation and the formation of attachment relationships. Parents should be encouraged to provide stable routines, and to respond consistently and appropriately to their infant's needs. Parents of toddlers must be aware that children of this age are in the important phase of developing communication and an autonomous self; toddlers have increased independence and will make new and potentially difficult demands—often in high-profile situations (e.g., tantrums in grocery stores). Interventions with parents of toddlers may focus on adequate supervision, linguistic stimulation, and the provision of clear commands and positive, consistent consequences for compliance and prosocial behavior. The preschool to school-age years are characterized by the development of self-concept and self-esteem. Behavioral control outside the home (e.g., school) is critical. The development of social networks and academic success continue to be important throughout childhood. These issues will need to be incorporated into individualized parenting skills programs.

Parents may benefit from the opportunity to discuss how children learn from watching their parents' behavior. Incorporation of examples from their own adult experiences can be useful in educating parents about the environmental influences on behavior. Parents can be taught methods for prompting the occurrence and increasing the frequency of their children's prosocial behavior. Such methods include monitoring behavior, giving clear commands, and applying principles of reinforcement (e.g., sticker charts, setting up token economies).

The manner in which these methods are presented and practiced may vary widely across treatment programs. The therapists can discuss and demonstrate a skill, practice a skill with a parent, supervise a parent practicing the skill with the child, or instruct a parent to use the skill at home and review the progress in subsequent sessions. Ideally, skills training in the use of mild, nonphysical discipline (e.g., time-out, removal of privileges, extinction, natural consequences) for inappropriate behavior (e.g., tantrumming, teasing) should follow training and mastery of the more positive management techniques.

Several parent-training manuals are available. Although some may not be designed specifically for use with maltreating parents, the basic intervention techniques are the same. Barkley's (1987) "Defiant Children" program and Forehand and McMahon's (1981) text are both very useful. Kelly's (1983a) book on the management of everyday child behavior problems is very direct and practical. Adaptation of basic techniques for working specifically with maltreating parents is reviewed by Walker and colleagues (1988) and Hansen and colleagues (1998).

If limited problem-solving skills are identified in the assessment, then problem-solving skills training must be incorporated into the treatment plan (Hansen *et al.*, 1998; V. M. MacMillan, Guevremont, & Hansen, 1988). Problem-solving training may be an effective intervention for dealing with the multiple and complex problems of maltreating parents (Hansen *et al.*, 1995). Problem-solving assessment and training may provide a framework for approaching the multifaceted difficulties of maltreating parents, including providing a model from which additional interventions or skill-training procedures might be introduced to broaden the parent's repertoire of potential solutions (Hansen *et al.*, 1989). A goal of problem-solving training would be to increase the identification and implementation of nonaggressive solutions and to decrease the tendency to use violence as a resolution technique. Problem solving in relation to child behavior management (e.g., selection of management strategy) would be tied directly to the parenting skills discussed earlier. General problem solving beyond child management issues may also be a focus. Treatment may address day-to-day problems such as from budgeting, scheduling appointments (especially important if multiple agencies are involved), planning meals, and organizing the running of a household.

Developing strategies for managing anger-arousing situations may also be a target. Interventions may include relaxation training, self-control and cognitive coping (Azar & Wolfe, 1989; Walker *et al.*, 1988). As an initial step in anger management, some parents may actually need to learn how to identify cues—physiological, behavioral and cognitive—related to arousal. An increased level of arousal may compromise a parent's ability to focus on and learn new management techniques. Therefore, it may be best to focus first on general strategies (e.g., generation of possible solutions, selection of solution, evaluation of solution) for less arousing issues (e.g., budgeting) before targeting situations that evoke anger or extreme frustration.

Intervening with maltreating families can be complicated even further in the presence of ongoing substance abuse (Bavolek & Henderson, 1990; Coleman & Straus, 1983). Substance abuse can compromise a parent's ability to adhere to treatment. Even the most basic adherence to treatment, attending the sessions, can be affected. In such cases, the substance abuse issues must be addressed before other components of treatment can be initiated. If a child's safety is at risk, temporary placement outside the home may be warranted until the substance abuse is brought under control.

Techniques for increasing the availability and utilization of supports will vary widely depending on the family's situation (Walker *et al.*, 1988). Better use of supports in the extended family should be explored. Existing supports in the community may be underutilized. Some families, having once attempted to engage with a community agency and having had a negative experience, may be unwilling to re-engage. The multiproblem nature of maltreating families may have earned them a reputation in the community as "difficult to work with" or "hopeless," and the therapist may need to act as a liaison between agencies if contact or cooperation have broken down.

An exception to the relatively narrow focus of much of the treatment research is Project 12-Ways, a multifaceted behavioral treatment program for abusive and neglectful parents (cf. Lutzker, 1984; Wesch & Lutzker, 1991). Treatment targets are varied, including child management and parent–child interactions, problem-solving skill, social support, stress reduction, self-control training, assertiveness, and problems of neglect (e.g., home cleanliness, safety). Evaluations have indicated that families receiving Project 12-Ways services showed generally lower recidivism rates and less frequent removal of children from the home than those who had not received such services. The project has been successfully imitated in other programs throughout the country (Hansen *et al.*, 1998).

Additional Interventions for Neglect

Neglect poses slightly different treatment issues than physical abuse. Compared with physical abuse, which tends to occur as discrete incidents, neglect is often more chronic and tends to be characterized by the lack of certain behaviors (e.g., lack of supervision) rather than inappropriate behaviors (e.g., aggression). Virtually any skill involved in running a household, such as planning meals or budgeting finances, or caring for children, such as attending to medical needs or facilitating development, can be targeted, operationalized, and shaped during treatment. In this area the need for individualized assessment and ongoing monitoring is perhaps most pressing. There has been surprisingly little attention to the treatment of neglectful families, with the exception of research from Project 12-Ways (e.g., Lutzker, 1984; Tertinger *et al.*, 1984; Watson-Perczel *et al.*, 1988).

Target areas for treatment may include cleanliness (e.g., Watson-Perczel *et al.*, 1988) or home safety (e.g., Tertinger *et al.*, 1984). For instance, home safety data from the HAPI (Tertinger *et al.*, 1984) may be used to identify and improve unsafe areas in the home. Parents may need education to provide general knowledge about home safety, such as which household products are poisonous, and assistance in developing realistic expectations for child behavior. Toddlers are very curious about their environment and may not simply "learn" not to put items into electrical sockets because the parents say not to do so. Rather, the parents may need to take additional precautions. It is important to note that economic factors may impact a parent's ability to carry out treatment recommendations. For example, a therapist may recommend that covers be put on all unused electrical sockets, but the parent may not be in a position to purchase the covers.

Stimulation training may be another area of intervention for neglectful families, particularly if a reduced frequency of positive parent–child interactions is observed in the assessment (Hansen & Warner, 1992; Lutzker, Lutzker, Braunling-McMorrow, & Eddleman, 1987). Certain components of general parenting skills training (e.g., Child's Game, Forehand & McMahon, 1981) provide good opportunities to promote positive, nondirective parent–child interaction.

Course and Prognosis

Research has documented that behaviorally based treatment programs can improve parenting knowledge, attitudes, skills, and behaviors, and result in fewer child injuries and reports to protective agencies (e.g., see Azar & Wolfe, 1989; Wolfe & Wekerle, 1993; Walker *et al.*, 1988, for reviews). Despite evidence for the efficacy of behavioral programs in the treatment of perpetrators of child abuse and neglect, several limitations of this approach have been identified. For example, other serious problems, such as substance abuse or severe parental psychopathology, may compromise the efficacy of behavioral treatments (Azar & Wolfe, 1989). Skills-training interventions require a high degree of adherence, in that parents must practice and implement new skills outside therapeutic sessions; however, the treatment adherence of physically abusive and neglectful families is notoriously poor (Azar & Wolfe, 1989; Hansen & Warner, 1994; Lundquist & Hansen, 1998). Session attendance, for example, is a very basic, though essential, measure of adherence. One treatment program found that maltreating families attended 72% of sessions scheduled in the home and 62% of sessions scheduled in the clinic (Hansen *et al.*, 1998; Malinosky-Rummell *et al.*, 1991).

A related issue is that many abusive families are not self-referred for treatment. The majority of reports of possible maltreatment are made by professionals, such as teachers, physicians, police, and social workers (NCCAN, 1988). Parents may not see their behavior as problematic and may not be willing participants in the assessment or treatment process. Court orders for treatment may increase the likelihood that parents may attend a session, but there are few data to suggest that such orders affect a parent's willingness to adopt new attitudes or to practice new skills outside sessions (Hansen & Warner, 1994). Even in cases where assessment has been ordered by the court, attendance at sessions can be very low. For example, Butler and colleagues (1994) found that 37% of mothers court-ordered for assessments failed to attend at least two thirds of their appointments.

Intervention programs for maltreating parents vary as to whether they report recidivism rates; the length of time following treatment during which recidivism is monitored also varies. Wesch and Lutzker (1991) examined recidivism rates of maltreating parents receiving Project 12-Ways services (i.e., in-home behaviorial intervention with multiple possible treatment targets). Recidivism was broadly defined as occurrence of abuse, neglect, or adoption or foster placement, or some combination. Recidivism rates were 56% prior to treatment, 13% during treatment, and 31% posttreatment. Parents who received services from the state protective service agency and other community programs (but not Project 12-Ways) had recidivism rates of 42% prior to treatment, 25% during treatment, and 25% posttreatment. In another individualized behavioral intervention program, physical abuse was reported in 22.6% of the families during the course of treatment and neglect was reported in 3.8% of the families (Hansen *et al.*, 1998). Following treatment completion, 21% of the cases were later reopened for maltreatment by Child Protective Services and 23% were re-referred to the intervention program. Other research has reported a recidivism rate of 16.8% across a 5-year follow-up period, with the greatest risk occurring within the first 2 years following treatment; neglect was the most common form of recidivism (Jones, 1995).

Overall, the research evidence suggests that treatment may result in changes in parental behavior (e.g., improved child-management skills) and reduce the likelihood of additional maltreatment. However, more treatment outcome research is needed. Research is needed with larger samples, proper randomization procedures, longer follow-up periods, better demonstration of treatment integrity and replicability, and incorporation of more multimethod assessments with psychometrically sound devices (Hansen *et al.*, 1998; Wolfe & Wekerle, 1993). In addition, more research is needed on the overall effects of treatment on parent–child relationships and child development (i.e., beyond child-management skills).

Summary

In recent decades, professional and societal awareness of the extent and seriousness of child physical abuse and neglect has increased dramatically. During this time much research evidence has accumulated that describes child maltreatment as a multidimensional problem with multiple causes that requires comprehensive, individualized treatment. The multiproblem nature of maltreating families presents a wide variety of assessment and treatment difficulties for clinicians and researchers. Despite the difficulties, we have learned much about the causes, consequences, assessment, and treatment of child physical abuse and neglect in recent years. However, because of the heterogeneity of the problem and the complexities of the research, we still have much to learn.

References

Abidin, R. R. (1986). *Parenting Stress Index* (2nd ed.). Charlottesville, VA: Pediatric Psychology Press.

Achenbach, T. M. (1991). *Manual for the Child Behavior Checklist/4–18 and 1991 profile.* Burlington: University of Vermont.

Ammerman, R. T., Cassisi, J. E., Hersen, M., & Van Hasselt, V. B. (1986). Consequences of physical abuse and neglect in children. *Clinical Psychology Review, 6,* 291–310.

Ammerman, R. T., Hersen, M., & Van Hasselt, V. B. (1988). *The Child Abuse and Neglect Interview Schedule (CANIS).* Unpublished instrument, Western Pennsylvania School for Blind Children, Pittsburgh, PA.

Ammerman, R. T., Hersen, M., Van Hasselt, V. B., Lubetsky, M. J., & Sieck, W. R. (1994). Maltreatment in psychiatrically hospitalized children and adolescents with developmental disabilities: Prevalence and correlates. *Journal of the American Academy of Child and Adolescent Psychiatry, 33,* 567–576.

Atkinson, L., & Butler, S. (1996). Court-ordered assessment: Impact of maternal noncompliance in child maltreatment cases. *Child Abuse & Neglect, 21,* 185–190.

Azar, S. T., & Rohrbeck, C. A. (1986). Child abuse and unrealistic expectations: Further validation of the Parent Opinion Questionnaire. *Journal of Consulting and Clinical Psychology, 54,* 867–868.

Azar, S. T., & Wolfe, D. A. (1989). Child abuse and neglect. In E. J. Mash & R. Barkley (Eds.), *Treatment of childhood disorders* (pp. 451–489). New York: Guilford.

Azar, S. T., Robinson, D. R., Hekimian, E., & Twentyman, C. T. (1984). Unrealistic expectations and problem-solving ability in maltreating and comparison mothers. *Journal of Consulting and Clinical Psychology, 52,* 687–691.

Barkley, R. A. (1987). *Defiant Children: A clinician's manual for parent training.* New York: Guilford.

Bauer, W. D., & Twentyman, C. T. (1985). Abusing, neglectful and comparison mothers' responses to child-related and nonchild–related stressors. *Journal of Consulting and Clinical Psychology, 53,* 335–343.

Bavolek, S. J., & Henderson, H. L. (1990). Child maltreatment and alcohol abuse: Comparisons and perspectives for treatment. *Journal of Chemical Dependency Treatment, 3,* 165–184.

Belsky, J., & Vondra, J. (1989). Lessons from child abuse: The determinants of parenting. In D. Cicchetti & V. Carlson (Eds.), *Child maltreatment theory and research on the causes and consequences of child abuse and neglect* (pp. 129–153). New York: Cambridge University Press.

Bousha, D. M., & Twentyman, C. T. (1984). Mother–child interactional style in abuse, neglect and control groups: Naturalistic observations in the home. *Journal of Abnormal Psychology, 93,* 106–114.

Butcher, J. N., Dahlstrom, W. G., Graham, J. R., Tellegen, A., & Kaemmer, B. (1989). *Minnesota Multiphasic Personality Inventory–2 (MMPI-2): Manual for administration and scoring.* Minneapolis: University of Minnesota Press.

Butler, S. M., Radia, N., & Magnatta, M. (1994). Maternal compliance to court-ordered assessment in cases of child maltreatment. *Child Abuse & Neglect, 18,* 203–211.

Cicchetti, D., & Lynch, M. (1995). Failures in the expectable environment and their impact on individual development: The case of child maltreatment. In D. Cicchetti & D. J. Cohen (Eds.), *Developmental psychopathology: Vol. 2. Risk, disorder and adaptation* (pp. 32–71). New York: Wiley.

Coleman, D. H., & Straus, M. A. (1983). Alcohol abuse and family violence. In E. Gottheil, K. A. Druley, T. E. Skoloda, & H. M. Waxman (Eds.), *Alcohol, drug abuse and aggression* (pp. 104–124). Springfield, MA: Thomas.

Derogatis, L. R. (1983). *SCL-90-R: Administration, scoring, and procedures manual–II.* Towson, MD: Clinical Psychometric Research.

DeRoma, V. M., & Hansen, D. J. (1994, November). *Development of the Parental Anger Inventory.* Paper presented at the meeting of the Association for the Advancement of Behavior Therapy, San Diego, CA.

Dowdney, L., & Skuse, D. (1993). Parenting provided by adults with mental retardation. *Journal of Child Psychology and Psychiatry, 34,* 25–47.

D'Zurilla, T. J., & Nezu, A. M. (1988, November). *Development and preliminary evaluation of the Social Problem-Solving Inventory.* Paper presented at the convention of the Association for the Advancement of Behavior Therapy, New York.

Eyberg, S. M., & Robinson, E. A. (1981). *Dyadic Parent–Child Interaction coding system: A manual* (Manuscript. No. 2582). San Rafael, CA: Social and Behavioral Sciences Documents, Select Press.

Eyberg, S. M., & Ross, A. W. (1978). Assessment of child behavior problems: The validation of a new inventory. *Journal of Clinical Child Psychology, 7,* 113–116.

Falshaw, L., Browne, K. D., & Hollin, C. R. (1996). Victim to offender: A review. *Aggression and Violent Behavior, 4,* 389–404.

Forehand, R., & McMahon, R. (1981). *Helping the noncompliant child: A clinician's guide to parent training*. New York: Guilford.

Frodi, A. M., & Lamb, M. E. (1980). Child abusers' responses to infant smiles and cries. *Child Development, 51*, 238–241.

Hansen, D. J., & Warner, J. E. (1992). Child physical abuse and neglect. In R. T. Ammerman & M. Hersen (Eds.), *Assessment of family violence: A clinical and legal sourcebook* (pp. 123–147). New York: Wiley.

Hansen, D. J., & Warner, J. E. (1994). Treatment adherence of maltreating families: A survey of professionals regarding prevalence and enhancement strategies. *Journal of Family Violence, 9*, 1–19.

Hansen, D. J., Pallotta, G. M., Tishelman, A. C., Conaway, L. P., & MacMillan, V. M. (1989). Parental problem-solving skills and child behavior problems: A comparison of physically abusive, neglectful, clinic and community families. *Journal of Family Violence, 4*, 353–368.

Hansen, D. J., Conaway, L. P., & Christopher, J. S. (1990). Victims of child physical abuse. In R. T. Ammerman & M. Hersen (Eds.), *Treatment of family violence: A sourcebook* (pp. 17–49). New York: Wiley.

Hansen, D. J., Pallotta, G. M., Christopher, J. S., Conaway, R. L., & Lundquist, L. M. (1995). The Parental Problem-Solving Measure: Further evaluation with maltreating and nonmaltreating parents. *Journal of Family Violence, 10*, 319–336.

Hansen, D. J., Warner-Rogers, J. E., & Hecht, D. B. (1998). Implementing and evaluating an individualized behavioral intervention program for maltreating families: Clinical and research issues. In J. R. Lutzker (Ed.), *Handbook of child abuse research and treatment.* (pp. 133–158). New York: Plenum.

Hecht, D. B., Hansen, D. J., & Chandler, R. M. (1996, August). Parental anger towards children: Assessment issues in child maltreatment. In L. Peterson (Chair), *Beyond parenting skills: Parent–child relationships and child maltreatment.* Symposium conducted at the American Psychological Association Convention, Toronto, Ontario, Canada.

Hill, H. M., Hawkins, S. R., Raposo, M., & Carr, P. (1995). Relationship between multiple exposures to violence and coping strategies among African-American mothers. *Violence and Victims, 10*, 55–71.

Jones, D. P. H. (1995). The outcome of intervention [Editorial]. *Child Abuse & Neglect, 19*, 1363–1377.

Kanner, A. D., Coyne, J., Schaefer, C., & Lazarus, R. S. (1981). Comparison of two modes of stress measurement: Daily hassles and uplifts versus major events. *Journal of Behavioral Medicine, 4*, 1–39.

Kaufman, J., & Zigler, E. (1989). The intergenerational transmission of child abuse. In D. Cicchetti & V. Carlson (Eds.), *Child maltreatment theory and research on the causes and consequences of child abuse and neglect* (pp. 129–153). New York: Cambridge University Press.

Kelley, M. L., Grace, N., & Elliott, S. N. (1990). Acceptability of positive and punitive discipline methods: Comparisons among abusive, potentially abusive, and nonabusive parents. *Child Abuse & Neglect, 14*, 219–226.

Kelly, J. A. (1983a). *Solving your child's behavior problems*. Boston: Little, Brown.

Kelly, J. A. (1983b). *Treating child-abusive families: Intervention based on skills-training principles*. New York: Plenum.

Kempe, C. H., & Helfer, R. (1972). *Helping the battered child and his family*. Philadelphia: Lippincott.

Kempe, C. H., Silverman, F. N., Steele, B. F., Droegemuller, W., & Silver, H. K. (1962). The battered child syndrome. *Journal of the American Medical Association, 191*, 17–24.

Kerig, P. K. (1995). Triangles in the family circle: Effects of family structure on marriage, parenting, and child adjustment. *Journal of Family Psychology, 9*, 28–43.

Lahey, B. B., Conger, R. D., Atkeson, B. M., & Treiber, F. A. (1984). Parenting behavior and emotional status of physically abusive mothers. *Journal of Consulting and Clinical Psychology, 52*, 1062–1071.

Lundquist, L. M., & Hansen, D. J. (1998). Enhancing treatment adherence, social validity, and generalization of parent-training interventions with physically abusive and neglectful families. In J. R. Lutzker (Ed.), *Handbook of child abuse research and treatment.* (pp. 449–471) New York: Pergamon.

Lutzker, J. R. (1984). Project 12-Ways: Treating child abuse and neglect from an ecobehavioral perspective. In R. F. Dangel & R. A. Polster (Eds.), *Parent training* (pp. 260–297). New York: Guilford.

Lutzker, S. Z., Lutzker, J. R., Braunling-McMorrow, D. B., & Eddleman, J. (1987). Prompting to increase mother–baby stimulation with single mothers. *Journal of Child and Adolescent Psychotherapy, 4*, 3–12.

Maccoby, E. E., & Martin, J. A. (1983). Socialization in the context of the family: Parent–child interaction. In E. M. Hetherington (Ed.), *Socialization, personality and social development: Vol. 4. Handbook of child psychology* (pp. 1–101). New York: Wiley.

MacMillan, H. L., MacMillan, J. H., Offord, D. R., Griffith, L., & MacMillan, A. (1994). Primary prevention of child physical abuse and neglect: A critical review: Part I. *Journal of Child Psychology and Psychiatry, 35*, 835–856.

MacMillan, V. M., Guevremont, D. C., & Hansen, D. J. (1988). Problem-solving training with a multiply distressed abusive and neglectful mother: Effects on social insularity, negative affect, and stress. *Journal of Family Violence, 3,* 313–326.

MacMillan, V. M., Olson, R. L., & Hansen, D. J. (1988, November). *The development of an anger inventory for use with maltreating parents.* Paper presented at the meeting of the Association for the Advancement of Behavior Therapy, New York.

MacMillan, V. M., Olson, R. L., & Hansen, D. J. (1991). Low and high deviance analogue assessment of parent-training with physically abusive parents. *Journal of Family Violence, 6,* 279–301.

Malinosky-Rummell, R., & Hansen, D. J. (1993). Long-term consequences of childhood physical abuse. *Psychological Bulletin, 114,* 68–79.

Malinosky-Rummell, R., Ellis, J. T., Warner, J. E., Ujcich, K., Carr, R. E., & Hansen, D. J. (1991, November). *Individualized behavioral intervention for physically abusive and neglectful families: An evaluation of the Family Interaction Skills Project.* Paper presented at the meeting of the Association for the Advancement of Behavior Therapy, New York.

Melton, G. B., & Limber, S. (1989). Psychologists' involvement in cases of child maltreatment. *American Psychologist, 44,* 1225–1233.

Milner, J. S. (1986). *The Child Abuse Potential Inventory: Manual* (2nd ed). Webster, NC: Psytec.

Milner, J. S. (1991). Additional issues in child abuse assessment. *American Psychologist, 46,* 80–81.

Milner, J. S. (1993). Social information processing and physical child abuse. *Clinical Psychology Review, 13,* 275–294.

Milner, J. S. (1994). Assessing physical child abuse risk: The child abuse potential inventory. *Clinical Psychology Review, 14,* 547–583.

Milner, J. S., & Chilamkurti, C. (1991). Physical child abuse perpetrator characteristics: A review of the literature. *Journal of Interpersonal Violence, 6,* 345–366.

Milner, J. S., Robertson, K. R., & Rogers, D. L. (1990). Childhood history of abuse and adult child abuse potential. *Journal of Family Violence, 5,* 15–34.

Muller, R. T., Fitzgerald, H. E., Sullivan, L. A., & Zucker, R. A. (1994). Social support and stress factors in child maltreatment among alcoholic families. *Canadian Journal of Behavioural Science, 26,* 438–461.

National Center on Child Abuse and Neglect. (1988). *Study of national incidence and prevalence of child abuse and neglect: 1986.* Washington, DC: U.S. Department of Health and Human Services.

National Center on Child Abuse and Neglect. (1994). *Child maltreatment 1992: Reports from the states to the National Center on Child Abuse and Neglect.* Washington, DC: U.S. Department of Health and Human Services.

National Center on Child Abuse and Neglect. (1996). *Third national incidence study of child abuse and neglect.* Washington, DC: U.S. Department of Health and Human Services.

O'Dell, S. L., Tarler-Benlolo, L., & Flynn, J. M. (1979). An instrument to measure knowledge of behavioral principles as applied to children. *Journal of Behavior Therapy and Experimental Psychiatry, 10,* 29–34.

Oldershaw, L., Walters, G. C., & Hall, D. K. (1989). A behavioral approach to the classification of different types of physically abusive mothers. *Merrill-Palmer Quarterly, 31,* 255–279.

Orme, T. C., & Rimmer, J. (1981). Alcoholism and child abuse: A review. *Journal of Studies on Alcoholism, 42,* 273–287.

Quamma, J. P., & Greenberg, M. T. (1994). Children's experience of life stress: The role of family social support and social problem-solving skills as protective factors. *Journal of Child Clinical Psychology, 23,* 295–305.

Reid, J. B. (Ed.). (1978). *A social learning approach to family intervention: Vol. 2. Observation in home settings.* Eugene, OR: Castalia.

Reid, J. B., Kavanagh, K., & Baldwin, D. V. (1987). abusive parents' perceptions of child problem behaviors: An example of parental bias. *Journal of Abnormal Child Psychology, 15,* 457–466.

Roehling, P. V., & Robin, A. L. (1986). Development and validation of the Family Beliefs Inventory: A measure of unrealistic beliefs among parents and adolescents. *Journal of Counsulting and Clinical Psychology, 54,* 693–697.

Sarason, I. G., Johnson, J. H., & Siegel, J. M. (1978). Assessing the impact of life change: Development of the Life Experiences Survey. *Journal of Consulting and Clinical Psychology, 46,* 932–946.

Schilling, R. F., Schinke, S. P., Blythe, B. J., & Barth, R. P. (1982). Child maltreatment and mentally retarded parents: Is there a relationship? *Mental Retardation, 20,* 201–209.

Schindler, F., & Arkowitz, H. (1986). The assessment of mother–child interactions in physically abusive and nonabusive families. *Journal of Family Violence, 1,* 247–257.

Siegel, J. M. (1986). The Multidimensional Anger Inventory. *Journal of Personality and Social Psychology, 51,* 191–200.

Spanier, G. B. (1976). Measuring dyadic adjustment: New scales for assessing the quality of marriage and similar dyads. *Journal of Marriage and the Family, 38,* 15–28.

Spielberger, C. D., Jacobs, G., Russel, S., & Crane, R. S. (1983). Assessment of anger: The State-Trait Anger Scale. In J. N. Butcher & C. D. Spielberger (Eds.), *Advances in personality assessment* (Vol. 2, pp. 159–187). Hillsdale, NJ: Erlbaum.

Spinetta, J. J., & Rigler, D. (1972). The child-abusing parent: A psychological review. *Psychological Bulletin, 77,* 296–304.

Stasiewicz, P. R., & Lisman, S. A. (1989). Effects of infant cries on alcohol consumption in college males at risk for child abuse. *Child Abuse & Neglect, 13,* 463–470.

Steele, B. F., & Pollack, C. V., (1974). A psychiatric study of parents who abuse infants and small children. In. R. G. Helfer & C. H. Kempe (Eds.), The battered child, 2nd ed. (pp. 3–21). Chicago: University of Chicago Press.

Stokes, T. F., & Osnes, P. G. (1989). An operant pursuit of generalization. *Behavior Therapy, 20,* 337–355.

Straus, M. A. (1979). Measuring intrafamily conflict and violence: The Conflict Tactics Scales. *Journal of Marriage and the Family, 41,* 75–88.

Straus, M. A., & Kantor, G. K. (1994). Corporal punishment of adolescents by parents: A risk factor in the epidemiology of depression, suicide, alcohol abuse, child abuse and wife beating. *Adolescence, 29,* 543–561.

Straus, M. A., Hamby, S. L., Boney-McCoy, S., & Sugarman, D. B. (1996). The Revised Conflict Tactics Scales (CTS2): Development and preliminary psychometric data. *Journal of Family Issues, 17,* 283–316.

Tertinger, D. A., Greene, B. F., & Lutzker, J. R. (1984). Home safety: Development and validation of one component of an ecobehavioral treatment for abused and neglected children. *Journal of Applied Behavior Analysis, 2,* 159–174.

Trickett, P. K., & Susman, E. J. (1988). Parental perceptions of child-rearing practices in physically abusive and nonabusive families. *Developmental Psychology, 22,* 115–123.

Vaillant, G. E. (1995). *The national history of alcoholism revisited.* Cambridge, MA: Harvard University Press.

Wahler, R. (1980). The insular mother: Her problem in parent–child treatment. *Journal of Applied Behavior Analysis, 13,* 207–219.

Walker, C. E., Bonner, B. L., & Kaufman, K. L. (1988). *The physically and sexually abused child: Evaluation and treatment.* New York: Pergamon.

Warner, J. E., & Hansen, D. J. (1994). Identification and reporting of physical abuse by medical professionals: A review and implications for research. *Child Abuse & Neglect, 18,* 11–25.

Warner, J. E., Ujcich, K., Ellis, J. T., Malinosky-Rummell, R., & Hansen, D. J. (1992, November). *Social validity of an individualized behavioral intervention program for physically abusive and neglectful families: Further evaluation of the Family Interaction Skills Project.* Paper presented at the conference of the Association for the Advancement of Behavior Therapy, Boston.

Watson-Perczel, M., Lutzker, J. R., Greene, B. F., & McGimpsey, B. J. (1988). Assessment and modification of home cleanliness among families adjudicated for child neglect. *Behavior Modification, 12,* 57–81.

Wekerle, C., & Wolfe, D. A. (1993). Prevention of child physical abuse and neglect: Promising new directions. *Clinical Psychology Review, 13,* 501–540.

Wesch, D., & Lutzker, J. R. (1991). A comprehensive 5-year evaluation of Project 12-Ways: An ecobehavioral program fro treating and preventing child abuse and neglect. *Journal of Family Violence, 6,* 17–35.

Widom, C. S. (1989). Does violence beget violence? A critical examination of the literature. *Psychological Bulletin, 106,* 3–28.

Wolfe, D. A. (1987). *Child abuse: Implications for child development and psychopathology.* Newbury Park, CA: Sage.

Wolfe, D. A. (1988). Child abuse and neglect. In E. J. Mash & L. G. Terdal (Eds.), *Behavioral assessment of childhood disorders* (2nd ed., pp. 627–669). New York: Guilford.

Wolfe, D. A., & Wekerle, C. (1993). Treatment strategies for child physical abuse and neglect: A critical progress report. *Clinical Psychology Review, 13,* 473–500.

Wolfe, D. A., Fairbank, J. A., Kelly, J. A., & Bradlyn, A. S. (1983). Child abusive parents' physiological responses to stressful and nonstressful behavior in children. *Behavioral Assessment, 5,* 363–371.

Wolfe, D. A., Edwards, B. E., Manion, I., & Koverola, C. (1988). Early intervention for parents at risk for child abuse and neglect: A preliminary investigation. *Journal of Consulting and Clinical Psychology, 56,* 40–47.

Zigler, E., & Hall, N. W. (1989). Physical child abuse in America: Past, present and future. In D. Cicchetti & V. Carlson. *Child maltreatment: Theory and research on the causes and consequences of child abuse and neglect* (pp. 38–75). New York: Cambridge University Press.

Relationship Aggression Between Partners

Alan Rosenbaum and Paul J. Gearan

Introduction

Relationship aggression is known by many names; battering, domestic violence, spouse abuse, dating aggression, and marital violence are the most common. Regardless of how it is named, it refers to aggression between partners involved in an intimate relationship. Although it is frequently attributed to the power differential between men and women, there is sufficient evidence that it occurs in same-sex relationships, both male and female. We also know that female to male aggression is as common as male to female aggression (O'Leary et al., 1989; Straus & Celles, 1986) although it has been convincingly argued that the meaning of female to male aggression is different and the consequences less damaging. This chapter is concerned with aggression by males toward females in the context of intimate heterosexual relationships.

Incidence and prevalence of this very common form of aggression have long been underestimated, especially by mental health professionals. Approximately a third of the married or dating population report having experienced some physical relationship aggression. Aggression in dysfunctional relationships is even more ubiquitous, yet frequently unreported to relationship therapists and thereby unrecognized. Despite its recent visibility in the press and the media, training in treatment of domestic aggression has not traditionally been part of the curricula of most therapists, and remains a specialization with few practitioners. In a variation of the don't ask, don't tell theme, therapists may not be assessing for behaviors that they feel ill equipped to treat. Patients, feeling stigmatized because they are either victims or perpetrators, may not be forthcoming about aggression, especially if they sense that the therapist is uncomfortable with the topic. Routinely assessing for the occurrence of relationship aggression, not surprisingly, produces incidence figures at or above those published in the literature.

Alan Rosenbaum • Department of Psychiatry, University of Massachusetts Medical Center , Worcester, MA 01655. *Paul J. Gearan* • Department of Psychiatry, University of Massachusetts Memorial Health Care System, Worcester, MA 01655.

Handbook of Psychological Approaches with Violent Offenders: Contemporary Strategies and Issues, edited by Van Hasselt and Hersen. Kluwer Academic/Plenum Publishers, New York, 1999.

When we think of relationship aggression the likely image is of a man physically battering a woman. Although battering connotes frequent, ongoing physical violence resulting in bruising or other injury, it is also applied when such aggression is infrequent and less severe. Gondolf (1988) classifies batterers into three categories; the largest of these is the "typical" batterer which includes more than half of all batterers. In contrast with the impression of the batterer as depicted by the media (news and entertainment), the typical batterer engages in less severe forms of aggression (grabbing, pushing, slapping), several times a year, on average. This is not to diminish the seriousness of this type of aggression, but to alert the therapist to the fact that just because the patient is not bruised and cowering, does not mean that there is not an aggression problem. In addition to physical aggression, relationship aggression subsumes verbal and emotional abuse, including yelling, swearing, name-calling, threats, and diminishing the self-esteem of the victim, as well as sexual abuse and the destruction of pets and property. Sexual abuse includes any unwanted sexual behavior, public sexual embarrassment, and sexual coercion. The profeminist construction of relationship aggression centers on power and control issues. Aggression, in this model, represents the male's way of controlling the woman. It is historically rooted in a patriarchal tradition in which it is not only the husband's right, but his obligation, to control his wife. Because he is responsible for her actions, he has the right to discipline her. The man is the head of the household and responsible for all decision making. Many abusive men, therefore, are controlling and jealous, restricting the woman's access to resources, monitoring her activities, and restricting her social interactions. The power to control is derived from the threat of physical aggression. Consequently, once physical aggression has occurred, it need not reoccur in order to exert its coercive force over the victim. The memory of the event coupled with the threat of recurrence is sufficient to maintain the power imbalance in the relationship. In addition, there are numerous nonphysical methods of coercion (e.g., isolation from family and friends, threats, withholding finances, use of demeaning language). Pence and Paymer (1993) have utilized the power and control wheel to depict the various coercive behaviors that occur in abusive relationships. In treating abusive relationships, it is necessary to focus on all of these forms of abusive behavior, not only on the physical.

The high incidence of relationship aggression belies the fact that most men are brought up believing that hitting a girl or woman is cowardly and unmanly. The factors that cause a man to violate this norm are the topic of much of the research literature on relationship aggression. Initially, researchers focused on the abuse victim, primarily because she was more accessible, and the population of shelter residents provided the early picture of the abusive male. With the advent of batterers' treatment programs has come an increase in research on batterers themselves. Interestingly, research on violent couples has produced very few findings of differences between battered women and their nonbattered peers. Batterers, on the other hand, are readily discriminated from nonbatterers on a host of variables.

Explanatory models of relationship aggression are as diverse as the population itself. The search for risk markers has focused on interpersonal, intrapersonal, sociocultural, and, more recently, physiological factors. Among the ecological factors associated with relationship aggression are socioeconomic status, level of educational attainment, occupational status, and race. Batterers are more likely to be underemployed, less well educated, members of minority groups, and of lower socioeconomic status (Saunders, 1993; Straus, Gelles, & Steinmetz, 1980). Despite these findings, it is generally recognized that relationship aggression occurs across the socioeconomic, racial, and ethnic spectrum (Saunders, 1993). Relationship aggression also occurs across a broad age range. Rates of dating aggression among high school and college age populations may exceed rates in adult married and dating populations; although battering may persist into middle or even old age, it is clearly less prevalent in older samples. Straus and colleagues (1980) reported that relationship aggression was three times more likely to occur in men younger than 30 years of age.

Individual and Couple Characteristics

While recognizing the role the sociopolitical, legal, and financial systems of a traditionally patriarchal society play in the creation of male aggression, existence of these influences fails to explain individual differences in the expression of relationship aggression. Increasingly, researchers have turned their focus to identifying the individual characteristics of batterers as a means of understanding how the aggression is produced.

One commonly replicated finding is that many batterers have witnessed interparental aggression (Caesar, 1988; Hotaling & Sugarman, 1986; Kalmuss, 1984; Murphy, Meyer, & O'Leary, 1993) when they were children. Batterers also tend to have a greater history of direct physical and emotional abuse than nonabusive men (Caesar, 1988; Else, Wonderlich, Beatty, Christie, & Staton, 1993; Hotaling & Sugarman, 1986; Marshall & Rose, 1988; Rosenbaum & O'Leary, 1981). Interestingly, witnessing violence generally seems to be a more powerful predictor of male aggression toward their female partners than being the direct victim of aggression as a child (Pagelow, 1984; Sugarman & Hotaling, 1989). Dutton & Golant (1995) invokes PTSD and borderline personality disorder as explanatory mechanisms that also have therapeutic implications. He focuses on the defective relationship between the batterer and both parents: the father because he is cold, distant, emotionally and physically abusive, and the mother because she is likely an abuse victim herself and therefore unavailable to nurture her son. In fact, batterers rarely describe a healthy, supportive, nurturing, loving relationship, especially with the father.

Given their abuse histories, it is not surprising that batterers also tend to have negative views of themselves. Depression is a commonly identified symptom among batterers (Dinwiddie, 1992; Maiuro, Cahn, Vitaliano, Wagner, & Zegree, 1988), and may also interact with other variables such as substance abuse and poor communicative abilities in the production of aggression. Rosenbaum (1986) found that abusive men tended to have undifferentiated sex-role identification in comparison with their nonviolent counterparts. In numerous studies, batterers were found to have defective self-esteem or poor self-concepts (Goldstein & Rosenbaum, 1985; Neidig, Friedman, & Collins, 1986; Telch & Lindquist, 1984). However, Prince and Arias (1994) found that the relationship between self-esteem and abusiveness may be moderated by other variables as well. Logistic regressions identified two groups of men with greater chances of relationship aggression than the base rate would predict: men who were low on self-esteem, low on the desirability of controlling events in their lives, and low on the perceived personal control; and men who were high on self-esteem, high on desirability of control, and low on perceived personal control. These two different types of batterers are consonant with distinctions of the expressive use of aggression by the former group and more controlled, instrumental aggression by the latter.

Elevated alcohol or drug use in partner-abusive men has been identified in a number of studies (Barnett & Fagan, 1993; Kantor & Straus, 1986; Tollman & Bennett, 1990; Van Hasselt, Morrison, & Bellak, 1985). Despite the preponderance of data indicating higher substance use in this population, the degree to which this is a contributing or causative factor in the production of aggressive behavior has been the subject of much debate. In their review of studies that examine the relationship between alcohol use and marital aggression, Kantor and Straus (1986) found that although the substantial majority of studies indicated general elevations in alcohol consumption by batterers in comparison with nonbattering control subjects, most aggressive episodes (74%) did not involve prior alcohol use. Alcohol, either because of its physiological effects, cognitive effects, or some combination, acts as a behavioral disinhibitor and may thereby increase the probability of aggressive behavior given other contextual or predisposing factors.

Poor communication skills, problem solving, and assertiveness, both generalized and spouse specific, have been identified as risk markers for partner abuse. When compared with their partners, many batterers exhibit inferior verbal skills (Ganley, 1981; Rounsaville, 1978). Correspondingly, Anglin and Holzworth-Munroe (1997) found that physically aggressive men produced less competent problem-solving strategies in response to both marital and nonmarital hypothetical situations. Batterers also display poor partner-specific assertiveness (Dutton & Strachan, 1987; Mauiro, Cahn, & Vitaliano, 1986; O'Leary & Curley, 1986; Rosenbaum & O'Leary, 1981). However, while Rosenbaum and O'Leary (1981) found batterers significantly lower in spouse-specific assertiveness than either discordant, nonviolent men or maritally satisfied men, O'Leary & Curley (1986) replicated only the significant distinction between batterers and maritally satisfied men.

Models that view human behavior as a function of the interaction between biological, social, and psychological elements are the rule, rather than the exception, yet in the domain of relationship aggression, biological factors have been all but ignored. Several studies have now suggested a relationship between traumatic head injury and an increased risk for relationship aggression (Rosenbaum & Hoge, 1989; Rosenbaum et al., 1994). Logistic regression analyses indicated that of the factors included, history of significant head injury was the best predictor of being a batterer and odds ratios indicated that the occurrence of a prior head injury increased the likelihood of relationship aggression almost sixfold (Rosenbaum et al., 1994). Serotonin (5-HT) has been implicated in both depression and impulsive aggression. Rosenbaum, Abend, Gearan, and Fletcher (1996) reported that among non-head-injured subjects, batterers had significantly lower levels of serotonergic activity than nonbatterers, as indexed by prolactin response to fenfluramine challenge. Finally, Gottman and colleagues (1995) compared the heart rate reactivity of batterers and nonbatterers in a conflictual interchange with spouses. They noted that a subsample of the batterers were vagal reactors, meaning that under stress conditions, they showed a decreased heart rate, contrary to what would be expected in a normal subject. However, the same pattern was apparently observed among the same percentage of nonbatterers (Jacobson, personal communication, 1995). The ultimate therapeutic utility of these findings remains to be demonstrated; however, biological adjuncts (such as the use of serotonin reuptake inhibitors) to more traditional forms of batterer treatment are already being explored.

The violent dyad has received substantial attention. In examining changes in the rates of relationship aggression from 1975 to 1985, Straus and Gelles (1986) noted that over that time span, overall rates of female to male aggression increased such that they exceeded the rates of male to female aggression and further, rates of the more severe forms of aggression were also higher for females to males than for males to females. Attachment theory's sine qua non status in explaining the qualities of a child's interpersonal relationships has also sparked adult analogs for romantic relationships. Holzworth-Munroe, Stuart, and Hutchinson (1997) applied some of these adult formulations in comparing batterers and nonbatterers. In comparison to nonviolent men, batterers reported significantly more anxiety about being abandoned in relationships and more anxious attachment to their wives than either maritally distressed or nondistressed nonviolent men. Batterers are often described as controlling, possessive, and jealous (Delgado & Bond, 1993), although there are questions as to the validity of this claim (Murphy, Meyer, & O'Leary, 1994), and similar statements have been made about abused women. Barnett, Martinez, and Bluestein (1995) found that batterers experienced significantly more jealousy than maritally satisfied, nonviolent men; however, maritally discordant but nonviolent men also evidenced these elevations. These findings underscore the necessity for inclusion of the discordant group in marital violence research to determine what factors may be associated with general, nonphysical conflict as opposed to actual physical abusiveness.

Violence is more prevalent in both racial and religious intermarriages (Rosenbaum & O'Leary, 1981), perhaps because of the greater opportunity for disagreement about deeply held, core beliefs. Regarding the role of socioeconomic, occupational, and educational status, Hornung, McCullough, and Sujimoto (1981) suggested that it is not absolute levels on these factors that is important, but rather discrepancies or incompatibilities between partners. It is easy to see how these factors might interact with individual characteristics such as defective self-esteem or poor impulse control to create a volatile environment ready to explode into aggression, given a spark of conflict.

Batterers have been distinguished from nonbatterers on a number of variables; however, increasingly research has focused on the complex nature of the interaction of these factors in the manifestation of aggression. Failure to identify a single batterer's profile and conflicting data over the significant contributions of many variables indicates that while there may be valid risk factors for men becoming aggressive in their relationships, batterers are a heterogeneous group. Furthermore, the inclusion of nonviolent but maritally discordant comparison groups in many recent studies has illuminated the relationship between these factors and relationship conflict versus physical aggression.

In summary, relationship aggression is a significant problem affecting at least a third of the married or dating population. It is even more significant if we consider only those individuals seeking therapy for relationship dysfunction. It has serious negative consequences for victims, perpetrators, and witnessing children. It also has high societal costs including law enforcement, judicial, and medical. It has been estimated, for example, that one in three women seeking care for any reason in hospital emergency rooms is battered (American Medical Association [AMA], 1992). This begs the question of what can be done to reduce, and ultimately eliminate, relationship aggression. Social and cultural changes addressing acceptability of violence toward women, gender equality issues, and sexualization of violence toward women in the media are clearly necessary but beyond the scope of this chapter. Our focus is on the psychological approaches to dealing with relationship aggression.

Treatment Issues

There is much controversy regarding whether batterers should be treated, and if so, how it should be accomplished. Many, especially among profeminists and battered women's advocates, argue convincingly that relationship aggression is a crime, not a condition, and should be treated via law enforcement and the legal system. Others argue for intervention, as opposed to treatment, and recommend educational programs, not unlike the approach commonly prescribed for drunk drivers. An important unanswered question is whether any program, therapeutic, educational, or penal is effective, and further, how effectiveness should be judged. At present, we have more questions than answers about these issues. Consequently, we identify the issues and discuss the current knowledge regarding each.

Issue: Is Battering a Psychological/Psychiatric Problem?

The battered women's movement and the proponents of profeminist approaches to batterers' treatment say it is not. In his preface to Gelles's *The Violent Home* (1972), Murray Straus articulates this position: "individual pathology is but a minor element. Few, if any, of the people he [Gelles] studied can be considered as suffering from any gross abnormality" (p. 16). However, Gelles interviewed only 14 men, did not use mental health professionals as interviewers, and did not use psychological assessments. A number of subsequent studies have and, although partner abuse does not constitute a specific psychopathological entity, it is clear that batterers display a wide spectrum of psychological disorders. Hamberger and Hastings (1991) evaluated batterers using the Millon (MCMI) and concluded that although batterers were a heterogeneous group and did not conform to a unified batterer profile, they showed significant elevations on borderline and antisocial characteristics. There is substantial support for the prevalence of borderline (Dutton & Starzomski, 1993; Else *et al.*, 1993; Hart, Dutton, & Newlove, 1993) and antisocial traits (Dutton, 1995; Else *et al.*, 1993; Hart, Dutton, & Newlove, 1993; Murphy *et al.*, 1993) among batterers. Batterers have been shown to have low self-esteem (Ball, 1977; Goldstein & Rosenbaum, 1985), excessive dependency needs (Wietzman & Dreen, 1982), depression, paranoia, and substance abuse problems (Faulk, 1974; Feazell, Mayers, & Deschner, 1984). Not surprisingly, antisocial personality disorder is often associated with batterers and recent work on heart rate reactivity is consistent with this (Gottman *et al.*, 1995). Irrespective of whether batterers exhibit psychopathology, behavioral models have always focused on maladaptive behavior in preference to medicalized syndromes. Rather than trying to "treat" mental "illness" behaviorists seek behavior change and have developed interventions for a wide range of undesirable behaviors. Conceptualized in this way, relationship aggression presents a worthy target for psychological intervention. The issue is not whether to treat, but how to treat most effectively.

Issue: To Arrest or Not

The arrest versus treatment controversy is a red herring. In a paper defending against criticism of their reactivity paper, Jacobson, Gottman, and Shortt (1995) made the statement: "Battering is primarily a public health problem, not a problem for psychotherapists" (p. 276). Can't public health problems be the domain of psychologists?

Who says arrest and psychotherapy are mutually exclusive? Initial enthusiasm that arrest alone was an effective deterrent to batterers (L. Sherman & Berk, 1984) has been moderated by numerous replications that have failed to support the initial claims of success (Dunford, Huizinga, & Elliot, 1990; Hirschel, Hutchison, & Dean, 1992; Sherman et al., 1992). In practice, batterers are rarely given sentences exceeding a few months, and it is hard to imagine how spending time in so misogynist an environment as jail would lead to reduction in either anger or aggression toward women. Legal remedies, arrest, and incarceration may play a role but are apparently inadequate unless combined with additional intervention. There is no question that relationship aggression is no less a crime than any other assault and battery, and there is no argument that arrest is the appropriate societal response to such behavior. The question is not whether to arrest, but whether arrest alone is effective in reducing violence against women and the evidence indicates that it is not. Whether to arrest and prosecute is a separate question from whether to treat. We can do either, or we can do both. Which is more effective is an empirical question.

Issue: The Format and Structure of Treatment—Options and Implications

After the question of whether relationship aggression should be treated, the issue that has received the most attention concerns treatment options. Most commonly, batterers are treated in cognitive-behaviorally oriented, time-limited, psychoeducational groups. Because judges are reluctant to impose indeterminate sentences, the time-limited or closed-ended format is a necessity of court-mandated treatment. Cognitive-behavioral approaches are well suited to short-term, time-limited group treatment. Treating batterers alone, as opposed to couple counseling, also emphasizes the point that the batterer is solely responsible for his aggressive behavior. Providing the victim with information about protecting her safety, the importance of using shelters, the police and legal resources if she is in danger, as well as encouragement and support in exiting the abusive relationship may present the couple's therapist with a conflict of interest. Treating the batterer in a group and referring the victim to the local shelter or women's group assures that she will get the necessary information and support, without compromising the therapeutic relationship with the batterer.

Treating relationship aggression in a couple counseling format poses two additional potential problems. There is the concern that bringing the couple together puts the woman at increased risk of violence. This is especially true if the couple is not cohabitating and meets solely for the therapy session. Further, couple counseling often exposes sensitive issues that may not be adequately resolved in session and may carry over into the parking lot or the ride home, where the therapist cannot monitor the levels of affect and defuse threatening situations. Recent research failed to find an increased risk to the woman in the couple counseling format (O'Leary, 1996); however, this study excluded more dangerous couples, where the risk might have been greater. A second problem concerns the fact that merely offering couple counseling sends the message that relationship aggression can be successfully treated and batterers rehabilitated, a message with which many would take issue. The counter argument that many battered women will remain in the relationship anyway ignores the fact that we may be holding out false hope to individuals already grasping at straws.

On the positive side, many of the strategies commonly taught in batterers' treatment programs may be more effective if they are properly presented to the female partner and she is cooperating in their implementation. A case in point is the time-out procedure, a critical component of many programs. Batterers are taught to monitor their level of angry affect and to take a time-out by leaving the situation when they feel they are in danger of aggressing. Batterers commonly report that their partners will try to prevent them from leaving and may physically block the door or grab the car keys. Ironically, many batterers aggress when blocked while trying to take a time-out. A likely reason for this problem stems from the fact that men tend to be conflict avoidant, whereas women are more likely to be conflict confrontive. She knows that if he leaves, the issue will go unresolved and he will have "had his way." Explaining the time-out to the woman, addressing her concerns by soliciting a pledge from the man that he will return to continue the discussion as soon as he can do so nonviolently, and encouraging her to use the time-out herself when she senses she may be in danger may facilitate the successful implementation of this strategy.

The empirical evidence supports the utility of couple counseling with this population. A number of couple programs have been in operation for many years and their effectiveness has been documented (O'Leary, 1996 ; O'Leary & Neidig, 1993). While one may not choose this treatment format, there seems to be little empirical evidence supporting its detractors.

Issue: Does Batterer's Treatment Work?

The short answer is "How do we define work?" Does reduction of aggression count or is cessation necessary? Since aggression is rarely a daily occurrence, even very aggressive couples may experience long nonviolent periods. The emotional distress derived from uncertainty as to when violence will occur may be more damaging than the actual aggression. While any reduction of aggression would be an improvement, the occurrence of any aggression, physical or not, is unacceptable and it is questionable whether a treatment that fails to completely eliminate aggression can be considered a success. How to assess outcome poses additional problems. The three most common methods are batterer self-report, victim report, and police or criminal records.

Methods of Measurement

Batterer report Follow-up interviews with batterers either immediately posttreatment or some time afterward are frequently reported. Interviews, either in person or by telephone, and paper-and-pencil questionnaires (often including some variation of the Conflict Tactics Scale [CTS; Straus, 1979]) completed either in person, or through the mail, and inquiring about aggression subsequent to group completion provide the outcome data. The veracity of such reports has been questioned not only because of general distrust of batterers, but also because of concerns that the batterer may fear that the recurrence of aggression will be reported back to the courts or probation department and result in further legal consequences. Even apart from such concerns, cognitive dissonance, social desirability, and the desire to please the therapist, concepts which often affect outcome reports of even nonaggressive patients might affect the validity of data obtained from perpetrators. These studies are also plagued by low participation rates creating a potentially significant reporting bias. At best, only about half of program participants are available to follow-up, with the number decreasing as a function of the length of the follow-up interval.

Victim report Victim report, most commonly by telephone interview, is typically viewed as more accurate than that of the batterer. As Hirschel, Hutchinson, & Dean (1992) noted, however, victim reports are seldom validated and there is no empirical support for the belief that they are many more accurate than perpetrator reports. In addition, victims are often unavailable as informants. Participation rates for victims range from a low of about 30% (Palmer, Brown, & Barrera, 1992) to a high of 76% (Dunford, 1992), and, as in the case with perpetrator reports, higher response rates correspond to shorter follow-up intervals. In many cases the batterer is no longer involved with the same woman, or possibly with any woman. In other cases he may have a new partner who is unfamiliar with his past history, creating a situation where he may be unwilling to give permission to contact her, and where contacting her without his permission would be an ethical breach. In any case, outcome studies relying on victim reports generate higher recidivism rates than studies relying on batterer reports. Studies comparing victim reports with perpetrator reports (within couple) have found only moderate levels of reliability (Jouriles & O'Leary, 1985).

Police or criminal records Criminal records containing arrests, convictions, and violations of protective orders provide the most objective measures of recidivism and the highest inclusion rates, since almost all group participants can be followed up. The main drawback is that many acts of aggression, especially verbal-emotional abuse and coercion, are never reported to the police. Further, perpetrators may move out of state and subsequently reoffend in another jurisdiction. Consequently, studies relying on police reports or criminal records significantly underestimate recidivism and produce inflated success rates for programs so evaluated. In fact, studies utilizing this outcome measure do generate the highest success rates, as compared with studies employing victim report or batterer self-report. This measure of outcome may be less useful in producing estimates of overall success rates for treatment, but more useful for evaluating specific aspects of treatment. For example, do longer programs produce less recidivism than shorter programs? If none of these methods of assessing outcome is without its flaws, perhaps the best approach to assessment would be a combination of them. Hamberger and Hastings (1988), for example, looked at all three indices and accepted any report of aggression as a negative outcome. Needless to say, such a strategy would tend to depress success rates.

Other measures Several investigators have evaluated the success of their programs by looking at pre–post changes on measures of behaviors associated with battering. Since batterers are often depressed, hostile, and have negative attitudes toward women, positive changes on measures of these variables have been taken as a measure of success. Studies employing couples will often consider positive changes in marital satisfaction in assessing treatment impact. The assumption is that changes in these dimensions will be associated with reductions in aggression. Since attitudinal changes do not always correspond to behavior change, the importance of change in associated behaviors must be demonstrated.

Follow-up interval As noted earlier, physical aggression in relationships is rarely a daily event and couples frequently experience long periods of nonviolence, even in the absence of treatment. Walker (1979) described this in her cycle of violence model, in which two of the three components of the cycle (the build-up and the postaggression period) were aggression free. Given this pattern, as well as the commonly observed "honeymoon period" that often accompanies participation in treatment, it is important to set follow-up intervals sufficiently long to enable discrimination between the positive effects of the treatment and the naturally occurring periods of nonviolence. The most common follow-up intervals (not including immediately posttreatment which is unacceptable) are 6 and 12 months. Shorter follow-up periods generally produce higher success rates.

Existing Outcome Data

Given the inconsistencies in how successful outcome is defined and assessed, it should not surprise us that the empirical outcome literature is inconsistent and inconclusive. Feldman and Ridley (1995) reviewed the outcome literature on batterers' treatment and divided the 30 studies surveyed into three methodological categories. The largest of the three, single group pre–post studies, included 20 studies which they characterized as (1) defining the sample as males having perpetrated at least one physical act of aggression against a female partner, as indexed by the CTS (Straus, 1979), interview, or police report; (2) utilizing a psychoeducational, cognitive-behavioral treatment approach (10–32 weeks in length); and (3) having a follow-up interval of 6–12 months. They concluded that these studies suggest that group treatment of batterers has a positive impact: "between one half and two-thirds of participants appear to cease acts of interpartner violence completely, while others substantially reduce their frequency and range of aggressive acts" (p. 335). The factors most consistently associated with recidivism were a history of alcohol and substance abuse problems, violence experiences in the family of origin (either as a victim or witness), and a previous criminal record (nonviolent).

The second category included six quasi-experimental, nonequivalent control group studies. These studies used either treatment dropouts or untreated controls. The three studies comparing treatment completers with treatment dropouts were inconsistent with one showing no differences in rates of recidivism (Edelson & Grusznski, 1988. Note: this reference contained two separate studies which produced different results), one showing completers to have a minimally lower rate of recidivism (Edelson & Grusznski, 1988), and one showing moderate differences (Hamberger & Hastings, 1988). Three studies compared treatment completers to untreated controls (Chen, Bersani, Myers, & Denton, 1989; Dutton, 1986; Waldo, 1988) and found significant and substantial differences in the recidivism rates of treated, as compared with untreated, subjects.

The third category included two experimental designs (employing control groups). In the first, Edelson and Syers (1990) compared three treatment models (education, self-help, and combined) and reported that based on partner reports at 6-month follow-up, the structured education and combined models both demonstrated significantly lower recidivism rates than the self-help group. In the second study (Harris, Savage, Jones, & Brooke, 1988) both conjoint group treatment and individual couples treatment demonstrated significant gains but did not differ from each other. These results were confirmed by O'Leary and Neidig (1993), who reported that both gender-specific treatment and conjoint group treatment demonstrated significant reductions in physical and psychological aggression, marital distress, and depressive symptomology.

While most of these studies offer hope that treatment of relationship aggression can be effective, our optimism must be tempered by the fact that these studies contain numerous methodological weaknesses and few represent experimental designs with random assignment to no-treatment control groups. The inherent dangers in relationship aggression preclude use of such designs; however, Harrell (1991) approximated such a comparison. She utilized a sample of batterers who had been adjudicated and either mandated into a batterers' treatment program or not. Although the decision rules utilized by judges in making dispositions was unknown, thus increasing the likelihood of a Berksonian bias, Harrell (1991) believed that the primary factor in referral decisions "appeared to be judicial approval of batterer treatment" (p. 3) and further that the two groups did not differ on severity of incident, the use of arrest, age, and alcohol or substance abuse. However, offenders referred to treatment were "more likely to be married to the victim, less likely to have a prior criminal record, and less likely to be unemployed" (p. 3). Results of this study were that there were no differences between treated and untreated offenders in rates of recidivism. There are several possible explanations for this in addition to the sampling problems. Several different programs were involved, differing in program length and content. Harrell also noted inconsistencies and delays in program operations. Further, as DeMaris and Jackson (1987) noted, there are greater opportunities for recidivism if the couple remains together and, as noted above, the treated group in this study was more likely to be married. Nevertheless, this is not the only study to cast doubt on the superiority of batterers' treatment over no treatment, and proponents of batterers' treatment are obliged to empirically demonstrate the value of the services they provide.

Outcome research on batterers' treatment may be flawed, but it is also in its early stages of development. If batterers are a heterogeneous population, as we believe them to be, then it is unlikely that any treatment will be effective for the whole population. Rather, different strategies may be necessary for different segments of the population. Such a prescriptive approach is beyond the scope of existing research in this area. Further, development of effective treatments for any problem is a dynamic process. It is not uncommon that early attempts at treatment are ineffective, but serve to inform the evolution of more effective interventions. Perhaps the question facing us is not whether batterers' treatment works, but what the effective components of existing treatments are, for which batterers, and how we might treat more effectively.

Issue: What Are the Strategies and Interventions That Typically Comprise Batterers Treatment Programs?

Interventions generally focus on the dual goals of attitude and behavior change. Among the attitudes targeted are the belief that there is a legitimate use of aggression in intimate relationships, external attributions for aggression (e.g. blaming others, including the victim), taking responsibility for one's behavior, negative attitudes toward women, patriarchal beliefs, and power and control issues. Most programs focus on the different forms of abusive-coercive behavior. Although the goal is often the elimination of physical aggression, programs are becoming increasingly sensitized to the fact that even if physical aggression ceases, the batterer may employ terroristic strategies that trade on previous violence and serve to maintain the batterer's control over the victim. The power and control wheel (Pence & Paymer, 1993) is often utilized by programs to raise consciousness regarding the effect that batterer behaviors may have on victims. A major interprogram difference concerns the degree to which power and control issues are emphasized, with the more profeminist programs focusing almost exclusively on power and control as the determinant of aggression.

Batterers have been identified as having traditional expectations regarding roles in the relationship (Tolman & Bennett, 1990), and failure by either partner to conform to these expectations has been associated with aggression. Exploration of role expectations and ideal–real discrepancies are discussed. Men are confronted with the choices that they have, namely to either attempt to negotiate changes with their partner, or to consider leaving the relationship. In many violent relationships, partners are so ill suited to each other and the ideal–real discrepancy is so large that dissolution of the relationship may be the best alternative. Two reasons batterers often have difficulty accepting this choice are that they have low self-esteem and fear that they will not find another mate, or that there are children involved. Other common strategies include empathy training and dealing with personal abuse histories and family of origin issues (Dutton & Golan, 1995; Gondolf, 1990).

Behavior change strategies include assertiveness training, communications training, anger management, relaxation, and stress reduction. Batterers are taught to identify cues that they are becoming angry and to use the time-out procedure. Many programs have a cognitive-behavioral orientation and also focus on identifying and replacing anger-provoking, inflammatory cognitions. Because alcohol and substance use is frequently associated with relationship aggression, most programs deal with these issues. Although alcohol–substance abuse cannot be adequately dealt with as a component of these groups, the effort is to raise consciousness about its relevance and to provide encouragement and referral for more intensive treatment.

Almost half of batterer treatment programs identify themselves as psychoeducational group approaches (Gondolf, 1990), which means that they share features of both a psychotherapy group and a didactic experience. About a quarter of programs are self-defined as management/control, didactic, or confrontational, or a combination, and an equal number are described as therapeutic (Gondolf, 1990). Management/control programs see their primary objective as protection of the victim and accomplish this through monitoring of the batterer and close communication between the program, the victim, and the legal system. Psychoeducational and therapeutic programs also have the objective of protecting the victim, but seek to accomplish this through successful treatment of the batterer, which is more effectively done if he views the treater as advocate, rather than as adversary. Psychoeducational and therapeutic programs may also be confrontive, and do not accept, tolerate, or endorse the use of aggression or coercion.

All treatment programs share the ultimate objective of eliminating aggression in intimate relationships. Although the woman is more often defined as the victim, aggression by either partner toward the other is unacceptable. There is great variability as to how to treat, but also a remarkable number of commonalties among programs. Structural differences include treatment length and duration, court versus self-referral, group versus individual treatment, couples versus gender specific treatment, psychoeducational versus therapeutic versus management/control, orientation (cognitive-behavioral, psychodynamic, family systems), training and professional status of treaters, and setting. According to the report of the American Psychological Association (APA) Presidential Task Force (1996) the most common intervention strategies are reeducation, resocialization, confrontation, and management/control, yet there are significant differences in the weight various programs place on each of these objectives. In terms of content, different programs touch many of the same bases but there is a great deal of variability regarding the emphasis and importance placed on each.

Summary

Relationship aggression is a sociolegal problem with significant public health implications. At a time when interpersonal aggression is our most significant social problem, the potential contributions of domestic aggression loom especially large. Evidence supports the detrimental impact not only on the participants, but also on witnessing children. Social change is essential, but unfortunately too slow and unpredictable to be depended on as an intervention strategy. Relationship aggression is a complex phenomenon; batterers and their victims are heterogeneous populations that cannot be simply and conveniently described. Conceptual schema range from criminal activity to psychological problem; proposed interventions range from incarceration to psychotherapy and neither conceptualizations nor proposed interventions are mutually exclusive. The psychological perspective is that relationship aggression is a crime, but that psychological constructs and interventions may be helpful in understanding and treating it.

Mental health professionals are in an excellent position to identify and intervene in cases of relationship aggression. Aggression is a common concomitant to relationship and family dysfunction, abuse victims are often depressed and anxious, and children of aggressive couples often display emotional and behavioral problems. All of these problems are likely to result in presentation to a mental health professional. Therapists need to be aware of the risk markers for aggression and also of the need to specifically assess for the occurrence of such aggression, as it is stigmatizing and may not always be identified as a presenting problem. Once the problem is identified, therapists must also be aware of the appropriate responses and interventions. In the case of the abuse victim it is essential to provide information and referral as an adjunct to treatment. Female victims need to be made aware of their legal rights and options, as well as of the location of shelter and advocacy services. Therapists must also be careful not to co-opt the autonomy of the victim and to respect her right not to make a report to the police. Unlike child abuse, there is not a mandatory reporting law for relationship aggression, and depriving the victim of her right to make choices is just another form of abuse.

Batterers' treatment or, more generically, intervention, has evolved both within and outside of the mental health professions. Although more frequently conducted from a psychoeducational or therapeutic perspective, didactic programs conducted by nonprofessional group leaders (sometimes ex-batterers) are not uncommon. Much of the research, however, has focused on time-limited, psychoeducational groups often employing cognitive-behavioral strategies and conducted by mental health professionals. Such programs are not offered as an alternative to legal intervention and, in fact, the combination of arrest and court mandated treatment appears to be superior to arrest alone. Although promising, the outcome literature on batterers' treatment is methodologically flawed and inconclusive. Intuitively, we might expect that any kind of treatment would be superior to no treatment, yet there is at least some evidence to the contrary. In this chapter, we have tried to view this literature developmentally and suggest that it is necessary to empirically evaluate whether batterers' treatment works from a more microscopic, prescriptive perspective. We need to discover what works and what does not, dispensing with ineffective components and either altering them or replacing them with more effective strategies. We have argued that batterers are a heterogeneous population and that different types of treatment may be required for different types of batterers. It is also possible, in fact likely, that some batterers may be untreatable and inappropriate for this type of intervention. At present, however, we cannot make these distinctions with an acceptable level of certainty. Much research is necessary to answer the many questions posed in this chapter.

ACKNOWLEDGEMENT

Preparation of this chapter was supported in part by an NIMH grant (MH 44812) to Alan Rosenbaum.

References

American Medical Association. (1992). Diagnostic and treatment guidelines on domestic violence. *Archives of Family Medicine, 1,* 39–47.
American Psychological Association. (1996). *Violence and the family.* Report of the American Psychological Association Presidential Task Force. Washington, DC: Author
Anglin, K., & Holzworth-Munroe, A. (1997). Comparing the responses of maritally violent and nonviolent spouses to problematic marital and nonmarital situations: Are the skill deficits of physically aggressive husbands and wives global? *Journal of Family Psychology, 11,* 301–313.
Ball, M. (1977). Issues of violence in family casework. *Social Casework, 58,* 3–12.
Barnett, O. W., & Fagan, R. W. (1993). Alcohol use in male spouse abusers and their female partners. *Journal of Family Violence, 8,* 1–25.
Barnett, O. W., Martinez, T. E., & Bluestein, B. W. (1995). Jealousy and romantic attachment in maritally violent and nonviolent men. *Journal of Interpersonal Violence, 10,* 473–486.
Caesar, P. L. (1988). Exposure to violence in the families-of-origin among wife-abusers and maritally nonviolent men. *Violence and Victims, 3,* 49–62.
Chen, H., Bersani, C., Myers, S. C., & Denton, R. (1989). Evaluating the effectiveness of a court sponsored abuser treatment program. *Journal of Family Violence, 4,* 309–322.
Delgado, A. R., & Bond, R. A. (1993). Attenuating the attribution of responsibility: The lay perception of jealousy as a motive for wife battery. *Journal of Applied Social Psychology, 23,* 1337–1356.
DeMaris, A., & Jackson, J. K. (1987). Batterers' reports of recidivism after counseling. *Social Casework, 68,* 458–465.
Dinwiddie, S. H. (1992). Psychiatric disorders among wife batterers. *Comprehensive Psychiatry, 33,* 411–416.
Dunford, F. W. (1992). The measurement of recidivism in cases of spouse assault. *Journal of Criminal Law and Criminology, 83,* 120–136.
Dunford, F. W., Huizinga, D., & Elliott, D. (1990). The role of arrest in domestic assault: The Omaha experiment. *Criminology, 28,* 183–206.
Dutton, D. G. (1986) The outcome of court-mandated treatment for wife-assault: A quasi-experimental evaluation. *Violence and Victims, 3,* 5–30.
Dutton, D. G., & Golant, S. K. (1995). *The batterer: A psychological profile.* New York: Basic Books.
Dutton, D. G., & Starzomski, A. J. (1993). Borderline personality in perpetrators of psychological and physical abuse. *Violence and Victims, 8,* 327–337.
Dutton, D. G., & Strachan, C. E. (1987). Motivational needs for power and spouse specific assertiveness in assaultive and nonassaultive men. *Violence and Victims, 3,* 145–156.
Edelson, J. L., & Grusznski, R. J. (1988). Treating men who batter: Four years of outcome data from the domestic abuse project. *Journal of Social Service Research, 12,* 3–22.

Edelson, J. L., & Syers, M. (1990). Relative effectiveness of group treatments for men who batter. *Social Work Research and Abstracts, 26*, 10–17.

Else, L., Wonderlich, S. A., Beatty, W. W., Christie, D. W., & Staton, R. D. (1993). Personality characteristics of men who physically abuse women. *Hospital and Community Psychiatry, 44*, 54–58.

Faulk, M. (1974). Men who assault their wives. *Medicine, Science, and the Law, 14*, 180–183.

Feazell, C. S., Mayers, R. S., & Deschner, J. (1984). Services for men who batter: Implications for programs and policies. *Family Relations, 33*, 217–223.

Feldman, C. M., & Ridley, C.A. (1995). The etiology and treatment of domestic violence between adult partners. *Clinical Psychology: Science and Practice 2*, 317–348.

Ganley, A. L. (1981). *Court-mandated counseling for men who batter: A three-day workshop for mental health professionals.* Washington, DC: Center for Women's Policy Studies.

Gelles, R. J. (1972). *The violent home.* Beverly Hills, CA.: Sage.

Goldstein, D., & Rosenbaum A. (1985). An evaluation of the self-esteem of maritally violent men. *Family Relations, 34*, 425–428.

Gondolf, E. W. (1988) Who are these guys? Toward a behavioral typology of batterers. *Violence and Victims, 3*, 187–203.

Gondolf, E. W. (1990). An exploratory survey of court-mandated batterer programs. *Response to the Victimization of Women and Children, 13*, 7–11.

Gottman, J. M., Jacobson, N. S, Rushe, R. H., Shortt, J. W., Babcock, J., LaTaillade, J. J., & Waltz, J. (1995). The relationship between heart rate reactivity, emotionally aggressive behavior, and general violence in batterers. *Journal of Family Psychology, 57*, 47–52.

Hamberger, J. K., & Hastings, J. E. (1988). Skills training for treatment of spouse abusers: An outcome study. *Journal of Family Violence, 3*, 121–130.

Hamberger, J. K., & Hastings, J. E. (1991). Personality correlates of men who batter and nonviolent men: Some continuities and discontinuities. *Journal of Family Violence, 6*, 131–147.

Harrell, A. (1991). *Evaluation of court-ordered treatment for domestic offenders: Final report.* Paper prepared for the State Justice Institute.

Harris, R., Savage, S., Jones, T., & Brooke, W. (1988). A comparison of treatments for abusive men and their partners within a family-service agency. *Canadian Journal of Community Mental Health, 7*, 147–155.

Hart, S. D., Dutton, D. G., & Newlove, T. (1993). The prevalence of personality disorders among wife assaulters. *Journal of Personality Disorders, 7*, 329–341.

Hirschel, D. J., Hutchison, I. W., & Dean, C. W. (1992). The failure of arrest to deter spouse abuse [Special issue: Experimentation in criminal justice]. *Journal of Research in Crime and Delinquency, 29*, 7–33.

Holzworth-Munroe, A., Stuart, G. L., & Hutchinson, G. (1997). Violent versus nonviolent husbands: Differences in attachment patterns, dependency, and jealousy. *Journal of Family Psychology, 11*, 314–331.

Hornung, C. A., McCullough, B. C., & Sujimoto, T. (1981). Status relationships in marriage: Risk factors in spouse abuse. *Journal of Marriage and the Family, 43*, 675–692.

Hotaling, G. T., & Sugarman, D. B. (1986). An analysis or risk markers in husband to wife violence: The current state of knowledge. *Violence and Victims, 1*, 101–124.

Jacobson, N. S., Gottman, J. M., & Shortt, J. W. (1995). The distinction between Type I and Type II batterers: Further considerations: Reply to Ornduff *et al.* (1995), Margolin *et al.* (1995), and Walker (1995). *Journal of Family Psychology, 9*, 272–279.

Jouriles, E. N., & O'Leary, K. D. (1985). Interspousal reliability of reports of marital violence. *Journal of Consulting and Clinical Psychology, 53*, 419–421.

Kalmuss, D. (1984). The intergenerational transmission of marital aggression. *Journal of Marriage and the Family, 46*, 11–19.

Kantor, G. K., & Straus, M. A. (1986, April). *The drunken bum theory of wife beating.* Paper presented at the National Alcoholism Forum conference on Alcohol and the Family, San Francisco.

Maiuro, R. D., Cahn, T. S., & Vitaliano, P. P. (1986). Assertiveness and hostility in domestically violent men. *Violence and Victims, 1*, 279–289.

Maiuro, R. D., Cahn, T. S., Vitaliano, P. P., Wagner, B. C., & Zegeree, J. B. (1988) Anger, hostility, and depression in domestically violent versus generally assaultive men and nonviolent control subjects. *Journal of Consulting and Clinical Psychology, 56*, 17–23.

Marshall, L. L., & Rose, P. R. (1988). Family of origin violence and courtship abuse. *Journal of Counseling and Development, 66*, 414–418.

Murphy, C. M., Meyer, S. L., & O'Leary, D. K. (1993). Family of violence and MCMI-II psychopathology among partner assaultive men. *Violence and Victims, 8*, 165–176.

Murphy, C. M., Meyer, S. L., & O'Leary, D. K. (1994). Dependency characteristics of partner assaultive men. *Journal of Abnormal Psychology, 103*, 729–735.

Neidig, P. H., Friedman, D. H., & Collins, B. S. (1986). Attitudinal characteristics of males who have engaged in spouse abuse. *Journal of Family Violence, 1*, 223–233.

O'Leary. K. D. (1996). Physical aggression in intimate relationships can be treated within a marital context under certain circumstances. *Journal of Interpersonal Violence, 11*, 450–452.

O'Leary, K. D., & Curley, A. D. (1986). Assertion and family violence: Correlates of spouse abuse. *Journal of Marital and Family Therapy, 12*, 281–290.

O'Leary, K. D., Barling, J., Arias, l., Rosenbaum, A., Malone, J., & Tyree, A. (1989). Prevalence and stability of physical aggression between spouses: A longitudinal analysis. *Journal of Consulting and Clinical Psychology, 57*, 263–268.

O'Leary, K. D., & Neidig, P. H. (1993, November). Treatment of spouse abuse. Poster presented at the Annual Convention of the Association for Advancement of Behavior Therapy.

Pagelow, M. D. (1984). *Family violence.* New York: Praeger.

Palmer, S. E., Brown, R. A., & Barrera, M. E. (1992). Group treatment program for abusive husbands: Long term evaluation. *American Journal of Orthopsychiatry, 62*, 276–283.

Pence, E., & Paymer, M. (1993). *Education groups for men who batter: The Duluth model.* New York: Springer.

Prince, J. E., & Arias, I. A. (1994). The role or perceived control and the desirability of control among abusive and nonabusive husbands. *American Journal of Family Therapy, 2*, 126–134.

Rosenbaum, A. (1986). Of men, macho, and marital violence. *Journal of Family Violence, 1*, 121–129.

Rosenbaum, A., & Hoge, S. K. (1989). Head injury and marital aggression. *American Journal of Psychiatry, 146*, 1048–1051.

Rosenbaum, A., & O'Leary, D. K. (1981). Marital violence: Characteristics of abusive couples. *Journal of Consulting and Clinical Psychology, 49*, 63–71.

Rosenbaum, A., Hoge, S. K., Adelman, S. A., Warnken, W. J., Fletcher, K. E., & Kane, R. L. (1994). Head injury in partner-abusive men. *Journal of Consulting and Clinical Psychology, 62*, 1187–1193.

Rosenbaum, A., Abend, S. L., Gearan, P. J., & Fletcher, K. E. (1996, May). *Serotonergic functioning in partner-abusive males.* Paper presented at the NAT Advanced Study Institute: The Biosocial Bases of Aggression, A. Raine, Director, Rhodes, Greece.

Rounsaville, B. (1978) Theories in marital violence: Evidence from a study of battered women. *Victimology: An International Journal, 3*, 11–31.

Saunders, D. G. (1993). Husbands who assault: Multiple profiles requiring multiple resources. In N. Hilton (Ed.), *Legal responses to wife assault.* Newbury Park, CA: Sage.

Sherman, L., & Berk, R. A. (1984, April). The Minneapolis domestic violence experiment. *Police Foundation Reports,* 1–8.

Sherman, L. W., Smith, D. A., Schmidt, J. D., & Rogan, D. P. (1992). Crime, punishment, and stake in conformity: Legal and informal control of domestic violence. *American Sociological Review, 57*, 680–690.

Straus, M. A. (1979). Measuring intrafamily conflict and violence: The Conflict Tactics (CT) Scales. *Journal of Marriage and the Family, 41*, 75–88.

Straus, M. A., & Gelles, R. J. (1986). Societal change and change in family violence from 1975 to 1985 as revealed by two national surveys. *Journal of Marriage and the Family, 48*, 465–479.

Straus, M. A., Gelles, R. J., & Steinmetz, S. K. (1980). *Behind closed doors: Violence in the American family.* New York: Anchor Books.

Sugarman, D. B., & Hotaling, G. T. (1989). Dating violence: Prevalence, context, and risk markers. In M. A. Pirog-Good & J. E. Stets (Eds.), *Violence in dating relationships: Emerging social issues* (pp. 5–11). New York: Praeger.

Telch, C. F., & Lindquist, C. U. (1984). Violent versus nonviolent couples: A comparison of patterns. *Psychotherapy, 21*, 242–248.

Tollman, R. M., & Bennett, L. W. (1990). A review of quantitative research on men who batter. *Journal of Interpersonal Violence, 5*, 87–118.

Van Hasselt, V. B., Morrison, R. L., & Bellak, A. S. (1985). Alcohol use in wife abusers and their spouses. *Addictive Behaviors, 10*, 127–135.

Waldo, M. (1988). Relationship enhancement counseling groups for wife abusers. *Journal of Mental Health Counseling, 10*, 37–45.

Walker, L. E. (1979). *The battered woman.* New York: Harper & Row.

Wietzman, J., & Dreen, K. (1982). Wife beating: A view of the marital dyad. *Social Casework, 63*, 259–265.

Elder Abuse

Rosalie S. Wolf

Introduction

With the passage of time, the concept of elder abuse has undergone various transformations. Initially, abuse and neglect of older adults was viewed in the context of protective services; next, framed as an issue of aging; then, family violence; and, most recently, crime. The multiple terms used to describe the person responsible for the violent act, "caregiver," "abuser," "perpetrator," and "offender," illustrate the different perspectives. As it turns out, each of the interpretations is more closely associated with one form of elder mistreatment than another (e.g., protective services with neglect) rather than representing an evolutionary process in the definition of the issue. Each provides a framework for intervention. The purpose of this chapter is to present information about perpetrators of elder mistreatment and approaches to intervention. (The word "perpetrator" is used to represent the person who is carrying out the abusive or neglectful action.)

Historical Background

Adult Protective Services (APS)

Intervention in cases of neglected or abused older adults was first articulated as "protective services" by the American Public Welfare Association in 1953 and reaffirmed as a legitimate public welfare role in the passage of the 1962 Public Welfare Amendments to the Social Security Act. Persons in need of protective services were "those who because of physical or mental limitations are unable to act in their own behalf; are seriously limited in the management of their affairs; are neglected or exploited, or, are living in unsafe or hazardous conditions" (District of Columbia Department. of Public Welfare [DCDPW], 1967, p. 12). Protective services included both a social and legal component; social services were defined as: "a range of agency

Rosalie S. Wolf • Institute on Aging, UMass Memorial Health Care, Worcester, Massachusetts 01605-2982.

Handbook of Psychological Approaches with Violent Offenders: Contemporary Strategies and Issues, edited by Van Hasselt and Hersen. Kluwer Academic/Plenum Publishers, New York, 1999.

services undertaken with or on behalf of an older client who, because of a physical or mental condition is unable to manage his money or carry on the activities of daily living and who has no one willing, and able to act on his behalf" (U.S. Department of Health, Education and Welfare [USDHEW], 1966, p. 7), and legal services as "actions by an agency which involve the readiness to use legal authority and procedures on behalf of an older person who cannot manage his money, or is exploited or is in danger" (USDHEW, 1966, p. 7). Under the legislation, the federal government increased its share (75%) of payment to state public assistance programs to provide for a "defined" list of social services and training activities in behalf of the needy aged, blind, and disabled. The amendments also authorized demonstration projects on protective services "to gain new knowledge about the functioning level of aged mentally impaired persons: to secure answers to some assumptions and questions around the practicality and efficaciousness of protective services; and to evaluate the effectiveness of a 'service unit' approach in the provision of protective services" (USDHEW, 1966, p. 9).

Although the demonstration projects failed to show the value of protective services in the lives of these older persons, proponents were successful in obtaining the passage of Title XX of the Social Security Act in 1974 that mandated and funded protective services for all persons 18 years and older without regard for income. By 1977, most states were providing adult protective services either through their departments of public welfare or under contract to other public or private agencies. Twelve states had passed protective services legislation. Increasingly, the program came under criticism. The questionable effectiveness of the program, high cost, potential infringement of civil rights, and stigma of public welfare led to "disenchantment" among both professionals and the public, and further development came to an end (Anetzberger, 1994).

Elder Abuse, Neglect, and Exploitation

The disclosure of "parent battering" at a Congressional hearing in 1978 and subsequent investigations and testimony awakened the nation and the media to a "new" problem of elder abuse. Victims were portrayed as very dependent, older persons (usually mothers) with physical and mental impairments mistreated by dutiful, but overburdened adult children (usually daughters). This reinterpretation of the problem of neglected and abused old persons from "adults in need of protective services" to "victims of elder abuse, neglect, and exploitation" gave new life to the adult protective services movement. It was not necessary to establish a new bureaucracy to meet the needs of elder abuse cases. The state systems were already in place.

Without model statutes on elder abuse to guide policy or program development, advocates for elder abuse legislation drew on their experiences with child and adult protective services. By 1985, 14 more states had passed adult protective services laws, and 9 states specific elder abuse laws. Within 8 years, all 50 states had protective legislation.

If a state program operates under adult protective statutes, it is more likely to limit its services to dependent adults, referring cases involving more functionally independent persons to other agencies such as the police, legal services, battered women's shelters, and the criminal justice system. For instance, the Colorado Adult

Protective Service manual (1988) states that "spousal abuse is not considered an adult protection issue unless one or both partners are disabled." Programs authorized under elder abuse legislation usually apply to any elderly victim.

Although Title XX of the Social Security Act (now administered in the form of the Social Service Block Grant to the states) still provides the legal mandate for adult protective services, it was the activity of aging advocates that had the most impact on federal policy. Much of the impetus for action on elder abuse in the early years came from the House of Representatives Select Committee on Aging (disbanded in 1994) and more recently from the Senate Special Committee on Aging. A decade-long effort to establish a federal policy on elder abuse was finally rewarded with the passage of an elder abuse prevention amendment to the Older Americans Act (OAA) in 1989. The reauthorization of the Act in 1992 not only placed the amendment into a new Title VII (Elder Rights) but also called for the creation of a National Center on Elder Abuse in 1992 under the aegis of the Administration on Aging. The prime contractor for the National Center was the American Public Welfare Association whose members are the state departments of social services and their adult protective services programs. Currently the National Center is housed at the National Association of State Units on Aging.

Family Violence and Elder Abuse

Consideration of elder abuse in the framework of family violence seemed obvious given its initial "discovery" during the Congressional family violence hearings and the work of family violence researchers. More than a decade ago, Finkelhor and Pillemer (1984) noted similarities between elder abuse, partner abuse, and child abuse. They all challenged and threatened cherished beliefs about the family. The victims often deny that mistreatment has occurred and resist help, and the perpetrator often has alcohol problems.

Despite similarities between elder abuse and other forms of family violence, the inclination had been to stress differences. Elder abuse advocates feared that following the child abuse model would infantilize the older person and result in infringement of his or her rights. Linkage with the battered women's movement was unlikely. Spouse abuse was a grassroots effort, antiprofessional, and strongly feminist, while the elder abuse was professionally motivated mainly by social workers. The initial formulation of elder abuse as caregiver stress did not fit the paradigm of the battered women's movement. However, as research later showed, the caregiver stress model was only one explanation for a much more complex phenomenon. Besides, spouse abuse was also a problem among the elderly and more prevalent than was evident from the state report statistics (Pillemer & Finkelhor, 1988).

The sharp line that had been drawn between elder abuse and the domestic violence model proved to be artificial and counterproductive. As early as 1988, elders were one of the groups eligible for services under the Family Violence Prevention and Services Act. To determine how the two groups might work together more effectively, the American Association of Retired Persons (AARP, 1993) sponsored a forum on the Older Battered Woman. As a result of that meeting, the Administration on Aging provided funds from its discretionary grant program to support six projects (1995–1997) to demonstrate collaboration between local domestic violence and battered women's shelters and adult and elder protective services.

Placing elder abuse under the rubric of family violence has allowed advocates and organizations working in the field to be part of more comprehensive policy and programmatic initiatives than was possible when abused elders were considered to be "adults in need of protective services." For example, the declaration of family violence as a public health issue has presented opportunities for closer ties between the health care establishment and family violence workers. The American Medical Association initiated a family violence project in 1992 that resulted in publication of diagnostic and treatment guidelines for both spouse and elder abuse; the calling of a national conference on family violence that included representation for the child, spouse, and elder abuse movements; and the creation of a coalition of physicians against family violence. Such recognition for elder abuse is very important, since physicians are believed to be in an excellent position to identify cases of elder abuse but few seem to be aware of the problem, where to report, or the services available. In contrast to the key role that physicians played in shaping the nation's response to child abuse, they were not involved in the development of the elder abuse movement.

Crime and Elder Abuse

Like the medical community, law enforcement and the criminal justice system were also not well informed or involved with protective service cases in the early years, partly due to their hands-off policy in domestic incidents, and also the tendency of older victims to deny abuse and to avoid pressing charges against a family member. The growing interest of law enforcement personnel in domestic violence issues has extended to elder abuse cases as well. One national police group (Police Executive Research Forum, 1994) has produced a training manual and many adult protective service and elder abuse agencies are providing training sessions for local law enforcement officers. A curriculum has also been designed for prosecuting attorneys that illustrates how caseworkers and attorneys can work together so that the needs of both the victim and the state are met (Reulbach & Tewksbury, 1994).

Linking family violence closer to the criminal justice system has created other opportunities for elder abuse programs. The Department of Justice's Office for Victims of Crime in 1992 sponsored a National Conference on Victimization of the Elderly that gave representatives from the criminal justice system, adult protective services, and elder abuse programs the chance to present information and discuss issues of common concern. The Office for Victims of Crime has also solicited ideas for their discretionary grants from family violence advocates and professionals, including those working on elder abuse.

In summary, the past 30 years have brought about changes in the way the problem of elder mistreatment has been perceived. Not all professionals in the elder abuse field approve of using abuse, family violence, or crime as conceptual frameworks for elder mistreatment. Some health practitioners (Fulmer & O'Malley, 1987) want to concentrate on intervention without having to use pejorative terms such as "abuse" and "neglect." They prefer to think of the cases as "inadequate care" situations, arguing that it is easier to decide what is "inadequate" or "adequate" care than "appropriate or inappropriate" behavior (Fulmer & O'Malley, 1987).

The family violence model with its emphasis on harm, intentionality, and responsibility has also been criticized (Phillips, 1988), as has the effort to "criminalize" elder abuse (Formby, 1992). Also, to avoid labeling victims and perpetrators, Johnson (1991) proposed "unnecessary suffering" as a construct for elder mistreatment. Rather than competing views of a single entity, the various interpretations reflect different aspects of a multidimensional problem, each of which suggests a different type of intervention.

Epidemiology

Definitions

Despite the different viewpoints on elder mistreatment, persons in the field generally agree that it is an act of commission (abuse) or omission (neglect), intentional or unintentional, and of one or more types: physical, psychological (emotional), or financial that produces unnecessary suffering, injury, pain, loss, or violation of human rights and decreased quality of life (Hudson, 1989). Whether the behavior is labeled abusive or neglectful may depend on its frequency, duration, intensity, severity, and consequences. Some confusion prevails because of differences in state definitions, particularly in how various manifestations might be categorized. For instance, sexual abuse appears as a separate type of abuse in 20 state statutes; in others, it is included in physical abuse. Most recently, some researchers (Gebotys, O'Connor, & Mair, 1992; M. F. Hudson, 1994; Moon & Williams, 1993) have questioned the statutory and professional definitions, suggesting that the older person's perception of the action, influenced by culture, values, and traditions, may be the salient factor in identification and intervention.

Prevalence: Victims and Perpetrators

Literature on elder mistreatment reveals four prevalence studies, completed several years ago and carried out in different countries. In the first, Pillemer and Finkelhor (1988) surveyed 2,020 community-dwelling, randomly selected elderly persons in the metropolitan Boston area about their experience with three types of maltreatment since they had reached 65 years of age. The methodology was based on two previous national family violence surveys (Straus, 1992) with additional questions related to unmet needs (neglect). Contact was made by telephone; if the older person could not respond, interviews were conducted with a proxy. Sixty-three persons reported being maltreated, which translated into a rate of 32 maltreated elderly per 1,000. The rate for physical violence was 20 per 1,000; verbal aggression, 11; and neglect, 4. If the rate were applied to the entire United States, it would represent almost 1 million victims. Fifty-eight percent of the perpetrators were spouses (23 wives and 14 husbands); 24%, adult children, and 18%, other persons (grandchildren, siblings, and boarders).

Using a similar methodology and instruments but adding financial exploitation, a Canadian–U.S. team conducted a national prevalence survey of elder mistreatment in Canada (Podnieks, 1992). Contact was also by telephone but did not include proxies, thereby eliminating persons from the sample who were unable to respond because of physical, mental, or cognitive deficits. Rate of victimization for Canada was 40 persons mistreated per 1,000 (financial abuse, 25 per 1,000; verbal aggression, 14; physical violence, 5; and neglect, 4). The total number of victims was 80, but some were subjected to more than one type of abuse. A full count of the abusers is not available in the report except by type of abuse. Friends, neighbors, and acquaintances were abusers in 40% of the financial exploitation cases; adult children, 28%; distant relatives, 24%; spouses, 4%; and relationship unknown, 4%. Ninety-two percent of the 26 perpetrators of verbal aggression and 9 of the 10 perpetrators of physical abuse were spouses; the others involved were relatives but not specified. No information was given regarding the perpetrators of neglect.

A third survey was conducted in a small, semi-industrialized town in Finland by a medical team (Kivelä, Kongäs-Saviaro, Kesti, Pahkala, & Ijäs, 1992) as part of a larger study on depression among older persons. Postal questionnaires, interviews, and clinical examinations were used to collect data from 1,225 persons. Again, the study excluded persons with severe physical disabilities or cognitive impairment. Three questions were used to elicit the information: one asked the respondents their opinion (yes or no) about types of abuse (physical, psychological, neglect, economic, and sexual); the second asked if they knew a person or persons who had been abused since he or she had reached retirement age; and the third asked if they themselves had been abused. Fifty-five persons reported having been mistreated. Spouses were abusers in 49% of the cases; adult children, 18%; other relatives, 18%, and friends, 15%. The rate was 2.5% of the men, 7.0% of the women, or an overall 5.7%.

Because of institutional concern about the rights of human subjects, a British team (Ogg, 1993) was unable to repeat the Boston–Canadian studies so instead added a few questions from them to an annual Omnibus Survey. Of the 593 individuals 65 years and older interviewed, 32 (5%) reported having been recently verbally abused by a close family member or relative; 9 (2%), physically abused; and 9 (2%), financial exploited. Again, persons unable to participate because of illness or severe disability were excluded. No information about abusers was obtained.

Results of the four studies are more similar than might be first apparent, especially if the proportion of persons financially exploited in the Canadian study is added to the Boston figures (Is there any reason to believe that the rate of financial exploitation would be higher in Canada than the United States?), suggesting a prevalence rate of about 5% across all studies. Although it appears that abuse is perpetrated more often by spouses than adult children, lack of sufficient data in the Canadian and British reports precludes a definitive statement to this effect.

Incidence

Tatara (1993) has developed a method for estimating incidence of abuse and neglect cases based on the reports received by the 50 states, but because of the great variation in criteria for reporting and definitions, the figures can be considered only approximations. In 1986, 117,000 reports were received nationwide. By 1991, reports had reached 227,000. Using the latter figure, Tatara calculated number of victims to be 735,000 nationwide. The 1996 reports totaled 293,000 (National Center on Elder Abuse, 1995). Of the substantiated cases, 36.7% involved adult children as abusers; 10.8%, other relatives; and 12.6%, spouses. The difference in the two types of studies (prevalence vs. incidence) as to spouse abuse among the elderly is rather dramatic. Pillemer and Finkelhor (1988) explain some of the difference by stating that an elder is most likely to be abused by the person with whom he or she lives, and many more elders live with spouses than with their children. However, some of the difference can be traced to the adult protective service criteria in some states that exclude spouse abuse unless one partner is disabled.

Theoretical Explanations

Many theoretical explanations have been proposed for elder mistreatment; four of the more likely are described here. The *situational* theory (Phillips, 1986), adapted from other forms of family violence, incorporates aging, structure, and caregiver factors. It proposes that lowering the stress and burden of caregiving will reduce the possibility of elder mistreatment and neglect. Another, advanced by Pillemer (1986), is *social exchange* theory based on the premise of reciprocity of rewards (benefits) and punishments (costs) in a relationship. When each individual contributes equally, a fair exchange exists; when one person becomes disabled or unwilling to reciprocate, the exchange is perceived as unfair. According to this view, caregivers who do not have the ability to escape or ameliorate the situation may become abusive (Wolf & Pillemer, 1989). However, a key concept in the social exchange perspective is that of *power*. Finkelhor (1983), in his attempt to identify common features of family abuse, noted that abuse can occur as a response to perceived powerlessness. He states that abusive acts may be carried out by abusers to compensate for their perceived lack or loss of power. Intervention in this model calls for changing the nature of the relationship, either decreasing the dependency of the victim or perpetrator or raising the cost of mistreatment to the perpetrator.

Symbolic interaction theory has been used by Steinmetz (1988) as a framework for her study of caregiver and care recipient interaction. Each person approaches the interaction with his or her own role definitions and expectations. If the behaviors match the roles and meanings that are assigned, the interaction continues; if there is a large discrepancy then conflict is more apt to arise. Intervention under these circumstances would require working with both the caregiver and care recipient to reach a more realistic appraisal of the situation, at the same time relieving the stress on the caregiver and increasing the coping skills of the care recipient.

Another perspective is provided by the *intra-individual dynamics* model that identifies family violence with the characteristics of the perpetrator. Although psychological or psychiatric explanations of family violence have been severely criticized (Gelles, 1993), personality styles or traits have been shown to be both correlated with and predictive of physical aggression in family violence (O'Leary, 1993). Anetzberger (1987) stated that the overall profile of the abusing adult offspring that emerged from her study suggested pathological individuals. The argument for including psychological issues is buttressed by the findings that a relatively large proportion of perpetrators have had histories of mental illness and alcohol abuse (Wolf & Pillemer, 1989). According to this model, intervention should focus on the perpetrator.

Risk Factors and Case Profiles

The theories have been useful in identifying possible risk factors although the number of studies remains relatively few (Anetzberger, 1987; Bristowe & Collins, 1989; Coyne, Reichman, & Bergib, 1993; Homer & Gilleard, 1990; Hwalek, Goodrich, & Quinn, 1995; Paveza *et al.*, 1992; Pillemer, 1986). Wolf, Godkin, & Pillemer (1984) examined 328 cases for differences among types of mistreatment (physical, psychological, financial, and neglect). Comparisons were made between those cases with the specific type of abuse and those in which that type was not present. Three distinct profiles were found. One was indicative of physical and psychological abuse. The perpetrators were more likely to have a history of psychopathology and to be dependent on the victim for financial resources. The victims were apt to be in poor emotional health but independent in activities of daily living. Since this type of abuse involved family members who were most intimately related and emotionally connected, it is likely that this type of maltreatment comes from longstanding pathological family and interpersonal dynamics that become more highly charged when the dependency relationship is altered, either because of illness (spouse) or financial needs (adult children).

A second profile represented the neglect cases. The victim was more likely to be widowed, very old, with cognitive and functional impairment and dependent on the perpetrator (caregiver). Neither psychological problems nor financial dependency were significant factors in the lives of these perpetrators. They did, however, consider the victim a source of stress. Financial exploitation cases presented still a third profile. The physical and mental state of the victims seemed to be relatively unimportant in these cases. The victims were generally widowed (unmarried) with few social supports. Perpetrators had financial problems and histories of substance abuse. It is easy to understand why, depending on case mix (some determined by the statute regulating protective services), the proportion of perpetrator types might vary.

The factors that seem the most predictive include the perpetrator's dependency on the victim, especially for financial support (physical abuse, financial exploitation); the perpetrator's psychological state (e.g., substance abuse, history of mental illness) (physical and psychological abuse); the victim's poor physical or cognitive status (neglect) and family social isolation (neglect). So far, evidence concerning two factors that are closely associated with child and spouse abuse, stressful life events and history of violence, is inconclusive. Lachs and Pillemer (1995) suggested that stressful life events and chronic financial strain may decrease the family's resistance and increase likelihood of abuse and a history of violence early in a spousal relation may foretell elder mistreatment in later life.

The only in-depth study of perpetrators was carried out more than a decade ago (Anetzberger, 1987). The sample consisted of 15 adult offspring who had physically abused an elder parent within the previous 18 months, referred by hospitals or adult protective services (APS) agencies. Anetzberger traces the etiology of physical abuse of elderly parents by these adult offspring to certain pathological personality characteristics, the acute stress in their lives, and their social isolation; also to the vulnerability of the elder parents and to the "prolonged and profound" intimacy between the adult offspring and elder parent. She divided the sample into three types. The first group was labeled "hostiles." They were aggressive, outspoken, angry at everyone, and hated authority. Contact with the elder parent was a very negative experience. They were also the most abusive of the three. The second group were the "authoritarians," the least likely to have any psychopathology but rigid in their expectations about the elder parent, critical, impatient, and generally unsympathetic to the elder's situation. The "dependents" were the third group, distinguished from the others by their financial dependency on the elder parent.

Case Examples

The following comments were taken from reassessment forms completed by caseworkers in a study of four elder abuse projects (Wolf & Pillemer, 1993). Caseworkers were asked to complete a reassessment at the time the case was closed or 6 months after intake, whichever was sooner. The particular question dealt with the reason for the perpetrator's abusive or neglectful behavior. Caregiver stress is the theme in the first three examples:

> Due to declining health, client has required more care. However, the perpetrator (spouse) feels the wife can do more for herself than she actually does or is willing to do. The husband has a history of alcohol abuse and when intoxicated is unable to fulfill caregiving responsibilities. He is also frustrated with increased caregiving responsibilities and may be unrealistically expecting his spouse to improve to the point where he will no longer need to provide the care.

> The perpetrator is not consciously abusing victim. She is stressed and overwhelmed in caring for him as she was before. But situation is not likely to change unless perpetrator is willing to accept outside help (which she has not yet been able to do.)

> The perpetrator (daughter) is very angry and rejects any psychological explanations of her mother's behavior. She frequently gets angry with her mother and yells at her to get her to do things she wants her to do. She feels that the things (ADLs) that her mother has difficulty doing stems from laziness primarily and not psychosis and dementia.

The next case deals with financial dependency:

> Perpetrator is dependent on client for financial support and housing. Perpetrator says she does not believe in medication and doctors. Client is somewhat demented (extent undetermined) and forgets to do what perpetrator asks. Perpetrator "gets upset."

In the last set of examples, the psychopathology of the perpetrator is very evident:

> Perpetrator has mental problems and is being treated for schizophrenia. Client's hearing is poor; if he doesn't respond to perpetrator, the perpetrator regards it as an insult and becomes very upset and yells at the client.

> Perpetrator has a history of mental illness (manic depressive), expresses frustration with client's lack of motivation to do even simple things and justifies her abusive behavior by saying "Well, no one was there to help me when my husband abused me."

> The main reason for the perpetrator's neglectful behavior is still her alcohol abuse.

> Perpetrator is diagnosed as paranoid schizophrenic; it appears that he has gone off of his medication. He demands attention from client, and uses outbursts and threatening behavior to isolate her from others.

> Longstanding history of emotional problems compounded by current drug abuse. Perpetrator is unable to care for himself due to emotional problems, social immaturity, and lack of impulse control. Inability to hold on to a job for long leads to his lack of self-esteem and a hateful dependency on his father.

> Perpetrator appears to have a severe characterological disorder (very likely borderline personality disorder) that appears responsible for her manipulative behavior. Client's low self-esteem due to tragic family history meshes with perpetrator's

behavior to create sadomasochistic relationship. Perpetrator is disabled for both psychological and physical reasons.

Intervention

Assessment

The goal of the assessment (Illinois Department on Aging, 1990) is to gather in-depth information about (1) the *client's* situation and functioning level as to the environment, physical health, activities of daily living, mental health, and social and economic resources; (2) the capacity of the client to make decisions about his or her own welfare as well as to understand the consequences of those decisions, (3) the level of risk to the client, and (4) the need for immediate interventions. Interviewing the suspected perpetrator is part of this process,

Generally, except for age, sex, and relationship to victim, states require that very little, if any, data on perpetrators be documented in the case files. In a survey of risk assessment instruments used by the state adult protective service agencies, Goodrich (1995) found that more than two thirds of the states did not require information on caregiving risk factors (e.g., lack of knowledge or skills, inappropriate reaction to stress, chronic fatigue, functional limitations), psychological state (e.g., alcohol and drug abuse, mental or emotional problems), and dependency (emotionally, financially dependent on victim). Several states, however, do include these data and numerically score the items to calculate the change in risk.

Social Services

The extent of involvement of adult protective service units with offender interventions ranges from none (Iowa and Oregon APS do only investigation, referring substantiated cases to social service agencies) to a full commitment to work within a family systems model that includes the perpetrator, as exemplified by the Illinois Elder Abuse Program. The Illinois Department on Aging contracts with local community-based agencies for adult protective services. Included in their practice guidelines is a detailed set of action steps for intervening with perpetrator types. In caregiver situations, a three-phase plan is used: providing relief or respite for the caregiver, education and support regarding the client's disease process and the demands on the caregiver, and interpersonal conflict resolution with the family.

In cases that involve domestic violence "grown old," the Illinois guidelines recommend an approach coordinated with a domestic violence program. They suggest working with the victim and also with the couple. (Unlike some APS units, Illinois elder abuse agencies accept spouse abuse cases without the requirement of disability.) Again, a detailed set of actions is outlined for the caseworker.

Intervention techniques with the dysfunctional abuser, another category, may involve working in the fields of substance abuse, mental health, and developmental disabilities. In these instances, it may be necessary to involve a counselor trained in these various fields to work with the family unit. The Illinois Department on Aging has produced a manual and curriculum for training caseworkers on *Improving Our Effectiveness in Working With Abusers* (Proctor, Hwalek, & Goodrich, 1993). Most state APS programs refer these situations to other community agencies.

Legal Services and Criminal Justice

Criminal prosecution has been an unlikely intervention in elder mistreatment cases, although with increased interest and involvement of law enforcement and the criminal justice system, this situation is changing. Most legal activity related to elder mistreatment is not addressed in the adult protective services or elder abuse acts but is part of the general civil and criminal codes of the states. However, nearly half the laws do have provisions making elder abuse a misdemeanor or a felony with penalties or fines that range from $500 to $10,000 and imprisonment from 90 days to 10 years.

Heisler (1991) made a strong case for involving the criminal justice system in elder abuse cases: It can stop the violence, protect the victim, protect the public, hold the offender accountable, rehabilitate the offender, communicate the societal intent to treat the conduct as a crime, and provide restitution to the victim. She noted that traditional methods and approaches for dealing with elder abuse may have discouraged victims and service providers from turning to the criminal justice system for help but she stated that new awareness, laws, and procedures enable the system to play a stronger part in deterring further violence, particularly as part of community-wide interdisciplinary efforts.

A number of legal instruments are available to caseworkers in adult protection situations. Included are guardianship, conservatorship, representative payee, and durable power of attorney. Most often they are used when the victim lacks capacity to make a decision or to handle their own affairs. Involuntary intervention is viewed as the last resort and is implemented in the least intrusive and restrictive way possible (Colorado Deptartment of Social Services, 1988). The victim in a threatening situation may obtain an order of protection or restraining order against the perpetrator. A civil commitment (mental commitment) allows for detaining the perpetrator on a short-term basis (e.g., 72 hours) in a facility for mental illness evaluation and treatment. Some states may also have an alcohol commitment that allows for both voluntary and involuntary commitment of persons who are intoxicated and dangerous to themselves or to others.

In the Wolf, Godkin, and Pillemer study (1984) of three model projects on elder abuse, orders of protection were sought in 26% of the cases, criminal action taken in 15%, involuntary commitment made in 12% and family court appearance in 10%. An analysis of the cases seen by four elder abuse projects (Wolf & Pillemer, 1994) revealed much lower usage of legal instruments: orders of protection, 10%; involuntary commitment, 4%; criminal action, 5%; and family court, 9%. Again, usage rates are dependent on the case mix. Sengstock, Hwalek, and Petrone (1989) looked at service patterns in 204 cases and noted that in only one or two cases were court work or protection orders provided. They stated that it was not known whether this situation resulted from the unavailability of such services, the workers' lack of awareness of the services, or their belief that such services would not be effective.

Approaches to Violent Offenders

Ramsey-Klasnik (1995) categorized offenders into two groups. Type I are individuals who are abusive or neglectful because they lack knowledge, competence, and resources to deal with the caregiving situation. Unless they have mental or physical impairments, or both, and are not able to comprehend the consequences of their actions, these offenders will usually agree to intervention. Ramsey-Klasnik placed the "well-intentioned, overwhelmed caregivers" in this group. The treatment in these cases most often is the provision of services. Type II are individuals with sadistic or abusive personalities who intentionally inflict pain and suffering and use the elder and his or her assets for their own benefit. These individuals are apt to deny the allegations and refuse services. Legal intervention may be necessary in these cases. Using this typology, some of the intervention strategies used with perpetrators are described in the following sections.

Type I: Victim Dependency and Caregiver Stress

Several studies have examined violent behavior in families caring for an Alzheimer patient, perhaps the most stressful of caretaking situations. A sample of caregivers and care recipients from a multisite Alzheimer's disease patient registry was interviewed to identify whether severe violent behaviors had occurred between the patient and the caregiver, other family members, and nonfamily members in the year since diagnosis, and the frequency of these behaviors (Paveza et al., 1992). The general prevalence of violent caregiver–patient dyads was 17%; 16% of patients were reported by caregivers to exhibit severe violent behavior toward the caregiver; and 5% of the caregivers were violent toward the patient. Mutual violence occurred in 4% of the families. Further analysis of the data found that neither cognitive nor functional impairment of the patient was predictive of abuse; rather it was caregiver depression and living arrangements (when patient resided with the immediate family but not with a spouse).

Coyne and his colleagues (1993) surveyed (by mail) 1,000 consecutive callers (caregivers of dementia patients) to a New Jersey–based toll-free telephone helpline for families of dementia patients. Almost 12% of the caregivers reported that they had on at least one occasion physically abused the demented patient in their care. When these caregivers were compared with the caregivers who had not been physically abusive, they were found to have been caring for the patient for more years and more hours per day, and the patients were functioning at lower levels. The caregivers also displayed higher levels of burden and depression.

One third (33%) of all caregivers reported having been physically abused at least once during the course of providing care after the diagnosis of dementia. These caregivers (in contrast to those who had not been abused) had also been providing care for longer periods to patients at a lower level of functioning. About 1 out of 11 caregivers (9%) said that the patient had been abusive before becoming demented. The authors propose that excessive caregiving demands and physically abusive behavior of the patient may lead to a higher risk of abuse in families with demented elders.

For a study of social supports and caregiving, Pillemer and Suitor (1992) interviewed 236 persons caring for a relative who had been diagnosed with dementia within the previous 6 months. Embedded within the battery of questions was a series of items about patients' disruptive behavior (Has the care recipient ever hit or tried to hurt you in any way?) and caregivers' violence or fear of violence (Have you ever been afraid that you might hit or try to hurt your relative and have you ever done so?). About 20% of the caregivers said that they "feared that they would become violent"; 6% said that they had actually done so; and 25% reported that the care recipient had become violent. When those who did fear becoming violent were compared with those who did not, the former were more likely to live in the same household as the care recipient, to have experienced disruptive behavior from the care recipient, and to have lower self-esteem. A comparison of those who feared becoming violent with those who actually did so revealed disruptive behavior of the care recipient and being the spouse as significant factors. Respondents who had experienced violence from the care recipient were more apt to have become violent themselves and to be the spouse rather than other caregiver relatives. The authors suggest that fear of violence results from an interplay among interactional stressors, caregiver characteristics, and contextual factors, a more complicated model than the simplistic one found in the elder abuse literature that depicts dependency leading directly to violence.

That abusive behavior is more apt to exist in families caring for an Alzheimer patient than in other families seems fairly certain given the findings from these three studies that use very different methodologies. Several ways of dealing with caregiver burden and stress in Alzheimer families have been reported in the literature, but not necessarily directed to abusive families. Haley (1983) has shown how caregivers were able to develop the skills necessary to manage problem behavior or increase their adaptive behavior so that family stress was reduced. Pinkston and Linsk (1984a, 1984b) also reported that family caregivers could use behavioral approaches successfully. Although the impact on caregiver burden was not measured, 89% of the caregivers in their research found the approach to be helpful. The assumption in these studies is that caregivers with greater control over troublesome behaviors will experience less distress. The direct effect of the training is simply to increase coping skills which, in turn, is hypothesized to decrease caregiver burden.

A small group of family caregivers of Alzheimer patients with mild to moderate decline was trained to carry out a cognitive stimulation program consisting of conversation, memory-provoking exercises, and problem-solving techniques. At the end of an 8-month period, caregivers in the treatment group maintained their mental health status and burden level over time while the caregivers in the nontreatment group showed an increase in perceived burden. Patient and caregiver groups did not differ significantly on any of the variables prior to treatment (Quayhagen & Quayhagen, 1988).

Making respite, day care, and other support services available to families to reduce the number of hours of caregiving per day is another strategy. Hooyman, Gonyea, and Montgomery 1985 used curtailment of an in-home chore service to study the impact of the program on caregivers. Slightly more than half the sample reported an increase in the amount of stress in their lives with the loss of the chore service. Marks (1987–1988) describes a cross-sectional study in which 25 families receiving in-home respite services were compared with 25 families on the waiting list. Substantial stress was seen among all the caregivers, but significantly less in those who were receiving the respite services. In a longitudinal study of a respite care program for families with Alzheimer's patients, Lawton, Brody, and Saperstein (1991) found no impact on the appraised burden, physical health, or mental health of the caregiver even among those caregivers who were originally the most stressed or most disadvantaged. Yet, some individual cases did show a positive outcome.

Mixed results have also been associated with other supportive services. Family caregivers of elderly community-dwelling dementia patients were randomly assigned to one of two support groups that met for 10 sessions (Haley, Brown, & Levine, 1987a). A third group was composed of persons on the waiting list. Participants in the support groups (one of which included stress-management techniques) did not show any greater improvement in social or psychological functioning than the waiting list controls although the support group members did rate the groups as helpful. Zarit, Anthony, and Boutselis (1987) compared the effect of two approaches, family counseling and support groups, for relieving stress and burden experienced by caregivers of dementia patients and also found no difference between the treatment groups and waiting list subjects.

None of these intervention studies specifically addressed caregivers who had abused their family member. Only one such project has been reported in the literature (Scogin et al., 1989). The initial intent of this project was to offer training to suspected or convicted abusers as an alternative to prosecution. Because the potential numbers of persons in this category was so small, the project was changed to train caregivers with high risk of abusive behavior as determined by a mental health screening interview. Eligibility was limited to caregivers of persons 55 years or older having no known psychosis or receiving psychiatric treatment at the time of entry into the program. Most participants were self-referrals. The standardized training model, used at five sites across the state, consisted of eight 2-hour sessions on adult development and aging, problem solving, stress and anger management, and community resources. Three groups comprised the sample: (1) immediate training ($n = 56$), (2) delayed training ($n = 16$), and (3) no training (controls, $n = 23$). Participants were assessed for anger, self-worth, perceived cost of providing care, and psychiatric symptoms on tested instruments. The results showed little change over time for either the anger or self-worth inventory but perceived social cost of providing care and psychiatric symptoms in the treatment sample decreased in comparison with the no treatment group (but only approached significance).

As Pillemer and Suitor (1992) have suggested, the relationships between victim dependency and aggressiveness and caregiver stress and violence may be much more complicated than the theoretical model guiding these studies. While there is some slight indication that stress on the caregiver could be reduced with training in behavior management, significant improvement in the mental health of the caregivers has not resulted from any of the various approaches described. Methodological problems were evident in most of the studies. Samples were self-selected, numbers of participants were small, and time frames were limited. Twelve or 16 hours of instruction may not be adequate. A single service, such as respite, may be helpful but only if used as part of a more comprehensive service package that involves both the caregiver and care recipient.

Type II: Abuser Dependency and Alcoholism

General Very few studies have been conducted with the Type II offender. They often do not remain in the household to be questioned or agree to receive services. Greenberg, McKibben, and Raymond (1990), using both qualitative and quantitative methods, investigated the characteristics of dependent adult children in 204 substantiated cases of elder abuse reported to the Wisconsin elder abuse program. Of the sample, 61% were sons, and 39%, daughters; average age was 43 years. Forty percent of the sons and 60% of the daughters were primary caregivers of their elder parents. With regard to type of abuse, 39% involved physical abuse; 20% financial exploitation; 21%, neglect; and 20%, multiple types. Among the group of offenders, those most apt to be financially dependent were younger, living with the elder parent, and chemically dependent. Of the 204 cases, 44% of the sons and 14% of the daughters had problems with alcohol or drugs. From the qualitative analysis of 14 financial dependency cases, the authors observed a pattern of "drinking, abuse, forcing the adult child from the household," then accepting the child back into the home, which they identified with parental overprotectiveness that overshadowed the abusive interactions and with a pattern of relationships characteristic of an alcoholic family system.

In the group of 204 offenders, 11% involved adult children with mental illness who were living with their elderly parents and were psychologically dependent on their parents for support, supervision, and companionship. Abusive acts tended to take place when the adult children had discontinued their medication. The authors noted from the qualitative analysis that many of the victims were suffering from major depression and other mental health problems. They recommended that elders be encouraged to accept outside help but did not offer any advice with regard to intervention with the perpetrators.

Vinton (1992), also using Wisconsin Elder Abuse Reporting System data, examined the service plans for 96 cases involving physically abusive caregivers of elderly persons with 266 cases of physical abuse, but not by a primary caregiver. Essentially, the comparison was between cases in which the victim is dependent on the caregiver and cases in which the abuser is dependent on the victim or Type I versus Type II. With regard to the service plans for the abusers, Vinton found that although 25% of the abusers who were caregivers and 34% of the other abusers were reported to have alcohol problems, only 3% in each group were referred for alcohol or drug treatment. She postulated that services for abusers are not in the treatment plans because (1) abusers will not utilize the services even if referred, (2) the services are lacking or scarce, (3) the absence of the abuser will leave the elder at risk of an out-of-home placement, and (4) service planning for abusers is regarded as less important or not part of their job.

Korbin, Anetzberger, Thomasson, and Austin (1991) selected a sample of individuals 60 years of age or older who had sought legal recourse as a result of maltreatment by an adult offspring. These cases were drawn from the Witness/Victim Service Center and Family Violence Program in one Ohio county (the type of cases that would not be accepted by the Ohio APS system). Although long-term problems with their adult offspring was a common among all the elders, they finally sought help because they could not control their adult child or ensure their own safety. The authors suggested that the lack of appropriate community facilities and housing for the chronically mentally ill may promote conscious or unconscious pressure on families to accept their offspring back into the household. Recommendations include counseling and emotional support for parents who elect not to shelter and care for financially dependent and problematic adult children.

Case examples In response to a question regarding factors related to intervention that had a significant impact on resolution, caseworkers in the study of four elder abuse projects (Wolf & Pillemer, 1993) recorded the following comments. The first set of examples include the cases in which social service and legal interventions appeared to be successful:

> 1) establishment of a therapeutic case manager-to-perpetrator relationship was essential, 2) limits set by Public Guardian on finances, 3) more inhome respite for perpetrator so his stress declined, and 4) adult day health care for victim.

After hooponopono (Hawaiian version of family therapy), the family gets along better and works together better. Family now recognizes the caretaker daughter's financial problems. Each child contributes additional money and support in terms of respite care. Caregiving daughter now able to work part-time outside of her mother's home and feels less stress from the care she does give to the client.

Outside intervention has helped this case as well as the presence of a volunteer on a weekly basis. Perpetrator sees [volunteer] advocate as being a friend to client who comes every week to check on client. Hopefully this restrains him from abusing client.

Apparently successful was 1) a restraining order to keep son (perpetrator) away from client and 2) informing probation officer before son was released from jail that he is to stay away from client or he would be re-incarcerated.

The next two examples illustrate the dilemma that abused parents face of parental responsibility and personal safety.

Perpetrator was arrested at time of report of physical abuse and was sentenced to 10 days in jail and one year probation. He was not to return to his father's (victim/client) home. Son was initially in the home after the abuse occurred, but was issued a "stay away" order one month after the abuse occurred. Client refused to have a restraining order against the son, although he was being helped by the victim witness program and encouraged to do this for his own protection. He also was reluctant to testify against his son in court. After sentencing, the client appeared to have a change of heart and wanted his son to return to his home "to take care of him until he dies." At the time of case closing, son had returned to father's home with the stipulation that he receive counseling and the client is aware he is still at some risk.

Individual counseling from social worker to help client trust mental health system and better understand mental illness. Lack of understanding/mistrust causes client to become protective of son, and there is more likelihood that she will allow him home. Client currently struggles with her wish for son to have supervision upon discharge and lack of legal mandates to impose this on son.

In approximately one quarter of substantiated cases, the victim refuses intervention. If time and caseload allow, the worker will try to maintain contact, to build trust, until help is accepted, as the worker describes in the following example. At other times, the only thing the worker can do is to withdraw from the case and wait until another episode of abuse or neglect occurs and the report for investigation is received. The second case typifies these situations.

A non-judgmental approach with the perpetrator is and will continue to be essential. There is not much room for the BIG INTERVENTION in this case, only for careful monitoring, rapport building over time, and on-going tactful exploration with the perpetrator and client as to how "things can be made better" for both of them.

This case is a good example in which the family system is so closed that case management outreach is ineffective. Unless another incident occurs in the future, there is very little opportunity for intervention.

An analysis of the cases seen by the three model elder abuse projects (Wolf & Pillemer, 1989) at case closing showed that about one third of them were resolved (discontinuation or alleviation of the mistreatment) "completely" with progress toward resolution noted for almost another third. Resolved cases were more likely to involve neglect whereas the unresolved cases were more apt to be physical abuse. For all three projects, the changes in "social or living situation" was rated as the most effective intervention and "changes in the circumstances of the perpetrator," the least successful strategy. Case resolution was more likely to occur when the victims were dependent and neglected than when they were more independent and physically abused.

In determining the effectiveness of interventions in the Illinois elder abuse program, Quinn, Hwalek, and Goodrich (1993) found that the cases most difficult to change were those involving abusers with substance abuse problems, inability to respond appropriately to stress, and financial dependence on the victim. Providing medical and psychiatric services to the abuser was significantly related to a reduction in the risk of abuse, neglect, or exploitation. Substance abuse of the perpetrator was the least likely factor to change over time. The research team strongly urged that funding be included for services to reduce chemical dependency among abusers if cases are to be resolved. Anetzberger (1987) also called for more involvement on the part of the mental health, mental retardation, and alcoholism service systems in the prevention and treatment of elder abuse. As she noted in 1987 and true today, few such service systems have become interested in elder abuse, and few prevention or treatment models have emerged from such systems.

Summary

One of the most hopeful signs in the campaign to broaden interest in and awareness of elder abuse and neglect is the development of coalitions that bring together representatives from the medical, mental health, legal, law enforcement, aging, financial, and religious organizations and battered women's shelters. Coalitions conduct a wide range of activities including case consultation, outreach and public awareness, education and training, advocacy, research, agency coordination, referral services, and legislation. They operate with varying degrees of formality, support, and sponsorship and represent state, regional, and local constituencies. Among the benefits are increased opportunities to identify community resources, more options for handling abuse cases, expanded knowledge on the part of the participating professionals, better chances to obtain new services, and greater likelihood of acquiring voluntary and in-kind support. Through the coalition, stronger linkages can be forged between adult protective services and elder abuse programs and mental health and substance abuse programs, law enforcement, and the criminal justice system. Rather than just focusing on elder abuse some communities have organized coalitions on family violence that include child, spouse, and elder abuse issues. In this model groups can learn from one another and work together to educate the community about family violence of all types. One such example is the Suffolk (New York) County Executive's Task Force on Family Violence which has a very active elder abuse committee.

The multidisciplinary team is another strategy that brings professionals together for a common purpose. As one of its functions, the San Francisco Consortium for Elder Abuse Prevention operates a multidisciplinary team that meets monthly to review cases referred through their consultation service or directly from member agencies. Membership includes representatives from case management, family counseling, mental health, geriatric medicine, civil law, law enforcement, financial management, and APS. Although no formal evaluation of this team (Wolf & Pillemer, 1994) has been carried out, members are enthusiastic about their experience and have expressed their impression of its benefits as helping both clients and service providers; avoiding situations where there are either too many agencies involved, or not enough; promoting more of a systems perspective rather than treating family members individually to the detriment of one member; introducing service providers brought in to deal with one case with the entire network; having all the resources "at your fingertips"; and deriving a care plan that best meets the needs of the elder.

The Illinois Department on Aging, after a demonstration project on multidisciplinary teams, now requires that all their 45 elder abuse agencies have a consultation team to deal with difficult cases, with representation from medical, legal, law enforcement, mental health, religious, and financial institutions.

Elder abuse as a concept has reflected changing values and attitudes in our society, beginning with the commitment in the sixties to meet the needs of older persons, later the growing attention to domestic abuse, and more recently the concern about violence and crime. Because it represents many types of behavior and victim–perpetrator relationships, elder abuse has easily been incorporated into these broader movements. The result has been greater awareness of elder abuse issues by medical, legal, and law enforcement personnel and domestic violence advocates. They have helped to legitimatize the elder abuse movement to the degree that was not possible when it was regarded exclusively as a public welfare or social service issue. However, the legacy of the public welfare days still remains when "protective services" were intended for those older persons who could no longer manage their own affairs because of mental impairments and had no family member to help them out. Self-neglect cases still comprise more than half the caseload of most state adult protective services programs with few resources allocated to serving perpetrators. Alcohol and drug abuse and mental illness are not easily treatable conditions that small, inadequately funded governmental agencies like APS can resolve. They are societal problems that require the active involvement of all segments of society.

References

American Association of Retired Persons. (1992). *Abused elders or battered women?* Washington, DC: AARP.

American Association of Retired Persons. (1993). *Abused elders or older battered women: Report on the AARP Forum October 29–30, 1992.* Washington, DC: AARP.

Anetzberger, G. J. (1987). *The etiology of elder abuse by adult offspring.* Springfield, IL: Thomas.

Anetzberger, G. J. (1994). Protective services and long-term care. In Z. Harel & R. Dunkle (Eds.), *Long term care: People and services.* New York: Springer.

Bristowe, E., & Collins, J. B. (1989). Family mediated abuse of non-institutionalized elder men and women living in British Columbia. *Journal of Elder Abuse & Neglect, 1*(1), 45–54.

Colorado Department of Social Services. (1988). *Adult protection services.* A training conference for adult protective services staff. Denver, CO.

Coyne, A. C., Reichman, W. E., & Bergib, L. J. (1993). The relationship between dementia and elder abuse. *American Journal of Psychiatry, 150*(4), 643–646.

District of Columbia Department of Public Welfare. (1967). *Protective services for adults: Report on protective services prepared for the DC Interdepartmental Committee on Aging.* Washington, DC.

Finkelhor, D. (1983). Common features of family abuse. In D. Finkelhor, R. J. Gelles, G. Hotaling, & M. Straus, (Eds.), *The dark side of families: Current family violence research.* (pp. 17–20). Beverly Hills, CA: Sage.

Finkelhor, D., & Pillemer, K. (1984, August). *Elder abuse: Its relationship to other forms of domestic violence.* Paper presented at the Second National Conference on Family Violence Research, Durham, NH.

Formby, W. A. (1992). Should elder abuse be decriminalized? A justice system perspective. *Journal of Elder Abuse & Neglect, 4*(4), 121–130.

Fulmer, T., & O'Malley, T. (1987). *Inadequate care of the elderly.* New York: Springer.

Gebotys, R. J., O'Connor, D., & Mair, K. J. (1992). Public perceptions of elder physical mistreatment. *Journal of Elder Abuse & Neglect, 4*(1–2), 151–172.

Gelles, R. J. (1991, May 2–3). *Review of theoretical models in family violence.* Paper presented at the National Institute on Aging Workshop on Family Conflicts and Elder Abuse, Bethesda, MD.

Gelles, R. J. (1993). Through a sociological lens: Social structure and family violence. In R. J. Gelles & D. R. Loseke (Eds), *Current controversies on family violence* (pp. 7–30). Newbury Park, CA: Sage.

Goodrich, C. S. (1995). *Survey of state risk assessment methodologies.* Worcester, MA: National Committee for the Prevention of Elder Abuse.

Greenberg, J. R., McKibben, M., & Raymond, J. (1990). Dependent adult children and elder abuse. *Journal of Elder Abuse & Neglect, 2*(1–2), 73–86.

Haley, A. (1983). A family-behavioral approach to the treatment of the cognitively impaired elderly. *Gerontologist, 23*(1), 13–15.

Haley, W. E., Brown, S. L., & Levine, E. G. (1987a). Experimental evaluation of the effectiveness of group intervention for dementia caregivers. *Gerontologist, 27*(3), 376–381.

Haley, W. E., Brown, S. L., & Levine, E. G. (1987b). Family caregiver appraisals of patient behavioral disturbance in senile dementia. *Clinical Gerontologist, 6*(4), 25-34.

Heisler, C. J. (1991). The role of the criminal justice system in elder abuse cases. *Journal of Elder Abuse & Neglect, 3*(1), 5–34.

Homer, A. C., & Gilleard, C. (1990). Abuse of elderly people by their carers. *British Medical Journal, 301,* 1359–62.

Hooyman, N., Gonyea, J. & Montgomery, R. (1985). The impact of in-home services termination on family caregivers. *Gerontologist, 25*(2), 141–145.

Hudson, M. F. (1989). Analyses of the concepts of elder mistreatment: Abuse and neglect. *Journal of Elder Abuse & Neglect, 1*(1), 5–25.

Hudson, M. (1991). Elder mistreatment: A taxonomy with definitions by Delphi. *Journal of Elder Abuse & Neglect, 3*(2), 1–20.

Hudson, M. F. (1994). Elder abuse: Its meaning to middle-age and older adults: Part II. Pilot results. *Journal of Elder Abuse & Neglect, 6*(1), 55–81.

Hwalek, M., Goodrich, C. S., Quinn, K. (1995). The role of healthcare and adult protective services.. In L. A. Baumhover & S. C. Beall (Eds.), *Abuse, neglect, and exploitation of older persons* (pp. 123–142). Baltimore: Health Professions Press.

Illinois Department on Aging. (1990). *Elder abuse intervention: Guidelines for practice.* Springfield, IL: Author.

Johnson, T. F. (1991). *Elder mistreatment: Deciding who is at risk.* Westport, CT: Greenwood.

Kivelä, S. L., Köngäs-Saviaro, P., Kesti, E., Pahkala, K., & Ijäs, M. L. (1992). Abuse in old age: Epidemiological data from Finland. *Journal of Elder Abuse & Neglect, 4*(3), 1–18.

Korbin, J. E., Anetzberger, G. J., Thomasson, R., & Austin, C. (1991). Abused elders who seek legal recourse against their adult offspring: Findings from an exploratory study. *Journal of Elder Abuse & Neglect, 3*(3), 1–18.

Lachs, M., & Pillemer, K. (1995). Abuse and neglect of elderly persons. *New England Journal of Medicine, 332*(7), 437–443.

Lawton, M. P., Brody, E. M., & Saperstein, A. R. (1991). *Respite for caregivers of Alzheimer patients.* New York: Springer.

Marks, R. (1987–88). Stress in families providing care to frail elderly relatives and the effects of receiving in-home respite services. *Home Health Care Services Quarterly, 8*(4), 103–130.

Moon, A., & Williams, O. (1993). Perceptions of elder abuse and help-seeking patterns among African-American, Caucasian American, and Korean-American elderly women. *Gerontologist, 33*(3), 386–395.

National Center on Elder Abuse. (1995). *Understanding the nature and extent of elder abuse in domestic settings.* Washington, DC: Author.

Ogg, J. (1993). Researching elder abuse in Britain. *Journal of Elder Abuse & Neglect, 52,* 37–54.

O'Leary, K. D. (1993). Through a psychological lens: Personality traits, personality disorders, and levels of violence. In R. J. Gelles & D. R. Loseke (Eds.), *Current controversies on family violence* (pp. 1–6). Newbury Park, CA: Sage.

Paveza, G. J., Cohen, D., Eisdorfer, C., Freeks, S., Semla, T., Ashford, V. W., Gorlick, P., Hirshman, R., Luchins, D., & Levy, P. (1992). Severe family violence and Alzheimer's disease: Prevalence and risk factors. *Gerontologist, 32*(4), 493–497.

Phillips, L. (1986). Theoretical explanations of elder abuse: Competing hypotheses and unresolved issues. In K. A. Pillemer & R. S. Wolf (Eds.), *Elder abuse: Conflict in the family.* (pp. 197–217). Dover, MA: Auburn House.

Phillips, L. (1988). The fit of elder abuse with the family violence paradigm, and the implications of a paradigm shift for clinical practice. *Public Health Nursing, 5,* 222–229.

Pillemer, K. (1986). Risk factors in elder abuse: Results from a case control study. In K.A. Pillemer & R. S. Wolf (Eds.), *Elder abuse: Conflict in the family* (pp. 239–264). Dover, MA: Auburn House.

Pillemer, K. & Finkelhor, D. (1988). Prevalence of elder abuse: A random sample survey. *Gerontologist, 28*(1), 51–57.

Pillemer, K., & Suitor, J. J. (1992). Violence and violent feelings: What causes them among family caregivers? *Journal of Gerontology, 47*(4), S165–S172.

Pinkston, E. M., & Linsk, N. L. (1984a) Behavioral family intervention with the impaired elderly. *Gerontologist, 24*(6), 576–583.

Pinkston, E. M., & Linsk, N. L. (1984b). *Care of the elderly: A family approach.* Elmsford, NY: Pergamon.

Podnieks, E. (1992). National survey on abuse of the elderly in Canada. *Journal of Elder Abuse & Neglect, 4*(1–2), 5–58.

Podnieks, E., Pillemer, K., Nicholson, J. P., Shillingon, T., & Frizzell, A. (1990). *National survey on abuse of the elderly in Canada: Final report.* Toronto, Ontario, Canada: Ryerson Technical Institute.

Police Executive Research Forum. (1994). *Improving the police response to domestic elder abuse.* Washington, DC: Author.

Proctor, J., Hwalek, M., & Goodrich, C. S. (1993). *Improving our effectiveness in working with abusers.* Springfield, IL: Illinois Department on Aging.

Quayhagen, M. P., & Quayhagen, M. (1988). Alzheimer's stress: Coping with the caregiving role. *Gerontologist, 28*(3), 391–396.

Quinn, K., Hwalek, M., & Goodrich, C.S. (1993). *Determining effective interventions in a community-based elder abuse system.* Springfield, IL: Illinois Department on Aging.

Ramsey-Klawsnik, H. (1995). Investigating suspected elder maltreatment. *Journal of Elder Abuse & Neglect, 7*(1), 41–68.

Reulbach, D., & Tewksbury, J. (1994). Collaboration between protective services and law enforcement: The Massachusetts model. *Journal of Elder Abuse & Neglect, 6*(1), 9–22.

Scogin, F., Beall, C., Bynum, J., Stephens, G., Grote, N. P., Baumhover, L. A., & Bolland, J. M. (1989). Training for abusive caregivers: An unconventional approach to an intervention dilemma. *Journal of Elder Abuse & Neglect, 1*(4), 73–86.

Sengstock, M. C., Hwalek, M., & Petrone, S. (1989). Services for aged abuse victims: Service types and related factors. *Journal of Elder Abuse & Neglect, 1*(4), 37–56.

Steinmetz, S. K. (1988). *Duty bound: Elder abuse and family care.* New York: Sage.

Straus, M. (1992). The Conflict Tactics Scales and its critics: An evaluation. In M. A. Straus & R. J. Gelles (Eds.), *Physical violence in American families* (pp. 49–74). New Brunswick, NJ: Transaction.

Tatara, T. (1993). Finding the nature and scope of domestic elder abuse with the use of state aggregate data: Summaries of the key findings of a national survey of state PAS and aging agencies. *Journal of Elder Abuse & Neglect, 5*(4), 35–57.

U.S. Department of Health, Education and Welfare. (1966). State letter No. 925. Subject: Four model demonstration projects . . . services to older adults in the public welfare program. Washington, DC: Author.

Vinton, L. (1992). Services planned in abusive elder care situations. *Journal of Elder Abuse & Neglect, 4*(3), 85–99.

Wolf, R.S., & Pillemer, K. A. (1989). *Helping elder victims: The reality of elder abuse.* New York: Columbia University Press.

Wolf, R. S., & Pillemer, K. (1993). The evaluation of four elder abuse projects. Worcester, MA: Medical Center of Central Massachusetts, Institute on Aging.

Wolf, R. S., & Pillemer, K. (1994). What's new in elder abuse programming? Four bright ideas. *Gerontologist, 34*(1), 126–129.

Wolf, R. S., Godkin, M. A., & Pillemer, K. (1984). *Final report: Three model projects on elder abuse.* Worcester, MA: University of Massachusetts Medical Center, University Center on Aging.

Zarit, S. H., Anthony, C. R., & Boutselis, M. (1987). Interventions with care givers of dementia patients: Comparison of two approaches. *Psychology and Aging, 2*(3), 225–232.

VI

SPECIAL TOPICS

Serial Arson and Fire-Related Crime Factors

Allen D. Sapp, Timothy G. Huff, Gordon P. Gary, and David J. Icove

Introduction

The information contained in this chapter is the result of ongoing research conducted by the National Center for the Analysis of Violent Crime (NCAVC) at the Federal Bureau of Investigation Academy in Quantico, Virginia. The NCAVC is a law-enforcement-oriented resource center that consolidates research, training, investigative, and operational support functions to provide assistance to law-enforcement agencies confronted with unusual, high-risk, vicious, or repetitive crimes. In 1986, a subunit was established within the Center to study arson and bombings. Representatives from the Bureau of Alcohol, Tobacco, and Firearms joined the Center staff to serve in the Arson and Bombing Investigative Services Subunit (ABIS). This arrangement is based on a concurrent investigative responsibility with the FBI in these areas. ABIS has the primary responsibility to provide assistance in arson, bombing, terrorism, and related violent crimes submitted to the NCAVC by federal, state, local, and foreign law enforcement agencies. The staff of the Center is joined by faculty from major universities, members of the mental health and medical professions, and other law enforcement representatives (NCAVC, 1992).

The ABIS Subunit has conducted a series of studies on serial arsonists (see Douglas, Burgess, Burgess, & Ressler, 1992; Huff, 1993, 1994; Icove & Estepp, 1987; Icove & Gilman, 1989; Icove & Horbert, 1990; Sapp & Huff, 1995; Sapp, Gary, Huff, & James, 1993, 1994; Sapp, Huff, Gary, Icove, & Horbert, 1994).

Allen D. Sapp • Department of Criminal Justice, Central Missouri State University, Warrensburg, Missouri 64093. *Timothy G. Huff* • Federal Bureau of Investigation, Arson and Bombing Investigative Services Subunit, National Center for the Analysis of Violent Crime, FBI Academy, Quantico, Virginia 22135. *Gordon P. Gary* • Bureau of Alcohol, Tobacco, and Firearms, Arson and Bombing Investigative Services Subunit, National Center for the Analysis of Violent Crime, FBI Academy, Quantico, Virginia 22135. *David J. Icove* • Tennessee Valley Authority, TVA Police, Knoxville, Tennessee 37902-1499.

Handbook of Psychological Approaches with Violent Offenders: Contemporary Strategies and Issues, edited by Van Hasselt and Hersen. Kluwer Academic/Plenum Publishers, New York, 1999.

Statement of Problem

This study arose from a concern about the extent of serial arson in the United States. Serial arson is an offense committed by firesetters who set three or more fires with a significant cooling-off period between the fires (Douglas *et al.,* 1992). Arson is a violent crime, often taking the lives of innocent people and causing tremendous financial losses in property. According to the Uniform Crime Reports produced by the FBI (1992), arsons in 1991 exceeded $1 billion in property loss. Arson is the second leading cause of deaths in residential fires (Federal Emergency Management Agency, 1988). Despite the huge losses in property and the deaths caused by arson, relatively little research has been conducted on arsonists. Most of the available research is in the form of clinical studies of very small numbers of arsonists. (See Geller, 1992, for an extensive review of the literature on arson studies in forensic psychiatry.) This study is intended to fill some of the gaps in knowledge about arsonists, particularly serial arsonists.

Definition of Terms

The following terms are used throughout the report and are defined here to facilitate understanding of the findings and conclusions of the research.

Arson

Arson is the willful and malicious burning of property (Douglas *et al.,* 1992). The criminal act of arson is divided into three elements (DeHaan, 1991):

1. There has been a burning of property. This must be shown to the court to be actual destruction, at least in part, not just scorching or sooting (although some states include any physical or visible impairment of any surface).
2. The burning is incendiary in origin. Proof of the existence of an effective incendiary device, no matter how simple it may be, is adequate. Proof must be accomplished by showing specifically how all possible natural or accidental cases have been considered and ruled out.
3. The burning is shown to be started with malice, that is, with the specific intent of destroying property (p. 324).

Arsonist

An arsonist is a person apprehended, charged, and convicted of one or more arsons (Douglas *et al.,* 1992).

Accelerant

Accelerants are any type of material or substance added to the targeted materials to enhance the combustion of those materials and to accelerate the burning (Douglas *et al.,* 1992).

TABLE 19.1
Arson Classification by Style and Type

Style	Single	Double	Triple	Mass	Spree	Serial
Number of fires	1	2	3	3 or more	3 or more	3 or more
Number of events	1	1	1	1	1	3 or more
Number of sites	1	2	3	2	3 or more	3 or more
Cool-off period	No	No	No	No	No	Yes

Classification of Arson by Style and Type

A variety of descriptive terms are added to the term arson in an attempt to communicate variations in arson behavior. Some commonly used terms are single, double, and triple arsons, as well as mass, spree, and serial arson. As reflected in Table 19.1, the style of the arson involves the number of fires set, the number of separate events occurring, the number of sites or locations involved, and whether or not there was a cooling-off period between the fires.

This classification by style and type is compatible with the classification used in the *Crime Classification Manual* (Douglas *et al.*, 1992). The terms single, double, and triple arsons are shown to be the number of fires set at one site at one time in a single event. The other three terms are somewhat more complex and are defined as follows:

Mass Arson

Mass arson involves an offender who sets three or more fires at the same site or location during a limited period of time (Douglas *et al.*, 992).

Spree Arson

Spree arson involves an arsonist who sets three or more fires at separate locations with no cooling-off period between the fires (Douglas *et al.*, 1992).

Serial Arson

Serial arson involves an offender who sets three or more fires with a cooling-off period between the fires (Douglas *et al.*, 1992).

Classification of Motivations of Arsonists

It is in the area of motives that most of the literature on firesetting and arson has concentrated. The literature also offers a number of classification schemes and typologies, most often based on motives. Geller (1992) offers an exhaustive review of that literature and identifies 20 or more attempts to classify arsonists into typologies. Several of the earlier typologies contributed significantly to the current understanding of the motives and profiles of arsonists (see Hurley & Monahan, 1969; Inciardi, 1970; Levin, 1976; Lewis & Yarnell, 1951; Robbins, 1967; Steinmetz, 1966; Vandersall & Wiener, 1970; Wolford, 1972). In more recent work, Sapp and colleagues (1993) followed the *Crime Classification Manual* typology (Douglas *et al.*, 1992) in their study of the motives of shipboard arsonists. Geller (1992) added another classification to the literature, more clinically focused than most of the others. He noted that arson may be associated with psychobiologic, medical, neurological, or mental disorders. Geller (1992) also separates juvenile firesetting and juvenile fireplay from arson by adults. The reference section includes research literature related to arson and motivations for arson.

Motive is defined as an inner drive or impulse that is the cause, reason, or incentive that induces or prompts a specific behavior (Rider, 1980). Through research, the NCAVC has determined that the identification of the offender's motive is a key element in crime analysis. This method of analysis is used by the NCAVC to identify personal traits and characteristics exhibited by an unknown offender. The NCAVC reviewed arson research literature and actual arson cases, and interviewed incarcerated arsonists across the nation. The following motive categories consistently appear and prove most effective in identifying offender characteristics:

1. Vandalism
2. Excitement
3. Revenge
4. Crime Concealment
5. Profit
6. Extremist

The motivations discussed in this chapter are outlined and described in the *Crime Classification Manual* (Douglas *et al.*, 1992). For purposes of reference and ease in cross-referencing, the motives are classified using the same numbering system used in the *Crime Classification Manual* (CCM).

200. Vandalism-Motivated Arson

Vandalism-motivated arson is defined as malicious or mischievous firesetting that results in damage to property. The most common targets are schools or school property and educational facilities. Vandals also frequently target abandoned structures and flammable vegetation.

210. Excitement-Motivated Arson

Offenders motivated by excitement include seekers of thrills, attention, recognition, and rarely, but importantly, sexual gratification. (The stereotypical arsonist who sets fires for sexual gratification is quite rare.)

Potential targets of the excitement-motivated arsonist run full spectrum from so-called nuisance fires to occupied apartment houses at nighttime. Firefighters are known to set fires so they can engage in the suppression effort (Huff, 1994). Security guards have set fires to relieve boredom and gain recognition.

220. *Revenge-Motivated Arson*

Revenge-motivated fires are set in retaliation for some injustice, real or imagined, perceived by the offender. Often revenge is also an element of other motives. This concept of mixed motives is expanded and further discussed later. The primary motive of revenge is further divided into four major subgroups.

221. Personal Revenge

The subgroup with this motive, as the name implies, strikes at an individual with the use of fire to retaliate for a personal grievance. This one-on-one retaliation may be a one-time occurrence and not the product of a serial arsonist. Triggering such retaliation may be an argument, fight, personal affront, or any of an infinite array of events perceived by the offender to warrant retaliation. Favorite targets include the victim's vehicle, home, or personal possessions.

222. Societal Retaliation

Perhaps the most dangerous of the revenge-motivated arsonists is the one who feels betrayed by society in general. This person generally suffers from a lifelong feeling of inadequacy, loneliness, persecution, or abuse and strikes out in revenge against the society perceived as having wronged him or her. The individual may suffer from a congenital condition affecting appearance or health. Targets are random and fire-setting behavior often escalates. All known cases involve serial arsonists.

223. Institutional Retaliation

Arsonists with retaliation against institutions in mind focus on such institutions as government, education, military service or services, medicine, religion, or any other entity reflecting and representing the establishment. Often these arsonists are serial arsonists, striking repeatedly at the institution or institutions against which retaliation is sought. The offender, in such cases, uses fire to settle grievances with the institution and to intimidate those associated with the institution. Buildings housing the institutions are the most frequently selected targets.

224. Group Retaliation

Targets for group retaliation may be religious, racial, fraternal (such as gangs or fraternal orders), or other groups. The offender tends to feel anger toward the group or members of the group collectively, rather than anger at a specific individual within the group. The target may be the group headquarters building, church, meeting place, or symbolic targets such as emblems or logos, regardless of what they are attached to. Arsonists motivated by group retaliation sometimes become serial offenders.

230. *Crime-Concealment–Motivated Arson*

Arson is the secondary criminal activity in this motivational category. The fire is set for the purpose of covering up a murder or burglary or to eliminate evidence left at a crime scene. Other examples include fires set to destroy business records to conceal cases of embezzlement and the many cases of auto theft arson where the fire is set to destroy evidence.

240. Profit-Motivated Arson

Arsonists in this category expect to profit from their firesetting, either directly for monetary gain or more indirectly to profit from a goal other than money. Examples of direct monetary gain include insurance fraud, liquidating property, dissolving businesses, destroying inventory, parcel clearance, or to gain employment. The latter is exemplified by a case of a construction worker wanting to rebuild an apartment complex he destroyed, or an unemployed laborer seeking employment as a forest fire fighter or as a logger to salvage burned timber.

Arsonists have set fire to western forests to rent their equipment as part of the suppression effort. In what may be the most disturbing of all, there are cases of parents murdering their own children for profit, with fire used to cover the crime. While this motive is uncommon, it is by no means unheard-of (Huff, 1994). Cases are documented where an insured child is murdered, but more commonly the parents wish to profit from getting rid of a perceived nuisance or hindrance: their own child.

Other nonmonetary reasons from which arsonists may profit range from setting brush fires to enhance hunting game, to setting fires to escape an undesirable environment as in the case of a serviceman (Sapp, Gary, Huff, & James, 1993, 1994).

250. Extremist-Motivated Arson

Arsonists may set fires to further social, political, or religious causes. Examples of extremist-motivated targets include abortion clinics, slaughterhouses, animal laboratories, fur farms, and furrier outlets. The targets of political terrorists reflect the focus of the terrorists' wrath.

Mixed Motives

Interviews conducted by the authors with incarcerated arsonists underscore the complexity of human behavior. When questioned about motives for their arsons, the arsonists indicated that while there was a primary motive (one of the six outlined earlier), there also often were secondary and supplementary motives as well. For example, the aspect of power must be considered. Many arsonists were the disenfranchised of our society. This is particularly true with the revenge arsonists who targeted society in general. It is clear that a part of their motive was to achieve a sense of power. But power considerations also apply to revenge arsonists of the other cited types. It is also apparent that power is an element in the extremist's motivation. Vandalism, it can be argued, also has an element of power. One could make a case, albeit less convincingly, that power also plays a role in other motivational categories.

Other researchers, most notably Lewis and Yarnell (1951), have asserted that revenge is present in all arsons to a greater or lesser degree. Motives for arson, like other aspects of human behavior, often defy structured, unbending definition. Strictly speaking, who can argue that vandals are not looking for excitement when they are engaging in their malicious mischief.? Add an element of power and revenge and one can see the problem of strict, unyielding classification. Fire investigators also should be aware that motivations may change, as in the case of an arsonist who initially set fires for revenge and later became an arsonist for hire, setting fires for profit.

The Serial Arsonist Project

The research involved the identification and interview of incarcerated serial arsonists. A total of 83 serial arsonists whose conviction was final, with no appeals pending, agreed to participate in the study. The subjects were free to participate in the study or not and free to answer or not answer any question posed. Subjects clearly understood that their participation would not benefit them in any manner. Many of the interviews were tape-recorded or videotaped. The convicted arsonists were interviewed using a comprehensive protocol to collect information on a variety of aspects of the arsonist's offenses, characteristics, and life history. The protocol was then analyzed to extract information on 168 variables that were encoded for computer analysis. The data were analyzed using descriptive statistics and cross-tabulations to examine relationships between variables.

The study involved two purposive samples. The first sample of 42 subjects representing one eastern and one western state were all interviewed a dozen years before the second sample. The second sample involved 41 subjects in several different state correctional systems who were interviewed in 1990–1992. The states were selected to provide a geographically representative sample of the United States. Similar protocols were used for the two samples. After data collection was completed, the two samples were compared to ensure that they were compatible and did not differ significantly on the critical variables. The samples were found to be compatible without significant differences and then were combined into a single sample for analysis.

Nearly 1,000 incarcerated arsonists' records were reviewed in the nearly three dozen facilities visited by the researchers. Those facilities included prisons, jails, and mental health facilities. Approximately 200 inmates were selected for interview. Of this number, some were unavailable for interview, some refused, and others did not cooperate. Some who cooperated were found not to be serial arsonists. The final sample for this study involved 83 serial arsonists, including 42 subjects from the earlier interviews and 41 from the more recent ones. The findings are presented here organized according to a motive-based analysis of the offenders.

Revenge-Motivated Arson

Revenge-motivated fires are set as a form of retaliation for some real or perceived wrong. The event or circumstance that is perceived as a wrong may have occurred months or years before the firesetting activity (Icove & Horbert, 1990). The broad classification of revenge-motivated arsonists is further divided into subgroups based on the target of the retaliation (Douglas *et al.*, 1992). Serial arsonists are more likely to direct their retaliation at institutions and society than at individuals or groups. In the study of serial arsonists conducted by the ABIS, 59% of the revenge-motivated arsonists directed their retaliation against society in general. Seven arsonists (20.6%) sought revenge against institutions of society. Five (14.7%) set personal revenge fires and 2 (5.9%) set fires to retaliate against a group.

Attributes of the Revenge-Motivated Serial Arsonist

The revenge-motivated serial arsonist is almost always a male, although 3 of the 5 women in this sample were classified as revenge-motivated arsonists. The arsonist is likely to be a White, single, male with an average of 10 years of education. His performance in school was fair to poor although he has an above average intelligence as measured by IQ tests. His sexual orientation is heterosexual. He has tattoos or other disfigurements. He has not served in the military and has a menial, laborer type of job.

Life History of the Revenge-Motivated Serial Arsonist

The revenge-motivated serial arsonist is likely to have a long history of institutionalization. He has a history of misdemeanor and felony arrests and has served time in juvenile detention, state prison, and county jails. He has a problematic psychological history and likely has been in a mental health institution for one or more stays.

He comes from a lower- to middle-class home with average, comfortable socioeconomic status. He was raised by both parents in a family that was often described as unstable. He is most likely to be a first- or second-born child, raised in a family atmosphere described as cold and distant. Although his relationships with young playmates is reported to be warm and friendly, his school environment was cold and distant.

History of Arsons by the Revenge-Motivated Serial Arsonist

The revenge-motivated serial arsonist sets an average of 35 fires before his career is ended by conviction and incarceration. The average age for setting the first fire is 15 years, generally older than most other serial arsonists. He is more likely to set fires in buildings other than residences, in vegetation, and in vehicles. He is least likely to set business fires. Almost all of his fires are set either outside a building or vehicle or inside when there is open entry to the vehicle or building. He very rarely breaks into a building to set a fire. The fires set by the revenge-motivated serial arsonist are intentional, premeditated, and targeted. Although he may sometimes set a fire impulsively, the target will be one that fits his personal target criteria, based on specific intentions to retaliate.

Societal Retaliation Serial Arsonist

Attributes of the Societal Retaliation Serial Arsonist

The societal retaliation serial arsonist is most likely to be male, although 2 of the 5 females included in this study were classified as societal retaliation arsonists. The arsonist is also likely to be White and single at the time of the offenses. Although not married at the time of the arson activity, the arsonist has previously been married one or two times. He has an education of 11 years with a school record of fair to poor performance. His intelligence is above average, as measured by IQ tests. He is unlikely to have served in the military services. He is employed, in jobs ranging from menial to skilled labor and has a generally stable employment record. His sexual orientation is heterosexual.

He is likely to have a juvenile record as well as a criminal history involving both misdemeanor and felony arrests. He probably has served at least one sentence in a state prison. He is very likely to have a problematic psychological history, often involving one or more suicide attempts.

Life History of the Societal Retaliation Serial Arsonist

The societal retaliation serial arsonist was most likely raised in a lower- to middle-class family with average to comfortable socioeconomic circumstances. He is likely to be the first-born child in a family where both parents were present, but in a home with chronic instability. He had poor relationships with his parents and his home atmosphere was cold and troubled. The school atmosphere was similarly reported to be cold and troubled and his relationships with younger playmates were often troubled as well.

History of Arsons by the Societal Retaliation Serial Arsonist

After starting to set fires at an average age of about $12\frac{1}{2}$ half years, the societal retaliation arsonist sets an average of 69 fires. He typically works alone and does not confide in anyone about his arsons. He sets fires in structures other than residences and businesses, and in vehicles and vegetation. He rarely selects residences or businesses as targets although buildings associated with government, education, religion, or other institutions may be selected. His fires are premeditated and intentional, although individual fires may be opportunistic in terms of selection of the target.

Personal Retaliation Serial Arsonists

Five of the serial arsonists in the ABIS study were classified as personal retaliation serial arsonists (Douglas *et al.*, 1992). The following discussion summarizes the observed traits and characteristics of the personal retaliation serial arsonist.

Attributes of the Personal Retaliation Serial Arsonist

All 5 personal retaliation serial arsonists were White, 4 males and 1 female. All 4 of the men had tattoos. One was married, 2 divorced, and 2 were single. The average educational level for the 5 personal retaliation arsonists was 7.75 years. Only one had reached the level of a General Education Development (GED) certificate. One had served in the military and 2 had been rejected for military service. All 5 had histories of misdemeanor and felony arrests. The 4 men had multiple misdemeanor arrests and multiple felony arrests. The female had only one misdemeanor arrest for petty theft but multiple felonies.

Life History of the Personal Retaliation Serial Arsonist

Only one personal retaliation serial arsonist had a foster home placement. However, all 5 had several stays in juvenile detention, state juvenile institutions, county jails, and state prisons. Two had also been in a mental health institution. All 5 had problematic psychological histories and 2 had attempted suicide. Four of the 5 had some type of permanent physical handicap or chronic medical condition. Two of the men were heterosexual, 2 were bisexual, and the female identified her sexual orientation as homosexual. They had generally stable work histories in jobs involving unskilled and skilled labor. The average IQ score was in the low normal range.

Two came from middle-class families and the remainder from lower-class families. Two families were described as advantaged or comfortable socioeconomically. The other three were either marginal or submarginal. Three of the five families were described as usually stable and two as chronically unstable. Three lived in families with both parents present, 1 with mother alone and 1 with other relatives. All 5 of the personal retaliation serial arsonists described their relationship with their mother as warm and close; however, 3 described their paternal relationship as hostile and aggressive. The family atmosphere was warm and friendly for 2, cold and troubled for 2, and sometimes one and then the other for the remaining member of the group. Similarly, there were mixed ratings given to playmates and school atmosphere.

History of Arson by the Personal Retaliation Serial Arsonists

The personal retaliation serial arsonists set their first fire at an average age of 23 years, although the range was from 7 years of age to 41 years. The personal retaliation arsonists set a total of 27 fires, an average of 5.3 each. The fires were set within one to two miles of the arsonist's home or workplace and were usually set after work or on days off and weekends. All were in areas with which the arsonist was well acquainted and all were committed alone. Target selection was based on directing the retaliation at a person. When open entry was not available, the arsonist either broke in or set a fire outside.

Feelings as the fire was being set were described as angry, mad, getting even, and revenge. Four of the fires were set in residences and four in vehicles that belonged to the person against whom the arsonist was retaliating. No fires were set in businesses.

Institutional Retaliation Serial Arsonists

In the ABIS study of serial arsonists, 7 were classified as institutional retaliation arsonists. This classification of arsonist targets institutions such as churches, government buildings, universities, educational facilities, or corporations (Douglas *et al.*, 1992).

Attributes of Institutional Retaliation Serial Arsonists

All 7 of the institutional retaliation serial arsonists were males. Five were White, 1 Black and 1 Hispanic. Four had tattoos and all 7 were single. Only 1 had a previous marriage. Their average educational level was 8.3 years of schooling. Six of the 7 had misdemeanor records and all 7 had felony records. Four of the 7 had previously served a felony sentence for aggravated arson.

Life History of Institutional Retaliation Serial Arsonists

Four of the 7 had records of juvenile detention and juvenile institutions. Three had mental health institution stays in their background and a history of psychological problems. All had served prison time. Three defined themselves as bisexual and 4 as heterosexual. Overall IQ scores were in the average intelligence range. Four of the institutional retaliation serial arsonists came from middle-class families and 3 from lower-class families. Four described their family atmospheres warm and friendly. The other 3 said their family atmosphere was cold and distant. School atmosphere was warm and friendly for 3 and cold and distant for 3. Playmates were described as warm and friendly.

History of Arsons by Institutional Retaliation Serial Arsonists

The average age of the institutional retaliation serial arsonist when he set his first fire was 16 years. The 7 arsonists set a total of 94 fires, an average of 13.4 each. The fires were generally set in institutional facilities within 1 to 2 miles of home or workplace. Several fires were set in institutions where the arsonists were living at the time. Feelings at the time of the fires were described as angry, mad, revengeful, and frustrated.

Group Retaliation Serial Arsonists

Group retaliation arsonists direct their retaliation against religious, racial, fraternal, or other groups. In the ABIS study of serial arsonists there were only 2 group retaliation serial arsonists. Both were male, 1 White, 1 Hispanic. Neither was married and neither served in the military services. Average educational level was 11 years. Only 1 had either a misdemeanor or a felony arrest record. Both, however, had an extensive history of stays in institutions, such as orphanages, foster homes, juvenile detention, and juvenile state facilities. Both had spent time in mental health institutions. Both had psychological histories that included suicide attempts.

Intelligence scores were in the average range. Both came from generally stable lower-class families and both lived with two natural parents. In both cases, the relationships with both the mother and father were described as cold and distant. Family atmosphere was cold and troubled as was the school atmosphere. Relationships with playmates were seen as warm and friendly. The two group retaliation arsonists set their first fires at ages 11 and 18. They set four fires each. One set the fires at work and at school, the other within one-half mile of home. Both walked to the scene of the fires. One set the fires alone; the other had an accomplice.

One described his fires as "gang activity" getting back at another gang. The other set his fires in an institution where he sought retaliation against other residents. Available materials were used by one arsonist, the other used gasoline. Matches were used to ignite the fires.

No deaths occurred from the fires set by the group retaliation serial arsonists. After setting the fires, both remained at the scene and then returned later to view the damage. They were not questioned for any fire before the ones they were arrested for setting. They offered no resistance on arrest and accepted full responsibility for their fires. They made no lifestyle changes and did not actively follow or become involved in the case after the fire. Alcohol and drug use were not noted in the group retaliation arsons. The fires remained consistent in frequency but increased in severity over time.

Excitement-Motivated Arson

Douglas and colleagues (1992) divided excitement-motivation arsonists into several subclassifications. Included are thrills-motivated, recognition-motivated, sexually motivated, and attention-motivated arsonists. The most common type of excitement-motivated arsonist found in this study was the thrills type, accounting for 17 of the 25 (68%) of the excitement category. One woman was classified as an excitement-motivated, thrills-seeking arsonist. The thrill seeker sets fires because he or she craves the excitement that is satisfied by firesetting (Douglas *et al.*, 1992, p. 170). Four (16.0%) of the excitement-motivated arsonists were classified as recognition seekers. These arsonists are sometimes described as the "hero" type, often remaining at the scene of the fire to warn others, to report the fire, or to assist in firefighting efforts. This type of arsonist craves the recognition and praise she or he receives for their efforts. Four (16.0%) of the others were attention seekers. These arsonists set fires to gain attention and to meet their needs for importance.

Attributes of the Excitement-Motivated Serial Arsonist

The typical excitement-motivated serial arsonist is a White male who is single. He is likely to have tattoos. He has an average 11 years of schooling and was an average student in academic performance. He has a felony arrest record and may have multiple felony arrests. He is less likely to have a misdemeanor record.

Life History of the Typical Excitement-Motivated Serial Arsonist

The typical excitement-motivated serial arsonist has an extensive record of institutionalization, having been in foster homes, juvenile detention, state juvenile centers, county jails, and state prisons. Most have a troubled mental health history as well, some with suicide attempts.

Usually, the excitement-motivated arsonist has a stable work background, usually in skilled and unskilled labor positions. He is most likely to have had a middle-class family described as average to comfortable in socioeconomic status. His relationship with his mother was likely to be warm and close but with his father, cold and troubled. He probably lived in a home with one or both parents present. His relationship with playmates ages 4 to 12 was reportedly warm and close, but the school atmosphere was described as cold and troubled. The family was usually stable but often described as troubled and cold.

History of Arsons by the Excitement-Motivated Serial Arsonist

The average excitement-motivated serial arsonist set his first fire at age 12 and set a total 40 fires. There is wide variation in the number of fires set by excitement-motivated serial arsonists, based on the subgroup classification. Excitement-thrills–motivated serial arsonists set 56 fires each while the excitement-attention–motivated serial arsonists set an average of only 4. The single excitement-sexual arsonist in the study set 40 fires. The excitement-recognition arsonists averaged 11 each.

The fires set by the excitement-motivated serial arsonist are typically within 1 to 2 miles of his home or workplace. All are set in areas with which he is familiar. Generally, he will walk to the scene of the arsons. Because he is not interested in hurting anyone, most targets are selected for minimal damage, except when the excitement-thrills arsonist is involved. In such cases, he is likely to set major conflagrations, involving businesses, residences, and other structures. When he sets a vegetation fire it is likely to be a major fire, as well. His motivation requires big fires to provide the thrills.

Excitement-Thrills Motivation

Attributes of the Thrills-Motivated Serial Arsonist

The typical thrills-motivated serial arsonist is a White male. He is single and never married. He has an average of less than 10 years schooling. His school performance was poor to average and he is unlikely to be engaged in any type of significant relationship with a woman at the time of his offenses. He is unlikely to have served in the military although he may have attempted to enlist but was rejected. He is likely to have misdemeanor arrests and almost certainly will have a record of felony arrests, probably multiple felony arrests.

Life History of the Thrills-Motivated Serial Arsonist

The typical excitement-thrills serial arsonist has an extensive history of institutionalization, ranging from foster home placements to prison. He has a history of juvenile detention and juvenile institutional placement. He has been in county jail at least once and is likely to also have a troubled mental health record and history. He is most likely to be heterosexual but nearly one third are bisexual or homosexual. He has a generally stable work history at unskilled and skilled labor positions.

The typical excitement-thrills serial arsonist came from a middle-class family where one or both of the natural parents were present. The family was described as socioeconomically comfortable and average and the family situation was stable. However, the family atmosphere is described as cold and troubled most of the time. His relationship with his mother was warm and close but the relationship with his father was cold and troubled. His relationship with playmates was warm and close but the school atmosphere was cold and troubled.

History of Arsons by the Thrills-Motivated Serial Arsonist

The typical excitement-thrills serial arsonist first set a fire at age 12. Subsequent to that fire he has set an average of 56 fires. Most were in residences and vegetation, but others targeted businesses, structures other than residences, and vehicles. All of the fires were set within 1 to 2 miles from his home or workplace, in areas with which he was very familiar. When he selected a target, it was premeditated and planned. If the building did not provide open entry, he would break in to set the fire. He set the fires alone and usually walked to the scene. When setting the fire, he had feelings of thrills, excitement, and power.

Excitement-Recognition Motivation

There were 4 serial arsonists who were classified as excitement-recognition motivated in the ABIS serial arson study. Since 4 cases are too few to develop "typical" profiles, the information that follows is based on summarizing the data from the 4 serial arsonists.

Attributes of Excitement-Recognition Serial Arsonists

All 4 of the excitement-recognition motivation serial arsonists were White males and all were single, never married. Three had tattoos and two had some type of permanent disfigurement. The four had an average educational level of 11.8 years of schooling with a range from 10 to 14 years. This group had the highest overall educational level of any of the motivational subgroups.

Life History of Excitement-Recognition Serial Arsonists

None of the 4 excitement-recognition serial arsonists had served in the military. One had multiple misdemeanor arrests and all 4 had prior felony arrests, including 1 with multiple arrests. They had unstable work histories, primarily at unskilled labor positions. Only 1 had a mental health hospitalization and 2 had troubled psychological records. Three of the 4 had spent no time in institutions as a juvenile. Three of the 4 excitement-recognition serial arsonists came from middle-class families where the father was described as cold and distant and the family atmosphere as troubled and cold. Both parents were present in two of the homes. One other lived with relatives other than natural parents and 1 lived in a foster home. The excitement-recognition serial arsonists reported childhood playmates as warm and friendly but the school atmosphere was seen as cold and troubled.

History of Arsons by Excitement-Recognition–Motivated Serial Arsonists

The 4 excitement-recognition–motivated serial arsonists set their first fire at an average age of 12 years and averaged 11 fires each before being arrested. All of the fires were set in areas with which the arsonists were familiar and all were within one to two miles of their home or workplace. Two walked to the scene of all of their fires while 1 drove a car and the other used public transportation.

The excitement-recognition–motivated serial arsonists set a total of 5 fires in residences, 16 in other structures, 14 in vegetation, and 10 in dumpsters, trash bins, and similar areas. None were set in vehicles or in businesses.

Excitement-Attention Motivation

A total of 4 of the serial arsonists in the ABIS study were classified as excitement-attention motivated. The arsonist sets fires to get attention and to be the center of concern of those around him. All 4 of the excitement-attention–motivated serial arsonists were White males. Symbolic perhaps of their need for attention, all 4 had tattoos. Two were single, 1 was married, and 1 was divorced. The average educational level of the 4 was 10 years. Academic performance was rated as average to poor. None had served in the military. Intelligence scores were in the average range.

Life History of the Excitement-Attention–Motivated Serial Arsonist

Three of the 4 excitement-attention–motivated serial arsonists had felony arrests and 2 had misdemeanor arrests on their record. Two had previous arrests for arson. Two had juvenile detention stays and 3 of the 4 had been in a mental health facility.

The usual work was in skilled and unskilled labor positions and they usually had a stable work history. Three came from a middle-class family and 1 from a lower-class family. The lower-class family was described as chronically unstable. Mothers were seen as warm and close while fathers were perceived as warm and close by 2 and cold and distant by 2 of the arsonists. In all 4, however, the family atmosphere was described as cold and troubled. Playmates were warm and close in relationships but school atmosphere was cold and troubled.

History of the Arsons Set by Excitement-Attention–Motivated Serial Arsonists

The average age for the first fire set by the excitement-attention–motivated serial arsonist was 18 years. The 4 excitement-attention–motivated arsonists set an average of 6.5 fires each. Only one was set in a residence. The others were set in other structures (15) and in trash cans, bins, and dumpsters (10). All were set close to the home or workplace of the serial arsonist, and all were set without accomplices. The targets were picked to "yield minimum damage." There was no intent to harm others or to create extensive damage.

Vandalism, Crime Concealment, Profit, and Other Motives

This section presents information on arsonists motivated by vandalism, profit, crime concealment, and other motives. Included are descriptions of arsonists and arson-related behavior drawn from the various ABIS studies and the *Crime Classification Manual.*

Vandalism-Motivated Arson

Vandalism-motivated arson is based on malicious and mischievous motivation that results in destruction or damage, or setting fires simply to destroy things. The serial arsonist study conducted by the ABIS included 6 willful and malicious mischief arsonists whose histories and cases were used to construct the "typical" arsonist discussed here.

Attributes of the vandalism-motivated serial arsonist The vandalism-motivated serial arsonist is typically a White male with some form of tattoo, scar or birthmark. Most have never been married and none had served in the military forces. The average educational level for vandalism-motivated serial arsonists was 11 years of schooling. His performance in school was fair to poor. He has average or below average intelligence as measured by IQ tests. His sexual orientation is heterosexual.

Life history of the vandalism-motivated serial arsonist The vandalism-motivated serial arsonist is likely to have a long history of institutionalization. Part of his childhood may have been spent in foster homes and in care of relatives. He has a history of multiple misdemeanor and felony arrests and has served time in juvenile detention, state prison, and county jails. He has a troubled psychological history and likely has been in a mental health institution for one or more stays. Suicide attempts and depression are often noted in the mental health histories of these arsonists.

Their usual occupations are unskilled laborer positions and service jobs. Their employment history is described as stable or generally stable. Most come from middle-class homes with average or comfortable socioeconomic conditions. The families are described as usually stable. Relationships with parents are described as warm and close with the mother, but cold and distant with the father. Most lived with one or both natural parents for most of their childhood. (In this study 4 of the 6 were third-born children in the family.) Relationships with school and young playmates were described as cold and troubled. Their families were very religious and involved in local church activities.

History of arsons by the vandalism-motivated serial arsonist The typical vandalism-motivated serial arsonist started firesetting at an early age. Fires may have been set before 6 years and the first arson fire was set at an average age of 8 years. The vandalism-motivated arsonist sets fires only in areas that he is well acquainted with and sets fires alone. Trash bins, dumpsters, and trash cans are his primary targets; however, he will set fires in unoccupied or vacant buildings, usually setting the fire outside the building unless there is open entry to the structure. Businesses will rarely be the target of a vandalism-motivated fire.

Vandalism-motivated serial arsonists set fires whenever the opportunity arises, but most will be set after work or school hours or on weekends. This likely time is based on opportunity, not a particular choice of the arsonist. Typically the fires will be set within one-half to one mile from home or work with the arsonists walking to the scenes of the arsons. An automobile may be used, if available, to travel to the scene of the offenses. If so, the vehicle likely will have average wear and tear and will have no special accessories, such as spotlights, citizen band radios, or scanners.

Crime-Concealment Motivations

Four of the serial arsonists were classified as crime-concealment motivated. According to the *Crime Classification Manual* (Douglas *et al.*, 1992), the arson is secondary to another crime and is set to hide or conceal the primary crime activity. In the 4 cases in this study, the primary crime was burglary. After burglarizing a business or a residence, the serial arsonists set fire to the structure to destroy the evidence of the burglary.

In another study at ABIS, arson-homicides are being studied (Sapp & Huff, 1995). Results suggest that crime concealment is a major factor in such crimes. Of 62 cases of arson-homicide studied, nearly one third involved a burglary, over one fourth a sexual assault, and nearly one fifth, a robbery as well as the arson-homicide (Sapp & Huff, 1995). Thus, 79% of the cases of arson-homicide involved an associated crime. In many of these cases, the primary purpose of the offender was likely to commit the associated crime with homicide and then arson as secondary and tertiary events after something went wrong in the primary event. If these arson-homicides are representative, the data would suggest that crime concealment may be the primary motive for the arson component of the crime (Sapp & Huff, 1995). The 4 cases in the serial arsonist study are not enough to develop typical profiles; therefore, the results will be reported with reference to the 4 cases only.

Attributes of the crime-concealment–motivated serial arsonist The four crime-concealment–motivated serial arsonists were all male, 2 White, 2 Black. All 4 had tattoos and 3 had never been married. The fourth was married and divorced. At the time of their crimes, 3 were living with a "significant other" and 1 was living alone. The 4 had an average educational level of 11 years of schooling with a range from 9 years to 12 years of schooling. Their academic progress and performance was described as average. None had served in the military, although 1 had applied and been rejected because of low scores on the written test. All 4 had multiple felony arrests and 3 of the 4 had misdemeanor arrests on their records.

Life history of the crime-concealment–motivated serial arsonist Unlike the other serial arsonists, crime-concealment arsonists were much less likely to have a childhood history of institutionalization. Only 1 had a juvenile record and none had been in orphanages, foster homes, or other institutions. Three of the 4 had a troubled psychological history, but none were diagnosed as chronically mentally ill. The 4 all had a generally stable work history, working at skilled and unskilled labor jobs.

The family histories of the crime-concealment–motivated serial arsonists were generally unremarkable. All 4 came from middle-class families enjoying average to comfortable socioeconomic status, although three of the families were described as chronically unstable. The three chronically unstable were families headed by a single parent, the father. The fourth arsonist also came from a single-parent family, but one headed by his mother. Relationships with mother and father were all described as warm and close. The family atmosphere was also described as warm and close. Childhood playmates were reportedly warm and close to the arsonists, who attended school in a friendly and warm atmosphere. All four families were described as moderately religious.

History of arsons by the crime-concealment–motivated serial arsonist The crime-concealment–motivated serial arsonists committed an average of only 5 arsons each, a total far below the average for the other types of serial arsonists. However, their overall firesetting behavior was similar to that of the other types. Two of the 4 first remember setting a fire at age 5 and 2 reportedly did not set a fire until age 13.

The crime-concealment–motivated serial arsonists set their fires close to home, all occurring no more than 10 miles from their home. They typically walked to the scene of the crime and subsequent arson designed to conceal the crime. Three of the 4 usually had an accomplice; 1 sometimes had two accomplices. All of the fires were set in areas with which they were well acquainted. Fires were set in residences, businesses, vehicles, and other structures to conceal thefts or to destroy evidence. Interestingly, all 4 reported setting one or two vegetation fires as juveniles.

Profit-Motivated Serial Arsonists

Four other serial arsonists were classified as profit-motivated arsonists. Arson for profit is a fire set for the purpose of achieving material gain either directly or indirectly. (Icove, Wherry, & Schroeder, 1998). The 4 serial arsonists in this study set fires for others for a price. They are called "torches for hire" in the criminal culture. Because there are only 4 cases, no attempt is made to offer a typical profile; instead, the 4 cases are discussed below.

Attributes of profit-motivated serial arsonist All 4 of the profit-motivated serial arsonists were White males. At the time of their offenses, 1 was single, 1 separated, and the other 2 divorced. Their academic achievement ranged from grade 5 to grade 12 with an average of 9 years of schooling. Their academic performance was described as poor to average.

Two of the 4 had served in the U.S. Army and both had moderate difficulty in adjusting to military life. Both received general discharges and neither progressed above the E-1 entry-level rank. Neither had any military criminal history. Three of the 4 had both misdemeanor and felony records, including one felony conviction for arson.

Life history of the profit-motivated serial arsonist The arson-for-profit offenders did not have extensive institutionalization in their backgrounds. Only 1 had ever been in a foster home and 2 had brief juvenile detention or juvenile institution stays. Despite their records, only 1 had served jail time and none had been incarcerated in a state or federal prison. None had any mental health record or history. Their work history was relatively stable, involving unskilled and skilled laborer positions.

Three of the 4 came from lower-class homes and 1 from a middle-class home. The middle-class home was described as advantaged, while the other three were reportedly average to marginally adequate. All four families were seen as usually stable. Relationships with the mother was described as warm and close while relationships with the father were mixed, ranging from warm and close to hostile and aggressive. One described his family atmosphere and school atmosphere as cold and troubled, but the others described theirs as warm and close.

History of arsons by the profit-motivated serial arsonist Two of the profit-motivated arsonists set their first fires at ages 12 and 14 while 2 others did not set their first one until ages 23 and 24. The profit-motivated serial arsonists set an average of 11 fires each. The profit-motivated arsons were set in preselected targets, often involving travel to the scene. The arsonists drove their car, rode public transportation, or, in a few cases, walked to the scenes of the fires. Their personal vehicles were described as average wear and tear to neglected and in poor condition. Three had an accomplice who accompanied them to the scene. Targets, preselected, involved primary businesses although one residence fire was included. Vehicles and other structures were also targeted on occasion.

Mixed Motives

Five of the serial arsonist exhibited mixed motives, sometimes behaving as though motivated by one type of motive and then at another time, by another. As an example of mixed motives, 1 serial arsonist set some fires for vandalism, later set several in revenge of a perceived wrong, and still later was hired to burn businesses for profit.

Mentally Disordered Motives

Five others had emotional problems (2), or blamed "evil spirits" (2) or religious fervor (1) as reasons for the arson activity. This group included one of the five females in the sample. None of these 5 arsonists exhibited patterns of behavior that allowed classification according to the *Crime Classification Manual* (Douglas *et al.*, 1992). For purposes of this study, we have classified the 5 offenders as having mentally disordered motives. When clinically evaluated, at least some of these 5 serial arsonists would probably be classified according to the psychobiological categories suggested by Geller (1992).

Other Motive-Related Considerations: Pyromania

Perhaps most conspicuous by its absence is any mention of pyromania in this discussion of motivations. The NCAVC has conducted considerable research on this subject and argues that there may not be such a thing. For an authoritative definition of the term, one must reject individual preference and refer to the American Psychiatric Association's *Diagnostic and Statistical Manual of Mental Disorders* (*DSM*) which has been the standard for psychological and psychiatric diagnoses for over 40 years. The current edition is the fourth (*DSM-IV;* American Psychiatric Association, 1994.) A review reveals that each edition of the *DSM* has treated this topic differently. *DSM-II* did not even list the "disorder." Pyromania, as a diagnosed personality disorder, has waxed and waned over the last 150 years or so. It cycles through the years as opinions vary. Perhaps there is a reason that something so nebulous successfully defies a solid definition. Perhaps pyromania does not exist as a "stand alone," solid disorder.

Could the firesetting impulses, characteristic of the various definitions of pyromania, be a manifestation of some other disorder? By the current *DSM-IV* definition, and some others, a pyromaniac cannot be psychotic. It is, therefore, easily argued that a firesetter using pyromania as a defense must know right from wrong. The so-called irresistible impulse to set fires may be just an impulse not resisted (Geller, Erlen, & Pinkas, 1986). Fire investigators are cautioned not to label a subject as a pyromaniac since this is a diagnosis to be made by a mental health professional. The authors have lectured to fire investigators, psychologists, and psychiatrists, asking each to define pyromania. Predictably, there were nearly as many definitions submitted as there were persons submitting them. In short, the term remains nebulous and defies clear definition. If there is such a person as a pyromaniac, he or she is a rare breed indeed.

ACKNOWLEDGMENTS

This research was partially funded by the Department of Justice, Federal Bureau of Investigation and the Federal Emergency Management Agency. The opinions expressed herein are those of the authors and do not necessarily represent the opinion of either the Department of Justice, the Federal Bureau of Investigation, or the Federal Emergency Management Agency.

References

American Psychiatric Association. (1994). *Diagnostic and statistical manual of mental disorders* (4th ed.). Washington, DC: Author.

DeHaan, J. D. (1991). *Kirk's fire investigation* (3rd ed.). Englewood Cliffs, NJ: Prentice-Hall.

Douglas, J. E., Burgess, A. W., Burgess, A. G., & Ressler, R. K. (1992). *Crime classification manual.* New York: Lexington Books.

DSM-IV. (1994). *Diagnostic and statistical manual of mental disorders.* Washington, DC: American Psychiatric Association.

Federal Bureau of Investigation. (Published annually). *Crime in the United States (Uniform Crime Reports).* Washington, DC: U.S. Government Printing Office.

Federal Emergency Management Agency. (1988). *Fire in the United States* (7th ed.). Emmitsburg, MD: Author.

Geller, J. L. (1992). Arson in Review: From profit to pathology. *Journal of Clinical Forensic Psychiatry, 15,* 623–645.

Geller, J. L., Erlen, J., & Pinkas, R. L. (1986). A historical appraisal of America's experience with pyromania—A diagnosis in search of a disorder. *International Journal of Law and Psychiatry, 9*(2), 201–229.

Huff, T. G. (1993, June). Filicide by fire—The worst crime? *Fire and Arson Investigator,* 3–5.

Huff, T. G. (1994, August). Fire-setting fire fighters: Arsonists in the fire department—Identification and prevention. *On Scene, International Association of Fire Chiefs,* 12, 14.

Hurley, W., & Monahan, T. M. (1969). Arson: The criminal and the crime. *British Journal of Criminology 9,* 4–21.

Icove, D. J., & Estepp, M. H. (1987, April). Motive-based offender profiles of arson and fire-related crimes. *FBI Law Enforcement Bulletin,* 17–23.

Icove, D. J., & Gilman, R. (1989, June). Arson reporting immunity laws. *FBI Law Enforcement Bulletin,* 14–19.

Icove, D. J. & Horbert, P. R. (1990). Serial arsonists: An introduction. *Police Chief, 57,*(12), 46–48.

Icove, D. J., Wherry, V. B., & Schroeder, J. D. (1978). *Contributing arson for profit: Advanced techniques for investigators,* (2nd ed.) (pp. 7–10). Columbus, Ohio: Battelle Press.

Inciardi, J. A. (1970, August). The adult firesetter: A typology. *Criminology, 8,* 145–155.

Levin, B. (1976, March). Psychological characteristics of firesetters. *Fire Journal,* 36–41.

Lewis, N. D. C., & Yarnell, H. (1951). *Pathological firesetting (pyromania)* (Nervous and Mental Disease Monographs No 82). New York: Coolidge Foundation.

NCAVC. (1992). *Annual report of the National Center for the Analysis of Violent Crime.* Washington, DC: National Center for the Analysis of Violent Crime, Federal Bureau of Investigation.

Rider, A. O. (1980). *The firesetter: A psychological profile.* Quantico, VA: FBI Academy, Federal Bureau of Investigation.

Robbins, E. (1967). Arson with special regard to pyromania. *New York State Journal of Medicine, 3,* 795–798.

Robbins, E. S., Herman, M., & Robbins, L. (1969). Sex and arson: Is there a relationship? *Journal of Medical Aspects of Human Sexuality, 3,* 57–63.

Sapp, A. D., & Huff, T. G. (1955). *Arson-homicides: Findings from a national study.* Washington, DC: National Center for the Analysis of Violent Crime, Federal Bureau of Investigation.

Sapp, A. D., Garry, G. P., Huff, T. G., & James, S. (1993). *Arsons aboard naval ships: Characteristics of offenses and offenders.* Washington, DC: National Center for the Analysis of Violent Crime, Federal Bureau of Investigation.

Sapp, A. D., Garry, G. P., Huff, T. G., & James, S. (1994). Motives of arsonists aboard naval ships. *Journal of Police and Criminal Psychology, 10*(1) 8–13.

Sapp, A. D., Huff, T. G., Gary, G. P. Icove, D. J., & Horbert, P. (1994). *A report of essential findings from a study of serial arsonists.* Washington, DC: National Center for the Analysis of Violent Crime, Federal Bureau of Investigation.

Steinmetz, R. C. (1966, September). Current arson problems. *Fire Journal,* 7–9.

Vandersall, T. A., & Wiener, J. M. (1970). Children who set fires. *Archives of General Psychiatry, 22*(January), 65–71.

Vreeland, R. G., & Waller, M. B. (1978). *The psychology of firesetting: A review and appraisal.* Washington, DC: U.S. Department of Commerce, National Bureau of Standards.

Wolford, M. R. (1972). Some attitudinal, psychological and sociological characteristics of incarcerated arsonists. *Fire and Arson Investigator,* 22, 1–26.

A Neurological Perspective

Frank A. Elliott

Introduction

Socioeconomic and environmental causes of criminal violence are so many, and the role of mental disorders so obvious, that they have been allowed to obscure the contribution of organic brain defects. This should no longer be acceptable in the courts or elsewhere. There is abundant evidence, collected over a century of research, that damage to specific structures in the brain can lead to recurrent attacks of destructive aggression in formerly equable individuals, that this and other disinhibited behaviors can also be associated with covert neurodevelopmental defects incurred before or after birth, and that the liability to violence in such individuals is usually increased by childhood exposure to social adversity, emotional deprivation, and physical or mental abuse, and is reinforced by criminal example.

On the other hand, worldwide ethnological studies have established that violent crime is relatively low in communities and societies that have retained their cultural taboos and constraints (Eibl-Eibesfeldt, 1979).

This chapter is not concerned with collective aggression or with the violent responses of psychotics to their delusions, illusions, and hallucinations, or to incidents of violence in the course of medical illness or intoxication as described by Tardiff (1992), but focuses largely on the small segment of the population that is responsible for over 70% of recurrent criminal violence.

Social and criminologic studies of the past commonly treated violence as a homogeneous entity, which it is not. Homogenization, as in some major studies of large cohorts, can lead to errors of interpretation in individual cases (Moffitt, 1993); what is needed is closer scrutiny of the etiology, pathology, and clinical features of the several types of violent aggression (Eichelman, 1992; Tardiff, 1992), as a guide to disposal, treatment, and prognosis.

Frank A. Elliott • Neurology Department, Pennsylvania Hospital, Philadelphia, Pennsylvania 19107.

Handbook of Psychological Approaches with Violent Offenders: Contemporary Strategies and Issues, edited by Van Hasselt and Hersen. Kluwer Academic/Plenum Publishers, New York, 1999.

A Neurologic Typology

Destructive interpersonal violence appears in at least two broad categories (predatory and affective) in both animals and man. They differ in their modes of expression, provoking stimuli, chemical and anatomical bases, prognosis, and treatment (Moyer, 1976; Valzelli, 1981), and each category can be subdivided according to etiology. However, tidy classification is often complicated by presence of multiple biological and social pathologies.

Predatory violence is cold, callous, and casual, and either planned or impulsive. It is carried out for profit—money, goods, power, sex (including the satisfaction of deviant sex) and getting rid of the opposition or of a witness to crime. It is the predominant form of aggression during epidemics of violence, and is found in both apparently normal individuals and psychopaths (the antisocial personality disorder). The latter is characterized by retardation of social and emotional development, without intellectual impairment. This view is supported by modern development psychology (Kegan, 1986) and by personal observations of this lifelong disorder. Compared with other male criminals, psychopaths commit a disproportionate number of crimes, which are also more violent (Hare & McPherson, 1984), but fortunately, the majority, though troublesome, are not violent. Some achieve political or commercial eminence.

The full personality profile includes a mask of superficial charm behind which lie inflated ideas of self-worth, incapacity for empathy, lack of remorse, manipulative behavior, a parasitic lifestyle, a need for stimulation, impulsivity, poor self-control, shallow affect, and social irresponsibility including multiple short-term sexual relationships. Marginal cases do not display the fully fledged mosaic and may present only fragments of the pattern. A particularly malignant combination of impulsivity, aggression, lack of empathy, and lack of foresight is not uncommon after severe head injury and encephalitis, and occurs in a subset of the Attention-Deficit/Hyperactive Disorder and other neurodevelopmental abnormalities. Cleckley (1982) and others have remarked that the psychopath has what seems to be a profound defect in understanding the meaning of emotionally charged words, such as evil, cancer, homicide, love, strangle, which evoke in them the same cortical EEG potentials as neutral words, such as table, life, children, and so on, implying a neurophysiological basis for their absence of guilt and lack of empathy for the disasters of others.

Psychopathy is usually classified as within psychiatric territory but has a neurobiological basis (Ratey, 1995). This is indicated by abnormal responses to neuropsychological tests designed to detect "organicity," nonspecific EEG abnormalities usually in the form of bilateral theta waves (in aggressive cases), a high P300 wave of event-related evoked potentials (E. Raine & Venables, 1988), resistance to aversive conditioning (and therefore failure to learn by experience), and defective skin conduction responses to significant social cues, which is consistent with bifrontal defect. (A. Damasio, Tramel, and M. Damasio, 1990) There is also a low level of serotonin metabolites in the spinal fluid, and low serotonin in the blood platelets of children with the aggressive conduct disorder, a common precursor of violence in adults. Minor neurological abnormalities are often present. Monroe (1978) carried out a detailed neurologic, neuropsychologic, psychiatric, and sociological study of 93 incorrigibly violent criminals in a maximum security institution. The personality profile of the group was that of the psychopath. Using a neurologic scale that included birth data, head injury, epileptoid mechanisms, brain insults, congenital stigmata (minor physical anomalies), hyperacousis, photophobia, motor strength, incoordination, and apraxia, there was a correlation at the .001 level between the neurological scale and violent behavior, and at the .05 level and beyond with a psychiatric history of overreactive emotional behavior, poor judgment, poor effort to improve, self-defeating actions, lack of responsibility, grandiose illusions, hyperchondriasis, and fugue states. There was a also a close correlation of antisocial traits in childhood and poor peer relations in adolescence.

A second type of predatory behavior includes many of the features of the psychopath, but starts in adolescence rather than childhood, increases rapidly in numbers and severity until the age of about 16, and then declines precipitously until the early 20s as the brain matures (Yakovlev & Lecours, 1967). It appears in epidemic form, like a highly contagious disease, in times of anomie and social change, as in Germany after World War I, in the United States since the 1960s, and in England, between 1950 and 1978. Indeed, violent interpersonal crime carried out by boys ages 14–16 increased 23-fold (Rutter & Giller, 1983). Moffitt (1993) found, from extensive studies in the United States and New Zealand, that in both countries antisocial behavior occurred in two groups of adolescents: those whose violence started early in childhood and persisted into adult life, and a much larger group whose criminal activities were limited to adolescence, who temporarily model the misbehavior of the psychopaths in their midst, which they perceive to be exciting, assertive, and profitable. It is logical to presume that their mimicry will extend to the examples set by TV and the movies. A meta-analysis prepared for the National Research Council by Comstock and Paik (1990), covering 188 studies, reported that the vast majority showed that exposure to TV violence resulted in increased aggressive behavior both at the time and over time.

Mimicry, which plays a major role in learning, has a neurophysiological basis. Normal in children, it diminishes with maturity, but can return in an exaggerated form in adults with lesions of the frontal lobe who display pathological dependency on environmental cues and a loss of personal autonomy (Lhermitte, Pillon, & Serdaru, 1986). Fortunately, mimicry in youth applies not only to antisocial behavior but also to the prosocial influences of role models whose example helps them to resist a criminogenic environment, as illustrated by Werner and Smith (1982) in their study of adolescent Hawaiians, in which some individuals proved to be "vulnerable but invincible."

Affective Aggression

The intermittent explosive disorder, formerly known as episodic dyscontrol is the most serious form of domestic violence. Its hallmark is recurrent attacks of intense rage, without reflective delay, sometimes accompanied by visible evidence of sympathetic discharge—sweating, piloerection, and pupillary dilatation. In the words of an observant witness who escaped a homicidal attack, "his eyes darkened and his mustache bristled." Kaplan (1899) described it as follows:

> [F]ollowing the most trivial and impersonal causes there is the effect of rage with its motor accompaniments. There may be the most grotesque gesticulations, excessive movements of the face and a sharp explosiveness of speech; there will be cursing and outbreaks of violence which are often directed towards things; there may or may not be amnesia for these events

afterwards. The outburst may terminate in an epileptic fit. There is an excessive reaction with inadequate adaptation to the situation, which is so remote from a well considered and purposeful act that it approaches a pure psychic reflex.

He described attacks in patients with head injury, psychosis, and arteriosclerosis.

The highly charged affect distinguishes it from the cold violence of predatory aggression and the habitual violence practiced as a means of survival in city slums and prisons (Wolfgang & Ferracuti, 1982). It is a cause of unpremeditated homicide and suicide, senseless attacks on strangers, bar fights, criminally aggressive driving, spouse and child abuse, and savage attacks on animals. Sometimes, particularly in women, aggression is verbal. Its contents are vindictive, profane, and out of character, and are often accompanied by salivation and a feline retraction of the upper lip. It is a form of child abuse, and can lead to criminal violence by provoking fatal retaliation on the part of a male who prefers to hit rather than argue.

The intermittent explosive disorder can exist on its own but usually accompanies psychological or neurological disorders—neuroses, posttraumatic stress disorder, psychoses, borderline disorders, trauma and acquired neurological diseases, neurodevelopmental abnormalities including mental retardation and autism, metabolic disorders including hypoglycemia, and exogenous and endogenous intoxications and toxaemias (Tardiff, 1992). It is usually associated with other less alarming forms of impulsive behavior (Bach-y-Rita, Lion, Climent, & Ervin, 1971), and appears to be linked to a failure of the central inhibitory mechanisms that normally control the expression (as opposed to the induction) of aggression (Gorenstein & Neuman, 1980).

A second type of affective violence, less common than the preceding, resembles the "sham rage" caused in animals by damaging the deep connections between the hypothalamus and the cortex, and it occurs as a single episode. Such rage "is excessive in degree, unfocused, cannot be interrupted, and does not fatigue" (Poeck, 1969). It can last for hours or days. The usual cause is a severe closed head injury, involving the orbito-frontal cortex, hippocampus, and anterior cingulate gyrus (Roberts, 1979). It has also resulted from damage to the midbrain by hemorrhage from an aneurysm (Poeck, 1969).

A typical example is as follows:

> A 30-year-old farmer was struck by lightning while riding a tractor. His scalp was badly burned, and his skull and one arm were fractured when he fell to the ground. Pulse and respiration failed but were immediately restored by a bystander. When he emerged from coma 3 weeks later he was delirious and violent, shouting, cursing, attempting to bite attendants, and throwing things. He had to be forcibly restrained, and did not respond to medication until he was given propranolol hydrochloride, as an experimental measure, whereupon his violence ceased though he did not appear sedated. Violence returned 2 days later when the propranolol was temporarily withdrawn (Elliott, 1977).

Clearly, such very sick patients are incapable of focused criminal violence, except by accident; their significance lies in the demonstration of the participation of the early mammalian and reptilian components of the human brain in atavistic behavior, extreme examples of which are the cannibalism by some serial murderers and the biting by patients with rabies.

A third type of affective violence appears in individuals who are not disinhibited, but overcontrolled (Megargee, 1982). They put up with intense provocation for a long time, but finally explode in an outburst of destructive fury in vengeance for past wrongs, minor or major, real or imagined. Blackburn (1968) examined 63 cases in a maximum security mental institution. Of the 38 most violent cases, only 8 had a previous criminal record, and no less than 31 out of the 38 were acquainted with their victims. There is no mention of neurological examination. They were intensively examined by neuropsychological tests, results of which were consistent with a diagnosis of an overcontrolled personality. Williams (1969) carried out electroencephalographic tests on 333 violent criminals and found that those guilty of a single major offense had only slightly more EEG abnormalities than the normal population, whereas 65% of violent recidivists had abnormal records; this has been confirmed by others (Stafford-Clark, 1959).

A well-known example is that of Charles Whitman who had a good record of self-control—altar boy, Eagle Scout, marine—but, when 25, he became obsessed with thoughts of killing which he recorded in a lengthy diary and reported to a psychiatrist. In it he expressed the hope that his case might help others in the same predicament and explained that he was going to kill his wife and mother to spare them embarrassment from what he proposed to do, which was to ascend the tower on the University campus in Houston and open fire on the public. He did so, killing 14 people and wounding 17 before he was shot in the head by a policeman. Autopsy revealed a malignant tumor, which from the histological evidence appeared to be from a temporal lobe, a conclusion which was supported by two other symptoms suggestive of temporal lobe pathology—hypergraphia and obsession with the moral aspects of his behavior. New evidence has recently been supplied by S. L. Brown (1994). The psychiatrist in charge of a state-ordered investigation of the massacre found that he and his mother had been oppressed and abused by his father, who forced him into a joyless and lonely childhood, the effects of which were obvious to his teachers at the time but gave no warning of what was to come.

In a fourth type of violence, the patient is obsessed with uncontrollable thoughts of death and killing, and may ultimately feel driven to carry them out. There were many such cases in the 1915–1925 epidemic of encephalitis lethargica, wherein compulsive movements and bizarre postures were also common. Sporadic cases of encephalitis due to other viruses are not uncommon in children today, with cognitive and emotional impairments, occasionally including criminal violence. Thus, a 10-year-old boy had mumps encephalitis, after which his personality was grossly altered, though his intellectual powers were unimpaired. He was given to attacks of rage, and to compulsive letter writing and endless moral introspection, all of which suggested temporal lobe pathology. He also had an obsession about women's breasts and a compulsion to fondle them, which he yielded to by stalking his victims home, breaking in, and raping them.

Obsessive-compulsive features, without rituals, were present in 21 recurrently violent subjects observed by the writer. There was covert evidence of neuropathology in 14; neurodevelopmental defects in 8; serious head injuries in 3; temporal lobe epileptic attacks in 1; encephalitis in 1; and temporal lobe theta in 1. Denckla (1989) reported neuropathological findings in 44 out of 54 cases of obsessive-compulsive disorder in children, and they were also present in 13 out of 19 cases seen by Hollander, Shiffman, and Liebowitz (1987). Interpersonal violence occurred, but rarely, in these studies. Published reports suggest that obsessions and compulsions play a role in some serial murderer's behaviors, who feel "driven" (Frazier, 1974).

Additional evidence of organic pathology in obsessional personalities has been provided by neuropsychological studies (Cox, Fedio, & Rapoport, 1989), and by imaging studies which showed hypermetabolism in the orbital gyrus and caudate nuclei (Baxter *et al.*, 1987), in the medical frontal cortex (Macklin *et al.*, 1991), and by the fact that clomipramine, which inhibits serotonin reuptake, has antiobsessional effects (Rapoport, 1989), and may therefor be expected to reduce compulsive violence. A diminished level of the serotonin metabolite 5HIAA has been found in the spinal fluid of nonviolent patients with the obsessive-compulsive disorder.

Sleep-related violence can be responsible for murder, homicide, suicide, assault, and child abuse. It can be neurogenic or psychogenic. The latter embraces dissociative disorders (fugues, multiple personality) and malingering, and neurological types include (1) disorders of arousal ("drunk with sleep"); (2) rapid-eye movement (REM) sleep disorders in which the normal active sleep paralysis of muscles is temporarily abrogated, allowing the subject to act out dreams, violent and otherwise; (3) sleep-walking (somnambulism) which occurs early in the night, when eye movements are normal and the subject is in a state of automation, without control of his or her behavior; and (4) nocturnal postepileptic automatism (Broughton *et al.*, 1994; Mahowald, Bundlie, & Schnenck, 1990). Somnambulism, often associated with a personal and familial history of sleep disorders, has been responsible for homicides, some of them extremely violent. It can be triggered by alcohol, soporific medications, and street drugs.

Clinical differentiation between REM disorders, somnambulism, psychiatric dissociative states, nocturnal seizure phenomena, and pathological intoxication, is often impossible without investigation in a sleep disorder center.

Epilepsy and Violence

It is generally accepted that, statistically, uncomplicated epileptics are no more liable to crime than the rest of the population, that planned aggression carried out for profit is inconsistent with the epileptic process, and that during postictal confusion the patient may violently resist attempts to restrain him or her and thus cause accidental injury. The same is true, occasionally, of persistent automatism following a temporal lobe seizure, so that from the forensic point of view it is unwise to plead that directed postictal aggression cannot occur (Gunn, 1991). In general, interictal violence is not due to the epilepsy per se, but to temporal lobe pathology which may be responsible for both the seizures and behavioral and emotional disorders (Blumer, 1991; Stevens & Hermann, 1981)

Nevertheless, the proportion of epileptics is greater in prisons and state hospitals than in the population at large. In Broadmoor, a British maximum security hospital for the insane, it was found that 2.7% of males and 2% of the females were epileptic (Wong, Lumsden, Fenton, & Fenwick, 1994), and in Philadelphia a random computer check disclosed that 3.4% of over 4,000 prisoners were receiving dilantin prescribed by physicians.

There is a link between temporal lobe pathology and sexual dysfunction. Global hyposexuality is common in temporal lobe epileptics and sexual perversions are not rare; they include transvestitism, voyeurism, fetishism, sadism, masochism, heterosexual and homosexual pederasty, and genital self-mutilation (Bear, Freeman &

Greenberg, 1984). Such deviations are likely to be associated with a history of hypoxia or brain damage at or shortly after birth (Kolarski, Freund, Machek, & Polak, 1967), and Langevin (1990) has reported high prevalence of morphologic defects in the temporal lobe, disclosed by computerized tomography, in persons given to deviant sexual practices. Unilateral destruction by stereotaxic surgery of the ventromedial hypothalamic nucleus has been successful in reducing or abolishing pedophilia in a small number of cases (Diekmann & Hassler, 1975; Roeder, 1966).

In many cases of criminal violence the diagnosis, prognosis, and treatment are complicated by multiple pathologies, psychological, sociological, and acquired or developmental neurobiological disorders, many of which are not clinically obvious and are likely to be missed by traditional neurological examination and by IQ tests (M. D. Levine, 1995). Let us consider the following case.

> A man, age 38, was given two life sentences for sexually assaulting and murdering two 12-year-old boys. Prior offenses included juvenile delinquencies from age 11, attempted rape on a 12-year-old girl, beating to death a 37-year-old aunt, and murder of a 4-year-old boy. Pedophilia and homosexuality dated from age 16 and persisted throughout adult life. The family history was turbulent but not criminal; a brother was epileptic. The prisoner had convulsions with severe cyanosis shortly after birth and was not expected to live; nocturnal convulsions returned at puberty, and then ceased. EEGs at that time, and since, have shown an epileptic spike focus in the left temporal lobe. Dilantin was prescribed by a distinguished psychiatrist, but was not given then or later. In addition to epilepsy the subject had neurodevelopmental disorders against a background of high intelligence and considerable artistic gifts. They included poor impulse control for both kindly deeds and criminal activities; explosive rage on minor provocation (including sudden loud noises in domestic altercations due to hyperacusis), defective audiomotor coordination, difficulty in spatial perceptions, as in copying plans on paper and painting pictures, and poor attention span. During his confinement he learned to control his temper and his "almost uncontrollable sexual drives" and has led a constructive life as artist, pest control officer, and peacemaker. But he does not consider that he should be paroled.

The Anatomical and Chemical Substrates of Violent Aggression

A century of experimental work with animals and clinicopathological studies in man has shown that the capacity to express and to inhibit violence is vested in a genetically ordered network of interconnected neuronal assemblies reaching bilaterally from the orbito-frontal cortex to the limbic system and midbrain, and that some of them are excitatory, some inhibitory, and some, such as the amygdala and hypothalamus, are both. A balance between excitation and inhibition, regarded by Sherrington (1925) as the fundamental operational principal of the normal nervous system, is often abrogated in criminal behavior. A second principle, that the temporal summation of subliminal sensory stimuli can evoke a reflex response, is often illustrated by explosive rage in response to repeated minimal provocations. The inhibitory equipment, destruction of which reduces the threshold of aggression, includes the orbitofrontal cortex, the septal area, medial muclei of the amygdala, the hippocampus, cingulate gyrus, head of caudate neclus, and ventromedial and ventrolateral nuclei of the hypothalamus (Valzelli, 1981; Weiger & Bear, 1988). In addition, mental symptoms, including rage, sometimes occur in children with pontine tumors (Cairns, 1950; Lassman & Arjona, 1967) and, rarely, in lesions of the palleo-cerebellum (Elliott, 1982). Poeck (1969) pointed out that areas concerned with inhibition greatly exceed those associated with excitation—a redundancy that helps explain why pathological aggression occurs less often in patients with a unilateral focal lesion, such as a tumor or a penetrating wound, than in bilateral diffuse conditions such as severe closed heady injury, encephalitis, alcoholic cerebral degeneration, neurodevelopmental disorders, the dementias, chronic degenerative disease (e.g., Huntington's disease), cardiorespiratory failure, and mental retardation. There is also an emerging body of evidence that, in animals, the cerebellum exerts an inhibitory influence on affective aggression and on limbic seizures (Moruzzi, 1958), while in man electrical stimulation of the anterior lobe of the cerebellum by a pacemaker can completely control—over prolonged periods—extreme violence in schizophrenics (Heath, 1977). Such stimulation has also been effective in stopping seizures and (in 2 cases) explosive interictal violence (Cooper, 1978). The cerebellum may also participate in cognitive processes; for instance, Kim, Ugurbil, and Strick (1994) demonstrated, by PET scan, activation of the cerebellum during the performance of an intellectual task. Supporting evidence has been reviewed by Leiner, and Dow (1989) and Schmahmann (1991).

The effects of a unilateral lesion in promoting violent responses to exogenous or endogenous provocation can be potentiated by existence of unsuspected covert neuropathology. Common examples are previous head injuries, and natal and perinatal asphyxia which results in unilateral or bilateral sclerosis of the medial aspect of the temporal lobes, including not only the hippocampus but also the hippocampal gyrus and amygdala. This is most often encountered as a complication of temporal lobe epileptics, who are also afflicted with antisocial behavior and emotional behavior Blumer, 1991; Scheibel, 1991).

The fundamental incapacity caused by a unilateral focal lesion can also be potentiated by psychological or social pathologies that in the presence of comparatively mild organic lesions can give rise to antisocial behaviors (Mednick & Christiansen, 1977; Rutter, 1980). Conversely, a stable social and family background can reduce the impact of neurological handicaps (Taylor, 1993; Werner & Smith, 1982).

Rarely can pathological lesions of the excitatory network abolish a lifelong history of intermittent explosive behavior. However, the writer has seen this happen to a habitually violent physician as a result of a minor stroke, which also caused unwonted childish behavior. Barrett and Hyland (1952) record the case of a woman with a lifelong history of explosive emotions who noticed an inability to get emotional as the first symptom of a pineal tumor which had spread to involve the posterior hypothalamus and anterior lobe of the cerebellum.

Similar control of explosive rages has often been obtained in children and adults by the surgical placement of small stereotactic lesions at various sites, notably in the amygdala and posterior hypothalamus (Sano, 1962), and also by unilateral temporal lobectomy. These treatments have been superseded by pharmacological agents in most cases.

The anatomical substrate is controlled by a complex system of chemical activators and inhibitors which, owing to the exponential growth of the cognitive neurosciences does not allow anything more than a brief summary here. Rapidly acting neurotransmitters produced by specialized neurones situated in or near the midline of the midbrain and medulla are distributed to receptor sites on neurones in the limbic system, basal ganglia, cortex, and cerebellum. Secondly, the system is under the influence of neuromodulators, which are slower acting than neurotransmitters. These hormones are of particular relevance to violent behavior. The neurotransmitters chiefly concerned with aggression are both activators (dopamine, norepinephrine and acetyl choline) and inhibitors (serotonin and gamma-amino-butyric acid). Norepinephrine activates affective aggression and reduces predatory violence. Acetyl choline activates both, and serotonin inhibits both. Dopamine enhances both (in animals). Low values of 5HIAA, a serotonin metabolite, have been found associated with impulsive behavior and emotionally charged aggression (including suicide) and in antisocial subjects. Low blood serotonin is found in children suffering from conduct disorder, which is often a precursor of violence later on.

The monoamines are subject to depredation by two enzymes, monoamine oxidase A and B. Low MAO activity is associated with disinhibition—impulsivity and aggression—and has been identified with assaultative behavior in a kindred of violent males, who displayed a point mutation in the structural gene for monoamine oxidase A (Brunner, Nelen, Breakefield, Ropers, & Van Oost, 1993).

The clinical evidence indicating an association between elevated levels of testosterone and aggression includes incidence of aggressive behavior, which often coincides with a tenfold increase of testosterone in boys at puberty, the dramatic reduction of sex crimes that follows castration in man, and the docility of castrated cattle (Moyer, 1976). Administration of antiandrogens has the same effect in man. Hawke (1950) quotes a group of sex offenders whose violence was reduced by castration but returned following the administration of large doses of testosterone. There also are reports of criminal violence carried out by formerly equable individuals who in their pursuit of athletic ambitions injected themselves with anabolic steroids over a considerable period (Volavka, 1995).

Despite these observations, scrutiny of all the evidence, human and animal, by a panel of the National Research Council failed to disclose any simple relationship between steroids and aggression, or between steroids and violence.

In women, the most common hormonal contributor to both verbal and physical aggression is premenstrual tension (or dysphoric) syndrome, which can have devastating and permanent effects on children exposed to it. It is thought to be due to an abnormally high estrogen–progesterone ratio, but is also aggravated by psychosocial factors to a degree that may obscure the hormonal factor. Multiple sources of aggravation have a multiplicative rather than an additive effect (Rutter, 1980).

Hypoglycemia, produced by excessive endogenous or exogenous insulin, was first recognized by Joslin in 1937. By 1947, Wilder and his colleagues at the Mayo Clinic had assembled a formidable list from the world literature of hypoglycemia-related crimes, from theft and arson to homicide and child abuse. It is produced by insulin overdosage, pancreatic insulinomas, an excessive fall of blood sugar after a carbohydrate meal, and an alcoholic hangover caused by the effects of alcohol on glucose metabolism (Kanarek, 1994; Virkkunen, 1986). It is particularly likely to produce violence in the intermittent explosive disorder, antisocial personality disorder, and those with organic brain defects. Let us consider a case illustration.

A respected citizen who was diabetic and had also developed occasional temporal lobe seizures in the middle life took an evening dose of insulin but omitted to dine because he had an engagement. While parking his car he got into an altercation with a policeman, whom he assaulted. He then drove around the parking lot in a pointless manner and attempted to run down another policeman, who shot him in the arm and so brought the chase to an end. When apprehended, he was belligerent and confused, and his blood sugar was found to be below 40 mgms. Confusion was abolished immediately by intravenous glucose; he subsequently had no recollection of anything he had done since leaving home.

The diagnosis is often missed if there is no clear-cut time relationship between food intake and hypoglycemia. It depends less on the history than on rigorous laboratory studies of blood glucose response to fasting and other provocations, and on blood insulin assays; it cannot be accurately diagnosed by a routine 3-hr glucose tolerance test. A fall of blood sugar induced under laboratory conditions can fail to induce the violence, which occurs under social circumstances; this, of course, can have forensic implications.

It is possible that fluctuations in frequency of violent behavior are related, inter alia, to diurnal, circadian, and seasonal variations in the level of neurotransmitters and neuromodulators; this would help explain not only the irregular episodicity of personal violence but also the seasonal alterations in the rates of homicide and suicide. Chemical systems are not immutable throughout life. Aside from the vulnerabilities to trauma and disease, there is recent evidence that in hamsters, at any rate, exposure to neglect or abuse in early life can induce permanent reduction in the hypothalamic output of vasopression.

Neurophysiological Correlations of Violent Behavior

Age

Pathological degrees of violent aggression can start with the tantrums of infancy, or a conduct disorder of childhood, and it may occur at any age in a previously stable individual following a serious head injury or other brain insult. In males a tenfold rise of testosterone levels during puberty is usually blamed for the usual increase in violent behavior in adolescence, but this is not the whole story since homicidal violence can start before puberty, and there is evidence in animals that androgens can both influence and be influenced by aggression (Miczek, Haney, Tidey, Jeffery, & Weerts, 1994). The current peak of criminal violence in normal adolescents is reached at about the 16th year, after which it falls precipitously over the next few years (Farrington, 1983; Moffitt, 1993). It is likely that the process of social maturation that occurs in the late teens and early 20s is related to completion of myelination, which is reached late in the third decade for the associative neocortex of the prefrontal, posterior parietal, and anterior temporal lobes (Kaes, 1907; Yakovlev & Lecours, 1967), and in the hippocampus (Benes, Turtle, Khan, & Farol, 1994). The question arises whether clumsiness, dyspraxias, and defective bimanual coordination, which are the most common of the covert developmental motor disorders in children, are due to the vulnerability associated with the relatively late maturation of the cerebellar cortex (Zecevic & Rakic, 1976) and the large cerebral commissures (Yakovlev & Lecours, 1967).

This timetable of complete maturational development differs widely from system to system, and there is clinical evidence that it can be modified in either direction by biological and environmental influences that can affect different systems and behaviors to an unequal degree (Glaser, 1981). Exposure in infancy and childhood to physical abuse and emotional neglect can permanently alter social and emotional development.

Sex

Most normal male individuals from cradle to grave are more prone to physical aggression than are most females, and pathological violence exhibited by individuals in the form of both affective and predatory aggression is far more common in males, who are also more prone to conditions that predispose to it: neurodevelopmental disorders, natal and perinatal injuries, and infections. Another difference, reported by Lindqvist and Allebeck (1990), is that (in Sweden) men with a major mental handicap were 5.5 times more likely than men with no disorder to be registered for a violent act, while women with a mental disorder were 24.8 times more likely than women without a disorder to be guilty of violent crime. Conversely, high intelligence has some protective value (Volavka, 1995).

An absolute distinction between the two sexes is the liability of women to the premenstrual dysphoric disorder that, in some individuals, is accompanied by attacks of extreme rage and violence; 60% of violent crimes committed by women are said to occur in the premenstrual week (Morton, Addition, Addison, Hunt, & Sullivan, 1953).

Genetics

Although there is ample evidence that selective breeding has been successfully used to promote aggressiveness in bulls for the bullring and in pit bulldogs, and has also produced, under laboratory conditions, aggressive mice, rabbits, guinea pigs, dogs, and dingoes, there has been reluctance to apply these lessons to the human condition. When violence "runs in the family" (a familiar explanation) it is commonly ascribed to intergenerational transfer of learned behavior. This may not be the whole truth. Thus, Stacey and Shupe (1983) found that in a sample of 150 male spouse batterers, 42% had *not* witnessed physical violence between their parents, 60% had not been physically obuselt, 59% had *not* been neglected, and 50% had *not* had an alcoholic father. In a group of 286 recurrently violent adults studied by Elliott (1982), 88 gave a history of violence in two or more generations. The modesty of this figure may be due to the composition of the sample, which was 95% Caucasian and mainly from middle and upper socioeconims classes, including one young woman who claimed that her family history of violence went back to an ancestor who was the first man to be hanged for murder in Massachusetts. Davenport (1915), in research sponsored by the Carnegie Institution, reported on family histories of 165 "wayward girls" in state institutions. In 79, who were neither epileptic nor psychotic, there had been violence in the family, involving both sexes in approximately half the siblings in each generation for two or more generations. Recently, a genetic defect was found in 5 male members of a highly aggressive kindred, who were guilty of arson, rape, aggression, and exhibitionism (Brunner *et al.*, 1993). They lacked monoamine oxidase A (MAOA). The female carriers were normal in behavior and intelligence. The defect was a point mutation in the structural gene for monoamine oxidase, which disturbs the chemical regulation of impulsive aggression.

Carey (1994), reporting for the National Research Panel on Violence, concluded that the data on the heritability of violence apply to important correlates of aggression and not to violence itself.

Neuropathological Correlates of Criminal Violence

The most convincing evidence of a close link between destructive personal violence and brain damage is provided by the occasional cases in which aggression occurs for the first time in a previously equable individual following damage by a tumor to structures which appear to exert an inhibitory influence on the repression of aggression: the orbito-frontal cortex (Strauss & Keschner, 1936), septal area (Zeman & King, 1958) anterior cingulate cortex in parasagittal tumors (Elliott, 1982), hippocampus (Malamud, 1967), medial amygdala nuclei (Vonderahe, 1944), anterior temporal lobe, ventromedial hypothalamus, anterior hypothalamus (Alpers, 1937), and, in children, the pons (Cairns, 1950, Lassman & Arjona, 1967). Rarely have lesions of the cerebellum been followed by attacks of rage. In the majority of tumor cases the subject is too sick to embark on criminal activities, but a small focal lesion in certain specific areas can give rise to violent behavior on mild provocation.

Severe head injuries (from falls, road accidents) are a much more common source of recurrent aggression. They were recorded in 10% of 469 cases in adults and children studied by Roberts (1979); the prevailing lesions in this type of case involve the orbito-frontal and anterior temporal cortex and are invariably diffuse and bilateral. Repeated minor trauma to the head, as occurs in jockeys and boxers, can also occasionally result in chronic irritability and attacks of rage on minor provocation.

From the forensic point of view it is necessary to remember, since head traumas is often used as an excuse, that the type of injury that can be held responsible for subsequent violence is usually severe enough to produce posttraumatic amnesia for 7 days or more and involves hospitalization.

Diffuse damage, as in closed head injury, is more likely than a focal lesion to produce behavioral disorders and cognitive impairment because the inhibitory equipment, both anatomical and chemical, is distributed bilaterally and diffusely. It occurs in encephalitis, meningitis, subarachnoid hemorrhage, chronic degenerative diseases (Alzheimer's and other dementias), Huntington's disease, arteriosclerosis, cardiopulmonary arrest, toxemias, and the important but often neglected neurodevelopmental disorders including mental retardation and marginal IQs.

Of these, individuals with neurodevelopmental disorders probably supply the largest pool of potentially violent subjects, but are often covert and easily missed by routine neurological examination and IQ tests (M. D. Levine, 1995). They were uncovered by Elliott (1982), for instance, in 40% of 286 recurrently violent subjects, who were specifically examined for them by using a long checklist based on studies of neurodevelopmental defects by Clements and Peters (1962), Clements (1966), Monroe (1978), Bach-y-Rita and colleagues (1971), and reviews by Barcley (1990), and Cantwell and Baker (1991). The search for neuropathology must cover conception, pregnancy, birth, infancy, childhood, adolescence, and beyond. The defects are often forgotten, and even more often denied (Ratey, 1995) or regarded as irrelevant. Common ingredients are attention deficit disorders (with or without hyperactivity), learning disorders (reading, language, writing, arithmetic), difficulties in higher cognitive functions and in social perceptions and skills, inability to learn common manual skills as in the use of tools, lack of athletic dexterity, disorders of working memory and remote and sequential memory (M. D. Levine, 1995), incapacity to assess time intervals and rhythms, and difficulties with spatial perceptions.

The pathological bases for some of these handicaps is known. In developmental dyslexias biopsy and autopsy materials have confirmed presence of multiple focal patches of maldevelopment of cortical architecture, which is clearly a defect of embryogenesis, and subcortical collections of neurons which imply faulty embryonic migration. There is also an abnormal symmetry of the temporal lobes (Galaburda, 1991). Cortical disorganization is also common in patients with temporal lobe epilepsy when associated with emotional or behavioral disorders, or when seizures do not respond to medication (Falconer & Cavannagh, 1959; Mathieson, 1975; Scheibel, 1991). Cortical dysplasia, with or without gross anatomical defects, also contributes to mental retardation. A physical basis for the attention-deficit/hyperactivity disorder in adults, dating from childhood, is provided by depression of glucose metabolism in multiple areas of the cortex during an auditory-attention test (Zametkin *et al.*, 1990).

A common defect is mesial temporal sclerosis, usually a sequel of perinatal asphyxia or severe infantile convulsions. Damage involves the hippocampus and may extend to the uncus, hippocampal gyrus, and amygdala, unilaterally or bilaterally (Scheibel, 1991). These are highly sensitive areas with respect to memory and aggression, but unilateral lesions can be asymptomatic.

The Clinical Evolution of Violence With Age

Longitudinal analyses of aggressive behavior have shown that its appearance in early childhood may predict criminal convictions for violence later in life, and that disinhibited violent behavior is usually accompanied by other, less dramatic, forms of impulsive behavior and lack of reflective delay in social activities: overdrinking, gambling, traffic offenses, sexual promiscuity, theft, truancy, and pathological lying (Bach-y-Rita *et al.*, 1971; Farrington, 1983; Robins, 1966).

The importance of scrutinizing the entire life history, from conception onward, was demonstrated in a unique study by Denno (1990) using the records of 987 subjects who were born at the Pennsylvania Hospital in Philadelphia between 1959 and 1962. This group was initially part of the National Collaborative Perinatal Project. Subjects were non-White and predominantly of low socioeconomic status. The sample (487 male and 500 female individuals) had been followed up from birth until the age of 22 years. It involved examination of the mothers as soon as they started attending the prenatal clinic. Pregnancies were supervised, as was labor and delivery. Each child was examined immediately after birth and at intervals thereafter. Researchers collected socioeconomic and family data when the mothers registered and at the child's 7th-year examination. School data were available, focusing on academic achievement during the ages of 13 to 14 years and on evidence of learning and behavioral disability during school attendance. Police records were collected for children ages 7–22. Much information was gathered from frequent home interviews with parents or caretakers. Each child was interviewed 16 times in all and was given pediatric examinations three times in the first 7 years. They all received selective intelligence tests at 7 years of age and achievement tests at the ages of 13 and 14 years. Lead levels were examined at 7 years.

This exercise carries with it the authority of facts recorded at the time, thus avoiding the dubious validity of retrospective questionnaires. Of 987 individuals, 151 became offenders by the age of 18 years, and nearly one quarter of these were arrested for violent crimes. Five percent of the male sample were chronic offenders, a figure that coincides with those in the study by Tracey, Wolfgang, and Figlio (1990) on a cohort of 10,000 male individuals born in Philadelphia in 1945, and with the results of their second study of 27,160 individuals born in 1958, approximately half of whom were male. In Denno's (1990) study, chronic offenders were responsible for 61% of the violent offenses. Neurologic differences between them and the control subjects included higher figures for neurodevelopmental disorders (attention deficit disorder, incoordination, articulation), head injury, and serum lead levels at 7 years. Denno concluded that "juvenile crime results from a variety of strong and independent biological and environmental influences. There appears to be a direct relationship of juvenile crime to familial instability and, most importantly, a lack of behavioral control associated with disorders of the central nervous system.

Similar findings were reported by Spreen (1989) in a longitudinal study of 203 children (average age 9) with learning difficulties (LD), compared with 52 controls, whom he followed until their mid 20s. He found that covert and overt neurological abnormalities were common in LD subjects. Those with LD but without neurological impairment fared worse than controls, those with minimal brain dysfunction did worse than those without it, and those with LD and definite brain damage did poorest of all as to temper outbursts, impulsivity, and fighting.

Another study, of 53 older delinquent males ages 11–16, 20% of whom had been convicted for violent crimes, and 51 nondelinquents, was carried out by M. Levine, Karniski, Palfrey, Meltzer, and Fenton (1985). Thirty-two areas were covered, including general health, seizures, trauma, neurodevelopmental defects, behavioral history, educational assessments and handicaps, attention, and the Wechsler Intelligence Scale for children. There was no socioeconomic difference between subjects and controls. The latter showed vulnerabilities, but delinquents displayed far more defects in the areas surveyed.

Continuity between birth injuries and subsequent aggression noted by Towbin (1971) and by D. O. Lewis, Pincus, and Glaser (1979) is especially noticeable when it is complicated by maternal neglect in the first year. A cohort of 4,269 males in Denmark was assessed for birth injury recorded at the time of delivery, maternal rejection in the first year, and violent crime at 18 years; 4.5% with both risk factors were responsible for 18% of the violent crime committed by the cohort.

Neuropathology in 161 Murderers

The chief psychiatrist of the California state prison at San Quentin has observed that my organic brain pathology is vastly under-diagnosed in the prison population and plays a much larger part in criminal behavior than was previously thought (Hicks, 1988, p.). This view was held by Thompson (1953), and is sustained by the following reports on child and adult murderers from seven prisons (including death row), state hospitals, and psychiatric, sociologic, and neurological clinics in teaching hospitals.

Raine and colleagues (1994) carried out a PET scan on 22 adult male murderers and 22 normal controls. They found lower glucose metabolism in murderers in the lateral and medial prefrontal cortex during a continuous performance tests, as compared with controls. Additional findings were a history of head injury "or other brain damage" in 10, epilepsy in 1, learning difficulty and hyperactivity in 1, schizophrenia in 3, passive aggression or paranoia in 2, abuse of psychoactive drugs in 2, and "unspecific bizarre circumstances suggesting mental impairment" in 5.

Frazier (1974) reported on a collaborative psychiatric study of 31 murderers in prisons and mental hospitals in six states. The sample was unusual in two respects: a predominance of middle- and upper-class subjects, and widespread denial of alcohol use at the time of the murder or murders. Twenty-three had killed 1 each, and 8 had killed a total of 68. Biological factors, including maturational and neurodevelopmental defects, were found to be as significant as socioenvironmental disadvantages; they included organic brain disorders in 6, temporal lobe epilepsy in 2, mental retardation in 2, brain tumor in 1, organic dementia in 4, episodic rages in 11, delayed neurological naturation in 5 (due to rubella in 1, prematurity in 1, and childhood diabetes in 1). Compulsive, "driven," behavior was recognized in 15. Parental brutality and deprivation were severe in 18. There was a history of repeated personal humiliation in 18, a sense of powerlessness in 15, and of personal inadequacy in 11.

Bender (1959), reporting on 36 cases of children under 16 years of age who had been responsible for an unintentional death, found organic brain disease with impulse disorder or epilepsy in 15, schizophrenic preoccupation with death or killing in the young children and psychopathy in adolescence in 13, and adverse home conditions in all. All cases were followed up for at least 5 to 25 years after the homicidal incident. The older boys, ages 11 to 15, had caused deaths by stabbing, repeated blows from a heavy object, or by shooting, in six cases. All of the subjects showed either schizophrenia, epilepsy, or significant brain damage.

In a study of 14 juvenile murderers (average age $16\frac{1}{2}$) who were condemned to death, all received comprehensive neurologic, EEG, neuropsychological, educational, and social evaluation by D. Lewis and colleagues (1988). Eight had suffered head injuries. There was a history of frequent lapses of consciousness in 9 (some of which were accompanied by "psychological" symptoms) and one of grand mal. Seven were or had been psychotic. Only 2 subjects had a full-scale IQ above 90. There was a history of prolonged brutal abuse in 12 and sodomy by relatives in 5. The authors wrote that the subjects' vulnerabilities were not recognized at the time of sentencing, although they could have been used in a plea for mitigation.

Merikangas (1981) examined 16 male murderers in a university behavioral neurology clinic and found abnormal neurological signs in 5, explicit brain damage in 4, epilepsy in 3, mental retardation in 5, psychopathy in 5, and other psychiatric disorders in 9. Forty-five percent had an abnormal EEG.

Elliott (1982) examined 13 murderers, from a series of 286 recurrently violent adults who were referred for neurological examination, largely by psychiatrists and attorneys. As in Frazier's (1974) study, middle- and upper-class subjects predominated. Average age of the murderers was 35.6 years, as against 26.6 years in the group as a whole. There was a history of severe head injury in 4, occasional psychomotor epileptic attacks in 5, temporal lobe spikes in 9, frontotemporal slowing in 4, neurodevelopmental defects in 4, pathological intoxication in 3, vascular malformation of the brain in 2, and somnambulism in 1. Four were obsessed with thoughts of death and felt driven to kill. There was a single case of a particularly vicious murder, by multiple knife wounds, of a supervisor by a normally hyperconscientous worker, who had no criminal record but harbored a list of insults and public ridicule and felt driven to exact vengeance. This he did in the presence of his coworkers. There were no symptoms or signs of past or present organic disorders or abnormal behavior, and the clinical picture was that of an overcontrolled personality (Blackburn, 1968; Megargee, 1982).

Thirty-one male murderers on death row were examined (while manacled) by Blake, Pincus, and Buckner (1993). The average age at the time of homicide was 32.7 (range 14 to 63) years. Only 1 subject exhibited obvious neurological impairment, and all but 1 had covert abnormalities that reflected brain damage or defects. A specific neurological diagnosis was possible in 20. Nine had evinced symptoms or EEG evidence, or both, of temporal lobe seizures, and 2 had a history of convulsive epilepsy. There was evidence of neurodevelopmental defects in the 11 cases of attention deficit disorder and suspected learning difficulties in 9. Mental retardation or borderline retardation (IQ less than 80) was present in 9. An unusual inclusion in this study was testing for presence of persistent infantile reflexes—the snout reflex, sucking reflex, and grasp reflex—which indicated frontal immaturity. Additional evidence of organicity was provided by abnormal magnetic resonance studies in 11 out of 21, and abnormal EEGs in 10 out of 21. Psychiatric diagnoses were paranoid schizophrenia in 8, dissociative disorders in 4, and depression in 9. Twenty-six had been subjected to severe and protracted physical abuse, including sexual abuse in 10.

Prevalence of developmental and acquired neurological disorders in these murderers was clearly higher than in the population at large. This applies to epilepsy and psychomotor symptoms (19%), head injury and other organic conditions (48%), learning and other neurodevelopmental disorders, (18%), and mental retardation (17%). Other complaints (lapses of consciousness and dissociative states, 13%) were difficult to categorize.

Summary

Many recent studies of violent criminals, other than the professional hit-man, have found neurological or neuropsychological defects, and additional evidence or pathology is being identified by electrophysiological investigation, CT scans, PET scans, magnetic imaging, and neurochemical studies. Nevertheless, most brain damaged individuals are not violent, and in those who are there is usually evidence of psychopathology, prolonged exposure to significant social adversity, or both. Thus, criminal violence appears to be the result of the confluence and interaction of multiple biological and environmental variables at a given moment or over a period; some of these variables are excitatory and some inhibitory. They include the behavior of the putative victim and the blood levels of alcohol and drugs in both the aggressor and he victim.

It has been pointed out that neurological disorders are seldom obvious in such cases. Aggressors usually look and sound normal. As Eric Fromm (1973) once remarked, "they don't wear the mark of Cain on their foreheads" (p. 432). The defects are often covert and are missed by cursory neurological examination and IQ examination. This is especially true of neurodevelopmental disorders, which are apt to go unrecognized and unaddressed as these subjects pass through schools, medical clinics, social services, and the courts.

Perhaps the most powerful inhibitory influences are prosocial cultural and religious constraints and social taboos. Historical examples over the centuries have illustrated the disastrous effects when individuals are weakened during periods of social disruption and anomie and when there is widespread erosion of personal integrity, a drying-up of compassion and altruism, uncontrolled material greed, corruption in high places, a lust for cruelty in entertainment, a descent of sexual mores to barnyard levels, and even a recourse to medieval demonology.

It is comforting to recall that through the centuries these epidemics have come to an end (Gurr, 1976). It is also encouraging that much progress has been made by pharmacological research, which has provided an impressive array of agents that not only can control specific types of violence (Miczek, Haney, et al., 1994; Volavka, 1995) but can make recalcitrant juvenile delinquents and criminals more accessible to psychotherapy by reducing their hostility (Eichelman, 1988). An early example was phenytoin which, in 1938, brought a measure of peace to the epileptic wards of state hospitals by controlling interictal violence. Later on, carbamexapine had an even wider sphere of activity as did antipsychotic agents and lithium for mania and depression; propranolol and other beta blockers for intermittent explosive disorder and violence in all organic cases, regardless of diagnosis (Miczek, Haney, et al., 1994); serotonergic agents for a variety of conditions, both organic and functional; antiandrogens to reduce the sex drive in sex offenders; and clomipramine to reduce aggressive thoughts (Rapoport, 1989).

Useful as they are for symptomatic control in subjects who can be supervised, whether in hospitals, prisons, clinics, or stable households, they cannot reach street criminals. The thrust of social and criminal studies, especially longitudinal investigations, is to reinforce the importance of prophylaxis by multimodal behavior therapies for the children and adolescents who gave early evidence of pathological aggression and neurological or neuropsychological deviance.

References

Alpers, B. J. (1937). Relation of the hypothalamus to disorders of personality: Report of a case. *Archives of Neurology and Psychiatry, 38,* 291–303.

Bach-y-Rita, G., Lion, J. R., Climent, C. E., & Ervin, F. R. (1971). Episodic dyscontrol: A study of 130 violent patients. *American Journal of Psychiatry, 127,* 1473–1478.

Barcley, R. A. (1990). *Attention deficit hyperactivity disorder: A handbook for diagnosis and treatment in psychiatric offenders.* New York: Guilford.

Barrett, H. J., & Hyland, H. H. (1952). Tumours involving the brainstem. *Quarterly Journal of Medicine, 21,* 265–284.

Baxter, L. R., Phelps, M. E., Mazziotta, J. C., Guze, B. H., Schwartz, B., & Selin, C. E. (1987). Local cerebral glucose metabolic rates in obsessive-compulsive disorders. *Archives of General Psychiatry, 44,* 211–218.

Bear, D. M., Freeman, R., & Greenberg, (1984). Behavioral alterations in temporal lobe epilepsy. In D. Blumer (Ed.), *Psychiatric aspects of epilepsy.* Washington, DC: American Psychiatric Press.

Bender, L. (1959). Children and adolescents who have killed. *American Journal of Psychiatry, 116,* 510–513.

Benes, F. M., Turtle, M., Khan, Y., & Farol, P. (1994). Myelination of a key relay zone in the hippocampal formation occurring in the human body during childhood, adolescence, and adulthood. *Archives of General Psychiatry, 51,* 477–484.

Blackburn, R. (1968). Personality in relation to extreme aggression in psychiatric offenders. *British Journal of Psychiatry, 114,* 821–828.

Blake, P. Y., Pincus, J. H., & Buckner, C. (1993). Neurologic abnormalities in murderers. *Neurology, 45,* 1641–1647.

Blumer, D. (1991). Epilepsy and disorders of mood. In D. S. Smith, D. M. Treiman, & M. Trimble (Eds.), *Advances in neurology* (Vol. 55, pp. 185–196). New York: Raven.

Broughton, R., Billings, R., Cartwright, R., Doucette, J., Edmeads, J., Edwards, N., Ervin, F., Orchard, B., Hill, R., & Turrell, G. (1994). Homicidal somnambulism: A Case report. *Sleep 17*(3), 253–264.

Brown, S. L. (1994). Title *National Geographic, 12*(6), 8–12.

Brunner, H.G., Nelen, M., Breakefield, x.o., Ropers, H.J & Van Oost B.A. (1993) Abnormal behavior associated when a pointmutation in the structional gene for monamine oxidage A. Science, 262, 578–580.

Cairns, H. (1950). Mental disorders with tumors of the pons. *Folia Psychiatry Neurology* (Netherlands), *53*, 193–203.

Cantwell, D. P., & Baker, L. (1991). *Psychiatric and developmental disorders in children with communication disorders.* Washington, DC: American Psychiatric Press.

Carey, G. (1994). Genetics and violence. In A. J., Reiss, K. Miczek, & J. A. Roth (Eds.), *Understanding and treating violence* (Vol. 2, pp. 21–58). Washington, DC: National Academy Press.

Cleckley, H. (1982). *The mask of sanity.* New York: New American Library.

Clements, S. D. (1966). *Minimal brain dysfunction in children* (National Institute of Neurology and Blindness Monograph No. 3). Washington, DC: U.S. Department of Health, Education, and Welfare.

Clements, S. D., & Peters, J. E. (1962). Minimal brain dysfunction in the school-age child. *Archives of General Psychiatry, 6,* 185–197.

Comstock, G., & Paik, H. (1990). *The effects of television on aggressive behavior.* Unpublished report to the National Academy of Science on Understanding and Control of Violent Behaviors (Vol. 1, p. 371). Washington, DC: National Academy Press.

Cooper, I. S. (1978). *Cerebellar stimulation in man.* New York: Raven.

Cox, C. S., Fedio, P., & Rapoport, J. C. (1989). Neuropsychological testing of obsessive-compulsive adolescents. In J. Rapoport (Ed.), *Obsessive compulsive disorders in children and adolescents.* Washington, DC: American Psychiatric Press.

Dalton, K. (1925). *The premenstrual syndrome.* Springfield, IL: Thomas.

Damasio, A. R., Tramel, D. T., & Damasio, M. (1990). Individuals with sociopathic behavior caused by frontal damage fail to respond automatically to social stimuli. *Behavioral Brain Research, 41,* 81–94.

Davenport, D. B. (1915). The feebly inhibited: Violent temper and its inheritance. *Journal of Nervous and Mental Diseases, 42,* 493–528.

Denckla, M. B. (1989). Title In J. Rapoport (Ed.), *Obsessive compulsive disorders in children and adolescents* (pp. 000–000). Washington, DC: American Psychiatric Press.

Denno, D. W. .(1990). *Biology and violence: From birth to adulthood.* New York: Cambridge University Press.

Diekmann, G., & Hassler, R. (1975). Unilateral hypothalamotomy in social delinquents: Report on 6 cases. *Confinia Neurologica, 37,* 177–186.

Eibl-Eibesveldt, I. (1979). *The biology of peace and war: Men, animals, and aggression.* New York: Viking.

Eichelman, B. (1988). Toward a rational pharmacotherapy for aggressive violent behavior. *Hospital and Community Psychiatry, 39*(1), 31–39.

Eichelman, B. (1992). Aggressive hebavior from woatory to chinie archieves of general psychology , 49, 488–492.

Elliott, F. A. (1977). Propranolol for the control of belligerent behavior following acute head injury. *Annals of Neurology, 1,* 488–491.

Elliott F. A. (1982). Neurological findings in adult minimal brain dysfunction and the dyscontrol syndrome. *Journal of Nervous and Mental Diseases, 170*(11), 680-687.

Falconer, M. A., & Cavannagh, J. B. (1959). Clinicopathological considerations of temporal lobe epilepsy due to small focal lesions. *Brain, 82,* 483–504.

Farrington, D. P. (1983). Offending from 10 to 20 years of age. In K. Vandusen & S. A. Mednick (Eds.), *Prospective studies of crime and delinquency* (pp. 17–38). Boston: Kluver-Nijhoff.

Frazier, S. H. (1974). Murder—Single and multiple. In S. H. Frazier (Ed.), *Research publications, Association for Research in Nervous and Mental Diseases.* Baltimore: Williams & Wilkins.

Fromm, E. (1973). *The anatomy of human destructiveness.* New York: Holt, Rinehart and Winston.

Galaburda, A. M. (1991). Neuropathological correlates of learning difficulties. *Seminars in Neurology, 11,* 20–27.

Glaser, G. H. (1981). Critical periods in brain development related to behavior, especially epilepsies. In J. R. Merikangas (Ed.), *Brain behavior relationships.* Lexington, MA: Lexington Books.

Gorenstein, E. E., & Newman, P. (1980). Disinhibitory psychopathology: A new perspective and a model for research. *Psychological Reviews, 87,* 301–315.

Gunn, J. C. (1991). Legal implications of behavioral changes in epilepsy. *Advances in Neurology, 55,* 461–472.

Gurr, T. R. (1976). The history of violent crime in Europe and America. In H. D. Graham, & T. R. Gurr (Eds.), *Violence in America: Historical and comparative perspectives.* Beverly Hills, CA: Sage.

Hare, R., & McPherson, L. M. (1984). Violent and aggressive behavior by criminal psychopaths. *International Journal of Law and Psychiatry, 7,* 35–50.

Hawke, C. C. (1950). Castration and sex crimes. *American Journal of Medical Deficiency, 55,* 220–226.

Heath, E. G. (1977). Modulation of emotion with a brain pacemaker. *Journal of Nervous and Mental Diseases, 165,* 300–317.

Hicks, P. S. (1988). Preface. In J. Morris, & W. T. Birnes (Eds.), *Serial killers.* New York: Dolphin Books.

Hollander, E., Shiffman, E., & Liebowitz, M. (1987, May). *Neurological soft signs in obsessional-compulsive disorder.* Poster presented at the 140th annual meeting of the American Psychiatric Association, Chicago.

Joslin, E. P. (1937). *Treatment of diabetes mellitus.* Philadelphia: Lea & Febiger.

Kaes, T. (1907). *Grosshirnrind des menschen in hihres fassengehalt: Ein gehirn anatomische atlas.* Jena, Germany: Fischer.

Kanarek, R. B. (1994). Nutrition and violent behavior. In *Understanding and preventing violence* (Vol. 2, pp. 515–540). Washington, DC: National Academy Press.

Kaplan, J. (1899). Kopftrauma und pschosen. *Allgemeine Psychiatrie, 56,* 292–297.

Kegan, R. G. (1986). Sociopathy, a developmental delay. In W. H. Reid, D. Dorr, & J. Walker (Eds.), *The child behind the mask.* New York: Norton.

Keschner, M., Bender, M. R., & Strauss, I. (1937). Mental symptoms in cases of subtentorial tumor. *Archives of Neurology and Psychiatry, 37,* 1–17.

Kim, S. G., Ugurbil, K., & Strick, P. L. (1994). Activation of cerebellar output nucleus during cognitive processing. *Science, 265,* 949–951.

Kolarski, A., Freund, K., Machek, J., & Polak, O. (1967). Male sexual deviation associated with early temporal lobe damage. *Archives of General Psychiatry, 17,* 735–743.

Langevin, R. (1990). Sexual anomalies and the brain. In W. L., Marshall, D. R. Laws, & H. Barbaree (Eds.), *Handbook of sexual assault: Issues, theories and treatment of the offender* (pp. 103–113). New York: Plenum.

Lassman, L. P., & Arjona, V. (1967). Pontine glioma in childhood. *Lancet, 1,* 913–915.

Leiner, H., Leiner, A. L., & Dow, (1989). Re-appraising the cerebellum: What does the hind-brain contribute to the fore-brain? *Behavioral Neuroscience, 103,* 998–1008.

Levine, M., Karniski, W. M., Palfrey, J. S., Meltzer, L., & Fenton, T. (1985). A study of risk factor complexes in early adolescent delinquency. *American Journal of Diseases of Childhood, 139,* 50–65.

Levine, M. D. (1995). Childhood neurodevelopmental dysfunctional learning disorders. *Harvard Mental Health Letter, 12,* 5–6.

Lewis, D., Pincus, J. H., Bard, S., Richardson, E., Pritchep, L. S., Feldman, M., & Yeager, C. (1988). Neuropsychiatric, psycho-educational and family characteristics of 14 juveniles condemned to death in the United States. *American Journal of Psychiatry, 145,* 584–589.

Lewis, D. O., Pincus, J. H., & Glaser, (1979). Violent juvenile delinquents: Psychiatric, neurological and abuse factors. *American Academy of Psychiatry, 18,* 307–319.

Lhermitte, F., Pillon, B., & Serdaru, M. (1986). Human anatomy and the frontol lobe: Imitation and utilization behavior. A neuro-psychological study of 75 patients. *Annals of Neurology, 19,* 326–334.

Linnoila, M., Virkunnen, M., Scheinen, M., Nuutila, A., Rimon, R., & Goodwin, F. (1983). Low cerebrospinal 5-hydroxy indoleacetic acid differentiates impulsive from non-impulsive violent behavior. *Life Sciences, 33,* 2609–2619.

Linqvist, P., & Allebeck, F. (1990). Schizophrenia and crime: A longitudinal follow-up of 644 schizophrenics in Stockholm. *British Journal of Psychiatry, 157,* 345–350.

Macklin, S. R., Harris, G. H., Pearson, G. D., Hohn-Saric, R., Jeffery, P., & Camargo, E. (1991). Elevated medical frontal blood flow in obsessive-compulsive patients in a Spekt study. *American Journal of Psychiatry, 148,* 1240–1242.

Mahowald, M. W., Bundlie, S. R., Hurwitz, T. D., & Schenck, C. H. (1990). Sleep violence: Forensic science implications: Polygraphic and video documentation. *Journal of Forensic Science, 35,* 413–430.

Malamud, N. C. (1967). Psychiatric disorders with intra-cranial tumors of the limbic system. *Archives of Psychiatry, 17,* 113–123.

Mathieson, G. (1975). Pathology of temporal lobe foci. In J. K. Penry, & D. D. Daly (Eds.), *Advances in neurology* (Vol. 11). New York: Raven.

Mednick, S. A., & Christiansen, K. (1977). *Biological bases of criminal behavior.* New York: Gardner.

Megargee, E. I. (1982). Psychological correlates and determinants of criminal behavior. In M. Wolfgang, & M. Weiner (Eds.), *Criminal violence*. Beverly Hills, CA: Sage.

Merikangas, J. R. (1981). *Brain–behavior relationships*. Lexington, MA: Lexington Books.

Miczek, K. A., Haney, M., Tidey, J., Jeffery, L., & Weerts, E. (1994). The neurochemistry and pharmacotherapeutics of aggression and violence. In A. J. Reis, & J. Miczek (Eds.), *Understanding and preventing violence*. Washington, DC: National Academy Press.

Moffitt, T. E. (1993). Adolescence-limited and life-course persistent anti-social behavior: A developmental taxonomy. *Psychological Reviews, 100*(4), 674–701.

Monroe, R. R. (1978). *Brain dysfunction in aggressive criminals*. Lexington, MA: Lexington Books.

Morton, J. H., Addition, H., Addison, R. G., Hunt, L., & Sullivan, H. A. (1953). A clinical study of pre-menstrual tension. *American Journal of Obstetrics and Gynecology, 65*, 1182–1191.

Moruzzi, G. (1958). Title In R. S. Dow, & G. Moruzzi (Eds.), *The physiology and psychology of the cerebellum* (pp. 000–000). Minneapolis: University of Minnesota Press.

Moyer, K. E. (1976). *The psychohistology of aggression*. New York: Harper.

Poeck, K. (1969). Pathophysiology of emotional disorders associated with brain damage. In P. J. Vinken, & G. W. Bruyn (Eds.), *Handbook of clinical neurology* (Vol. 3). Amsterdam: North Holland.

Raine, A., Bauchsbaum, M., Stanley, J., Lottenberg, S., Abel, M., & Stoddard, J. (1994). Selective reductions in prefrontal glucose metabolism in murderers. *Biological Psychiatry, 36*, 368–373.

Raine E., & Venables, P. H. (1988). Enhanced P3 evoked potentials and psychopathy. *International Journal of Psychophysiology, 8*, 1–16.

Rapoport, J. L. (1989). The biology of obsessions and compulsions. *Scientific American, 260*, 83–89.

Ratey, J. J. (Ed.). (1995). *Neuropsychiatry of personality disorders*. Cambridge, MA: Blackwell.

Reich, W. (1974). *The impulsive character and other writings*. New York: Viking.

Roberts, A. H. (1979). *Severe accidental head injury: An assessment of long-term prognosis*. London: Macmillan.

Robins, L. N. (1966). *Deviant children grown up*. Baltimore: Williams & Wilkins.

Roeder, F. D. (1966). Stereotactic lesions of the tuber cinerium in sexual deviation. *Confinia Neurologica, 27*, 162–163.

Rutter, M. (1980). *Changing youth in a changing society*. Cambridge, MA: Harvard University Press.

Rutter, M., & Giller, G. (1983). *Juvenile delinquency: Trends and perspectives*. New York: Guilford.

Sano, K. (1962). Sedative neurosurgery: With special reference to posterior-medial hypothalamotomy. *Neurologie Medico-Chirg, 4*, 112–142.

Scheibel, A. B. (1991). Are complex partial seizures a sequel of temporal lobe dysgenesis? In D. B. Smith, D. M. Treiman, & M. R. Trimble (Eds.), *Advances in neurology* (Vol. 55). New York: Raven.

Schmahmann, J. D. (1991). An emerging concept: The cerebellar contribution to higher function. *Archives of Neurology, 48*, 1178–1187.

Sherrington, C. S. (1925). On the nature of reflex excitation and inhibition. *Proceedings of the Royal Society, 97B*, 519–545.

Spreen, O. (1989). The relationship between learning disorders and neuropsychology: Some results and observations. *Journal of Clinical and Experimental Neuropsychology, 11*(1), 117–140.

Stacey, W., & Shupe, H. (1983). *The family secret*. Boston: Beacon.

Stafford-Clark, D. (1959). The foundations of research in psychiatry. *British Medical Journal, 2*, 1199–1204.

Stevens, J. R., & Hermann, B. P. (1981). Temporal lobe epilepsy, psychopathology, and violence: The state of the evidence. *Neurology, 31*, 1127–1132.

Strauss, I., & Keschner, M. (1936). Mental symptoms in tumor of the frontal lobe. *Archives of Neurology and Psychiatry, 35*, 572–596.

Tardiff, K. (1992). The current state of psychiatry in the treatment of violent patients. *Advances of General Psychiatry, 49*, 493–499.

Taylor, D. C. (1993). The roots and role of violence in development. In P. J. Taylor (Ed.), *Violence in society*. London: Royal College of Physicians.

Thompson, G. M. (1953). *The psychopathic delinquent and criminal*. Springfield, IL: Thomas.

Towbin, A. (1971). Organic causes of minimal brain dysfunction: Peri-natal origins of minimal cerebral lesions. *Journal of the American Medical Association, 217*, 1207–1214.

Tracy, P. E., Wolfgang, M. E., & Figlio, R. M. (1990). *Delinquency careers in 2 birth cohorts*. New York: Plenum.

Treiman, D. M. (1986). Epilepsy and violence: Medical and legal issues. *Epilepsia, 27* (Suppl. 2), S77–S104.

Valzelli, L. (1981). *Psychobiology of aggression and violence*. New York: Raven.

Virkkunen, M. (1986). Reactive hypoglycemic tendency among habitually violent offenders. *Nutrition Reviews, 44* (Suppl. 1), 94–103.

Volavka, J. (1995). *Neurobiology of violence*. Washington, DC: American Psychiatric Press.

Vonderahe, A. R. (1944). The anatomic substratum of emotion. *New Scholasticism, 18*, 79–95.

Weiger, W. A., & Bear, D. M. (1988). An approach to the neurology of aggression. *Journal of Psychiatric Research, 22*(2), 85–98.

Werner, E. E., & Smith, R. (1982). *Vulnerable but invincible. A study of resilient children*. New York: McGraw-Hill.

Wilder, S. (1947). Sugar metabolism and its relation to criminology. In R. M. Lindner, & R. V. Seliger (Eds.), *Handbook of correctional psychology*. New York: Philosophical Library.

Williams D. (1969). Neural factors related to habitual aggression: Consideration of deficiencies between habitual aggression and those who have committed crimes of violence. *Brain, 92*, 503–520.

Wolfgang, M. E., & Ferracuti, F. (1982). *The subculture of violence*. Beverly Hills, CA: Sage.

Wong, M. T., Lumsden, S., Fenton, G. W., & Fenwick, P. B. G. (1994). Epilepsy and violence in mentally abnormal offenders in a maximum security mental hospital. *Journal of Epilepsy, 7*, 253–258.

Yakovlev, P. I., & Lecours, A. R. (1967). The myelogenetic cycle of regional maturation of the brain. In A. Minkowski (Ed.), *Regional development of the brain in early life* (pp. 3–70). Philadelphia: Davis.

Zametkin, A. J., Nordahl, T. E., Gross, M., King, A. C., Semple, W. E., Rumsey, J., Hamberger, S., & Cohen, R. M. (1990). Cerebral glucose metabolism in adults with hyperactivity of childhood onset. *New England Journal of Medicine, 323*, 1361–1366.

Zecevic, M., & Rakic, P. (1976). Differentiation of Purkinje cells and their relationship to other components of developing cerebellar cortex in man. *Journal of Comparative Neurology, 167*, 27–48.

Zeman, W., & King, F. A. (1958). Tumor of the septum pellucidum and adjacent structures with abnormal affective behavior: An anterior midbrain structure syndrome. *Journal of Nervous and Mental Disease, 127*, 490–503.

21

Psychiatric Assessment of the Violent Offender

Otto Kausch and Phillip J. Resnick

Introduction

This chapter addresses the psychiatric assessment of potentially violent persons who come into contact with the legal system. We discuss the process of psychiatric risk assessment in general, and then examine the specific contexts of civil commitment, release of insanity acquittees, and probation. Finally, we use stalkers as a specific example of the risk assessment process. Throughout this chapter, the emphasis is on practical, rather than theoretical, considerations.

Psychiatric Assessment of Risk Factors

Although psychiatrists are often asked to predict violent behavior, they have not demonstrated the ability to do this well (Monahan, 1996). They typically overpredict violence by 40% to 95% (false-positives). Rather than attempting to predict violent acts, psychiatrists should assess the risk for violence (Wack, 1993). In general, the number of risk factors is proportional to the risk of future violent behavior. Some risk factors, such as antisocial personality disorder, are particularly ominous (Hare & McPherson, 1984). Although there are also a variety of demographic factors associated with violence (Resnick & Kausch, 1995), no helpful interventions are possible to modify them. We focus primarily on dynamic risk factors, that is, those that are amenable to some form of intervention.

Otto Kausch and Phillip J. Resnick • Department of Psychiatry, Case Western Reserve University, Cleveland, Ohio 44106.

Handbook of Psychological Approaches with Violent Offenders: Contemporary Strategies and Issues, edited by Van Hasselt and Hersen. Kluwer Academic/Plenum Publishers, New York, 1999.

Past Violence

The best predictor of future violence is a history of past violence (Klassen & O'Connor, 1988). The probability of further assault increases with each additional prior act (Shah, 1978). Understanding the forces that led to past violent acts improves the clinician'sability to evaluate the current risk of violence, and also helps the clinician develop recommendations for preventing future violence. Thus, it is important to learn as much as possible about past violent acts. When reviewing a detailed history of past violent acts, following checklist may be helpful (Wack, 1993):

a. Circumstances and age of onset
b. Types of violent behaviors
   - violent crimes
   - hospitalizations for violence
   - spouse or child abuse
   - fights in school or bars
   - violent highway disputes
c. Severity and frequency of violence
d. Types and usage of weapons
e. Characteristics of the violence (e.g,, impulsivity, level of planning, rituals)
f. Situational factors, known triggers
g. Mental status characteristics related to the behavior (delusions, hallucinations, organic problems)
h. Substance abuse
i. Medication compliance
j. Offender's coping strategies for anger, frustration, depression, and so on

In addition to obtaining detailed information from the offender, the psychiatrist should routinely obtain collateral information. Collateral information includes the victim's account of past violence, accounts from witnesses, and information from family members. Other potential sources of information are police reports, military records, school records, and hospital charts.

If the individual has been found not guilty by reason of insanity (NGRI) for an identified event, then it is important to note all of the details. Who said what? What was the degree of injury? What were the defendant's thoughts and feelings before, during, and after the act? An offender's inability to identify thoughts and feelings is a poor prognostic sign (Ball, Dotson, Brothers, Young, & Robbins, 1992).

In reviewing an offender's history, the psychiatrist should look for patterns of violence. For example, was the violent act instigated by an insult that caused the individual to feel disrespected? Has violence occurred only in the presence of psychotic symptoms, such as paranoid delusions? Is there a pattern of family violence, nonfamily violence, or both (Straznickas, McNeil, & Binder, 1993)? Violence limited to family members tends to be less severe (Shields, McCall, & Hanneke, 1988). Was past violence the result of affective or predatory aggression (Meloy, 1987)? Affective aggression results when an individual experiences a threat and reacts emotionally. Predatory aggression is planned and carried out with emotional detachment (or sadistic pleasure). Predatory violence is the hallmark of the psychopathic character.

Mental Illness

Studies done in the first half of this century suggested that mentally ill persons were no more violent than other citizens in the community (Brown, 1985). More recent studies, however, have shown that mentally ill persons are, in fact, more violent. This material is well summarized in Torrey's (1994) review of the literature (see also Monahan, 1992).

S. C. Wessely, Castle, and Douglas (1994) found an association between schizophrenia in men and violent crime. Paranoid schizophrenics often commit the most serious crimes because of their ability to plan and their retention of some reality testing.

Depressed persons may become violent due to despair. Mothers may project their own unacceptable psychotic symptoms onto their children. Mothers contemplating suicide may decide to take their young children with them to heaven because they cannot bear to be separated from them (Resnick, 1969).

A high percentage of manic offenders engage in assaultive or threatening behavior, but serious violence is rare (Binder & McNiel, 1988; Higgins, 1990). Manic persons show less criminality and substantially less homicidality than schizophrenic individuals. Manic offenders are most likely to respond violently to any form of limit setting (Tardiff & Sweillam, 1980).

In assessing persons with mental illness, the psychiatrist should inquire about current medications and compliance with medications. If there is a history of noncompliance with medications, the examiner should attempt to ascertain the reasons. Amador, Straus, Yale, and Gorman (1991) found a relationship between medication noncompliance and lack of insight into mental illness. Thus, it is useful to question a mentally ill subject about his or her insight into mental illness and understanding of the role of medications in preventing relapse.

The psychiatrist should look for patterns of victim selection. In the community, the most likely victims of violence by psychiatric patients are family members (Estroff & Zimmer, 1994). A chaotic, crowded family environment is more likely to precipitate violence (Mulvey & Lidz, 1984). In addition, financial dependence on family members by persons with chronic mental illness is associated with a greater risk of violence toward them (Estroff, Zimmer, Lachicotte, & Benoit, 1994). In a case where the choice of victims seems to have been rooted in a specific delusion, it is important to find out if the delusion applied only to that person or to a group of persons.

Psychotic Symptoms

The violent behavior of the mentally ill is often a "rational" response to irrational beliefs (Junginger, 1996). Persecutory delusions are more likely to be acted on than other types of delusions (S. Wessely, Buchanan, & Reed, 1993). Paranoid persons with delusions often commit violence that is well planned and consistent with the delusion. The violence is usually directed at a specific person who is perceived as persecuting the subject. Offenders with persecutory delusions may resort to violence or even homicide in an effort to protect themselves (D'Orban & O'Connor, 1989; Straznickas *et al.*, 1993). Paranoid symptoms may result from personality traits, mental illness such as paranoid schizophrenia or delusional disorder (Boxer, 1993), or substance abuse (Regier, Farmer, & Rae, 1991).

In assessing the risk potential in a paranoid offender, it is critical to ask what he would do if confronted by the perceived persecutor. If asked whether he feels homicidal, the subject may honestly answer, "No." However, he may be prepared to kill to protect himself. The psychiatrist should specifically ask the offender if he perceives himself to be singled out or mistreated. If so, does he carry a grudge or have any revenge fantasies?

Paranoid offenders may present as hostile, suspicious, sensitive to slights, or fearful. If fearful, it is important to assess the degree of fear because increasing fear may precipitate violence. Evidence of fear resulting from persecutory delusions may include changes of residence, long journeys to evade persecutors, barricading oneself into a room, carrying weapons for protection, and asking the police for protection from persecutors.

Systematized delusional beliefs that are logically elaborated increase the risk of violent crime (Hafner & Boker, 1982). Persons who previously acted on delusions are more likely to engage in violent behavior (Junginger, 1995). Those who actively seek information to confirm or refute a delusional belief are more likely to report subsequent psychotic action (Buchanan *et al.*, 1993). Persons with delusional misidentification syndromes may be more dangerous than those with other psychoses (Silva, Leong, & Weinstock, 1992).

Once one accepts the fact that delusions are experienced as real, one can better understand the emergence of violent responses by individuals who either fear imminent harm or experience external forces as overriding their personal control. "Threat/control-override" symptoms associated with increased aggression include (Link & Stueve, 1994):

a. Feeling dominated by forces beyond one's control
b. Believing that thoughts are being put into one's head
c. Believing that there are people who wish one harm
d. Believing that one is being followed

Persons who reported delusional symptoms involving perceived threat or control override, or both, were twice as likely to engage in assaultive behavior as those with other psychotic symptoms (J. Swanson, Borum, Swartz, & Monahan, 1994). Individuals with threat/control override symptoms combined with alcohol or drug use disorders were especially prone to violent behavior (i.e., 8 to 10 times more likely to commit violence than those with no disorder).

Psychotic patients with command hallucinations are at increased risk for violence (Junginger, 1990, 1995). The rate of compliance with command hallucinations varies in different studies from 10% to 80%. The likelihood of obeying commands is increased if the voice is familiar and if there is a hallucination-related delusion (Junginger, 1990). For example, a man who hears a voice telling him to kill his mother is more likely to act on it if he has a delusional belief that his mother is a witch. The psychiatrist should carefully inquire about the presence of command hallucinations. If they are present, the examiner should ask about the individual's past ability to resist the commands, his currently perception of his ability to resist the commands, and his coping strategies for putting the voices out of his mind.

In the presence of hallucinations and delusions, violence may result indirectly through disturbed moods such as fear, anger, sadness, or anxiety (Buchanan *et al.*,

1993; Kennedy, Kemp, & Dyer, 1992). Fear or anger are the emotions that most often precede the threatening or assaultive behavior of offenders diagnosed with delusional disorder (Kennedy *et al.*, 1992).

Personality Traits

Personality traits associated with violence include impulsivity, low frustration tolerance, and an inability to tolerate criticism. Such individuals are often self-centered, drive automobiles recklessly, and tend to dehumanize others (Reid & Balis, 1987).

Antisocial personality is heavily represented in offender populations, with rates as high as 45% in jail groups (Petrich, 1976). In contrast, the overall prevalence of Antisocial Personality Disorder in community samples is about 3% in males and about 1% in females (DSM-IV, p. 648; American Psychiatric Association, 1994). Criminals with antisocial personalities are much more likely to use violent and aggressive behavior (Hare & McPherson, 1984). Those with antisocial personalities typically commit violence with revenge as a motive, or during periods of heavy drinking. This violence is cold and calculating and lacks the emotionality common among nonpsychopaths (Williamson, Hare, & Wong, 1987). Antisocial personality disorder increases the risk of homicidal behavior in both men and women (Eronen, Hakola, & Tiihonen, 1996). A combination of low IQ and antisocial personality is particularly ominous (Heilbrun, 1990).

Substance Abuse

Violence is highly associated with drug and alcohol use. J. W. Swanson, Holzer, Ganju, and Jono (1990) demonstrated that individuals in the community with a pattern of drug or alcohol abuse are 12 times more likely to be violent than persons without such problems. When drugs or alcohol are combined with other psychopathology, the combination is more volatile than either alone. Alcohol intoxicated individuals are involved in the majority of violent crimes, including murders, assaults, sexual assaults, and family violence (Brain, 1986; Collins, 1981; Murdoch, Pihl, & Ross, 1990; Pernanen, 1976, 1981). PCP is the hallucinogen most strongly associated with violence (Budd & Lindstrom, 1982). Stimulants, such as amphetamines and cocaine, increase the risk of violence due to disinhibition, grandiosity, and a tendency toward paranoia (Honer, Gewirtz, & Turey, 1987).

The psychiatrist should note whether the offender has insight into how substance abuse has contributed to past acts of violence, and determine the offender's strategies for managing without drugs or alcohol during times of stress.

Weapons

The psychiatric examination should assess the offender's access to deadly weapons. According to recent data released from the Centers for Disease Control and Prevention (Gun deaths on rise, 1996), the proportion of homicides from gunfire in the United States jumped 18% in 10 years. Firearms are now used in almost three quarters of all homicides. The offender should be asked if he has ever owned a gun and if he owns one now. Did he ever threaten or injure a person with a gun? How recently was it acquired? Does he keep the gun loaded? Recently moving a gun may be an ominous sign. For example, if a paranoid individual has recently moved a handgun from a closet shelf to under the bed, he is at greater risk for killing someone in misperceived self-protection.

Stress

The examiner should inquire about the number and severity of personal stressors in the offender's life. It is helpful to know how the offender has coped with stressful events in the past. Does he act impulsively? Does he talk out problems or hold them inside, building up resentment until he is ready to "blow up?" Does the offender have supportive family or friends to help him cope with stress?

"Organic" Factors

Brain injury should be considered in the differential diagnosis of violent behavior. Bryant, Scott, Golden, and Tori (1984) found that brain-damaged prison inmates committed violent crimes more frequently than those without brain damage. Formerly normal individuals may develop explosive rages after a brain insult (Krakowski, Convit, Jaeger, Lin, & Volavka, 1989). Both delirium and dementia can lead to violence. Kalunian, Binder, and McNiel (1990) found that geriatric patients with organic brain disease were more assaultive than those with any other diagnosis. An association between aggression and epilepsy, especially partial complex seizures, has been noted, although this relationship remains controversial. (Devinsky & Bear, 1984; Pincus & Tucker, 1985).

The psychiatrist should carefully look for signs of cognitive impairment and brain damage. If a screening examination such as the mini-mental status examination (Folstein, Folstein, & McHugh, 1975) is abnormal, a more complete neuropsychological evaluation may be in order to determine the precise level of impairment (Strub & Black, 1993).

Medical illnesses associated with violent behavior include hypoxia, electrolyte imbalances, hepatic disease, renal disease, systemic infections, thyroid disease, and poisoning by heavy metals. Specific brain diseases that can result in violence include viral encephalitis, AIDS, tuberculosis, syphilis, fungal meningitis tumors, and Wilson's disease (Tardiff, 1992). One should suspect a physical etiology when persons engage in impulsive acts of aggression without adequate provocation. This is especially true when the behavior is inconsistent with their usual character style.

The offender should be evaluated for signs of intoxication. On physical examination, physiologic signs of intoxication include dysarthria (seen with alcohol, barbiturates, and phencyclidine [PCP]), incoordination and unsteady gait (seen with alcohol, barbiturates, and hallucinogens), nystagmus (seen with alcohol, barbiturates, and PCP), dilated pupils (seen with amphetamine, cocaine, hallucinogens, and anticholinergics), flushing (seen with alcohol), perspiration (seen with amphetamine, cocaine, and hallucinogens), dry skin and mucous membranes (seen with anticholinergics and antihistamines), tachycardia (seen with amphetamines, cocaine, hallucinogens, and anticholinergics), and elevated blood pressure (seen with amphetamines, cocaine, and PCP) (Reid & Balis, 1987).

Assessment of Violent Threats

All threats should be taken seriously and details fully elucidated. Understanding how a violent act will be carried out and the expected consequences for the offender helps in assessing the degree of danger. In addition, fully facing the consequences of his or her act may help the offender to elect an alternative coping strategy. For example, an offender may be focused on revenge against his wife due to her infidelity. When confronted with the likelihood of spending many years in prison, he may decide to leave his wife instead.

Offenders' threats are an important element to be taken into account in the process of assessing the likelihood of dangerous behavior. If threats are made in the context of longstanding delusional beliefs that have not been acted on over several years, the danger may be quite low. When an offender expresses a threat or homicidal ideas, the clinician ought to consider the following questions:

a. What is the magnitude of the intended harm?
b. Why is the threat being made now?
c. What does the threatener want?
d. How likely is the threat to induce violent behavior by the intended victim?
e. How serious is the intent behind the threat?
f. How developed is the plan for executing the violence?
g. Is the threat absolute and without alternative courses of action?
h. Is the threat based on likely or unlikely contingencies?
i. Does the offender have a lethal weapon in mind?
j. How available is the weapon of choice?
k. How accessible is the potential victim?
l. How soon is the offender likely to carry out his threat?
m. Has the offender already taken any action toward fulfillment of the threat?
n. Has the offender shown a recent decrease in his ability to control violent impulses?
o. Has the offender been violent under similar circumstances in the past?
p. Is the offender likely to be disinhibited by substance abuse?
q. Is the offender willing to undergo the consequences of his violent act?
r. Has the offender been able to form a therapeutic alliance with a therapist?

Civil Commitment

All psychiatrists are expected to be familiar with the civil commitment statutes in their state. Civil commitment statutes vary from one jurisdiction to another, but usually have several elements in common. Commitment statutes are based on the legal doctrines of *parens patriae* and the police power of the state. Under *parens patriae* the state may take responsibility for those who are unable to care for themselves. In recent years, however, the emphasis has been on police power, using civil commitment to prevent imminent harm to self or others (Appelbaum, 1994). In the end, physicians do not commit patients; they assist the court in deciding whether or not to commit.

In the United States, involuntary patients are entitled to be maintained in the least restrictive treatment environment (*Lake v. Cameron*, 1966; Slobogin,1994). Some states have provisions for outpatient civil commitment (R. D. Miller, 1988). Even if a state has an outpatient civil commitment statute, however, it may be difficult to enforce. In Ohio, for example, some county probate judges honor outpatient commitment while others restrict it to insanity acquittees.

The threshold question in civil commitment is the presence of mental illness, which is generally defined by statute. Some jurisdictions define the term more broadly than others. In Ohio, mental illness is defined as "a substantial disorder of thought, mood, perception, orientation or memory that grossly impairs judgement, behavior, capacity to recognize reality or ability to meet the ordinary demands of life" (Ohio Revised Code, 1989, p. 172). This is a fairly broad definition and allows for considerable latitude.

The first task in deciding whether an offender is eligible for civil commitment is determining whether the person actually has a mental illness. For practical reasons, persons who show equivocal signs of mental illness and a high potential for violence are usually admitted from emergency rooms to hospitals for a limited time. It is then the job of the inpatient psychiatrist to do a complete assessment. During this evaluation period, the psychiatrist must decide whether the admission is due to a true mental illness or to drugs, alcohol, antisocial behavior, or personality difficulties not related to mental illness. If the doctor concludes that there is no mental illness, the potentially violent individual cannot be kept in the hospital against his will.

Case Example

A 34-year-old homosexual man with AIDS and no prior psychiatric history was admitted after complaining of depression and suicidality. Neuropsychological testing showed no evidence of AIDS dementia. Shortly after admission, the patient was no longer depressed or suicidal. However, he was noted to be manipulative and theatrical. He told his psychiatrist in a very dramatic manner that the staff at another hospital in town had ignored his needs. He had thoughts of going back there with a gun and "shooting the place up." He said he did not need to be in the hospital and demanded to be discharged. A forensic consultation was requested. The consultant noted features of a personality disorder, but no evidence of psychosis. The patient said he had only been "kidding" when he had made the statement about shooting up the other hospital, but he remained upset with the staff there. He still wanted to be discharged, but agreed to outpatient therapy. The consultant offered the opinion that the patient was not civilly committable and recommended discharge with outpatient follow-up.

Civil commitment statutes usually require that due to the mental illness, a person be a danger to self or others, or be unable to care for his basic physical needs. There must be a causal relationship between the mental illness and any dangerousness. Thus, a schizophrenic offender would not be civilly commitable if his mental illness were in full remission, even if he intended to kill an acquaintance because of a gambling debt.

Release of Insanity Acquittees

For a thorough review of this issue, see Chapter 23 on release decision making. Insanity acquittees are usually retained in the hospital by the same civil commitment provisions that are used for nonforensic patients. However, the commitment criteria are often broadly construed to allow the courts to err on the side of community safety. This allows forensic patients at high risk for violent behavior to be kept in the hospital even after a lengthy period of remission of mental illness. However, the U.S. Supreme Court has held that insanity acquittees may not be detained in the hospital if they have no mental illness, even if they remain dangerous (*Foucha v. Louisiana*, 1992).

Insanity acquittees are usually released from the hospital on conditional release. They remain civilly committed to the hospital while being allowed to live in the community as the least restrictive treatment alternative (Slobogin, 1994). If patients violate the conditions of their release, they may be returned to the hospital by the court. Release plans for insanity acquittees include a variety of supports to ensure that the patient receives close follow-up care to minimize risk in the community.

Although this system sounds good in theory, limited resources make it difficult to implement in practice. For example, the hospital may recommend a 24-hour group home placement for a patient with poor insight, residual illness, and persistent problems with substance abuse. However, the county to which the individual is released may not have any 24-hour supervised group homes. Even if there are supervised group homes available, they may refuse to accept forensic patients because of bias. The hospital staff is then placed in the unenviable position of deciding whether to compromise on safety issues by recommending a less supervised setting, or offering the opinion that even though the patient no longer needs to be in the hospital, there is no available placement in the community. Economic pressures to decide one way or the other will vary, depending on who pays for the cost of hospital care.

The job of evaluating insanity acquittees for release is demanding and fraught with peril. If a released insanity acquittee subsequently commits a violent act, it reflects poorly on the hospital, the state department of mental health, and the judge who authorized the release. The story may be splashed across the headlines and create community outrage. Fingers are pointed and people ask, "How could you let someone out who had already proven himself to be violent?"

Although there is a substantial body of research literature concerning factors associated with an increased risk of violence, there is little guidance in the scientific literature about the actual process of making release decisions (Werner & Meloy, 1992). There have been some early attempts to develop standardized instruments, such as the Eisner Scale (Eisner,1989). Nonetheless, a certain level of risk is inherent in all release decisions. The psychiatrist can only point out the areas of danger and ways to minimize risk. The actual decision to release is a public policy issue reflecting the level of risk the community is willing to assume.

When evaluating patients for possible release, a psychiatrist should perform a thorough violence risk assessment. In addition, he should evaluate other areas of potential dangerousness, such as the risk of arson or sex offenses. The following specific factors should be considered:

a. The offense for which the person was found not guilty by reason of insanity (NGRI) may not truly reflect his potential danger. This is especially true when mental illness and psychopathy co-exist (Meloy, 1988). For example, an individual may have been found NGRI for a relatively trivial offense, but be intent on covert retribution against those he dislikes, due to his antisocial personality. Hence, the psychiatrist should have a detailed knowledge of an individual's past criminal history, including crimes unrelated to the NGRI offense.

Unfortunately, this information is sometimes difficult for mental health clinicians to obtain.

If an insanity acquittee is returned to the hospital after an assault resulting from antisocial tendencies, it becomes more difficult to make release decisions. The assault risk will remain even when the mental illness is in remission. Since psychopathy is generally not amenable to mental health intervention, no improvement can be expected. Nonetheless, the mental health providers are likely to be held responsible for any violent outcome. If such individuals are kept in the hospital for long periods of time, they often become predatory toward more vulnerable patients and cause severe disruption to the hospital milieu.

b. The psychiatrist should consider the risk of patients being absent without leave (AWOL), both in the hospital and on conditional release in the community. If an individual on conditional release fails to keep appointments and stops his medication, he may again become actively mentally ill and dangerous. One important reason that patients go AWOL from civil hospitals is a sense of hopelessness about having their release approved by the court.

c. Compliance with psychotropic medication is a significant factor in reducing violence in the community. Cohen, McEwen, Williams, Silver, and Spodak (1986) found that 36% of released insanity acquitees who took their medication regularly were readmitted to the hospital within 5 years of release, compared with 92% of those who did not comply with medication recommendations.

d. Long-term violence in the institution, or the absence of it, does not necessarily predict community violence (Monahan, 1981; Quinsey & Maguire, 1986).

e. Patients should demonstrate an ability to handle increasing levels of responsibility before conditional release. The following options are possible:
  • Transferring patients from a maximum security hospital to a civil setting. The risk of escape from the civil hospital should be assessed when this is done.
  • Transferring patients to a less structured ward within the hospital;
  • Allowing patients a variety of limited privileges on hospital grounds;
  • Allowing supervised community passes. In addition, one can vary the ratio of staff-to-patient supervision.
  • Allowing community passes supervised by responsible family members;
  • Lengthening the duration of passes.
  • Random screening in the hospital for the use of drugs and alcohol, especially on return from community passes

f. The patient's social support system in the community should be ascertained. Some research on this topic has produced counterintuitive findings, however. One study found that the more friends a released patient reported having in the community, and the more time he spent with those friends, the more likely he was to commit a violent act (Klassen & O'Connor, 1985). Thus, friends may function more as instigators of violence than as supports to prevent violence. Further, family members of persons with serious mental illness are at increased risk for being targets of violence (Estroff *et al.*, 1994).

g. The quality of aftercare should be considered. The ability of the community mental health agency to provide frequent and consistent case management supervision is vital (Dvoskin & Steadman, 1994). Responsible and knowledgeable staff must be available in group homes. They must be able to recognize signs of early decompensation, covert drug and alcohol use, and other potentially dangerous behavior (e.g., prostitution, gambling, and bringing unsavory acquaintances into the home). Inadequate supervision can be disastrous. One of the authors recently evaluated a case in which a group home employee provided cocaine to several group home residents in exchange for being allowed to film them raping another group home resident.

Probation

Psychiatrists may be called upon by judges prior to sentencing to evaluate defendants for possible probation rather than incarceration. Alternatively, probation officers may request evaluations directly to help them understand problems encountered in working with their probationers. Referral issues include assessment for the presence of mental illness, the need for immediate hospitalization, and the defendant's treatability and prognosis.

If a drug dependent offender is unwilling to enter a substance abuse program, the psychiatrist might point out that the man has a treatable substance abuse problem, but is a poor candidate for treatment due to his lack of insight and poor cooperation. It is not useful to recommend any form of treatment that is not actually available in the community. The defendant's ability to pay for treatment may determine eligibility for some programs. Many communities, for example, lack specialized treatment for sex offenders unless the individual can pay personally or through insurance.

In making treatment recommendations, the psychiatrist's job is to provide the court with data and possibilities, but not to try to influence the decision (Melton, Petrila, Poythress, & Slobogin, 1987). Thus, recommendations may be phrased, "If the court decides to grant probation, then . . ."

Special programs may be helpful in reducing recidivism in chronically mentally ill offenders. This population of patients is frequently readmitted to hospitals and jails. The two factors that contribute most to recidivism are noncompliance with psychotropic medications and substance abuse. Repeatedly sending such persons to jail helps little and adds to the stigma of all mentally ill persons.

Some mentally disordered offender programs have been successful in keeping chronically mentally ill persons both out of jail and out of the hospital. To be eligible for one such program in Cleveland, Ohio, the offender must have a psychotic disorder and a felony conviction. Offenders accepted into the program are placed on probation rather than in prison. The offender is jointly followed by a case manager from a mental health agency and a specially trained probation officer. Conditions of probation are similar to those required for patients on conditional release. The most common conditions are that the offender must take all prescribed medication, keep all appointments with mental health providers, and be subject to random alcohol and drug screens. If the offender violates a specified condition, he may be returned to jail.

Parole

Psychiatrists may be called upon to evaluate incarcerated defendants who are being considered for release from prison. The most common referral issues are (a) the need for civil commitment to a psychiatric hospital on the expiration of sentence; (b) a general prediction of dangerousness. Since psychiatrists are not able to reliably predict dangerousness (Resnick & Kausch, 1995), the preferred approach is to do a thorough risk assessment, noting possible interventions for dynamic risk factors. For those conditions not amenable to treatment, suggestions might still be made regarding provisions that may minimize the chances of harm to the community. The psychiatrist should not recommend for or against parole, leaving this decision to the correctional authorities.

Case Example

A psychiatrist evaluated an offender with schizophrenia who was well controlled with antipsychotic medication. He had a long history of documented pedophilic behavior. Still, he denied any sexual interest in children now or in the past, saying he had been "railroaded by the system." The psychiatrist pointed out the documented evidence supporting a sexual disorder and made a diagnosis of pedophilia in addition to the schizophrenia. He recommended that if the board saw fit to grant parole, the following conditions of parole should be imposed: The offender should live in a 24-hour supervised apartment, attend a weekly sex offender group, and submit to any medications recommended by the outpatient doctor, including possible injectable hormone medication in addition to his neuroleptic medication. The psychiatrist was informed by the outpatient team that no supervised beds were available due to funding cuts. The psychiatrist declined to change his recommendation due to the degree of risk.

As noted in the above example, the psychiatrist must maintain the integrity of his clinical judgment and not concede to political pressure based on financial considerations. While it is important to maintain a good relationship with community agencies and be open to alternate treatment plans, community safety must not be compromised. If there is a bad outcome after the psychiatrist agrees to alter his recommendation, it would be difficult to defend his actions in a resulting lawsuit.

Stalking

Stalking is a behavior rather than a diagnosis. Like other behaviors, it may be prompted by a variety of motivations and underlying conditions (McHugh & Slavney, 1983). Stalking is also an offense in most jurisdictions. California became the first state to enact a criminal law against stalking, in 1990, following several highly publicized homicides (Morin, 1993). Legally, the definition of stalking varies from one jurisdiction to another. Elements may include such behavior as following, loitering in the victim's vicinity, approaching the victim repeatedly, telephoning, sending letters, interfering with personal property, and threatening (Mullen & Pathe, 1994b). Another element in the legal definition may be an intention to cause distress or harm. The impact on the victim may also be specified (i.e., the behavior would cause a reasonable person, in the victim's circumstances, serious concern for his safety).

Crime categories such as Menacing by Stalking and Aggravated Trespassing permit police to make an arrest based on "reasonable cause" without requiring a warrant. In Ohio, for example, a written statement by the alleged victim is sufficient to demonstrate "reasonable cause."

Categories of Stalkers

Domestic Violence

The largest group of stalkers is ex-husbands and ex-lovers who refuse to accept the ending of the relationship, or who seek retribution for rejection or infidelity (Mullen & Pathe, 1994b). Although this population has not been well studied (Kurt, 1995), it appears that most of the psychopathology involves personality disorders and substance abuse disorders. In 1990, 30% of the 4,399 women killed in the United States were murdered by their boyfriends or husbands (B. Miller, 1993). In contrast, about 4% of the men killed were slain by girlfriends or wives. Approximately 90% of women killed by their husbands or boyfriends are stalked prior to their deaths (Morin, 1993).

A history of domestic violence is often present in these relationships. Typically, stalking occurs after the wife tries to break off the relationship. The husband is unwilling to accept the end of the relationship. He often has a history of being controlling, narcissistic, and jealous. He may follow and harass his ex-wife. He may send threatening letters. He may harass his estranged wife at work. He may break into her house and destroy her belongings. He may be violent toward her privately or in public. He may rape his ex-wife. He may harass or assault the ex-wife's new lover. The end result may be the murder of the ex-wife, and sometimes the suicide of the perpetrator (see, e.g., B. Miller, 1993).

A subgroup of these stalkers engages in workplace violence (Resnick & Kausch, 1995). Murder on the job is the leading cause of fatal injuries for women and the third leading cause for men. In one study, 16% of murders of women on the job were committed by spouses and other intimates, compared to 5% by coworkers (Levin, Hewitt, & Misner, 1992).

Erotomania

This condition is listed in *DSM-IV* as a delusional disorder (American Psychiatric Association, 1994). Kraepelin (1921) classified the disorder as a subtype of paranoia. The condition was originally described as a delusional belief, held by a woman, that a man of higher social station is secretly madly in love with her. Although she may have had only fleeting contact with him, she believes that he communicates with her through subtle means. Any disavowals of affection by the pursued are interpreted by the patient as a test of her love. When men suffer from erotomania (Taylor, Mehandra, & Gunn, 1983), they are more likely to be seen in forensic contexts (Goldstein, 1987).

Some authors have broadened the concept of erotomania to include a group of persons who have a preoccupying, morbid infatuation with the victim, in addition to those who have a delusion of being loved by the victim (Meloy, 1989). Segal (1990) suggested that this group is actually more prevalent than the delusional erotomanic group. Mullen and Pathe (1994a) provided a comprehensive summary of the diagnostic and nosological issues of morbid infatuation, and provided case examples that highlighted the dangerousness of these individuals.

Celebrities are often the target of erotomanics. Dietz, Matthews, Duyne, and colleagues (1991) found that 16% of 214 subjects who wrote to celebrities had erotomanic delusions. Eleven subjects believed they were married to the celebrity. Among 100 subjects who wrote to senators and congressmen, 5 had erotomanic delusions and 2 believed they were married to the politicians (Dietz, Matthews, Martell, *et al.*, 1991).

Violence can be a feature of erotomania and morbid infatuation. The violence may be directed toward (a) the beloved; (b) persons standing between the perpetrator and the beloved; (c) a symbolic third person, as in the case of John Hinckley (Caplan, 1987). In a letter written to the *New York Times* after he was acquitted by reason of insanity, Hinckley said: "My actions on March 30, 1981, have given special meaning to my life and no amount of imprisonment or hospitalization can tarnish my historical deed. . . . I . . . committed the ultimate crime in hopes of winning the heart of a girl. It was an unprecedented demonstration of love" (quoted in Goldstein, 1987, p. 269).

Pathological Jealousy

This condition is also classified in *DSM-IV* as a delusional disorder. The syndrome can be primary or secondary to other psychoses (Mooney, 1965). It has also been referred to as the "Othello Syndrome" (Todd & Dewhurst, 1955). The jealousy is irrational, rather than excessive. Onset can occur from the late teens to the 60s. Males predominate and are more likely to be homicidal and suicidal (Cobb, 1979). There is often coexisting alcohol dependence, and the jealousy is increased during periods of intoxication.

Case Example
A married man, 39 years old, was admitted to a mental hospital in May, 1951, as the direct result of disorderly behavior arising from delusions concerning his wife's fidelity. During the previous year, he had rendered his wife (a virtuous woman) miserable by repeatedly accusing her of infidelity on an enormous scale. He would use field glasses to spy on her from afar, and, after pretending to leave the house, he was wont to reenter surreptitiously in an attempt to trap her with a lover. Furthermore, he would search the house with meticulous care for evidence of her infidelity, and tax his children with aiding and abetting their mother in her lechery. He threatened several men in the neighborhood with violence because he suspected them of a liaison with his wife. . . . He often expressed regret that he could not make his wife perpetually pregnant to keep her "fully occupied," and spent half the night attempting to assuage (by one means or another) the insatiable lust with which he thought she was consumed. Moreover, he frequently threatened her with violence and once seized her by the throat. (Todd & Dewhurst, 1955)

Paraphilias

There are two ways in which paraphilias can be associated with stalking behavior. First, the stalking may facilitate the crime, or be a means of observing and choosing potential victims. Second, stalking may be a part of the erotic fantasy sequence that forms the core of the paraphilia. This fantasy may be acted out to enhance the sexual arousal of the paraphile.

Case Example
The patient is now 40 years old and of average intelligence (WAIS 108). He was admitted to a special hospital at the age of 25 following the murder of a

woman. . . . By the age of 16 his fantasy had come to include kidnapping the girls in order to take them to his imagined hideaway, there to torture them. His methods of kidnap included hypnosis chloroform, pretending to be invisible, and blows to the head to render them unconscious. At this age he began also to carry out several pieces of previously fantasized controlling behavior—snatching a girl's handbag, taking a female librarian's pen, and hiding a wooden Indian club in some rocks in order to "kidnap" an attractive girl on a route which he knew she took. From the age of 16 he would regularly follow girls in the street and he used the anxiety he produced in these girls as fantasy material for later self-masturbation. He said, "The climax of the fantasy would be when I caused the maximum amount of fear and disgust and I told her I would kill her or describe what I was going to do, or stabbing them." (MacCulloch, Snowden, Wood, & Mills, 1983)

Clinical Evaluation of Stalkers

Because the stalker may well try to pretend normality or allege coincidence, the psychiatrist should seek collateral sources of information and attempt to interview the victim. The evaluator should examine the past legal history, looking for a previous pattern of stalking behavior. This may include prior arrests for menacing, telephone harassment, or domestic violence. Evidence of a paraphilia may be gleaned from a history of sexual offenses. The examiner should review the psychiatric history, looking for stalking behavior as part of the illness pattern.

The psychiatrist should examine the usual risk factors for violence, such as past violence, paranoia, substance abuse, and access to lethal weapons. The evaluator should focus especially on:

a. Social isolation
b. The offender's ability to manage anger
c. The presence of depression, llingness to die, suicidality, and feelings that there is nothing to live for
d. Insight into the reality of the relationship, or lack of relationship, with the potential victim
e. Revenge fantasies
f. Grudges against the victim and any person standing between the victim and the offender
g. Jealous feelings
h. Dysfunctional personality traits, especially paranoia, narcissism, and antisocial features
i. Evidence of a paraphilia

Conclusion

The psychiatric evaluation of violent offenders requires a detailed knowledge of the risk factors associated with violence. Psychiatrists are especially skilled in examining those risk factors associated with mental illness and psychopathology. The referral issue will determine the focus and scope of the evaluation. Oliver Wendell Holmes observed, "Every year, if not every day, we have to wager our salvation upon some prophesy based upon imperfect knowledge." In performing psychiatric evaluations of violent offenders, we certainly have imperfect knowledge. Nonetheless, we provide an important service by doing careful evaluations to reduce the risk of violence in the community.

ACKNOWLEDGMENTS

Portions of this material are taken from Resnick, P. J., and Kausch, O. (1995). Violence in the workplace: Role of the consultant. *Consulting Psychology Journal: Practice and Research, 47*, 213–222. Copyright 1995 by the Educational Publishing Foundation and the Division of Consulting Psychology. Adapted with permission.

References

Amador, X. F., Straus, D. H., Yale, S. A., & Gorman, J. M. (1991). Awareness of illness in schizophrenia. *Schizophrenia Bulletin, 17*, 113–132.
American Psychiatric Association. (1994). *Diagnostic and statistical manual of mental disorders* (4th ed.). Washington DC: Author.
Appelbaum, P. S. (1994). *Almost a revolution* (pp. 17–70). New York: Oxford University Press.
Ball, E. M., Dotson, L. A., Brothers, L. T., Young, D., & Robbins, D. (1992, October). *Prediction of dangerous behavior*. Paper presented at the Annual Meeting of Psychiatry and the Law, Boston.
Binder, R. L., & McNiel, D. (1988). Effects of diagnosis and context on dangerousness. *American Journal of Psychiatry, 145*, 728–732.
Boxer, P. A. (1993). Assessment of potential violence in the paranoid worker. *Journal of Occupational Medicine, 35*, 127–131.
Brain, P. F. (1986). *Alcohol and aggression*. New York: Croom Helm.
Brown, P. (1985). *The transfer of care: Psychiatric deinstitutionalization and its aftermath*. London: Routledge & Kegan Paul.
Bryant, E. T., Scott, M. L., Golden, C. J., & Tori, C. D. (1984). Neuropsychological deficits, learning disability, and violent behavior. *Journal of Consulting and Clinical Psychology, 52*, 323–324.
Buchanan, A., Reed, A., Wessely, S., Garety, P., Taylor, P., Grubin, D., & Dunn, G. (1993). Acting on delusions: II. The phenomenonolgical correlates of acting on delusions. *British Journal of Psychiatry, 163*, 77–81.
Budd, R. D., & Lindstrom, D. M. (1982). Characteristics of victims of PCP-related deaths in Los Angeles County. *Journal of Clinical Toxicology, 19*, 997–1004.
Caplan. L. (1987). *The insanity defense and the trial of John W. Hinckley, Jr*. New York: Dell.
Cobb, J. (1979). Morbid jealousy. *British Journal of Hospital Medicine, 21*, 511–518.
Cohen, M., McEwen, J., Williams, K., Silver, S., & Spodak, M. (1986). *A base expectancy model for forensic release decisions*. Alexandria, VA: Research Management Associates.
Collins, J. J., Jr. (Ed.). (1981). *Drinking and crime*. New York: Guilford.
Devinsky, O., & Bear, D. (1984). Varieties of aggressive behavior in temporal lobe epilepsy. *American Journal of Psychiatry, 141*, 651–655.
Dietz, P. E., Matthews, D. B., Duyne, C. V., Martel, D. A., Parry, D. H., Stewart, T. M., Throuda, D. R., Warren, J., & Crowder, J. D. (1991). Threatening and otherwise inappropriate letters to Hollywood celebrities. *Journal of Forensic Sciences, 36*, 185–209.
Dietz, P. E., Matthews, D. B., Martell, D. A., Stewart, T. M., Hrouda, D. R., & Warren, J. (1991). Threatening and otherwise inappropriate letters to members of the United States Congress. *Journal of Forensic Sciences, 36*, 1445–1468.
D'Orban, P., & O'Connor, A. (1989). Women who kill their parents. *British Journal of Psychiatry, 154*, 27–33.
Dvoskin, J. A., & Steadman, H. J. (1994). Using intensive case management to reduce violence by mentally ill persons in the community. *Hospital and Community Psychiatry, 45*, 679–684.
Eisner, H. R. (1989). Returning the not guilty by reason of insanity to the community: A new scale to determine readiness. *Bulletin of the American Academy of Psychiatry and the Law, 17*, 401–413.

Eronen, M., Hakola, P., & Tiihonen, J. (1996). Mental disorders and homicidal behavior in Finland. *Archives of General Psychiatry, 53*, 497–504.

Estroff, S. E., & Zimmer, C. (1994). Social networks, social support, and violence. In J. Monahan, & H. J. Steadman (Eds.). *Violence and mental disorder*. Chicago: The University of Chicago Press, pp. 259–295.

Estroff, S. E., Zimmer, C., Lachicotte, W. S., & Benoit, J. (1994). The influence of social networks and social support on violence by persons with serious mental illness. *Hospital and Community Psychiatry, 45*, 669–679.

Folstein, M. F., Folstein, S. E., & McHugh, P. R. (1975). Mini-mental state: A practical method for grading the cognitive state of patients for the clinician. *Journal of Psychiatric Research, 12*, 189–198.

Foucha v. Louisiana. (1992). 112 S. Ct. 1780.

Goldstein, R. L. (1987). More forensic romances: De Clerambault's syndrome in men. *Bulletin of the American Academy of Psychiatry and the Law, 15*, 267–274.

Gun deaths on rise. (1996, June 7) *Cleveland Plain Dealer*, p. 12-A.

Hafner, H., & Boker, W. (1982). *Crimes of violence by mentally abnormal offenders: A psychiatric and epidemiological study in the Federal Republic of Germany*. Cambridge, England: Cambridge University Press.

Hare, R. D., & McPherson, L. M. (1984). Violent and aggressive behavior by criminal psychopaths. *International Journal of Law and Psychiatry, 7*, 35–50.

Heilbrun, A. B. (1990). The measurement of criminal dangerousness as a personality construct: Further validation of a research index. *Journal of Personality Assessment, 54*, 141–148.

Higgins, J. (1990). Affective psychoses. In R. Bluglass & P. Bowden (Eds.), *Principles and practice of forensic psychiatry*. Edinburgh, Scotland: Churchill Livingstone.

Honer, W. E., Gewirtz, E., & Turey, M. (1987). Psychosis and violence in cocaine smokers. *Lancet, 1*, 451.

Junginger, J. (1990). Predicting compliance with command hallucinations. *American Journal of Psychiatry, 147*, 245–247.

Junginger, J. (1995). Command hallucinations and the prediction of dangerousness. *Psychiatric Services, 46*, 911–914.

Junginger, J. (1996). Psychosis and violence: The case for a content analysis of psychotic experience. *Schizophrenia Bulletin, 22*, 91–103.

Kalunian, D. A., Binder, R. L., & McNiel, D. E. (1990). Violence by geriatric patients who need psychiatric hospitalization. *Journal of Clinical Psychiatry, 51*, 340–342.

Kennedy, H. G., Kemp, L. I., & Dyer, D. E. (1992). Fear and anger in delusional (paranoid) disorder: The association with violence. *British Journal of Psychiatry, 160*, 488–492.

Klassen, D., & O'Connor, W. (1988). Predicting violence in schizophrenic and nonschizophrenic patients: A prospective. *Journal of Community Psychology, 16*, 217–227.

Klassen, D., & O'Connor, W. A. (1988). A prospective study of predictors of violence in adult male mental health admissions. *Law and Human Behavior, 12*, 143–158.

Kraepelin, E. (R. M. Barkley, trans.). (1921). *Manic-depressive insanity and paranoia*. Edinburgh, Scotland: Livingston.

Krakowski, M., Convit, A., Jaeger, J., Lin, S., & Volavka, J. (1989). Neurologic impairment in violent schizophrenic patients. *American Journal of Psychiatry, 146*, 849–853.

Kurt, J. L. (1995). Stalking as a variant of domestic violence. *Bulletin of the American Academy of Psychiatry and the Law, 23*, 219–230.

Lake v. Cameron. (1966). 124 U.S. App. D.C. 264, 364 F. 2d 657.

Levin, P. F., Hewitt, J. B., & Misner, S. T. (1992). Female workplace homicides. *American Association of Occupational Health Nurses Journal, 40*, 229–236.

Link, B. G., & Stueve, C. A. (1994). Psychotic symptoms and the violent/illegal behavior of mental patients compared to community controls. In J. Monahan & H. Steadman (Eds.), *Violence and mental disorder: Developments in risk assessment* (pp. 137–159). Chicago: University of Chicago Press.

MacCulloch, M. J., Snowden, P. R., Wood, P. J. W., & Mills, H. E. (1983). Sadistic fantasy, sadistic behavior and offending. *British Journal of Psychiatry, 143*, 20–29.

McHugh, P. R., & Slavney, P. R. (1983). *The perspectives of psychiatry*. Baltimore: Johns Hopkins University Press.

Meloy, R. (1987). The prediction of violence in outpatient psychotherapy. *American Journal of Psychotherapy, 41*, 38–45.

Meloy, R. (1988). Violent and homicidal behavior in primitive mental states. *Journal of the Amererican Academy of Psychoanalysis, 16*, 381–394.

Meloy, R. (1989). Unrequited love and the wish to kill: Diagnosis and treatment of borderline erotomania. *Bulletin of the Menninger Clinic, 53*, 477–492.

Melton, G. B., Petrila, J., Poythress, N. G., & Slobogin, C. (1987). *Psychological evaluations for the courts*. New York: Guilford.

Miller, B. (1993, April 18). Stalking. *Chicago Tribune Magazine*, 14–20.

Miller, R. D. (1988). Outpatient civil commitment of the mentally ill: An overview and an update. *Behavioral Sciences & the Law, 6*, 99–118.

Monahan, J. (1981). *The clinical prediction of violent behavior* (DHHS Publication No. ADM81-921).Washington, DC: U.S. Government Printing Office.

Monahan, J. (1992). Mental disorder and violent behavior: Perceptions and evidence. *American Psychologist, 47*, 511–521.

Monahan, J. (1996). Violence prediction: The last 20 and the next 20 years. *Criminal Justice and Behavior.*

Mooney, H. B. (1965). Pathologic jealousy and psychochemotherapy. *British Journal of Psychiatry, 111*, 1023–1042.

Morin, K. S. (1993). The phenomenon of stalking: Do existing state statutes provide adequate protection? *San Diego Justice Journal, 1*, 123–162.

Mullen, P. E., & Pathe, M. (1994a). The pathological extensions of love. *British Journal of Psychiatry, 165*, 614–623.

Mullen, P. E., & Pathe, M. (1994b). Stalking and the pathologies of love. *Australia and New Zealand Journal of Psychiatry, 28*, 469–477.

Mulvey, E. P., & Lidz, C. W. (1984). Clinical considerations in the prediction of dangerousness in mental patients. *Clinical Psychology Review, 4*, 379–401.

Murdoch, D., Pihl, R. O., & Ross, D. (1990). Alcohol and crimes of violence: Present issues. *The International Journal of Addictions, 25*, 1065–1081.

Ohio Revised Code. (1989). 5122. 01(B).

Pernanen, K. (1976). Alcohol and crimes of violence. In B. Kissin & H. Begleiter (Eds.), *The biology of alcoholism* (Vol. 4, pp. 351–443). New York: Plenum.

Pernanen, K. (1981). Theoretical aspects of the relationship between alcohol use and crime. In J. J. Collins (Ed.), *Drinking and crime* (pp. 1–69). New York: Guilford.

Petrich, J. (1976). Rate of psychiatric morbidity in a metropolitan county jail population. *American Journal of Psychiatry, 133*, 1439–1444.

Pincus, J. H., & Tucker, G. J. (1985). Limbic systems & violence. In *Behavioral neurology*. 13th ed., (pp. 84–89). New York: Oxford University Press.

Quinsey, V., & Maguire, A. (1986). Maximum security psychiatric patients: Actuarial and clinical prediction of dangerousness. *Journal of Interpersonal Violence, 1*, 143–171.

Regier, D. A., Farmer, M. E., & Rae, D. S. (1991) Comorbidity of mental disorders with alcohol and other drug abuse: Results from the epidemiological catchment area (ECA) study. *Journal of the American Medical Association, 264*, 2511–2518.

Reid, W. H., & Balis, G. U. (1987). Evaluation of the violent patient. *American Psychiatric Association Annual Review, 6*, 491–509.

Resnick, P. J. (1969). Child murder by parents: A psychiatric review of filicide. *American Journal of Psychiatry, 126*, 73–83.

Resnick, P. J., & Kausch, O. (1995). Violence in the workplace: Role of the consultant. *Consulting Psychology Journal: Practice and Research, 47*, 213–222.

Segal, J. H. (1990). [Letter to the editor]. *American Journal of Psychiatry, 147*, 820–821.

Shah, S. A. (1978). Dangerousness: A paradigm for exploring some issues in law and psychology. *American Psychologist, 33*, 224–238.

Shields, N. M., McCall, G. J., & Hanneke, C. R. (1988). Patterns of family and nonfamily violence: Violent husbands and violent men. *Violence and Victim, 3*, 83–97.

Silva, J. A., Leong, G. B., & Weinstock, R. (1992). The dangerousness of persons with misidentification syndromes. *Bulletin of the American Academy of Psychiatry and the Law, 20*, 77–86.

Slobogin, C. (1994). Involuntary community treatment of people who are violent and mentally ill: A legal analysis. *Hospital and Community Psychiatry, 45*, 685–689.

Straznickas, K. A., McNeil, D. E., & Binder, R. L. (1993). Violence toward family caregivers by mentally ill relatives. *Hospital and Community Psychiatry, 44*, 385–387.

Strub, R. L., & Black, F. W. (1993). *The mental status examination in neurology* (3rd ed). Philadelphia: Davis.

Swanson, J., Borum, R., Swartz, M., & Monahan, J. (1996). *Criminal Behavior & Mental Health, 6*, 307–329.

Swanson, J. W., Holzer, C. E., Ganju, V. K., & Jono, R. T. (1990). Violence and psychiatric disorder in the community: Evidence from the epidemiologic catchment area surveys. *Hospital and Community Psychiatry, 41*, 761–770.

Tardiff, K. (1992). The current state of psychiatry in the treatment of violent patients. *Archives of General Psychiatry, 49,* 493–499.

Tardiff, K., & Sweillam, A. (1980). Assault, suicide, and mental illness. *Archives of General Psychiatry, 37,* 164–169.

Taylor, P., Mahendra, B., & Gunn, J. (1983). Erotomania in males. *Psychological Medicine, 13,* 645–650.

Todd, J., & Dewhurst, K. (1955). The Othello syndrome. *Journal of Nervous and Mental Disease, 122,* 367–374.

Torrey, E. F. (1994). Violent behavior by individuals with serious mental illness. *Hospital and Community Psychiatry, 45,* 653–662.

Wack, R. C. (1993). The ongoing risk assessment in the treatment of forensic patients on conditional release status. *Psychiatric Quarterly, 64,* 275–293.

Werner, P. D., & Meloy, J. R. (1992). Decision making about dangerousness in releasing patients from long-term psychiatric hospitalization. *The Journal of Psychiatry & Law, 20,* 35–47.

Wessely, S., Buchanan, A., & Reed, A. (1993). Acting on delusions: I. Prevalence. *British Journal of Psychiatry, 163,* 69–76.

Wessely, S. C., Castle, D., & Douglas, A. J. (1994) The criminal careers of incident cases of schizophrenia. *Psychological Medicine, 24,* 483–502.

Williamson, S., Hare, R. D., & Wong, S. (1987). Violence, criminal psychopaths and their victims. *Canadian Journal of Behavioral Science, 19,* 454–462.

The Neuropsychology of Aggression

Katrina R. Rayls and Wiley Mittenberg

Introduction

Neuropsychology is the study of the relationship between brain function and behavior. More specifically, the clinical neuropsychologist attempts to determine the biological understructure of specific behaviors by assessing changes in emotion, cognition, and personality that occur as a result of brain pathology. By utilizing standardized neuropsychological tests to examine brain functions, the clinical neuropsychologist can diagnose the type, location, and velocity of central nervous system disease and, more important, address the effect that such a disease has on a patient's adaptive capabilities.

In addressing the neuropsychology of aggressive behavior, it is important to note that some degree of aggressive behavior is necessary to survive in the environment and, like most other survival skills, is represented both neuroanatomically and chemically (Elliott, 1992). It is therefore likely that neurologic dysfunction in the neuroanatomical structures concerned with aggression can lead to dysfunction in the presentation of aggressive behavior or violent behavior (Volkow & Tancredi, 1987). This reasoning is supported by the observation that aggressive and violent behaviors are common in patients with neurological disorders (Silver & Yudofsky, 1987).

Violent behavior can be caused by a variety of factors including environmental stressors, mental illness, substance abuse, brain dysfunction, or a combination of these (Langevin, Ben-Aron, Wortzman, Dickey, & Handy, 1987). In the field of psychology, brain dysfunction is too frequently overlooked as a possible contributing factor in violent behavior (Bach-y-Rita, Lion, & Climent, 1971). It is, however, imperative to determine whether brain dysfunction is underlying the aggressive behavior for several reasons. These include the impact such dysfunction has on treatment, the prediction of future violence potential, and the determination of insanity or incompetence to stand trial. Neuropsychological assessment of individuals who have

Katrina R. Rayls • Department of Psychiatry, Medical University of South Carolina, Charleston, South Carolina 29401. *Wiley Mittenberg* • Center for Psychological Studies, Nova Southeastern University, Fort Lauderdale, Florida 33314.
Handbook of Psychological Approaches with Violent Offenders: Contemporary Strategies and Issues, edited by Van Hasselt and Hersen. Kluwer Academic/Plenum Publishers, New York, 1999.

expressed violent behavior can assist in diagnosis, location of the underlying neuropathology, and determination of prognosis.

Because of the multiple neuroanatomic bases of aggressive behavior, and the diversity of pathologies that may affect these structures, both brain structure and function must be examined to gain an understanding of the neuropsychology of aggression and violence.

Functional Neuroanatomy of the Central Nervous System

Frontal Lobe

The frontal lobe is the largest of all of the lobes of the brain and comprises about one third of the hemispheric surface (Carpenter, 1991). In an evolutionary sense, the frontal lobes are the last brain area to have developed (Lezak, 1995). In accordance with this, analogous structures are frequently much smaller or absent in lower mammals. The frontal lobes are slow to mature developmentally and slow to attain full functional capacity (Majovski, 1989). Due to the slow process of neuronal migration full structural and functional development is not concluded until early adulthood. In young children, this immaturity is commonly responsible for the inability to obey certain verbal instructions or inhibit behaviors (Majovski, 1989). Such behaviors parallel those seen in patients with frontal lobe dysfunction.

The three principal divisions of the frontal lobes are the precentral region, the premotor region, and the prefrontal region (including the orbital frontal cortex). The primary division of interest in the understanding of aggressive behavior is the prefrontal region. This area of the frontal lobe appears to be responsible for behavioral inhibition, attention, and emotional states (Kolb & Whishaw, 1990). As mentioned earlier, the frontal lobes are more prominent in the human nervous system but less evolved or nonexistent in lower mammals. In such lower mammals, instinctual behavior prevails and little control is manifested over innate impulses. The frontal lobes, connected to underlying instinctual and emotional centers, allow humans to monitor or modulate emotional states and behaviors (Fuster, 1980).

Parietal Lobe

The parietal lobe is the region of the cerebral cortex underlying the parietal skull bone. Generally, the right parietal lobe is specialized for visuospatial evaluation including depth perception, orientation in space, or visual perception of common or familiar objects (Kolb & Whishaw, 1990). The left parietal lobe is specialized for language functions such as writing, reading, arithmetic, and fluent speech. Because of these specialized functions, the parietal lobe is not involved in the central nervous system's role in aggressive behavior. However, the parietal region is often affected in disorders that are associated with aggression such as Alzheimer's dementia (see later section).

Temporal Lobe

In an evolutionary sense, the temporal lobe and its underlying structures are the oldest part of the human brain (Kolb & Whishaw, 1990). The outer surface, or temporal cortex, is responsible for auditory sensation and perception, storage of verbal and visual memories, language, and affective comprehension. The underlying structures of the temporal lobe, commonly referred to as the limbic system, are highly similar in humans and lower mammals. These structures are associated with such functions as memory mediation and emotional responsiveness (Elliott, 1987; Kolb & Whishaw, 1990; Lezak, 1995).

The Limbic System

The limbic system is composed of several distinct but connected structures. One such structure, the hippocampus, has a primary role in memory functioning and does not appear to directly influence aggressive behavior. The amygdala, another structure in the limbic system, does seem to have a direct relationship to aggressive behavior. Evidence for this comes from numerous human and nonhuman studies. Electrical stimulation of the amygdala most frequently results in aroused attention, fear, rage, and aggressive reactions (Carpenter, 1991). Stimulation or destruction of the amygdala also has an effect on norepinephrine levels in the brain. Drug studies examining the effects of norepinephrine levels on behavior indicate that it is closely associated with aggressive behavior (Eichelman, 1987). Surgical removal of the amygdala in both animals and humans consistently produces disturbances of emotional behavior. The most common symptoms of amygdala removal are known collectively as the Kluver–Bucy syndrome. These include placidity and an absence of fear, rage, or aggression, hypersexuality, hyperorality, and social initiation (Carpenter, 1991; Kolb & Whishaw, 1990). Bilateral lesions which can occur with diseases such as herpes simplex encephalitis or trauma produce similar symptoms (Elliott, 1992; Greenwood, Bhalla, Gordon, & Roberts, 1983; Lezak, 1995).

Based on these observations, amygdalectomy, or surgical removal of the amygdala, has been performed in over 500 cases across several countries for the treatment of violent criminals. In Japan, India, Thailand, and Sweden, 134, 132, 100, and 50 cases have been reported, respectively. This surgery has been demonstrated to be adequately effective in reducing aggressive behavior, with a success rate of 75% to 85% (Goldstein, 1974). This surgery, however, also frequently results in the emergence of Kluver–Bucy syndrome and is not favored in the United States.

Another neural structure located subcortically and connected to the amygdala is the hypothalamus. The hypothalamus is related to and serves to regulate many visceral activities. Autonomic functions such as water balance, weight regulation, temperature regulation, sugar and fat metabolism, and sleep–wake cycles are all related to hypothalamic processes (Carpenter, 1991). Disruption in the functioning of, or destruction in this area causes an imbalance in drive states resulting in such symptoms as anorexia, hyperphagia, or impaired sleep–wake cycles. Thus, the hypothalamus may play a role in eating and sleeping disorders.

The hypothalamus controls many sympathetic and parasympathetic responses through its many connections to other subcortical and cortical regions. Stimulation of this region results in increased metabolic and somatic activities characteristic of emotional stress, combat, or flight. Lesions in this region, or interruption of the cortical connections with the hypothalamus, reliably induce unprovoked rage attacks in humans and other animals (Goldstein, 1974).

In the surgical studies described earlier, the damage or stimulation is anatomically precise, affecting only very specific areas. Damage to the human brain due to trauma or disease, however, more typically involves whole regions, such as the temporal or frontal lobes. Two behavioral syndromes are described in the *Manual of the International Classification of Diseases and Related Health Problems* (World Health Organization [WHO], 1992) and are associated with an increased probability of criminal violence: orbital-frontal lobe syndrome and temporal lobe syndrome.

Abnormalities Related to Aggressive and Violent Behaviors

Orbital-Frontal Lobe Syndrome

The orbital or basal frontal cortex plays an important role in the inhibition of impulses and emotions. (Kolb & Whishaw, 1990; Lezak, 1995; Malloy, Bihrle, Duffy, & Cimino, 1993). Personality changes are predominant when this area is damaged but gross cognitive functions such as intelligence may remain intact (Silver, Hales, & Yudofsky, 1992). These personality changes are collectively referred to as orbital-frontal lobe syndrome and frequently produce impulsivity and a release of emotional impulses including violent or aggressive behaviors in response to trivial irritations (Cummings, 1985; Silver & Yudofsky, 1987; Silver et al., 1992). These patients routinely display a lack of foresight or planning that can lead to a failure to appreciate the consequences of their behavior.

Inadequate utilization of feedback from the environment to monitor behavior is typically observed in patients with frontal lobe damage (Kolb & Whishaw, 1990). Perseveration, or the senseless repetition of stereotyped behavior, is also a common manifestation of frontal lobe syndrome. This phenomenon is observed on standardized tests such as the Wisconsin Card Sorting Test and Verbal Fluency tests. The patient will often report mistakes in the face of continuous corrective feedback and may even verbalize that their responses are wrong but continue to make errors (Kolb & Whishaw, 1990; Majovski, 1989; Milner, 1964). There is an apparent disconnection between language and behavior; thus, environmental feedback fails to inhibit behavior (Lezak, 1995). In violent criminal behavior, perseveration can take the form of senselessly repetitive stabbings or gunshots (Elliott, 1992).

Blumer and Benson (1975) have suggested that patients with orbital-frontal lobe damage tend to exhibit what they have termed "pseudopsychopathology." These patients exhibit such symptoms as disinhibition, uncharacteristic lewdness, sexual promiscuity, and increased motor behavior (Kolb & Whishaw, 1990; Silver & Yudofsky, 1987; Silver et al., 1992). They often display apathy, irritability, dyscontrol of anger or aggressive behavior, or an exacerbation of preexisting behavioral traits. They may present a lack of concern for the consequences of their behavior by demonstrating increased risk taking, unrestrained use of drugs or alcohol, indiscriminate selection of foods, and gluttony (Lezak, 1995; Silver & Yudofsky, 1987; Silver et al., 1992). Several published case histories demonstrate these behavioral and personality abnormalities. The most widely cited is that of Phineas Gage, first reported by Harlow in 1868 (Kolb & Whishaw, 1990). An explosion sent an iron bar through the front of his head affecting only his frontal lobes. His behavior reportedly changed after the accident from "average and persistent" to "impulsive and audacious" (Blumer & Benson, 1975).

On standardized tests, orbital-frontal damage most commonly results in disorientation to time and memory impairments. Attentional abilities are often reduced.

The patient may also display anosmia, or the inability to smell, due to damage to the olfactory nerves which run underneath the orbital-frontal regions (Kolb & Whishaw, 1990). This symptom may first appear as an inability to taste food. As mentioned earlier, intelligence may often remain intact following injury to the frontal-orbital region; however, more sophisticated and sensitive neuropsychological tests will detect other forms of cognitive damage.

Temporal Lobe Syndrome

The second major syndrome associated with uncontrollable aggression is the temporal lobe syndrome. Damage to the temporal lobes frequently involves the underlying subcortical structures including the amygdala and the hypothalamus. As discussed earlier, damage in this area may result in unprovoked rage or exaggerated anger in reaction to minimal frustration or provocation. For example, in *Torsney v. the City of New York* (1979) (Beresford, 1980), a New York policeman shot and killed an unarmed boy. At the trial, a forensic psychiatrist successfully demonstrated that the policeman had suffered a temporal lobe seizure which grossly interfered with his functioning. Further, because he was not aware of wrongdoing at the time of the crime, the policeman could not be held accountable for his conduct (Beresford, 1980). Another case example of this type of compulsive aggression is the case of Charles Whitman. He had a compulsion to take a gun into a tower in Austin, Texas, and kill people. He recorded this compulsion in his diary and told his psychiatrist about it. So that they would not be saddened by what he was about to do, he killed his mother and wife before acting on his compulsion. He killed 13 people before being shot by police. He was found on postmortem examination to have a temporal lobe glioma, a specific type of rapidly growing brain tumor, located in the temporal lobe (Elliott, 1987).

Given the legal responsibilities of psychologists with potentially dangerous patients, knowledge of such potential organic factors is essential (Hamstra, 1987). Psychologists are required to protect third parties from violence by their patients, and failure to do so may result in legal action against the psychologist. For example, in a 1985 Supreme Court case, *Peck v. the Counseling Service of Addison County*, the therapist was held liable for failing to warn a patient's father about property destruction (Stone, 1986). The patient suffered from temporal lobe epilepsy and burned down his father's barn after informing the therapist of his nebulous intentions. The therapist felt confident that the patient would not act out his anger, and was successfully sued by the patient's father. These cases demonstrate an obvious need for psychologists to understand and consider the presence of organic dysfunction in order to recommend the appropriate patient treatment, medical or otherwise. This understanding and consideration is also imperative when making decisions regarding the prediction of dangerousness in patients who have expressed aggressive ideation.

On formal examination, temporal lobe syndrome is characterized by impairment of memory and intelligence. Psychiatric symptoms, such as auditory or visual hallucinations, are also common in these patients. The temporal lobes contain primary and secondary auditory and visual association areas (Carpenter, 1991). Damage to these areas may result in erroneous activation of auditory or visual memories that are stored in the temporal lobes or perceptive distortions in stimuli (Lezak, 1995). Such malfunctions may produce unusual auditory or visual perceptions that are difficult to distinguish from those reported by psychiatric patients experiencing hallucinations.

Other psychiatric symptoms, such as paranoia, anxiety, and associated delusions, also commonly occur as a result of temporal lobe damage. These symptoms frequently occur between seizures, interictally, in patients with temporal lobe epilepsy (Koch-Weser, Garron, & Gilley, 1988). Panic attacks may also be associated with abnormal electrical activity in the temporal lobe, and are effectively treated with anti-seizure drugs (e.g., Xanax).

Temporal and frontal lobe syndromes can result from a variety of neuropathological processes. In order to identify violence that has a neuropychologic basis it is necessary to appreciate the more prevalent disorders that lead to aggressive behavior.

Head Trauma

Head trauma is the most frequent cause of brain damage in the United States (Kurtzke, 1984). One of the most frequent causes of head trauma is injury sustained in motor vehicle accidents (Silver *et al.*, 1992), which frequently results in contusions to frontal, temporal, and subcortical regions. These areas are most susceptible to damage, primarily because of the nature of the swift impact against the bones of the skull. As discussed earlier, damage to these areas of the brain commonly results in behavioral and mood disturbances, frequently agitation and aggression (Franzen & Lovell, 1987; Kwentus, Hart, Peck, & Kornstein, 1985).

The immediate effects of a concussion are apparent during hospitalization. Patients commonly display a period of acute confusion shortly after they return to consciousness; this confusion can last from days to weeks (Lezak, 1995); it is frequently characterized by incoherence, uncooperativeness, motor restlessness, agitation, incomprehension, and resistive and assaultive behavior (Eames, 1990). Posttraumatic aggression or agitation is extremely common, and is most often a result of frontal and subcortical temporal damage (Franzen & Lovell, 1987). Longer periods of unconsciousness and memory impairment predict more severe agitation (Fichera, Mittenberg, Zielinski, Rayls, & Tremont, 1995). Further, patients who display aggressive behavior immediately following the injury are more likely to be irritable, violent, disinhibited, and emotionally labile after recovery due to permanent orbital frontal and subcortical damage, (Fichera *et al.*, 1995).

The long-term emotional and behavioral deficits that result from head injury can be severely debilitating and can affect every area of social activity, work activity, and relations with family members. In a study investigating the long-term effects of head injury, Thomsen (1984) found that 65% to 80% of patients with severe head injuries had personality changes that persisted for up to 15 years postinjury and affected the patient's ability to hold jobs for any length of time, interact appropriately with others, and resume their previously held role in the family. The aggressive tendencies of these patients may even be acted out on family members. For example, Rosenbaum and Hoge (1989) found that of 31 consecutive male patients referred for wife battering, 61.3% had histories of severe head injury. This rate far exceeds the prevalence of head injuries in the population at large, suggesting a strong link between head injury and aggressive behavior (Rosenbaum & Hoge, 1989).

Because of their injuries and the resulting emotional and behavior disturbances, namely aggression, these patients may later find their way into the criminal justice system. For example, Lewis, Pincus, Feldman, Jackson, and Bard (1986) examined a sample of death row inmates in five different states. All of the 15 inmates examined had histories of severe head injuries due to trauma including automobile accidents, physical batterings, and falls (Lewis *et al.*, 1986). In another study, 14 juveniles were examined who were condemned to death in the United States in 1986 (Lewis *et al.*, 1988). A history of head trauma was found in all 14. These results suggest that criminal violence is often a result of central nervous system dysfunction. Such dysfunction, however, is often overlooked as a contributing factor in criminal violence cases. The identification of neuropsychological impairment may constitute a mitigating factor in sentencing, determination of insanity at the time of the crime, or decisions regarding the ability of the offender to aid in his own defense (Lewis *et al.*, 1986). History alone is not sufficient to constitute a mitigating factor, due to the wide range of possible injuries and residual deficits. However, neuropsychological examination can objectively document the presence or absence of frontal or temporal lobe syndromes that result from head trauma and may be essential in the determination of criminal insanity, criminal responsibility, and rehabilitative prognosis in such patients.

Epilepsy

Epilepsy is an excessive, uncontrolled discharge of electrical impulses from neurons in the brain associated with a disturbance of consciousness (Adams & Duchen, 1992). Epilepsy is a symptom rather than a disease and may be caused by any of a large number of neuropathological processes such as head injury, vascular disorder, brain tumors, infections such as encephalitis and neurosyphilis, or toxic reaction (Bigler, 1988; Kolb & Whishaw, 1990; Reitan & Wolfson, 1992). Seizure disorders are classified as idiopathic when they appear to arise spontaneously and in the absence of other central nervous system dysfunction.

Abnormal, excessive, electrical discharges in the brain, occurring in epileptic patients, can lead to unprovoked stimulation of the structures discussed earlier, including the orbital-frontal lobe, amygdala, and hypothalamus, and this results in aggressive or violent behavior. Stimulation of these structures most commonly occurs due to temporal lobe epilepsy. Grand mal and petit mal seizures, which are generalized, may also result in stimulation of these structures due to the widespread electrical discharge of this type of seizure over the entire brain. Temporal lobe epilepsy, grand mal, or petit mal seizures can result from any of the causes of epilepsy just mentioned. Further, children who exhibit petit mal (absence seizures), or akinetic seizures (drop attacks) often develop temporal lobe epilepsy or grand mal seizures as adults (Bennett & Krein, 1989). Electrical activity in the brain is abnormal in epileptic patients between seizures as well as during the seizure, and their behavior may reflect this abnormality.

Patients with epilepsy involving the temporal lobes demonstrate a variety of pathological behaviors such as irritability, anger outbursts, obsessional traits, and verbosity (Bear, Levin, & Blumer 1982; Waxman & Geschwind, 1975). According to Lezak (1995), every type of behavioral disorder occurs with greater frequency in epileptic patients than in the general population. These patients often display organically based psychiatric disorders including auditory or visual hallucinations and delusions. Electrical activity in the temporal lobes also mimics the symptoms of such psychiatric disorders as schizophrenia and manic-depression, making epilepsy a vital differential diagnosis in these cases (Lezak, 1995). Neuropsychological testing can document dysfunction of the temporal lobes. Test results will reveal memory impairment, intellectual reduction, attentional impairment, and other neuropsychological symptoms (Dodrill, 1981).

Alzheimer's Disease

Alzheimer's disease is a brain disorder characterized by a progressive dementia that occurs in middle or late life. The disease affects an estimated 7% of the population ages 65 and older (Terry & Katzman, 1983). Pathologic characteristics of Alzheimer's disease include degeneration of specific nerve cells in the brain and the presence of neuritic plaques and neurofibrillary tangles, most predominantly in the temporal and parietal lobes (Mckahn *et al.*, 1984). These patients frequently exhibit organically based behavioral disturbances, emotional disorders, and personality changes which tend to advance in severity as the disease progresses.

Aggression is one of the behavioral disturbances commonly reported by the caregivers of Alzheimer's disease patients (Rubins, Mace, & Lucas, 1982). In a recent study of 170 Alzheimer's disease patients, Deutsch, Bylsma, Rovner, Steele, and Folstein (1991) reported that episodes of physical aggression occurred in 30% of cases, and that these incidents of violent behavior were significantly associated with the presence of hallucinations and delusions. Further, the authors found that psychotic symptoms, hallucinations, and delusions occur in 40% of all Alzheimer's disease patients. The authors conclude that Alzheimer's disease patients may become aggressive because of mistaken beliefs, or delusions of persecution, reference, or jealousy (Deutsch *et al.*, 1991).

On neuropsychological examination, Alzheimer's disease is recognized by the presence of memory impairment, due to temporal lobe dysfunction, and intellectual reduction (Mckahn *et al.*, 1984). Other common symptoms that will be apparent on examination include an inability to name common objects, copy geometric designs, or perceive depth; symptoms associated with the degeneration of the parietal lobes.

Metabolic Conditions

Metabolic activity in various regions of the brain reflect the functional activity of separate neuronal systems (Carpenter, 1991). Violent behavior has been associated with certain metabolic abnormalities in the central nervous system, most recognizably, endocrine system dysfunction. Aggressive behavior is related to changes in hormonal levels, and has been specifically linked to alterations in sexual hormonal quantities. In women, this is most strikingly seen during the premenstrual phase (Goldstein, 1974). The behavioral pattern commonly observed, which includes verbal or physical violence, is termed premenstrual syndrome, and in a minority of women results in attacks of rage (Elliott, 1987). Several studies have investigated the link between violent crimes and premenstrual syndrome and found that anywhere from 40% to 80% of women charged with violent crimes committed their offenses during the premenstrual week (Cummings, 1985; Elliott, 1987; Goldstein, 1974).

Other metabolic conditions have been connected to violent behavior including hypoglycemia, elevated testosterone levels, Sanfilippo syndrome, Speilmeyer–Vogt syndrome, and phenylketonuria (Elliott, 1987; Goldstein, 1974). In a study by Volkow and Tancredi (1987), 4 psychiatric patients with a history of violent behavior were evaluated using electroencephalogram (EEG), computed tomography (CT scan), and positron emission tomography (PET). Three of these patients showed EEG abnormalities, 2 showed CT scan abnormalities, and all 4 of these cases showed evidence of blood flow and metabolic abnormalities using the PET scan. These results demonstrate the difficulty and complexity of detecting central nervous system dysfunction and indicate that brief psychiatric or neurologic screenings may not result in accurate or beneficial results. Neuropsychological examination can aid in the determination of metabolic dysfunction by detecting global mental disturbances, particularly those involving attentional and memory functions, reasoning, and judgment abilities (Lezak, 1995).

Developmental Disorders

Aggressive activity is sometimes noted in both mentally retarded patients and adults suffering from Attention-Deficit/Hyperactivity Disorder (Cummings, 1985; Silver & Yudofsky, 1987). A survey of mentally retarded patients over the age of 40 found that behavior disorders, most often verbal abusiveness or aggression toward self, others, and objects, were the most standard problems and were of a persistent nature (Day, 1985). Studies examining adults who began suffering from Attention-Deficit/Hyperactivity Disorder as children reveal that an abnormally large number are involved in delinquent behavior or develop sociopathic or explosive personality disturbances (Wender, Reimherr, & Wood, 1981). Based on these findings, it appears that developmental disorders represent another group of diagnoses that should be considered when examining a patient who has exhibited violent behavior.

An exhaustive evaluation is necessary to diagnose the presence of central nervous system dysfunction that may be precipitating violent or aggressive behavior. It is meaningful to examine neurobehavioral history, neuropsychological test results, and laboratory test results.

Diagnosis

In the evaluation of patients who exhibit violent behavior, it is imperative to first obtain a thorough neurobehavioral history. As discussed earlier, significant neurologic histories are often overlooked. Obviously, one should inquire about neurologic disease such as epilepsy or brain tumor. However, the examiner should be especially attentive to histories of trauma or insult, developmental difficulties earlier in life, or general medical conditions that may lead to neurologic dysfunction.

The neuropsychological correlates of brain pathology are well established based on the deficits observed in patients with brain dysfunction. Therefore, neuropsychological testing is particularly important in determining if impaired central nervous system functioning is related to the person's abnormal behavior. A complete examination of cognitive functions requires multiple assessment measures to survey many discrete functional areas including intelligence and memory, as well as more specific functions such as sensation, perception, language, learning, attention, concept formation, and judgment. Tests may be chosen to examine specific areas of interest. For example, the Wechsler Memory Scale–Revised may be used to assess memory functions, or the Wisconsin Card Sort Test may be employed to examine frontal lobe functioning. Test batteries such as the Halstead–Reitan Battery and the Luria–Nebraska Test Battery that include a variety of specific subtests, are also commonly utilized.

Regardless of the diagnostic procedures chosen, the results serve to diagnose the presence of cortical dysfunction and to provide an accurate and unbiased estimate of the person's cognitive capacity (Kolb & Whishaw, 1990). This information, then, is used to facilitate patient care and to uncover neuropsychological syndromes that otherwise may have been disregarded.

Laboratory tests also play a vital role in the diagnosis and understanding of violent behavior. Electroencephalography (EEG) is used to detect abnormal electrical activity that leads to the stimulation of brain areas that contribute to violent behavior. Brain imaging techniques, most commonly computed tomography (CT) and magnetic resonance imaging (MRI), play a significant part in discovering the etiologies of behavioral disorders including space occupying lesions, vascular disease, and degenerative processes (Daniel, Zigan, & Weihberger, 1992). Newly developed techniques such as positron emission tomography (PET), which provides information on glucose metabolism, may also prove valuable in determining sources of dysfunction (Hamstra, 1987). Unfortunately, although these tests are able to identify many brain abnormalities, they are not yet reliable in the detection of microscopic lesions or functional deficits that may arise as a result of unobservable damage. Therefore, it is imperative to evaluate a patient utilizing a combination of procedures including neurobehavioral history, neuropsychological testing, and laboratory tests.

Two psychiatric diagnoses are applicable to patients who exhibit violent behavior due to brain disease. These are detailed in the *Diagnostic and Statistical Manual of Mental Disorders*, 4th edition (*DSM-IV*; American Psychiatric Association, 1994). Personality Change Due to a General Medical Condition, Aggressive Type (diagnostic code 310.1) is characterized by a persistent personality disturbance that is due to the direct physiological effects of a medical condition. Frequent symptoms include affective instability, poor impulse control, outbursts of rage, and aggression grossly out of proportion to any precipitant. These patients tend to exhibit labile mood and may express paranoid ideation. Personality Change Due to a General Medical Condition, Aggressive Type can be caused by a variety of neurological conditions including head trauma, epilepsy, Alzheimer's disease, endocrine disorders affecting the central nervous system, or any other brain disease that affects the orbito-frontal or subcortical temporal areas.

Intermittent Explosive Disorder (diagnostic code 312.34) is characterized by the occurrence of discrete episodes of failure to resist aggressive impulses that result in serious assaultive acts or destruction of property. The degree of aggressiveness expressed during an episode is clearly out of proportion to the stressor, and there are no signs of generalized impulsiveness or aggressiveness between episodes. This diagnosis can be made only after other disorders that may cause aggressive behavior are ruled out (e.g., Borderline Personality Disorder, Conduct Disorder, Manic Episode, and Antisocial Personality Disorder). Intermittent Explosive Disorder may be associated with a history of neurologic conditions or developmental difficulties.

With regard to medico-legal issues, patients diagnosed with Personalty Change Due to a General Medical Condition, Aggressive Type or Intermittent Explosive Disorder may be incompetent to stand trial. For example, in the state of Florida competency to stand trial requires an understanding by the person of what they are accused of and of the legal process, the ability to disclose the facts of the alleged crime and cooperate with their attorney, the ability to assist in preparing a defense and to challenge prosecution witnesses, and the ability to behave appropriately in court. Patients with neuropsychological impairments including intellectual impairment, memory impairment, or reasoning and judgment difficulties may be considered incompetent by this legal definition.

In the question of competency to stand trial, it must further be established that the patient may not be restored to competency at a later time following the appropriate medical treatment or sufficient recovery period. For example, cognitive impairments following head trauma may continue for up to 2 to 3 years; however, any residual impairments remaining after this time are considered permanent (Kolb & Whishaw, 1990). If the patient's deficits are considered permanent and they cannot be restored to competency, the patient will not stand trial.

Patients who are found not to have been able to tell right from wrong at the time of the crime or who did not understand the nature or the consequences of their actions may be considered insane at the time of the crime. This is frequently the case in patients who suffer from mental diseases such as intractable epilepsy, Alzheimer's disease, and severe head injury. Patients with orbito-frontal or subcortical temporal damage may act involuntarily or without an understanding of what they are doing. In these cases, the patient will be found not guilty by reason of insanity.

Although the abridgment of criminal responsibility in cases of brain dysfunction could lead to many legal abuses, clinicians have a responsibility to investigate and identify neuropsychological factors related to aggression and criminal violence. The detection of brain dysfunction underlying violent behavior is not only of value in the courtroom, but also in the determination of an appropriate course of treatment for such patients.

References

Adams, J. H., & Duchen, L. W. (1992). *Greenfields neuropathology*. New York: Oxford University Press.

American Psychiatric Association. (1994). *Diagnostic and statistical manual of mental disorders* (4th ed.). Washington, DC: Author.

Bach-y-Rita, G., Lion, J. R., Climent C. E., Jr., & Ervin, F. R. (1971). Episodic dyscontrol: A study of 130 violent patients. *American Journal of Psychiatry, 217*, 1472–1478.

Bear, D., Levin, K., Blumer, D., Cletham, D., & Ryder, J. (1982). Interictal behaviour in hospitalized temporal lobe epileptics: Relationship to idiopathic psychiatric syndromes. *Journal of Neurology, Neurosurgery, and Psychiatry, 45*, 481–488.

Bennett, T. L., & Krein, L. K. (1989). The neuropsychology of epilepsy: Psychological and social impact. In C. R. Reynolds & E. Fletcher-Janzen (Eds.), *Handbook of clinical child neuropsychology* (pp.409–418). New York: Plenum.

Beresford, T. P. (1980). [Letter to the editor]. *Neurology, 30*, 1339.

Bigler, E. D. (1988). *Diagnostic clinical neuropsychology*. Austin: University of Texas Press.

Blumer, D., & Benson, D. F. (1975). Personality changes with frontal and temporal lobe lesions. In D. F. Benson & D. Blumer (Eds.), *Psychiatric aspects of neurologic disease* (pp. 62–79). New York: Grune & Stratton.

Carpenter, M. B. (1991). *Core text of neuroanatomy* (4th ed.). Baltimore: Williams & Wilkins.

Cummings, J. L. (1985). *Clinical neuropsychiatry*. Orlando, FL: Grune & Stratton.

Daniel, D. G., Zigun, J. R., & Weinberger, D. R. (1992). Brain imaging in neuropsychiatry. In S. C. Yudofsky & R. E. Hales (Eds.), *The American psychiatric press textbook of neuropsychiatry* (2nd ed., pp. 165–186). Washington, DC: American Psychiatric Press.

Day, K. (1985). Psychiatric disorders in the middle aged and elderly mentally handicapped. *British Journal of Psychiatry, 38*, 449–456.

Deutsch, L. H., Bylsma, F. W., Rovner, B. W., Steele, C., & Folstein, M. F. (1991). Psychosis and physical aggression in probable Alzheimer's disease. *American Journal of Psychiatry, 148*, 1159–1163.

Dodrill, C. (1981). Neuropsychology of epilepsy. In S. B. Fiskov & T. J. Boll (Eds.), *Handbook of clinical neuropsychology*. New York: Wiley.

Eames, P. (1990). Organic bases of behavioural disorders after traumatic brain injury. In R. L. Wood (Ed.), *Neurobehavioural sequelae of traumatic brain injury* (pp. 18–33). Bristol, PA: Taylor & Francis.

Eichelman, B. (1987). Neurochemical bases of aggressive behavior. *Psychiatric Annals, 17*, 371–374.

Elliott, F. A. (1987). Neuroanatomy and neurology of aggression. *Psychiatric Annals, 17*, 385–388.

Elliott, F. A. (1992). Violence. The neurologic contribution: An overview. *Archives of Neurology, 49*, 595–603.

Fichera, S. M., Mittenberg, W., Zielinski, R. E., Rayls, K., & Tremont, G. (1995). Frontal and subcortical contributions to the severity of post-traumatic agitation. *Archives of Clinical Neuropsychology*, pp. 321–326.

Franzen, M. D., & Lovell, M. R. (1987). Behavioral treatments of aggressive sequelae of brain injury. *Psychiatric Annals, 17*, 389–396.

Fuster, J. M. (1980). *The prefrontal cortex*. New York: Raven.

Goldstein, M. (1974). Brain research and violent behavior: A summary and evaluation of the status of biomedical research on brain and aggressive violent behavior. *Archives of Neurology, 30*, 1–35.

Greenwood, R., Bhalla, A., Gordon, A., & Roberts, J. (1983). Behavior disturbances during recovery from herpes simplex encephalitis. *Journal of Neurology, Neurosurgery, and Psychiatry, 46*, 809–817.

Hamstra, B. (1987). Neurobiological substrates of violence: An overview for forensic clinicians. *Journal of Psychiatry and the Law, Fall/Winter*, 349–373.

Koch-Weser, M., Garron, D. C., Gilley, D. W., & Bergen D. (1988). Prevalence of psychologic disorders after surgical treatment of seizures. *Archives of Neurology, 45*, 1308–1311.

Kolb, B., & Whishaw, I. Q. (1990). *Fundamentals of human neuropsychology* (3rd ed.). New York: Freeman.

Kurtzke, J. F. (1984). Neuroepidemiology. *Annals of Neurology, 16*, 265–277.

Kwentus, J. A., Hart, R. P., Peck, E. T., & Kornstein, S. (1985). Psychiatric complications of closed head trauma. *Psychosomatics, 26*, 8–17.

Langevin, R., Ben-Aron, M., Wortzman, G., Dickey, R., & Handy, L. (1987). Brain damage, diagnosis, and substance abuse among violent offenders. *Behavioral Sciences and the Law, 5*, 77–94.

Lewis, D. O., Pincus, J. H., Feldman, M., Jackson, L., & Bard, B. (1986). Psychiatric, neurological, and psychoeducational characteristics of 15 death row inmates in the United States. *American Journal of Psychiatry, 143*, 838–845.

Lewis, D. O., Pincus, J. H., Bard, B., Richardson, E., Prichep, L. S., Feldman, M., & Yeager, C. (1988). Neuropsychiatric, psychoeducational, and family characteristics of 14 juveniles condemned to death in the United States. *American Journal of Psychiatry, 145* (5), 584–589.

Lezak, M. D. (1995). *Neuropsychological assessment* (3rd ed.). New York: Oxford University Press.

Majovski, L. (1989). Higher cortical functions in children. In C. R. Reynolds & E. Fletcher-Janzen (Eds.), *Handbook of clinical child neuropsychology* (pp. 41–67). New York: Plenum.

Malloy, P., Bihrle, A., Duffy, J., & Cimino, C. (1993). The orbitomedial frontal syndrome. *Archives of Clinical Neuropsychology, 8*, 185–201.

Mckahn, G., Drachman, D., Folstein, M., Katzman, R., Price, D., & Stadlan, E. M. (1984). Clinical diagnosis of Alzheimer's disease: Report of the NINCDS–ADRDA work group under the auspices of Department of Health and Human Services task force on Alzheimer's disease. *Neurology, 34*, 939–944.

Milner, B. (1964). Some effects of frontal lobotomy in man. In J. M. Warren & K. Akert (Eds.), *The frontal granular cortex and behavior* (pp. 313–334). New York: McGraw-Hill.

Reitan, R. M., & Wolfson, D. (1992). *Neuroanatomy and neuropathology: A clinical guide for neuropsychologists* (2nd ed.). Tucson, AZ: Neuropsychology Press.

Rosenbaum, A., & Hoge, S. K. (1989). Head injury and marital aggression, *American Journal of Psychiatry, 146*, 1048–1051.

Rubins, P. V., Mace, N. L., & Lucas, M. J. (1982). The impact of dementia on the family. *Journal of the American Medical Association, 248*, 333–335.

Silver, J. M., & Yudofsky, S. C. (1987). Aggressive behavior in patients with neuropsychiatric disorders. *Psychiatric Annals, 17*, 367–370.

Silver, J. M., Hales, R. E., & Yudofsky, S. C. (1992). Neuropsychiatric aspects of traumatic brain injury. In S. C. Yudofsky & R. E. Hales (Eds.), *The American Psychiatric Press textbook of neuropsychiatry* (2nd ed., pp. 363–396). Washington, DC: American Psychiatric Press.

Stone, A. A. (1986). Vermont adopts *Tarasoff*: A real barn burner. *American Journal of Psychiatry, 143*, 352–355.

Terry, R. D., & Katzman, R. (1983). Senile dementia of the Alzheimer type. *Annals of Neurology, 14*, 497–506.

Thomsen, I. V. (1984). Late outcome of very severe blunt head trauma: A 10–15 year second follow-up, *Journal of Neurology, Neurosurgery, and Psychiatry, 47*, 260–268.

Volkow, N. D., & Tancredi, L. (1987). Neural substrates of violent behaviour: A preliminary study with positron emission tomography. *British Journal of Psychiatry, 151,* 668–673.

Waxman, S. G., & Geschwind, N. (1975). The interictal behavior syndrome of temporal lob epilepsy. *Archives of General Psychiatry, 32,* 1580–1586.

Wender, P. H., Reimherr, F. W., & Wood, D. R. (1981). Attention deficit disorder ("minimal brain dysfunction") in adults. *Archives of General Psychiatry, 38,* 449–456.

World Health Organization. (1992). *Manual of the international classification of diseases and related health problems* (10th rev.). Geneva, Switzerland: Author.

23

Prediction of Dangerousness and Release Decision Making

Norman G. Poythress, Jr.

Introduction

Although personality disorders (e.g., antisocial personality) and substance use-abuse disorders are fairly common in offender populations, most offenders do not suffer from major mental disorders (e.g., schizophrenia, affective disorders, other psychoses) (Teplin, 1991). Similarly, most persons with major mental illness are not prone to serious violence (Swanson, 1994). Nevertheless, our society is particularly sensitized to issues surrounding the treatment, management, and release from confinement of persons whose history reveals both criminal behavior and mental disorder. Consequently, a variety of special legal rules, some quite elaborate, have been established to govern the return of offenders with mental illness to the community. Such rules inevitably, but to varying degrees, involve clinical judgments about such issues as the stability of symptoms, likely compliance with community-based treatment, risk for future violence, and the type and extent of supervision needed in the community. Therefore, the mental health professionals responsible for these judgments are often under close scrutiny by the public, the press, and the legal system itself.

This chapter reviews major issues in the literature on release decision making and synthesizes suggestions from diverse sources into a coherent set of recommendations for forensic clinicians to follow. We first consider the contexts in which release decisions occur and the tensions experienced by mental health professionals who participate in such decisions. In the section on policy development, we consider administrative issues in the development of hospital policies to guide release decision making. The next section deals with substantive matters related to such policies, including staffing, assessment, decision rules, and documentation. The final section considers issues in the implementation of release decisions.

Norman G. Poythress, Jr. • Department of Mental Health, Law & Policy, F.M.H.I.—University of South Florida, Tampa, Florida 33612-3899.

Handbook of Psychological Approaches with Violent Offenders: Contemporary Strategies and Issues, edited by Van Hasselt and Hersen. Kluwer Academic/Plenum Publishers, New York, 1999.

473

Criminal Justice Psychiatric Release Decisions: Contexts and Tensions

There are three primary criminal justice contexts in which judgments by mental health professionals weigh considerably in the potential release to the community of offenders who are mentally ill. These include bail and bond decisions, end-of-sentence releases from prison, and hospital discharge of persons acquitted not-guilty-by-reason-of-insanity (NGRI). After describing briefly each of these contexts, we consider sources of tension and conflict in release decision making with these criminal justice clients.

Pretrial Bail and Bond Decisions

At the pretrial stage, some offenders are adjudicated incompetent to stand trial and are ordered to receive psychiatric treatment to restore competence. Most commonly, this treatment is provided in maximum security, state forensic psychiatric hospitals, or forensic units in state civil hospitals. When their illness is in sufficient remission that competence is judged "restored," these defendants are returned to court so that prosecution may proceed. At this point, they may be released from custody pending trial, and the opinions of the treating mental health staff may inform the courts' decisions about these defendants' requests to be placed on bond.

End-of-Sentence Discharge

Psychiatric judgments are also relevant to release decisions regarding convicted offenders who are residing in mental health units at the time that their sentences expire. These mental health units may be in the prison system itself, although some jurisdictions provide for the transfer of their most severely mentally ill inmates to hospitals operated by state mental health departments. Although these individuals cannot be detained any longer under the authority of their sentence, neither can clinicians discharge them "willy-nilly" simply because their sentence has expired. These inmates' combined criminal and mental health histories will often dictate that clinicians consider whether to file a petition with the probate court for involuntary psychiatric hospitalization (civil commitment) upon completion of sentence. The legal criteria for involuntary hospitalization in all states include that the person is currently mentally ill, and as a result of that illness poses a significant risk of harm to others (Monahan & Shah, 1989).[1]

Not-Guilty-by-Reason-of-Insanity: Community Placements

The offender population of greatest concern and notoriety consists of those persons acquitted not-guilty-by-reason-of-insanity (NGRI) at trial. The overwhelming majority of NGRIs have been diagnosed with a major psychosis (Steadman et al., 1993), and the NGRI acquittal confirms a "causal" relationship between the person's mental illness and his or her index crime. Persons acquitted NGRI are usually committed for involuntary treatment subsequent to their trials, on commitment criteria that are arguably less stringent than those in the usual civil commitment context (Jones v. United States, 1983).[2] Their eventual release from involuntary inpatient treatment is ultimately premised on the judgment of the mental health professionals having responsibility for their treatment. In an increasingly more conservative political climate (LaFond & Durham, 1992), the final authority for NGRI release into the community often resides with the original committing criminal court, with the forensic treatment staff providing recommendations and conditional release plans for NGRI clients who remain under the court's jurisdiction.

This chapter focuses primarily on issues that arise in the areas of end-of-sentence discharge and NGRI community placements, predominately the latter. Although some of the liability issues discussed in the following sections may apply in an indirect way to mental health judgments that inform courts' bail and bond decisions (see *Hicks v. United States, 1975;* Miller, Doren, Van Rybroek, & Maier, 1988), the return to court of persons whose competence to stand trial has been restored focuses much more on functional abilities for future participation in the adjudication process and less frequently on risk assessment and community management issues.

Sources of Tension in Release Decision Making

Discharge decisions returning mentally ill persons from the criminal justice system to the community occur in a highly politicized environment. As a result, clinicians involved in these decisions may experience pressure from a variety of sources. Generally, these pressures reflect tension between the rights and mental health needs of the individual client on the one hand, and community safety and social control concerns on the other.

With respect to clients' rights and needs, clinicians will recognize a substantial number of cases in which stability of symptoms is fairly rapidly achieved, with further progress beyond stabilization dependent on the clients' involvement in activities outside the institution. The limited programming available in corrections or forensic institutions, which are often underfunded and poorly staffed in terms of rehabilitative services, may have little if any beneficial effect. For these clients, protracted confinement represents only the opportunity for clients to become disgruntled, resentful, and institutionalized. Thus, both professional ethical considerations and the legal responsibility to provide treatment that is in these clients' best interests may urge clinicians toward community placement and treatment as soon as is clinically feasible.

Elsewhere in the system, however, these primary rehabilitative considerations may be countered by negative attitudes toward criminal justice mental health clients and an incentive structure that discourages discharging such clients into the community. One major concern is the fear of malpractice suits. Where bad outcomes (postrelease aggression in the community) do occur, clinicians may face civil charges for "negligent release" and legal and financial liability for the violent acts of their former clients (Poythress & Brodsky, 1992; Smith, 1994). Negative publicity regarding the management and control of these clients can cost clinicians and hospital administrators their jobs and damage the credibility of entire programs, even in the absence of actual aggression by the client (Reichlin & Bloom, 1993). The fear of malpractice suits may lead to conservative and defensive clinical practice (Simon, 1992) that results in substantially longer stays in forensic hospitals than would appear appropriate based on the clinical considerations alone (Poythress & Brodsky, 1992; Steadman, 1985).

Although judges enjoy, by judicial immunity, protection from these kinds of malpractice liability concerns, they may be reluctant to place mentally ill defendants on bond or approve conditional release plans for NGRI clients because they are elected officials. They may be unwilling to risk loss of popularity with the electorate that might result from postrelease aggression by these individuals in the community. Awareness of the judiciary's conservative stance may result in mental health professionals' postponing the proposal of discharge or conditional release beyond the point that these recommendations are initially clinically appropriate.

Mental health professionals in institutions serving criminal justice mental health clients may also find resistance among community service providers to whom responsibility for these clients passes once community placement is approved. The history of chronic mental illness, the history of criminal justice involvement, or both, may foster the view of these clients as poor treatment risks that these agencies would prefer not to have foisted upon them (Miller & Fiddleman, 1984). Absent good working relationships with community providers, hospital clinicians may question whether the necessary degree of community supervision and aftercare is available to support a recommendation for community placement. To induce community agencies to work cooperatively with these clients, it may be necessary to work toward system changes that provide additional funding for special programs (e.g., forensic case management) or the assurance of liability protection in the event of bad outcome cases (Leverette, Bloom, & Williams, 1994).

Finally, although less formally, clinicians may feel pressured by any of several advocacy groups to approach release decision making in ways consonant with those groups' interests. Such groups may include advocates for the clients themselves (e.g., National [or local] Alliance for the Mentally Ill [NAMI]) or spokespersons for the victims of criminal activity (e.g., Victims of Crime and Leniency [VOCAL]).

Whatever the net influence of the various forces and pressures that may influence clinical decision making, clients' readiness for hospital release needs to be continuously monitored and judgments about discharge readiness must be made. We now turn to administrative issues regarding establishing policies to govern such judgments and decisions.

Policy Development: Administrative Considerations

Whether to Have Explicit Policies Concerning Risk Assessment and Release

Before discussing the intricacies of hospital discharge policies, perhaps it is necessary to consider a prior question of whether to have explicit policies at all. Considering this issue strictly from a liability perspective, Monahan (1993) described the rationale for *not* having an explicit release decision policy:

> [I]t is counterproductive to draft exemplary guidelines . . . if the guidelines are merely to be filed in some cabinet or entombed in a staff handbook, never to be read. Again, *it is much better to have no policies at all than to have policies that are not followed in actual practice.* If one has no formal policies regarding risk, one can always try to argue after the fact that there were implied policies or understandings about how high-risk patients were to be handled. . . . On the other hand, when clear and reasonable policies have been formulated and committed to writing by the agency itself, and those policies were violated in the case that gave rise to a tort action, the ballgame is over. (p. 247; italics in original).

Monahan's analysis is correct as it pertains to legal strategy governing cases that result in a tort claim (e. g., for negligent release). However, it does not follow that having no policies is the best course of action. There are several reasons that favor development of policies to govern risk assessment and discharge decision making.

First, having no written policy (and arguing "implied" policies) offers no great protection in court. This defense may be easily eroded by plaintiff's attorney's cross-examinations, which are likely to reveal considerable variability as to what constituted those "implied" procedures in the minds of various staff members, suggesting to the jury that "implied procedures" constitutes "no procedures." Second, this whole rationale is premised on planning for the rare (albeit potentially catastrophic) event. Although recent studies (Lidz, Mulvey, & Gardner, 1993; Steadman *et al.*, 1994, Table 3) indicate that persons with mental illness discharged to the community are more frequently aggressive than earlier studies indicate, aggression resulting in serious injury is still very infrequent. Even when such aggression occurs, it will not necessarily be of the type that gives rise to a negligence suit. Third, and most important, are the lost benefits that having well considered policies would provide. These include the capacity for appropriate and uniform risk assessments and release decisions (Weiner & Wettstein, 1993), reduction in the fear and uncertainty with which clinical staff might otherwise approach these tasks, and a potential template for the demonstration and documentation of *diligence*, not negligence, in the clinical process culminating in the decision to release.

In summary, although a rationale for having no explicit policies regarding risk assessment and release can be advanced, on balance the benefits of having explicit policies (and following them) outweigh the potential benefits of having no policies. We next consider procedures for developing and validating such policies.

Recommended Procedures for Risk–Release Policy Development

It has been argued elsewhere that policies governing risk assessment and release decision making should not be developed by internal staff alone, but should include input from legal and mental health consultants outside the hospital's own staff (Monahan, 1993; Poythress, 1990). Legal experts may identify particular issues regarding assessment, monitoring, or documentation that have been identified as problematic in previously reported negligence cases. Clinical experts may advise on the most current research and clinical procedures for approaching the risk assessment and risk management tasks. Incorporating these experts' suggestions into substantive policy provides the best assurance that the hospital's practice will be consistent with contemporary standards of care. Use of outside consultants provides a mechanism for demonstrating that special attention has been given to these important issues. While many (if not most) hospital policies may be developed by in-house staff and forwarded for review and approval by the medical staff committee, the use of consultants demonstrates sensitivity to the complexity of issues in risk assessment and special care in crafting the release decision process—in a word, *diligence*.

A second step in policy development has been recommended for psychiatric hospitals that provide services to previously violent or potentially aggressive clients (Poythress, 1987). This step involves arranging for peer review of the proposed policy by an independent panel of clinicians with expertise in the areas of risk assessment and discharge planning. This process allows for independent suggestions regarding substantive policy; the peer review panel may suggest additional or alternative actions to those proposed by the policy development group. It also provides two benefits from a liability management perspective. First, simply obtaining an independent peer review is a further demonstration of diligence with respect to risk assessment and discharge planning issues; most other hospital policies would not be subjected to this additional layer of review. Second, the peer review panel provides an independent assessment of the hospital's standard of care, and one that has been formulated outside the context of ongoing liability litigation. Assuming that the proffered policy has met with the panel members' approval (or has been modified to address their concerns), their review constitutes a preemptive strike against claims that may arise later, alleging failure to practice with due care.

Substantive Issues in Risk–Release Policy Development

Policies regarding risk assessment and release may be organized around a number of substantive issues. Here we consider five primary factors: (1) staffing and training, (2) procedures for risk assessment and risk management, (3) deliberation guidelines, (4) documentation, and (5) relationships with aftercare providers.

Staffing and Training

Hospital policies governing risk–release procedures should specify the staff responsible for various components of the process. Initial judgments regarding risk level, risk management, and discharge readiness properly should fall to the treatment team responsible for the client's care. Two main considerations with respect to staffing include basic credentials and specialty training.

Because of the potential political and legal ramifications of risk–release decisions, essential tasks should not be assigned to residents, interns, or more peripheral treatment team members. The attending psychiatrist or other designated treatment team leader should be responsible for coordinating the risk assessment, risk review, and development of a discharge plan. Coordination implies a team effort, and (as discussed later) treatment team members of various professional disciplines (nursing, psychology, social work) may be assigned specific tasks. Ideally, these staff will have terminal degrees in their respective fields and will have met state licensure or certification requirements.

This level of credentialing should be considered necessary, although not sufficient, for primary participation in risk–release decision making. Treatment team members responsible for risk–release decisions should also have received training on topics such as the violence prediction literature, empirical correlates of aggression, risk reduction–management techniques, and so on, and regular (e.g., annual) updates or refresher training on such topics should be conducted and documented for all staff (Monahan, 1993). Relatively few medical school or graduate professional programs offer courses of instruction specifically on these issues. Yet, there is an extensive and burgeoning literature that ought to inform clinical judgments about risk and release. Exposure to this literature will enable treatment teams to make more competent and appropriate decisions or recommendations regarding discharge. From a liability management perspective, absence of such knowledge or training would certainly leave the hospital and its staff more vulnerable in the aftermath of a bad outcome.

Procedures for Risk Assessment–Risk Management

A specific risk protocol, and procedure for developing that protocol, should be outlined in hospital policy; it should indicate the information to be gathered, by whom, in what form, and specify the person or persons responsible to review and synthesize various elements of the protocol.

Specifying the appropriate elements of a risk protocol is no small task. As Lidz and Mulvey (1984) have noted, "no consensus exists about the best way to assess . . . dangerousness. . . . The problem, of course, is that this voluminous literature is both overwhelming and disjointed" (p. 380; cites omitted). Despite this daunting assessment, there are some excellent sources of information on risk factors in persons with mental illness (Hodgins, 1993; Lidz & Mulvey, 1984; Monahan, 1981; Monahan & Steadman, 1994). Further, the literature reveals some general consensus regarding important domains of information that should be tapped as well as some user-friendly forms that have been developed to assist in the risk–release judgment process.

Information About Risk

Prominent researchers have identified four broad domains of information that may inform judgments about risks. These include (1) dispositional factors (e.g., demographic, fixed personality variables), (2) historical factors (e.g., social history, mental hospitalization history, criminal justice history), (3) contextual factors (e.g., perceived stress, social and support networks, access to weapons), and (4) clinical factors (e.g., diagnosis, type and severity of specific symptoms, substance use) (Steadman *et al.*, 1994, p. 303). Table 23.1 summarizes some of the key findings from research on factors within each of these domains.

The conceptual distinction between static and dynamic risk factors may be helpful in guiding risk–release decisions. Static factors include correlates of risk that cannot be changed or manipulated to any significant degree. Some dispositional factors (e.g., age), personality traits (e.g., psychopathy), and historical factors (e.g., number of prior incidents of violence) have been correlated with recidivism, but there is nothing a clinician can do to "manage" them; similarly, historical events cannot be undone (Steadman *et al.*, 1994). Dynamic factors, on the other hand, are those factors related to risk that can be affected by clinical or other management techniques. These may include environmental factors (e.g., social networks, support structure, access to weapons) or clinical factors (e.g., symptom type and severity, drug or alcohol effects). While static factors may be thought of as informing judgments about baseline risk (relatively speaking, the level of risk an individual poses), dynamic (I do not mean here "psychodynamic") factors are those key elements that can be impacted and around which a risk management plan will be developed.

As noted earlier, there is no professional consensus as to how risk assessments should be performed. Given the ample length of time available to prison mental health or forensic hospital units to develop information on the types of clients considered here, multiple sources of information should be tapped. Primary sources of information may include the state attorney's office, which can provide reports containing details and descriptions of past behavior that led to police intervention; records of prior treatment, particularly involuntary commitments, that may describe behavior that resulted in the probate court's determination of "dangerous to others";

TABLE 23.1
Correlates of Violence

A. Dispositional factors
  1. Demographics
    a. Gender
      MALES posing a higher risk of violence is a more robust finding in studies limited to serious expressions of violence (e. g., felony arrest reports). Studies using self- and collateral report measures have found a higher incidence of violence among women (Lidz, Mulvey, & Gardner, 1993; Steadman *et al.*, 1994) including studies of domestic violence (Bland & Orn, 1986; O'Leary *et al.*, 1989). The greater frequency among women is primarily in relatively minor forms (hitting, slapping, shoving), while men are at greater risk for more lethal expressions of violence.
    b. Age
      YOUTH is associated with higher risk, and greatest risk is in late adolescence to early adulthood. Some studies suggest a decrease in aggressive behavior after age 40; this "burn-out" phenomenon may not hold for psychopaths (Hare, McPherson, & Forth, 1988).
  2. Personality Traits
    a. Antisocial Personality Disorder (APD)
      APD is significantly associated with criminality in adults. The presence of APD, substance abuse, or both, mediates the association between major psychoses and crime (see part D.2) (Robins, 1993).
    b. Psychopathy
      Psychopathy, as measured by the Psychopathy Checklist–Revised (PCL-R), is related to but distinguishable from APD as defined in *DSM-IV* (American Psychiatric Association, 1994) (Hare, Hart, & Harpur, 1991). PCL-R scores are positively associated with parole failure (Hart, Kropp, & Hare, 1988; Serin, Peters, & Barbaree, 1990) and with violence recidivism in correctional and forensic populations (Hare & Hart, 1993). PCL-R scores may be a better predictor of violence than is a diagnosis of APD (Harris, Rice, & Cormier, 1991).
B. Historical factors
  1. Arrest history
    The single most robust predictor of future violence is a history of multiple prior offenses (Monahan, 1981).
  2. Conduct disorder and delinquency
    Conduct disorder (CD) is associated with adult criminality, primarily through its association with delinquency and adult disorders (APD, substance abuse) (Robins, 1993).
  3. Age of onset
    Early onset of violent behavior (prior to age 13) is a significant predictor of delinquency careers and adult criminality (Patterson & Yoerger, 1993; Tolan, 1987).
C. Contextual factors
  1. Weapon availability
    The lethality of violence is enhanced by the availability of weapons. Clinical factors associated with increased propensity for weapons accumulation include (1) paranoid features and (2) use of stimulants (amphetamines) (Meloy, 1993).
  2. Social support
    Social networks may serve as a buffer against life stresses, thus aiding in adjustment or coping. Due in part to increased availability, family members may be at increased risk for violence victimization, especially where there is a prior history of domestic violence (Gondolf, Mulvey, & Lidz, 1990). Risk for violence toward significant others may be enhanced when those persons are involved in setting limits (Straznickas, McNeil, & Binder, 1993) or are perceived by the individual to be threatening or hostile (Estroff & Simmer, 1994).
  3. Victim availability
    Higher risk for persons with history of violence toward a broad range of victims, or multiple assaults on a narrow class of victims who remain available (e.g., significant others).
D. Clinical factors
  1. Major psychoses
    There is a modest association between *current diagnosis* of major psychosis (bipolar disorder, schizophrenia) and violence in the community; recent data suggest a risk multiplier of about 6 compared

TABLE 23.1 (*Continued*)

to the risk posed by undiagnosed persons (Swanson, Holzer, Ganju, & Jono, 1990). Having been diagnosed previously for major psychosis or having been hospitalized previously for same is *not* an indicator of increased risk (Swanson, 1994). The presence of current active symptoms explains the relationship between psychosis and violence (Link, Andrews, & Cullen, 1992). Specific psychotic symptoms associated with enhanced risk include persecutory delusions (inducing perceived threat) and thought insertion-control (inducing perceived loss of internal controls) (Link & Stueve, 1994).

2. Substance abuse
   There is a stronger association between substance abuse and violence in the community (relative risk factor 12 to 16 times) than between psychosis and violence. Substance abuse diagnosis also moderates the relationship between major mental disorder and crime (see A.2.a).

Note. Data from *Psychological Evaluations for the Courts: A Handbook for Mental Health Professionals and Lawyers* (2nd ed., Table 9-4, pp. 287–288, by G. B. Melton, J. Petrila, N. G. Poythress, and C. Slogobin, 1997, New York: Guilford. Copyright 1997 by Guilford Press. Adapted with permission.

family members, who may provide details regarding juvenile history or adult domestic violence; and the client him- or herself. Prior psychiatric treatment records and criminal justice information should be requested routinely and soon after admission to the forensic unit; notations of these requests (and timely follow-up requests when information is not forthcoming) should be made to document the hospital's diligence in seeking relevant third-party information. Social history and family background information should be gathered routinely, and documentation forms may be structured to ensure inquiry into issues relevant to risk assessment (e.g., juvenile record, domestic violence).

The hospital policy on risk assessment should also indicate a method for bringing this information together in a coherent form for the treatment team or ultimate decision maker. As Weiner and Wettstein (1993) have noted, "This information . . . should not be buried in the chart among the rest of the clinical, administrative, and financial data" (p. 254). I have recommended elsewhere (Poythress, 1989) that an integrated report, termed a "Violent Behavior Analysis" be prepared by an assigned clinician. This report should be based on a review of the third-party information described earlier and interviews with the client to flesh out these and other (unreported) instances of significant violence. Each instance should be scrutinized for precipitants, methods, victim characteristics, contextual factors, contribution of substance use, relationship (if any) to active clinical symptoms, and so forth.

A form such as that shown in Figure 23.1 may facilitate coding of potentially relevant information about each event and the subsequent analysis for factors or themes that recur across events. Forms such as this, and the synthesized report based on the completed forms, aid in several ways. First, they encourage separate documentation of all independent violent events known to the staff. Second, they encourage a systematic and uniform approach to documentation and assessment. Third, they facilitate analysis and the reduction of what may otherwise be an unwieldy collection of narrative reports. And finally, they make evident to any external reviewer of the record that the risk assessment involved a focused, deliberate, and organized effort.

Other treatment team members may be assigned the responsibility of developing additional reports synthesizing particular information relevant to risk assessment–risk management. For example, a treatment team nurse may be assigned to summarize pertinent information regarding inpatient behavior, such as incidents of significant ag-

<u>VIOLENT EPISODE REPORT</u>

PATIENT NAME: _____ FILE NO.: _____

EPISODE DATE: _____   LOCATION:_____

METHOD OF DISCOVERY: _____

INFORMATION SOURCE:_____

A.   **VIOLENT EPISODE SCENARIO:**

B.   **DISPOSITIONAL FACTORS AT TIME OF EPISODE:**

   PATIENT'S AGE: _____   LIVING WITH FAMILY: _____   EMPLOYED: _____

   ALCOHOL/DRUG(OPIATE) ABUSE: _____

   MEDICATIONS: _____   TAKING THEM: _____

   MENTAL DISORDER (DX): _____

   APPARENT MOTIVATION: _____

   DELUSIONAL/HALLUCINATING/OTHER SYMTOMS PRESENT: _____

   _____

   RECENT TRAUMATIC EVENT: _____

   APPARENT MENTAL STATE: _____

   _____

   OTHER: _____

C.   **SITUATIONAL FACTORS AT TIME OF EPISODE:**

   PROVOKED BY VICTIM: _____   EXHORTED BY OTHERS:_____

   DRUG/ALCOHOL INVOLVED: _____   WEAPON USED: _____

   EASILY ACCESSABLE:_____ OCCURRED DURING COMMISSION OF ANOTHER CRIME:_____

   VICTIM'S RELATIONSHIP TO PATIENT: _____

   OTHER: _____

D.   **CIVIL/LEGAL OUTCOME OF THIS EPISODE:** _____

   _____

E.   **COMMENTS/ANALYSIS:**

FIGURE 23.1. Form to facilitate coding in violent behavior analysis.

gression (e.g., from hospital incident reports) and medication compliance; a social worker may be asked to report on family or other community resources and supports, and the client's history (if any) of participation and compliance in outpatient treatment. This set of specially developed reports is then available to the treatment team to guide its recommendations or decisions regarding release and placement.

Information About Risk Management

For purposes of risk management the most pertinent information will usually be the dynamic factors related to prior instances of violent behavior. Indeed, risk assessment (as opposed to a categorical "prediction of dangerousness") is premised on the notion that violence is often the result of interactions between person and situation (environment). Thus, best judgments about violence recidivism are conditional ones based on best estimates about the future status of environmental and personal factors (e.g., changes in clinical status, occurrence of stressful events). Although the future status of these factors cannot be foretold with certainty, the risk management plan should specify the safeguards or controls that will be implemented to minimize the recurrence of symptoms or situations that, in the past, have been associated with expressions of violence.

Although it is beyond the scope of this paper to discuss comprehensively all of the issues in risk management, it may be helpful to consider briefly the premises of three general types of plans discussed by Monahan (1993). These include incapacitation, target hardening, and intensified treatment.

Incapacitation involves constructing barriers that prevent the anticipated expressions of violent behavior. Of course, the decision to *not* release is the most extreme form of incapacitation; the hospital staff may decide that the risk is too high and that controls are too weak to justify recommending discharge. In this instance, denying release or petitioning the appropriate authority for extended commitment would be appropriate actions. However, lesser forms of incapacitation may also be considered. For example, if concerns are only in relation to a particular potential target or victim, the discharge plan could provide for a supervised residential placement (e.g., halfway house, adult congregate living facility) in an area geographically remote from the potential victim's residence. With day-to-day supervision of the client's activities available, the physical distance between client and victim serves to prevent the feared aggression. If prior conflicts between client and family members have been around specific control issues (e.g., management of the client's Social Security or other support checks), responsibility for those issues may be transferred to another person (e.g., professional guardian or corporate entity), thus removing the family members from "at-risk" roles that have contributed to prior expressions of violence.

Incapacitation can also target specific violence-related behaviors or contextual factors. The prescription and careful monitoring of disulfiram (antabuse), for example, may help prevent recurrent episodes of alcohol abuse with which aggressive behavior has been associated historically. Placement in a supervised residential setting and required participation in a day treatment program may help limit access to "bad company" or a gang of peers who may have previously exhorted the client to act aggressively.

Target hardening refers to alerting and preparing persons at risk for the client's return to the community. One obvious action here is to plan to notify concerned persons (e.g., persons that the client has previously threatened or injured) at the point that community release is approved. Notification may include the location of the intended residence, the neighborhood of which concerned persons can then avoid in order to minimize the risk of unintended contact. If the client will live with a family member whom he or she has previously assaulted, living arrangements may call for responsible relatives (e.g., siblings, aunts, uncles) to take up temporary residence with the client and at-risk family member. This may provide sufficient support for the at-risk family member to permit the client to return home and attempt reconciliation and reintegration with the family.

Various forms of intensified treatment may be considered when it is judged clinically that the client may not comply fully with the prescribed regime. The use of depot medications, where appropriate, relieves the client from having to take regularly oral medications. When medication is not available in injectable form, additional monitoring (family members, mental health outreach teams) may be incorporated into the treatment plan to ensure that the necessary supervision of medication is available. When drug abuse is a concern, frequent but random drug screening should be considered to monitor for possible relapse.

Deliberation Procedures

The designated decision makers should have available to them the current medical record, collateral or third-party information, and special reports developed (described earlier) to inform their deliberations regarding risk and release. Further issues that a hospital's risk–release policies should address include the nature of decision rule or rules, the provisions (if any) for second-level review, and the authority of clinical review entities versus that of hospital administration.

Decision Rule

It was suggested earlier that decisions about release be made by a team of licensed professionals who have received training specifically on issues related to risk–release decision making. It is further recommended that the policy include an explicit decision rule that defines the decision process. The decision rule employed by the team may vary depending on the type of release requested and whether or not there are provisions for second-level review. The latter issue (second review) will be discussed in the next section.

For persons involuntarily committed under court authority to forensic mental health units, several graduated release issues are possible. Although the discussion thus far has focused on release to some community setting, treatment teams and review boards may also pass judgment on requests for supervised or unsupervised grounds privileges, escorted or unescorted day trips to the community, trial (overnight) visits to the community, or transfer from forensic to a less secure, civil hospital. Again, there are no hard and fast rules for approaching these various decisions, and current practices vary from one state to another. Whatever rules are decided on, they should be rational and implemented consistently. One arrangement is to require the full team of designated clinicians to participate in all decisions that involve release from hospital custody. Thus, any unescorted pass, family-supervised community visit, or discharge to civil unit or community placement might require full team deliberations, while staff-supervised activities (e.g., staff escorted grounds pass or community visit) might be relegated to a subcommittee (e.g., three persons) of the team. Within either of these contexts, an explicit decision rule (e.g., majority, two-thirds, or unanimous) should be indicated. When the requested status change (e.g., escorted pass, release) is denied by the reviewing authority, the basis or rationale for the denial should be made explicit and should identify further accomplishments or treatment gains needed to justify such requests in the future. As discussed in the section on documentation, a number of user-friendly forms, review guides, and decision tables have been developed that may facilitate a systematic review and discussion of the database and aid in making careful, consistent decisions.

Hierarchical Review

A number of authorities (Schwartz & Pinsker, 1987; Simon, 1992; Weiner & Wettstein, 1993) recommend the involvement of outside consultants in these important decisions. Others suggest a more formal, hierarchical review process in which the original treatment team's decision is subject to review by an independent panel of staff who are not involved directly in the client's treatment (Dudley, 1978; Travin & Bluestone, 1987). These review panels might be composed of the hospital clinical director, discipline (psychiatry, psychology, social work, nursing) chiefs, senior members from other treatment teams in the hospital, or some combination. Such consultations or hierarchical reviews can be structured as either optional (e.g., only in cases where doubts exist about the client's level of risk) or automatic (i.e., all requests that involve release from custody, regardless of perceived risk).

Logically, requests for status changes should not go forward to a review panel unless the initial review team has given its approval for the requested change. Any policy providing for elective or optional review should indicate the circumstances in which the review should be sought. Travin and Bluestone (1987) suggest the following criteria for invoking an optional review process: (1) There is a history of extreme violent or threatening behavior resulting in injury preceding the current admission; (2) there is a history of violence toward family members, or an unwillingness of family to have the patient return home (or both); (3) there is a history of rapid decompensations associated with violence in a noncompliant patient who also abuses either alcohol or drugs; (4) there is a history of arrests, incarcerations, or involvements with the criminal justice system for repeated violent acts; (5) there is a history of repeated assaultive, disruptive, or threatening behavior while on the ward in the hospital; or (6) there is a history of unremitting psychosis with agitation, hostility, disorganization, paranoid delusions, and command hallucinations to harm self or others, despite intensive inpatient treatment.

Review panel members, of course, should have basic credentials and special training on risk–release issues that is at least equivalent to that required of the first-level decision maker. The consultant or review panel should have available the same clinical database (hospital record, collateral information, special reports) used by the initial review team; it should also have the liberty to conduct its own interview of the client and to question treatment team members about clinical, risk assessment, and risk management issues. As with the first-level review, the risk–release policies should specify the decision rule by which the review panel makes its judgment. When the review panel denies an activity or status change that was recommended by the initial review team, the basis for the denial should be clearly indicated in a way that aids the treatment team in planning further treatment.

Clinical Versus Administrative Authority

A final issue to be considered is the locus of ultimate authority in release decision making. The structure recommended earlier suggests that the decision of the hierarchical review panel should prevail over or "trump" the decision of the initial review team. However, should the final authority rest with this clinical body, or should it reside with the hospital administration?

In some instances, this will be a somewhat moot point. In a number of jurisdictions, the committing criminal court retains jurisdiction over persons committed after an NGRI acquittal and no release (conditional or otherwise) can be implemented without the court's approval. In other cases (release from civil commitment for prison inmates committed at end of sentence; NGRI release in jurisdictions where courts do not retain jurisdiction), however, the hospital will have the ultimate authority. Different models are available here, and variations exist across states in terms of the allocation of authority. Some may place the final authority with the clinical decision maker; others may give the review team or review panel recommendation power only, yielding in the final analysis to the decision of the hospital administrator.

There are advantages and disadvantages associated with each of these models. The clinical model emphasizes the clinical needs of the particular client who is the subject of review, but it may be less sensitive to other (i.e., political) factors that might be considered in such decisions. The administrative model provides an additional layer of review and ultimately spreads the responsibility (and liability) for the decision somewhat more broadly. However, it also reduces somewhat the authority of the senior clinical staff and may result in significant frustration for both clients and clinicians when administrators veto recommendations for status change that have survived successive clinical and consultant or panel reviews. This is particularly relevant where administrators may have difficulty specifying the further clinical progress that needs to be demonstrated in order to justify approval in future review. Acknowledging that rationales for either model may be advanced, it is recommended here that the risk–release policy allocate only recommendation power to the initial review team and consultant or review panel, leaving the ultimate decision authority with hospital administration. This recommendation is based on the view that these kinds of release decisions do ultimately and inevitably involve social, moral, and political issues that stand somewhat outside a purely clinical decision-making framework. Therefore, an administrative authority is most appropriate in the final analysis.

Whatever model is chosen, however, written policy should make clear the respective authorities of clinical and administrative staff. Where the clinical model is selected, the policy should clearly delegate final authority for release decision making and implementation to the clinical decision process. Where the administrative model is selected, clinical reports and summaries should be framed in terms that make recommendations, and communications with courts and other outside authorities should be under administrative letterhead and signature.

Documentation

Although all clinical documentation is important, that pertaining to risk–release decision making is particularly so. Those who participate in the risk assessment and release decision-making process must have the pertinent information before them. Further, it must be in a form that facilitates comprehension and interpretation, in order to make consistent, fair, and well-informed judgments. From a liability perspective, in the event of aggressive behavior postrelease that results in claims of "negligent release," the quality of documentation in the medical record is the best, if not the only, defense. We consider briefly several facets of risk–release documentation.

Requests for Third-Party Reports

As noted earlier, several kinds of third-party information (police reports describing prior instances of violent behavior, previous medical records, family member reports) may inform the risk assessment. However, one cannot be assured that information will necessarily be forthcoming simply because it has been requested. Further, some information may be privileged and obtainable only with written permission of the client (e.g., records of prior treatment), which may be denied by some clients. Thus, the clinical record should show that reasonable efforts were made to obtain the relevant information, even if not all such information was ultimately obtained. This means documenting written requests to district attorneys' offices, prior treatment providers, and so on, and follow-up FAX or phone requests when necessary. If desired information is not obtained, the record should make clear that it was not for lack of effort on the hospital's part.

Issues Considered and Deliberated by the Review Team or Review Panel

As discussed previously, a wide range of issues may be considered in risk assessment and the development of risk management plans. The special reports and kinds of forms recommended earlier may be of some use in initial development. However, it is also important to document what the review team or panel considered in reviewing such reports and the clinical record as a whole.

A number of user-friendly forms have been recommended to aid in the documentation of the release decision process. Marra, Konzelman, and Giles (1987) developed a "Dangerousness Assessment Sheet" that lists eight categories of risk elements for clinicians to weigh. These include

1. History of dangerous behavior (juvenile and adult)
2. Institutional record
3. Stressors, means to violence
4. Victim and environmental issues
5. Mental disorder
6. Psychological testing
7. Actuarial scales
8. Moderator variables

Based on information in the clinical record, third-party data, and special reports, the review team members enter global judgments (High, Medium, Low) for each category indicating their assessment of the level of risk posed by the client.

A somewhat different measure was developed by Eisner (1989), who suggested ratings on 15 aspects of behavior (e.g., signs of illness, institutional behavior, substance abuse) using 5-point scales with descriptors anchoring each rating. A third alternative was developed by Kroll and Mackenzie (1983), who suggested a structured decision table for analyzing the risk of releasing a patient, depending on which, and how many, of 17 questions are answered in the affirmative from the clinical data.

The utility of devices such as these has been well summarized by Kroll and Mackenzie (1983):

> The use of decision trees, decision tables, linear models and other strategies, although not a perfect solution, helps to organize and integrate clinical information and place it in better perspective.... The use of ... a decision table ... ensures that significant factors, pointing toward or away from risk, will not be overlooked and that the clinician will not suffer from information overload when faced with more than five or six salient variables. (pp. 31, 33–34).

Such devices not only ensure that "all the bases are touched," but they help to illuminate differences of opinion or judgment that may occur among members of the decision team or panel.

Decision Rationale

Devices such as rating forms or decision tables may also facilitate the writing of the narrative report. If the review team or panel's decision is to deny the request, then uniformly low ratings or areas of uncertainty and disagreement may provide clues to treatment planning. The rationale for denial should describe additional behavior change or treatment progress that the reviewing body would like to see in order for such requests to have a better chance of meeting with favorable review in the future.

If the decision is to approve the requested activity or status change, then significant differences of opinion should be discussed in a narrative report that ultimately explains the team or panel's decision and the risk management plan for dealing with problems that persist (Simon, 1992). The standard of care for clinical practice does not require that clinicians always be correct in their prognostications and judgments about clients' future behaviors. However, it does require careful, informed, and diligent decision making. Thus, the narrative report should build on the special reports and review guides (summary forms, tables, or ratings) to yield a description of the team or panel's decision process and the risks–benefits analysis that has been conducted.

Client Exit Interview

A final piece of documentation, primarily for liability protection, is suggested in cases where approval is given to release clients whose violent histories are closely associated with psychiatric symptoms. Given this condition, clinicians will presumably not recommend or approve release unless the symptoms of concern are presently well controlled. As a protection against arguments from hindsight in bad outcome cases (e.g., "The hospital released the person when he was still symptomatic"), a videotaped exit interview with the client has been recommended (Poythress, 1990). This interview should be conducted by a treatment team member who covers with the client relevant historical information and current mental status issues, including current symptoms, attitude toward treatment, willingness to comply with aftercare planning, and so forth. This preserves a live, dynamic record of the patient "as he was at the time of discharge" which may serve well should litigation arise around claims of premature release.

Implementation of Release Decisions

Once final approval has been obtained to move forward with the release of the forensic client into the community, transfer of treatment responsibility and continuity of care is the major implementation issue. Where possible, it is recommended that actual physical contact between the client and community aftercare provider be arranged prior to discharge. This may be accomplished in any of several ways. Geographic proximity to the hospital permitting, one way is to invite the appropriate representative of the community agency (e.g., the case manager or social worker) to attend treatment team meetings in the hospital prior to discharge. This permits the client to meet his or her social worker or case manager and to begin associating treatment obligations to this new person. Simultaneously, the social worker or case manager may begin to learn about the client, his or her history, and the particular facets of the case that will become the focus of scrutiny and management in the community. This alliance may be further developed prior to final discharge via trial visits in the community that include the client visiting the community agency. These practices may facilitate continuity of care and compliance once the discharge is effected.

Some authorities (e.g., Simon, 1992) also recommend that the releasing hospital call the community agency on the day of the first scheduled appointment postrelease to ensure that the client showed up. If the client misses the appointment, then recommended procedures include (1) contacting the client by phone to request that he come in immediately, (2) enlisting the aid of a responsible relative if the client cannot be persuaded to come in, (3) sending a mobile unit (treatment team) to the client's residence if family cannot be persuaded to bring him in, and (4) requesting police assistance in bringing the client in for his appointment.

Whether any or all of these suggestions will be feasible in any given case, however, will vary depending on geography, resources, and conditions of the release. Some forensic hospitals or mental health units will not have their own mobile mental health teams to send out into the community. And in some instances, discharge may be to towns or cities at great distances from the hospital, making on-site visits by mobile mental health units impractical. In such cases, the hospital may need to prevail on local service providers (e g., community mental health centers) to try to establish contact with the client. If hospital release has been a "conditional release" with the court's approval, with provisions for revoking the release for failure to comply with the release plan, then it may be easier to involve the police in bringing the client in for the initial appointment. However, in jurisdictions where the release is "outright," then there may be no legitimate legal or administrative leverage that can be brought to bear on a client who refuses to keep his aftercare appointments.

Summary

Psychiatric release decisions involving criminal justice system clients pose special challenges to mental health professionals who provide services to these individuals. Whether these clients in fact pose a greater risk to society than do other criminal justice clients is an open empirical question. However, it is clear that public perceptions about the "criminally insane" have given rise to legal safeguards and procedures that limit mental health professionals' discretion in making discharge decisions. Both clinical considerations (the clients' mental health needs) and social and legal influences (protecting the public, avoiding malpractice claims) affect clinicians in discharging their duties. We have taken the position in this chapter that these duties can best be met through the development and careful implementation of a well-conceived, structured policy that provides for a systematic and detailed risk assessment–risk management plan that is subjected to both clinical and administrative review. This process affords the greatest assurance that these important decisions will be clinically sound, consistent, and fair, and will allow for consideration of both individual client and societal interests in the treatment of criminal justice mental health clients.

Notes

1. In most states, risk of harm to self may also justify involuntary hospitalization. In some states, inability to meet basic needs (i.e., being "gravely disabled") may also warrant commitment. This chapter deals exclusively with considerations of harm to others.
2. See note 1 and accompanying text. In *Jones* the Supreme Court held that being found NGRI of any offense (in *Jones*, attempted theft of a windbreaker) satisfies the "dangerousness" criterion for commitment. Further, the state must meet a "clear and convincing" burden of proof in civil commitment, while *Jones* held that only "a preponderance" standard must be met in the commitment of persons acquitted as NGRI.

References

Bland, R., & Orn, H. (1986). Family violence and psychiatric disorder. *Canadian Journal of Psychiatry, 31*, 129–137.

Dudley, H. (1978). A review board for determining the dangerousness of mentally ill offenders. *Hospital and Community Psychiatry, 29*, 453–456.

Eisner, H. R. (1989). Returning the not guilty by reason of insanity to the community: A new scale to determine readiness. *Bulletin of the American Academy of Psychiatry and the Law, 17*, 401–413.

Estroff, S. E., & Zimmer, C. (1994). Social networks, social support, and violence among persons with severe, persistent mental illness. In J. Monahan & H. J. Steadman (Eds.), *Violence and mental disorder: Developments in risk assessments* (pp. 259–295). Chicago: University of Chicago Press.

Gondolf, E. W., Mulvey, E. P., & Lidz, C. W. (1990). Characteristics of family and nonfamily assaults. *Hospital and Community Psychiatry, 41*, 191–193.

Hare, R., McPherson, L. M., & Forth, A. E. (1988). Male psychopaths and their criminal careers. *Journal of Consulting and Clinical Psychology, 56*, 710–714.

Hare, R. D., & Hart, S. D. (1993). Psychopathy, mental disorder and crime. In S. Hodgins (Ed.), *Mental disorder and crime* (pp. 104–118). Newbury Park, CA: Sage.

Hare, R. D., Hart, S. D., & Harpur, T. (1991). Psychopathy and the DSM-IV criteria for antisocial personality disorder. *Journal of Consulting and Clinical Psychology, 59*, 391–398.

Harris, G. T., Rice, M. E., & Cormier, C. A. (1991). Psychopathy and violence recidivism. *Law and Human Behavior, 15*, 625–637.

Hart, S. D., Kropp, P. R., & Hare, R. D. (1988). Performance of male psychopaths following conditional release from prison. *Journal of Consulting and Clinical Psychology, 56*, 227–232.

Hicks v. United States. 511 F. 2d 407 (1975).

Hodgins, S. (1993). *Mental disorder and crime.* Newbury Park, CA: Sage.

Jones v. United States. 103 S. Ct. 3043 (1983).

Kroll, J., & Mackenzie, T. B. (1983). When psychiatrists are liable: Risk management and violent patients. *Hospital and Community Psychiatry, 34*, 29–37.

LaFond, J. Q., & Durham, M. L. (1992). *Back to the asylum: The future of mental health law and policy in the United States.* New York: Oxford University Press.

Leverette, M., Bloom, J. D., & Williams, M. H. (1994). Tort liability coverage for community providers who serve insanity acquittees. *Hospital and Community Psychiatry, 45,* 933–935.

Lidz, C. W., & Mulvey, E. P. (1984). Clinical considerations in the prediction of dangerousness in mental patients. *Clinical Psychology Review, 4,* 379–401.

Lidz, C. W., Mulvey, E. P., & Gardner, W. (1993). The accuracy of predictions of violence to others. *Journal of the American Medical Association, 269,* 1007–1011.

Link, B. G., & Stueve, A. (1994). Psychotic symptoms and the violent/illegal behavior of mental patients compared to community controls. In J. Monahan & H. J. Steadman (Eds.), *Violence and mental disorder: Developments in risk assessments* (pp. 137–159). Chicago: University of Chicago Press.

Link, B. G., Andrews, H. A., & Cullen, F. T. (1992). The violent and illegal behavior of mental patients reconsidered. *American Sociological Review, 57,* 275–292.

Marra, H. A., Konzelman, G. E., & Giles, P. G. (1987). A clinical strategy to the assessment of dangerousness. *International Journal of Offender Therapy and Comparative Criminology, 31,* 291–299.

Meloy, R. (1993, January). *Assessment of violence potential.* Workbook distributed at workshop on risk assessment, Orlando, FL.

Melton, G. B., Petrila, J., Poythress, N. C., & Slogobin, C. (1997). *Psychological evaluations for the courts: A handbook for mental health professionals and lawyers* (2nd ed.). New York: Guilford.

Miller, R., & Fiddleman, P. (1984). Outpatient commitment: Treatment in the least restrictive alternative. *Hospital and Community Psychiatry, 35,* 147–151.

Miller, R. D., Doren, D. M., Van Rybroek, G., & Maier, G. J. (1988). Emerging problems for staff associated with the release of potentially dangerous forensic patients. *Bulletin of the American Academy of Psychiatry and the Law, 16,* 309–320.

Monahan, J. (1981). *Predicting violent behavior: An assessment of clinical techniques.* Beverly Hills, CA: Sage.

Monahan, J. (1993). Limiting therapist exposure to *Tarasoff* liability: Guidelines for risk containment, *Psychologist, 48,* 242–257.

Monahan, J., & Shah, S. A. (1989). Dangerousness and commitment of the mentally disordered in the United States. *Schizophrenia Bulletin, 15,* 541–553.

Monahan, J., & Steadman, H. J. (1994). *Violence and mental disorder: Developments in risk assessments.* Chicago: University of Chicago Press.

O'Leary, K. D., Barling, J., Arias, I., Rosenbaum, A., Malone, J., & Tyree, A. (1989). Prevalence and stability of physical aggression between spouses: A longitudinal analysis. *Journal of Consulting and Clinical Psychology, 57,* 263–268.

Patterson, G. R., & Yoerger, K. (1993). Developmental models for delinquent behavior. In S. Hodgins (Ed.) *Mental disorder and crime* (pp. 140–172). Newbury Park, CA: Sage.

Poythress, N. G. (1987). Avoiding negligent release: A risk-management strategy. *Hospital and Community Psychiatry, 38,* 1051–1052.

Poythress, N. G. (1989). *Discharge decisions: Standards of care and management of liability risks.* Invited address to conference sponsored by Division of Forensic Mental Health, Massachusetts Department of Mental Health, Auburn, MA.

Poythress, N. G. (1990). Avoiding negligent release: Contemporary clinical and risk management strategies. *American Journal of Psychiatry, 147,* 994–997.

Poythress, N. G., & Brodsky, S. L. (1992). In the wake of a negligent release law suit: An investigation of professional consequences and institutional impact on a state psychiatric hospital. *Law and Human Behavior, 16,* 155–173.

Reichlin, S. M., & Bloom, J. D. (1993). Effects of publicity on a forensic hospital. *Bulletin of the American Academy of Psychiatry and the Law, 21,* 475–483.

Robins, L. N. (1993). Childhood conduct problems, adult psychopathology and crime. In S. Hodgins (Ed.), *Mental disorder and crime* (pp. 173–193). Newbury Park, CA: Sage.

Schwartz, H. I., & Pinsker, H. (1987). Mediating retention or release of the potentially dangerous patient. *Hospital and Community Psychiatry, 38,* 75–77.

Serin, R. C., Peters, R. D., & Barbaree, H. E. (1990). Predictors of psychopathy and release outcome in a criminal population. *Psychological Assessment: A Journal of Consulting and Clinical Psychology, 2,* 419–422.

Simon, R. I. (1992). *Clinical Psychiatry and the law* (2nd ed.). Washington, DC: American Psychiatric Association.

Smith, S. R. (1994). The legal liabilities of mental health institutions. *Administration and Policy in Mental Health, 21,* 379–394.

Steadman, H. J. (1985). Insanity defense research and treatment of insanity acquittees. *Behavioral Sciences and the Law, 3,* 37–48.

Steadman, H. J., McCreevy, M. A., Morrissey, M. P., Callahan, L. A., Robbins, P. C., & Cirincione, C. (1993). *Before and after Hinckley: Evaluating insanity defense reform.* New York: Guilford.

Steadman, H. J., Monahan, J., Appelbaum, P. S., Crisso, T., Mulvey, E. P., Roth, L. H., Robbins, P. C., & Klassen, D. (1994). Designing a new generation of risk assessment research,. In J. Monahan & H. J. Steadman (Eds.), *Violence and mental disorder: Developments in risk assessments* (pp. 297–318). Chicago: University of Chicago Press.

Straznickas, K. A., McNeil, D. E., & Binder, R. L. (1993). Violence toward family caregivers. *Hospital and Community Psychiatry, 44,* 385–387.

Swanson, J. W. (1994). Mental disorder, substance abuse and community violence: An epidemiological approach. In J. Monahan & H. J. Steadman (Eds.), *Violence and mental disorder: Developments in risk assessments* (pp. 101–136). Chicago: University of Chicago Press.

Swanson, J. W., Holzer, C. W., Ganju, V. K., & Jono, R. T. (1990). Violence and psychiatric disorder in the community: Evidence from the Epidemiologic Catchment Area surveys. *Hospital and Community Psychiatry, 41,* 761–770.

Teplin, L. A. (1991). The criminalization hypothesis: Myth, misnomer, or management strategy? In S. A. Shah & B. D. Sales (Eds.), *Law and mental health: Major developments and research needs* (NIMH; DHHS Publication No. (ADM) 91-1875, pp. 149–184). Washington, DC: U.S. Department of Health and Human Services.

Tolan, P. H. (1987). Implications of age of onset for delinquency risk. *Journal of Abnormal Psychology, 15,* 47–65.

Travin, S., & Bluestone, H. (1987). Discharging the violent psychiatric inpatient. *Journal of Forensic Sciences, 32,* 999–1008.

Weiner, B. A., & Wettstein, R. M. (1993). *Legal issues in mental health care.* New York: Plenum.

Alcohol, Drugs, and Interpersonal Violence

Linda J. Roberts, Caton F. Roberts, and Kenneth E. Leonard

Introduction

There is a large body of research suggesting a strong empirical relationship between violent acts and alcohol and other drug use. Many studies report that well over 50% of violent offenses—homicide, assault, rape—are accompanied by the consumption of alcohol, drugs, or both, by perpetrators and victims (see Collins, 1989; Greenberg, 1981; Murdoch, Pihl, & Ross, 1990; Pernanen, 1991; Reiss & Roth, 1993). While there are strong public perceptions embracing and reinforcing this link (Fagan, 1990; MacAndrew & Edgerton, 1969), the empirical association may be akin to the emperor's clothes—less substantial than apparent, however revealing. Without a careful analysis and interpretation of the meaning of the empirical relationship, it is easy for lay and professional audiences alike to draw the premature and unwarranted conclusion that alcohol and drugs are a primary cause of violent crimes.

The purpose of this chapter is to provide an integrative overview of the empirical and theoretical literatures on the etiological links between alcohol, drugs, and interpersonal violence. We critically review the literature that purports to establish the empirical association between alcohol or drug use and violence and examine the available evidence for various explanatory models of the association. The empirical literature we review can be divided into three types of studies: epidemiological studies based on offender and general population samples, experimental studies looking at main effects of drugs and alcohol on aggression, and, finally, multifactorial studies that attempt to examine interactions and moderating variables in more complex casual models. Each of these approaches has inherent limita-

Linda J. Roberts • Department of Child and Family Studies, University of Wisconsin, Madison, Wisconsin 53706. *Caton F. Roberts* • Department of Psychology, University of Wisconsin, Madison, and Mendota Mental Health Institute, Madison, Wisconsin 53706. *Kenneth E. Leonard* • Research Institute on Addictions, and Department of Psychiatry at the State University of New York at Buffalo Medical School, Buffalo, New York 14203-1016.

Handbook of Psychological Approaches with Violent Offenders: Contemporary Strategies and Issues, edited by Van Hasselt and Hersen. Kluwer Academic/Plenum Publishers, New York, 1999.

tions, and it is only through summation and integration of these divergent approaches that we come closer to achieving an understanding of the alcohol, drug, and violence etiological web. In the concluding section of the chapter, we address pragmatic issues related to alcohol and drug use and the violent offender including risk assessment and treatment.

Although we discuss the association between illicit drugs and violence, our primary focus is on alcohol. Alcohol is more widely used than other substances, has a substantially larger body of research literature, and is without question the psychoactive substance that is most consistently and uniquely associated with violent behavior (Reiss & Roth, 1993; Miczek *et al.*, 1994). It is only at the level of experimental evidence that we focus on specific drugs (e.g., opiates, cocaine, barbiturates) other than alcohol since isolating the effects of a specific substance on violent episodes is extremely difficult given the prevalence of polysubstance use in the population of drug users. While many alcohol users rarely if ever use other drugs, most drug users use multiple drugs, frequently in combination with alcohol (Chaiken & Chaiken, 1982; Wish & Johnson, 1986). Understanding the mechanisms of action of these drugs and how they may interface with violent acts is complicated when the neuropsychopharmacologic properties of the drugs occur within a context of polysubstance intoxication. Further, although we review epidemiological studies of "other drug use," limitations of this summary categorization must be fully acknowledged. "Other drugs" refers to a panoply of drugs with widely divergent neuropsychopharmacologic properties, dependence liabilities, legal sanctions, and contexts of use. It would be imprudent, in light of the diversity of "other drugs," the prevalence of polysubstance use, and the high rates of polydrug use with alcohol, to make any conclusions about the underlying mechanisms connecting violence and substance use for the "other drug" category as a whole.

What Role Do Alcohol and Drugs Have in Violent Episodes? Overview of Etiological Models

Numerous theoretical models have been proposed to explain the association of alcohol and drugs with violence (see Goldstein, 1985; Graham, 1980; Ito, Miller, & Pollock, 1996; Pernanen, 1981). There are at least three major explanatory models, which although not mutually exclusive, for heuristic purposes can be considered conceptually distinct explanations of the substance use–violence association.

Acute Effects Model

From this perspective, it is the acute intoxicating effects of a substance that lead to violent or aggressive behavior. The mechanism of effect may be either direct, for example, the drug activates an aggression-specific brain mechanism, or indirect, for example, the substance alters perceptual and cognitive information processing in a way that contributes to violent responding. It should be noted that even from a direct effects perspective, a substance may have a direct effect on violence without necessarily leading to indiscriminant violence on every occasion of use. It is, for example, conceivable that a substance could directly impact a specific brain mechanism and effect a reduction in the threshold necessary to evoke aggression. In such a scenario, aggression would not be an invariant outcome of use of the substance independent of situation.

Third Factor Model

In this model, the association between violence and alcohol or drug use is actually spurious because both are caused by a shared "third factor," most usually an individual difference factor that leads to both drug or alcohol use or abuse and to the propensity to engage in violent acts. Most important in this respect is the constellation of background characteristics associated with a hostile disposition, antisocial personality disorder (Widiger & Trull, 1994), or the "general deviance syndrome" (Osgood, Johnston, O'Malley, & Bachman, 1988). However, individual differences of a more transitory nature (e.g., stress, marital distress) could also result in both increased drug or alcohol use and violent behaviors.

Acquisition Model

This model suggests that the relationship between violence and alcohol or drug use is driven by the social, cultural, and contextual factors associated with acquiring or using the intoxicants. This model is most applicable to substances that either have addictive properties that create strong motivational states for acquiring the substance, or are illegal and part of an illegal distribution system. In the case of illegal drugs, users place themselves in social contexts where violence is more likely, or even normative, due to the drug distribution system. Illicit drug use occurs in a context in which violence is routinely used to achieve desired ends, such as acquiring a drug, maintaining an expensive drug habit, or enforcing the implicit rules of an illegal drug distribution system. Goldstein (1985) has differentiated between concepts of economic-compulsive violence (where drug users resort to violent crime to support their lifestyles) and of systemic violence (where violence is normatively integrated with and intrinsic to cultural systems of drug distribution and use). With respect to alcohol, the focus has been more on alcohol use contexts or settings that have aggression-eliciting properties. The obvious example is the violent barroom context. Bars in which violence occurs usually provide a number of aggression-instigating conditions and individuals who choose to frequently attend such bars are likely to manifest characteristics that also promote aggressiveness. Consequently, aggression may be a likely event in such contexts independent of alcohol consumption.

Although acquisition models describe important dimensions of causation (see Cervantes, 1992, for related research), our review is focused principally on an evaluation of the available evidence supporting either the acute effects or the third variable models. To anticipate, this review concludes that the extant empirical evidence provides support for the indirect acute effects model (for alcohol and some benzodiazepines only), but that a more comprehensive understanding of the causal processes underlying the substance use–violence connection requires a multifactorial model that accounts for individual difference, situational, and macrosocial or cultural factors.

Epidemiological Studies of Alcohol and Drug Use and Violence

Research on the Global Association of Alcohol and Drug Use with Violent Acts

Offender Population Studies

The vast majority of epidemiological studies on the association of alcohol and drug use with violence have relied on samples that are convenient to identify and access, such as treatment populations or offenders incarcerated in jails or prisons. These studies have consistently identified high rates of both alcohol and drug abuse in offender populations (for reviews see Collins, 1993; Greenberg, 1981; Reiss & Roth, 1993; Wish & Johnson, 1986; Wright, 1993). For example, the New York Department of Correctional Services measured alcohol abuse with the Michigan Alcoholism Screening Test in a 1991 survey and found that 29% of 23,084 newly committed state prisoners received scores suggestive of alcohol abuse. Data from the 1991 Survey of Inmates of State Correctional Facilities (U.S. Department of Justice, 1993) indicate that 41% of violent offenders reported daily drinking in the year prior to their offense. Estimates are that 20%–40% of individuals convicted for homicide or assault are alcoholics (Greenberg, 1981).

Interpreting any of these descriptive statistics as indicative of the role of drug or alcohol use in violent offending is problematic for a number of reasons. First, while the rates of alcohol and drug use in offender populations are high, to be suggestive of a link between substance use and violence, it should be established that rates for violent offenders are higher than those of a comparison group of nonviolent individuals. Comparisons are often made to general population rates of alcohol and drug use (see Collins, 1993; Roizen & Schneberk, 1977) with the conclusion that offender rates are considerably higher. For example, while drinking is a daily activity for 7.5% of the general population (U.S. Department of Health and Human Services, 1995), as noted previously, it was found that 41% of violent offenders in state prisons reported a daily drinking pattern prior to their arrest. However, offender populations are not comparable to the general population and it is not clear what an appropriate comparison group should be (Greenberg, 1981; Roizen, 1993). When Roizen and Schneberk (1977) compared offender alcohol use in the previous year to general population samples that were similar to prison populations in age and gender the discrepancies in rates were substantially reduced. These presumably would be reduced further were the samples to be matched more closely on other relevant demographic variables such as race, socioeconomic status, employment, and so on, that may also be associated with alcohol or drug use. Further, although data indicate a high prevalence of drug and alcohol use among perpetrators of violent crime, similar or even higher rates have been found for nonviolent offenders (Welte & Miller, 1987). These findings suggest that there is not a unique association between habitual substance use and violent offending. Patterns of drug and alcohol use may be associated with or have causal implications for deviant behavior more generally rather than specifically with regard to violence.

A further difficulty in interpreting the relationship between offenders' alcohol or drug use and violent acts is that arrested or incarcerated individuals may not be representative of the universe of violent actors, and the violent behaviors that result in arrest or incarceration may not be representative of all violent acts. By comparing

1-year prevalence reports of victimization from a representative sample of men and women in Thunder Bay, Canada, with official police records in the same time period, Pernanen (1991) found that only 4% of the violent events reported by interviewed adults had a corresponding police record. We calculated a similar statistic based on self-report data collected in the 1991 National Household Survey of Drug Abuse (NHSDA; reported in Tables 1 and 2 of Harrison and Gfroerer, 1992). The percentage of the NHSDA population that reported engaging in any violent crime was 7% while the percentage reporting being booked for a violent crime was 0.4%, indicating that approximately 6% of violent events in the sample resulted in an arrest. Only a small fraction of the violent episodes that occur in our society result in arrest and incarceration and the incidents that do result in arrest cannot be considered to be "randomly" selected. That a violent act comes to the attention of police may itself be related systematically to alcohol and drug involvement. Intoxicated offenders may be more easily caught by police and individuals with records of alcohol or drug abuse, or types of crimes that involve alcohol or drug user, may be treated differentially by the criminal justice system (Greenberg, 1981; Pernanen, 1981), though empirical support for these speculations has not been presented. Nonetheless, these methodological critiques suggest that association between alcohol and violent crime may be overestimated by data based on incarcerated offenders (extensive methodological critiques of the alcohol and violence literature may be found in Greenberg, 1981; Roizen, 1982), or, at least, that such estimates are not known to represent validly the parameters of association in the much larger relevant population of nonarrested or nonimprisoned violent actors in our society.

General Population Studies

Although research examining alcohol, drugs, and violence in the general population has been rare, there have been two recent studies that have examined this issue. The Epidemiology Catchment Area (ECA) project (L. N. Robins & Regier, 1991) is a large, multisite epidemiological study of the prevalence of psychiatric disorders in the general population. The NIMH Diagnostic Interview Schedule, a structured diagnostic interview designed to yield the phenomenological and behavioral data required for scoring symptom criteria and deriving *DSM-III* diagnoses, was administered to more than 17,000 community respondents in five diverse urban settings in the United States in the course of the ECA study. Swanson (1993, 1994) reported on some specific limited information on violence that was fortuitously collected in the ECA interviews at two study sites (Durham, NC, and Los Angeles, CA) with about 7,000 subjects, allowing calculation of lifetime and 1-year violence-perpetration prevalence indices and their covariation with alcohol abuse and dependence, substance abuse, and major mental disorders. The 1-year prevalence of violent interpersonal episodes in the general population with no alcohol abuse or major mental disorders was 2%. Persons with only major mental disorders and no alcohol abuse disorders showed violence-prevalence rates of 6.8%; persons with alcohol abuse or dependence disorder and no major mental disorder had prevalence rates of 15.3%; and persons with dual diagnoses of major mental disorder plus alcohol disorders showed violence-perpetration prevalence rates of 19.6% (Swanson, 1993, 1994). Logistic regression models designed to test systematic hypotheses demonstrated that the conditional effects of young age, male gender, and low socioeconomic status were significantly associated with violence. However, when statistical controls were entered for mental disorders and alcohol disorders the effects of male gender and low socioeconomic status were markedly diminished, whereas controls for sociodemographic variables only marginally reduced the effects of the disorder variables. Swanson concludes from this that the increased risk for violence perpetration seen in younger low-SES males may be largely attributable to the substantially increased prevalence of alcohol abuse and psychiatric comorbidity in this group.

Violence prevalence estimates are also available in the NIDA-sponsored National Household Survey of Drug and Alcohol Abuse (NHSDA; 1993). Since 1971, the NHSDA survey has tracked patterns of legal and illegal drug use among the general household population. For the first time, in 1991, questions were added to the survey to assess both self-reported criminal behavior and criminal actions that resulted in arrest and formal criminal charges. Harrison and Gfroerer (1992) have used these data to estimate violence-perpetration prevalence rates for different categories of drug use for adults ages 18–49. Violence involvement among individuals with no drug or alcohol use in the previous year was 2.7%, while it was 6.3% among those who drank at least monthly, 14.6% among those who used alcohol and marijuana, and 26.1% among those who used alcohol, marijuana, and cocaine. However, a similar pattern of results was found for property offenses (e.g., stealing, damaging or destroying property, breaking and entering). The rates of engaging in property crime were 1.7% for individuals with no alcohol or drug use, 3.8% for those who used alcohol, 8.0% for those who drank monthly, 13% for those who used alcohol and marijuana, and 24.7% for those who used alcohol, marijuana, and cocaine.

For a number of reasons, general population studies of *marital* violence are particularly important in elucidating the link between violence and alcohol, and, to some extent, other drugs and violence. First, family violence is underrepresented in offender and prison populations because there is a negative relationship between the closeness of the relationship between perpetrator and victim and the likelihood of arrest and conviction (Greenberg, 1981). General population samples represent the only route to representative information about violence between intimates. Fortunately, such population studies have been carried out, most notably, the National Family Violence Survey conducted in 1975 with 2,143 families and the National Family Violence Resurvey conducted in 1985 with 6,002 families (see Straus & Gelles, 1990, for comprehensive treatment of the methodology and results of the surveys).

As documented by these surveys, marital violence is extremely common in our society, and for women, it represents the single greatest cause of injury—ranking higher than automobile accidents, muggings, and rapes combined (Stark & Flitcraft, 1988). Most violence (56%) against women is perpetuated by husbands, family members, or male friends (U.S. Bureau of the Census, 1992). Straus, Gelles, and Steinmetz (1980), using data from the 1975 survey, reported that the lifetime prevalence of marital aggression was approximately 30% with 15% reporting aggression in the preceding year. The 1-year prevalence rate for husband-to-wife aggression has been estimated between 11% (Kennedy & Dutton, 1987) and 22% (Meredith, Abbott, & Adams, 1986), with significantly higher rates reported among premarital and early marriage samples (Leonard & Senchak, 1993; McLaughlin, Leonard, & Senchak, 1992; O'Leary, Barling, Arias, Rosenbaum, Malone, & Tyree, 1989). For example, the Buffalo Newlywed Study (BNS; Leonard & Senchak, 1993) recruited couples as they applied for their marriage license and followed them in the early years of their marriage.

Based on a sample of 541 couples, prevalence of husband aggression in the first year of marriage based on a positive report by either spouse was 38%.

Finally, the research on marital violence is particularly relevant to advancing our understanding of the alcohol or drug and violence relationship because of the methodological sophistication characterizing current research in this area (Collins & Messerschmidt, 1993). While most work on the relationship between alcohol or drugs and violence has been descriptive or limited to bivariate correlations, research on alcohol and marital violence has utilized longitudinal designs, appropriate comparison groups, and mutivariate approaches allowing for an examination of the combined, unique, and interaction effects of theoretically important variables. (Methodological critiques and reviews of the early work on the association of alcohol and marital violence are not reviewed here but may be found in Hamilton & Collins, 1981; Leonard, 1993; Leonard & Jacob, 1988).

Several systematic studies have found that alcohol use, particularly heavy or problem drinking, are related to the likelihood of marital violence (Coleman & Straus, 1979; Heyman, O'Leary, & Jouriles, 1995; Kantor & Straus, 1987; Leonard & Senchak, 1993, 1996; Leonard, Bromet, Parkinson, Day, & Ryan, 1985; Pan, Neidig, & O'Leary, 1994). Coleman and Straus (1979), for example, reported a 1-year prevalence of severe marital violence of 30% among men who got drunk very often, but only 5% among men who occasionally got drunk, and 2% among those who never got drunk. In a national sample of 11,870 male U.S. army personnel from 38 bases, Pan and colleagues (1994) found that having an alcohol problem significantly increased likelihood of both mild and severe forms of husband-to-wife aggression. Further, in a number of these recent studies, the predictive relationship was found to hold even after controlling for sociodemographic and personality variables that could have produced a spurious relationship. In the Buffalo Newlywed study, husband's premarital drinking was a strong prospective predictor of husband-to-wife physical aggression 1 year later after controlling for premarital aggression, marital conflict styles, perceived power, husband's history of violence in family of origin, and husband personality characteristics, including hostility (Leonard & Senchak, 1996). Drug use has also been found to be a strong unique predictor of marital aggression, particularly severe marital aggression (Kantor & Straus, 1989; Pan *et al.*, 1994).

Comment

Despite consistently high prevalence rates for habitual heavy alcohol and drug use in offender populations, several methodological weaknesses in these studies make definitive statements about the empirical association difficult. Stronger evidence for the association is found in general population studies such as the ECA and NHSDA studies: alcohol and drug users engage in violent acts at a higher rate than the general population. However, this pattern was not found to be unique to violent crime. It may be that any causal influence of alcohol and drug use patterns involve deviant or criminal behavior more generally, rather than a specific effect only on violent behavior. The data are also consistent with the third variable explanatory model and the existence of a "general deviance syndrome" that may explain the link between alcohol or drug use and violence; individuals who are likely to engage in one form of deviance (heavy alcohol or illicit drug use) are also likely to engage in other forms of deviant behavior, including interpersonal violence and property crime. Correlational studies show that early-onset aggression in boys is a significant predictor of both heavy drinking in early adulthood and of violent offending and general criminality (Pulkinnen, 1983). The literature in psychiatric epidemiology demonstrates, in fact, that substantial proportions of substance abusers show aggressive, violent, and otherwise deviant behavior before the onset of their substance abuse, suggesting that the association between substance abuse and aggression may, in some persons, simply represent co-manifestations of premorbid personality characteristics such as irritability, impulsivity, hyperactivity, anger dyscontrol, lack of empathy, and so forth (Hechtman, Weiss, & Perlman, 1984; Muntaner, Nagoshi, & Jaffe, 1989; L. Robins, 1966).

In the alcohol and marital aggression area, rigorous methodologies have been used that suggest a somewhat different picture, although it is unclear whether results would generalize to other types of violence. Alcohol use, particularly heavy problem drinking, contributes to the prospective prediction of marital aggression over and above competing variables, such as a family history of violence and personality. Although a spurious relationship cannot be completely discounted since not all theoretically relevant variables have been examined, the observed relationship may reflect a causal process and may be related to acute consumption of alcohol (Leonard, 1993). However, event-based studies of the proximal predictors of aggression are critical to further document the relationship between intoxication and violence and to help specify the underlying causative mechanisms that may be operative.

Event-Based Studies

Because the studies reported thus far have not determined whether alcohol or other drugs were consumed at the time of the violent act, they do not allow us to draw any conclusions about the effects of intoxication per se on violent behavior. If the goal is to evaluate the acute-effects explanatory model, *event-based* data are required that attempt to establish the extent to which intoxication occurred immediately prior to a specific violent act. In other words, it is critical to differentiate between the alcohol and drug use as *distal variables* (e.g., a history of substance abuse, typical patterns of use, dependence characteristics, and diagnostic status) on the one hand, and the *proximal* or acute effects of the substance (e.g., short-term physiological, cognitive, affective, and behavioral alterations) on the other.

To provide a basis for evaluating the acute-effects explanatory model, data collection efforts must be extremely precise (e.g., amounts consumed, time elapsed between consumption and violent act, type of drug or type of alcoholic beverage) and clearly establish intoxication at the time of the act. There is a paucity of research that incorporates multiple assessments of substance use collected with the specificity required to determine level of intoxication at the time of the violent act and a proliferation of studies that do not provide a precise specification of what the assessed drug or alcohol variable actually represents. For example, the Drug Use Forecasting (DUF) system, established by the National Institute of Justice, has been collecting voluntary interview data as well as urine specimens from arrestees giving a fairly accurate picture of illicit drug use in the arrestee population. The arrestees' data are collected anonymously and the response rate is high; approximately 95% of the arrestees approached agree to the interview and 80% of those agree to also provide the specimen, which is then tested for ten illicit drugs. Since the program's inception in 1987, the proportion of drug using offenders among those arrested has never fallen below 60% and has reached 85%; positive tests are most often for cocaine or marijuana, with about 20% of arrestees testing positive for more than one illicit substance (U.S. Department of Justice, 1996).

Although the DUF program collects an impressive array of data from arrestees, interpreting the meaning of the data is formidable. Drug use testing is done at the time of arrest, but the arrest may or may not occur in temporal proximity to the violent event; arrestees are asked if they used alcohol within 72 hr before committing the alleged crime, therefore leaving open the question of intoxication at the time of the crime; drug testing results suggest that cocaine and marijuana are the most prevalent illicit substances used prior to an arrest, but the testing covers differing time periods for different drugs—marijuana (and PCP) can be detected for several weeks after use while positive results for the other drugs tested refer to the preceding 24–48 hr.

Similar problems are evident in the large body of event-based research relying on alcohol and drug use data collected for other purposes, such as court or police records or emergency room intake reports. In this literature, alcohol or drug presence is derived from data that are collected unsystematically; there are no specific instructions given in any of these settings on whether to indicate drug or alcohol use, much less on *how* to report it. Moreover, it is not always clear that the substance use reported actually occurred prior to the violent event. Thus, there is great imprecision in these reports. Findings, however, are fairly consistent with respect to the proximal association of alcohol and violent crime: alcohol use is present in a substantial number (7%–85%; most studies reporting a figure greater than 60%) of homicides, rapes, and assaults (for reviews see Collins, 1989; Greenberg, 1981; Murdoch *et al.*, 1990; Pernanen, 1976, 1991; Roizen, 1993).

Perpetrator Reports of Alcohol and Drug Use at the Time of the Violent Event

Although subject to retrospective and self-presentation biases, perpetrator reports of alcohol and drug use at the time of the violent act offer an important complement to estimates based on official records. Offender populations have been surveyed regularly about their alcohol and drug use at the time of their offense by the Bureau of Justice Statistics. The most recent data currently available involves a 1991 nationally representative survey of 13,986 state prison inmates (U.S. Department of Justice, 1993). According to self-report, 49% of violent offenders were under the influence of alcohol or drugs at the time of the offense for which they were incarcerated. Again, it is important to compare this proportion with the proportion of offenders who committed crimes not involving violence but who reported being "under the influence" of alcohol or drugs at the time. In this same survey, the comparable figure for inmates who had committed property offenses was 53%—slightly higher than for violent crimes.

However, as can be seen in Table 24.1, when the data are examined separately for alcohol and drugs some important differences emerge. First of all, drugs are less commonly used at the time of a violent crime than is alcohol. Although robbery is categorized by the BJS survey as a violent offense, if robbery is excluded, the relationship between violent offending and alcohol use is stronger yet. Alcohol is two to four times more likely to be involved in interpersonally violent offenses (homicide, assault, rape) than are drugs. This pattern is not repeated with property offenses. Fur-

TABLE 24.1

Percentage of State Prison Inmates Reporting Being Under the Influence of Drugs or Alcohol at the Time of the Offense

Type of Offense	Alcohol only	Drugs only	Alcohol and Drugs
All offenses	18	17	14
Violent offenses	21	12	16
Homicide	25	10	17
Sexual assault	22	5	14
Robbery	15	19	18
Assault	27	8	14
Property offenses	18	21	14
Drug offenses	8	26	10
Public order offenses	31	10	9

From: Bureau of Justice Statistics, *Survey of State Prison Inmates, 1991* (p. 26), 1993, Washington, DC: U.S. Department of Justice.

ther, drinking before criminal violence is more likely than drinking before nonviolent criminal behavior, again especially when robbery is excluded from the category of violent offenses. Among those who reported drinking prior to the offense, the average amount was nearly nine ounces of ethanol (equivalent to about 18 drinks) suggesting, on average, very heavy drinking at the time of the offense. These findings essentially replicate Welte and Miller's (1987) analysis of the BJS's 1978 survey of jail inmates and 1979 survey of state prison inmates.

Not surprisingly, inmates with drug offense convictions were the most likely to report being under the influence of a drug (other than alcohol) at the time of the offense. Inmates with property offense convictions were also more likely to report being under the influence of drugs than inmates with violent offenses. As with the alcohol data, these findings mirror Welte and Miller's (1987) earlier report. Thus, there is no suggestion in the data that drug use evidences an association with violence in particular, and there is little reason to suspect a causal role for the acute effects of the psychoactive agent. Providing limited support for the economic-compulsive model of the drugs and violence association, in the 1991 BJS inmate survey, more than a quarter of inmates sentenced for robbery, burglary, or larceny reported committing the crime to get money for drugs, as did 12% of those sentenced for a violent crime.

Again, limitations of data based on the offender population for estimating the alcohol or drug–violence nexus should not be overlooked. Although the descriptive data deriving from such studies are often of utility and interest, selection biases are introduced in offender samples that substantially constrain generalizability. Offender data may not generalize to actual violent acts since many criminally violent acts are not reported and do not lead to arrests and conviction. Different types of crimes may have different likelihoods of resulting in an arrest, and intoxication itself may lead to different rates of arrest. Further, the data from any one source are unlikely to be representative of all offender types (Collins & Messerschmidt, 1993). Jail detainees differ from state correctional populations which differ from federal prison populations. For example, 1 in 3 state prisoners reported being under the influence of alcohol at the time of the offense leading to incarceration, compared to 1 in 10 federal prisoners (Wright, 1993).

Victim Reports of Perpetrator's Alcohol and Substance Use

An alternative to estimates of the event-based association between alcohol or drugs and violence based on perpetrator reports are general population studies of violent victimization. In these surveys, the "victim" provides an assessment of the presence or absence of alcohol or drug use by the perpetrator. There are a number of limitations inherent in this approach. The victim often will not have adequate information to make a judgment about presence or absence of alcohol or drugs, much less the quantity consumed or degree of intoxication. Given the strong association of substance use and violence in the public mind, victims' reports of the association may represent little more than further evidence for this schema. Nonetheless, these studies provide yet another perspective on the association, one that is not subject to the same self-presentation biases as the perpetrator's perspective and one that goes beyond the confines of the arrested, incarcerated, or treatment populations.

Pernanen (1991) has recently completed a victimization survey based on a general probability sample of 933 adults in a medium-sized Canadian city. Respondents were asked to report on victimizations since age 15, as well as victimizations in the past year. The 1-year incidence rate was 10% for both male and female respondents, while the victimization rate since age 15 was somewhat higher for males, 60%, as compared to 44% for females. In more than half (51%) of the violent incidents, the perpetrator was perceived by the victim to have been drinking. It is important to note that over half of the violent incidents reported by women involved incidents with their spouse (only 12% of male reports involved conflicts with the spouse).

The Bureau of Justice Statistics National Crime Victimization Survey asks victims about their perceptions of the perpetrator's use of alcohol and drugs. In 30% of violent victimizations in 1992, victims reported that their assailant was under the influence of either drugs or alcohol or both; 18% were seen as using alcohol only, 4.3% drugs only, and 6.1% both (U.S. Department of Justice, 1994). In 50% of cases, the victim reported not knowing whether or not the offender was under the influence of drugs or alcohol. In instances of rape, this percentage was somewhat lower (38%) but still substantial.

The most comprehensive study on sexual victimization to date was the Ms. Foundation project led by Mary P. Koss in 1987 (Koss, Gidycz, & Wisniewski, 1987; Koss, Dinero, Seibel, & Cox, 1988), even though the project was limited to college students. The project, which consisted of a questionnaire administered to a nationally representative sample of 6,159 college students at 32 institutions in the United States, indicated that 54% of women reported experiencing some form of sexual abuse since age 14; 27% had experienced an incident that met the legal definition of rape, including attempted rapes (15% reported rapes, 12% attempted rapes). Although incidents described in these studies met the legal definition of rape, they clearly differ from the rape incidents studied in samples of arrested and convicted offenders. Only 57% of the women who had been raped according to the definition used in the Koss study labeled their experience as rape. Regardless of the appropriate label for the incidents, these data significantly augment our understanding of sexually violating events in the general population. Koss and colleagues (1988) reported that of respondents who had experienced rape events, 73% of the perpetrators were believed by the victim to have used alcohol or other drugs prior to the assault. There was a trend in the data for fewer perpetrators to be using drugs or alcohol depending on closeness of the relationship between the respondent and the perpetrator; 76% of the men were perceived to be drinking in stranger rapes, 84% on casual dates, 55% on steady dates and 42% with a spouse or family member. Unfortunately, no information is available in the Koss survey on the amount or timing of the drug or alcohol use and, like all of the data reviewed in this section, the available data do not help establish the role of alcohol or drug use in these rape events.

Perpetrator and Victim Reports of Alcohol and Substance Use Prior to Marital Violence

As in studies of other types of violence, in the marital violence literature the evidence regarding the effects of alcohol or drug use proximal to the violent event is relatively sparse. In Pernanen's (1991) Canadian study, 44% of victims of marital abuse indicated that the offending spouse had been drinking. By victim (wife) report, the rate was very similar (40%) in the BNS study. However, the rate for husbands reporting on their own drinking prior to their aggressive act was substantially lower, 25%, and comparable to the 22% rate that Kantor and Straus (1989) report. Rates of perpetrator alcohol and drug use prior to marital aggression appear to be somewhat lower than the reported rates for other types of violent acts and offenses (Leonard, 1993). Further, unlike the violence literature more generally in which it is likely that both offender and victim have been drinking, when violence is perpetrated against wives, the wife is unlikely to be drinking (Leonard, 1993).

Comment

With respect to drugs other than alcohol, there is little evidence in the studies reviewed of an empirical association between acute use and violent offending in particular (although there is some evidence of a connection with criminal offenses in general) giving little reason to suspect a causal relationship based on the psychopharmacological effects of the drugs on the likelihood of interpersonal violence. However, as we suggested earlier, because "other drug" use represents such an array of diverse substances, it is difficult to draw conclusions from empirical analyses at this level of generality. Lack of an association overall may mask a strong relationship between a specific drug and violent offending. However, since polysubstance use is so ubiquitous in offender populations, it is difficult to make definitive statements about the association broken down by specific substances. What little experimental data we have on the specific drugs (reviewed in the next section) remain the best evidence we have to support or refute the acute-effects model of substance use and violent behavior.

The empirical association between acute alcohol consumption and violent events, on the other hand, appears to be substantiated by the existing data. While each data source we reviewed has serious methodological limitations, the fact that alcohol consumption is consistently found to be involved in violent acts whether reported by perpetrator, victim, or archival record lends some credence to the validity of the empirical association. The meaning of the association, however, remains elusive. For example, while a large percentage of violent offenders are reportedly under the influence of alcohol at the time of their offense, a high percentage of victims are also reported to be under the influence (alcohol and drug effects on victimization are not reviewed here; see Pernanen, 1991; Testa & Parks, 1996). This may mean that the association between acute consumption and violence may be artifactual rather than causal—the association may describe only where and when the violence took place (Murdoch *et al.*, 1990; see Fagan, 1993, for discussion of setting or context effects). However, it may also be that alcohol consumption, in particular, influences both per- petration of violence and victimization, perhaps as a result of its impact on the social interactions of the perpetrator and victim. It is worth noting in this regard that Leonard (1984) found that high levels of aggression were most likely to occur in a lab- oratory analog study of aggression when two intoxicated individuals were interact- ing as compared with the situation when one sober and one intoxicated individual or two sober individuals were interacting.

It is also important to recognize that the distinction between proximal and distal effects of alcohol is often not possible to draw, owing to both methodological limita- tions and the empirical covariation between proximal and distal measures of use: An individual intoxicated at the time of a violent act is also likely to be a regular or chronic alcohol user. Therefore, when the correlational data suggest a strong associa- tion between acute alcohol use and violence this may simply reflect the association between chronic use (or other third variables) and violence rather than implicating the psychopharmacological properties of the substance as a causal mechanism.

A further difficulty in interpreting the prevalence rates for acute alcohol con- sumption relating to violence lies in the difficulty of specifying a null hypothesis (Greenberg, 1981; Leonard & Jacob, 1988; Roizen, 1982). While these prevalence rates suggest the *potential* significance of the acute effects of alcohol, prevalence rates alone cannot establish a causal role without an appropriate "benchmark": the proportion of similar individuals in similar contexts ingesting similar amounts but *not* involved in violent acts (Reis & Roth, 1993). That is, violence and alcohol intoxication may co- occur by chance, and it is unclear what degree of co-occurrence would be expected in the absence of a relationship. Although in-depth examination of violent episodes would greatly enhance our understanding of the dynamics and causal processes in- volved in interpersonal violence, research published in this area to date is not yet suf- ficiently sophisticated to contribute to etiological inferences.

Experimental Studies of the Effects of Alcohol and Other Drugs on Aggressive Behavior

In this section we review briefly the scientific data from experiments with ani- mals and humans that relate to questions of acute and chronic causal effects of alcohol and drugs on aggressive mammalian social behavior. After the threshold questions of acute effects of substance use on aggressive behavior are addressed, we examine the- oretical perspectives on the mechanisms of effect for alcohol and briefly review some of the variables that might influence the alcohol–violence relationship.

Effects of Alcohol

Animal Experiments

Acute doses of alcohol have been demonstrated to result in reliable increases in aggressive responding, as seen, for example, in abnormal attack and threat behaviors, in fish, mice, rats, cats, dogs, and primates (Miczek *et al.*, 1994). The magnitude of al-cohol-induced increase in aggression is related to the biphasic dose–effect curve: Very low doses of alcohol (0.1–0.6 g/kg) increase aggression in response to provoking cir-cumstances; at high doses (1.2–1.6 g/kg) the initiation of aggressive threat and attack behaviors decreases relative to low doses, and extremely high doses (> 2.4 g/kg) lead to sedation (Miczek *et al.*, 1994). Most experimental work with animals has focused on the acute effects of alcohol that are observed during the early phase of drug action when motor-activating, euphoric, arousing effects are evident; this work does not in-form our knowledge concerning aggressive responding in later phases of alcohol pharmacology action. Peterson and Pohorecky (1989) studied chronic intoxicating doses of alcohol (3 daily doses) administered to male rats, and reported that chronic intoxication led to remarkably more severe, injurious attack behaviors in resident–intruder interactions; apparently the more typically ritualized forms of aggression in such situations is disrupted by chronic alcohol intoxication.

Human Experiments

Several studies have explored the effect of alcohol on human aggression through the use of laboratory analogs of aggression. The most widely used with regard to al-cohol and drug effects has been the competitive reaction-time paradigm designed by Taylor and colleagues wherein subjects are provided an opportunity to aggress against a perceived opponent by delivering electric shock of variable intensity (for re-views, see Taylor, 1993; S. P. Taylor & Chermack, 1993; S. P. Taylor & Leonard, 1983; useful meta-analytic summaries are provided by Bushman & Cooper, 1990; Ito *et al.*, 1996). In these experiments, subjects are typically administered sufficient alcohol to achieve blood alcohol content (BACs) in the .10 range, thus providing generalizabil-ity to the definitions of legal intoxication in most states.

The data from these research programs have shown generally (a) that alcohol in-duces higher levels of aggression—higher shock intensities selected by subjects—than those seen in either placebo-drinks or no-beverage control conditions (e.g., Shuntich & Taylor, 1972); and (b) that high doses of alcohol (e.g., BAC = 0.10 vs. 0.03) are associated with subjects' behaving more aggressively (e.g., S. P. Taylor & Gam-mon, 1975). Bushman and Cooper (1990) completed a meta-analysis of 30 available experimental studies using human subjects that had examined psychological ques-tions concerning the causal relationship between alcohol administration, the belief that one had received alcohol, and aggression. Results of these pooled experimental effects and aggregate comparisons showed that research participants who received alcoholic beverages behaved significantly more aggressively than did participants who did not receive alcohol.

With respect to the belief that one has been administered alcohol, it is commonly believed in our culture that alcohol consumption leads to a disinhibition of aggres-sion (Critchlow, 1986; Roizen, 1983). When "placebo" effect-sizes were computed and analyzed, wherein participants who (erroneously) believed that they were given al-cohol were contrasted with those who actually received alcohol, results showed that alcohol predicted increased aggressive responding whereas the belief that one had re-ceived alcohol was not significantly predictive (Bushman & Cooper, 1990). Bushman and Cooper also included a set of careful tests of the effects of the so-called "anti-placebo" experimental conditions in which participants were led to believe they had not received alcohol when in fact they had. The statistical analysis of the studies that had used such control conditions showed no significant effect of alcohol on aggressive responding. Because the belief that one had ingested alcohol was systematically controlled in these antiplacebo conditions, Bushman and Cooper concluded that the theoretical hypothesis that alcohol affects aggression directly was unsupported by existing research. In other words, in human beings there are factors beyond the pure pharmacologic effects on neural tissue that must be invoked to explain the causal relation between alcohol and aggressive responding. Therefore, it appears that beliefs alone, and alcohol alone, cannot explain the experimental data concerning the alcohol–aggression link in human beings. Instead, it appears that direct pharmacologic effects cannot be entirely and reasonably separated in human beings from the psychopharmacologic effects on related, mediating, cognitive and social information processing.

The conclusion that alcohol has a robust main effect on human aggression, across diverse controlled observational conditions, was also reached by Ito and colleagues (1996) in their recent meta-analysis based on 49 studies. They reported further that the alcohol–aggression effect obtains even when nonaggressive response alternatives are available. Alcohol–aggression effect sizes were larger in studies where nonaggressive response options were unavailable, thus lending some credence to Gustafson's (1993) criticism that alcohol's effect on aggression is limited when access to nonaggressive behavioral alternatives is provided. However, the availability of nonaggressive response alternatives did not eliminate significant alcohol–aggression effects in Ito and colleagues' (1996) analysis.

Effects of Drugs Other Than Alcohol

Cannabis

Attack and threat behaviors across a wide variety of animal species and experimental preparations are diminished, and submissive and flight reactions are augmented, by acute administration of cannabis extracts or delta-9-tetrahydrocannabinol (THC, the primary psychoactive ingredient in marijuana and hashish; Miczek *et al.*, 1994). In humans, high doses of THC are associated with reduced aggression relative to low doses and no-drug control conditions (S. P. Taylor, Vardaris, *et al.*, 1976); and THC reduces hostility in staged social settings (Salzman, Van Der Kolk, & Shader, 1976).

Opiates

Acute administration of opiates (morphine, heroin, methadone) leads to decreases in diverse forms of aggressive responses in animals and human beings (Miczek *et al.*, 1994). Opiates have high abuse potential because of their effects on subjective well-being and euphoria, along with their propensities for creating physiological dependence. During withdrawal from chronic opiate use, animals demonstrate chronic and prolonged aggressiveness that parallels observations and reports of human opiate-dependent users. The consensus conclusion from drug researchers is that in humans, the phase of withdrawal from chronic opiate use creates a state of vulnerability toward being provoked into aggressive defensive behaviors and aggressive instrumental acts designed to procure resources to maintain drug habits. However, no evidence supports the idea that acute doses of opiates induce aggressive responding (Miczek *et al.*, 1994).

Amphetamines and Cocaine

Miczek and colleagues' (1994) comprehensive review paper concludes that across the majority of experimental conditions and animal species, acute doses of amphetamines do not increase offensive aggressive behavior. This comports with studies of human subjects which demonstrate that, unlike alcohol, high doses of amphetamines do not influence rate nor intensity of aggressive responding in competitive experimental tasks (Beezley, Gantner, Bailey, & Taylor, 1987). However, chronic abuse of amphetamine is known to precipitate, in predisposed users, a form of amphetamine psychosis characterized by intense paranoid delusions and accessory hallucinatory responses which at times lead to secondary effects of violent, occasionally homicidal, acts driven by the amphetamine-induced psychotic beliefs and affects (Ellinwood, 1971).

In animal studies, acute doses of cocaine have been associated with increased defensive behaviors, but disruption rather than augmentation of territorial aggression responses. Chronic treatment with cocaine also does not increase aggressive responding in animals (Miczek *et al.*, 1994). Most human acts of aggression associated with cocaine use appear to be secondary to the violence that is integral to the culture of drug users and dealers (DeLaRosa & Soriano, 1992; Goldstein, 1985, 1989; Martinez, 1992; Reis & Roth, 1993).

Benzodiazepines

Experiments with humans demonstrate that acute administration of diazepam (commonly known as Valium, one of the benzodiazepines administered as anxiolytic medication) has aggression-inducing effects in male and female subjects (Gantner & Taylor, 1988; Wilkinson, 1985). S. P. Taylor and Chermack (1993) report, however, that not all benzodiazepines appear to increase aggression. Similarly, in animal studies, both diazepam and chlordiazepoxide (Librium), but not all benzodiazepines, seem to share with alcohol a biphasic effect on aggression where low doses increase and high doses suppress frequencies of threat and attack behaviors (Miczek, Weerts, & DeBold, 1993).

Comment

The preceding review of the experimental literature leads to the conclusion that there is not a viable psychopharmacological causal link between the acute use of most illicit drugs of abuse and aggression, except insofar as some substances can occasionally trigger aggression-inducing psychotic states of mind (e.g., amphetamine or phencyclidine psychosis) or withdrawal syndromes. The evidence does, on the other hand, support a causal link between aggression and the acute administration of alcohol and some benzodiazepines. However, that same evidence is not consistent with a direct effect model wherein the pharmacology of alcohol and benzodiazepines stimulates brain mechanisms that invariably disinhibit aggressive or violent responding. An indirect effects model is a better fit with existing data, but a theoretical understanding of the underlying neurobiological and psychological mechanisms that account for the indirect effects remains to be developed.

The Complexity of the Alcohol–Violence Relationship

Despite existence of a robust experimental alcohol-induced aggression effect across a range of controlled conditions with animals and persons, analysis of the same experimental work also demonstrates convincingly that there are remarkable interindividual differences in the observed effects of alcohol that are masked by the reporting of group statistics: Some, but not all, experimental subjects demonstrate clear alcohol-induced increases in aggression, while other individuals show either no effect of alcohol or even decreases in aggressive responding at the same alcohol doses. Alcohol appears to have complex, variable, and nonspecific effects on neuronal activity and behavior that lead to aggression by some persons on some occasions in association with some dosages. Variable effects are consistent with what we know about alcohol effects on social behavior in general (see Steele & Josephs, 1990). MacAndrew and Edgerton (1969), convincingly made this point: "The same man in the same bar, drinking approximately the same amount of alcohol, may, on three nights running, be, say, surly and belligerent on the first evening, the spirit of amiability on the second, and morose and withdrawn on the third" (MacAndrew & Edgerton, 1969, p. 15).

Although there are numerous theoretical perspectives describing the potential role of cognitive processing deficits in facilitating aggressive responding under conditions of alcohol intoxication (e.g., Pihl, Peterson, & Lau, 1993; Steele & Josephs, 1990; S. P. Taylor & Chermack, 1993; S. P. Taylor & Leonard, 1983) they generally converge in specifying a disruption in social information processing as the final common pathway. Alcohol is seen to alter perception and thought such that the intoxicated perceiver cannot process simultaneously and effectively, numerous stimulus inputs or cues. Instead, attention is narrowed to salient impinging cues. This attentional processing deficit leaves the intoxicated person less capable of reasoning about and responding to socially relevant but nonsalient or peripheral cues.

When an alcohol-impaired individual is in an environment that contains salient provoking cues for the instigation of aggression, that person will be more disposed not to attend to internal and external cues that are relevant to the inhibition of aggression. The sober individual who is faced with the same salient instigating cues has the cognitive resources to be able to attend to, access, process, and respond to cues (e.g., situational dangers, norms, internal cautionary moral prohibitions) that signal the importance of behavioral inhibition. Inhibitory cues often require more cognitive processing than instigating cues. These inhibitory cues are substantially less available to the intoxicated actor, hence they exert proportionately less controlling influence on the end-products of social judgment and behavior.

In addition to the cognitive effects on increasing the salience of instigative cues and decreasing the salience of inhibitory cues, research shows that alcohol has other psychopharmacologically induced social-information processing effects. The fact that alcohol can increase negative mood states (Robbins & Brotherton, 1980), and that it stimulates anxiolytic receptors and hence decreases fear of punishment (Pihl *et al.*, 1993), indicate that anxiety and other mood effects may play related roles in making inhibitory social meanings less salient and relevant to the aroused and provoked intoxicated individual. Other mediating social-information processing effects may exist as well. Sayette, Wilson, and Elias (1993) studied an aggression analogue (hypothetical responses to a videotaped provocation) in an experiment designed to test the effects of alcohol on four component functions (cue encoding, cue interpretation, response generation, response selection) proposed to be involved in social-information processing. Results showed that alcohol intoxication was associated with choosing aggressive responses to a mild provoking stimulus, even when basic social information appeared to be encoded, perceived, and interpreted in a fashion similar to sober subjects. Moreover, alcohol intoxication resulted in failure to generate socially competent responses to the interpersonal conflict, failure to recognize and select socially competent responses from available response alternatives, and a disposition to respond to an initial failure in conflict negotiation with aggressive rather than conflict de-escalating behaviors.

Lang (1993) has argued that progress in understanding the effects of drinking on behavior "will be greatest if the pursuit of generalizations that apply to all drinking by any person in any situation at any time is abandoned" (p. 124). To advance our understanding of the mechanisms through which alcohol induces aggression, it is important to identify what is known about relevant factors that are associated with and may mediate or moderate the effects of alcohol on social behavior. Although there are many factors that have been found to influence the alcohol–violence relationship, in this section we will briefly describe how differences in biobehavioral dispositions, cognitive beliefs and expectations, and setting variables interact with alcohol in its relations to aggressive responding.

Individual Differences in Biobehavioral Dispositions

Individual differences in the effects of alcohol on aggression are common in animal experiments (Miczek *et al.,*1993). In squirrel monkeys, alcohol doubled the rates of aggressive displays and overt actions in high-status individuals but not in low-status animals, suggesting that social rank appears to be a factor moderating alcohol's aggression-inducing effects (Winslow & Miczek, 1985). The fact that subordinate monkeys do not demonstrate large alcohol-induced increases in aggressive behavior is inconsistent with a direct-effect, pure disinhibition model of the pharmacologic action of alcohol. Individual history of aggressive behavior also appears to be a relevant moderating and predictive factor: In rodents and monkeys, the rates of threat and attack behaviors more than doubled in alcohol-intoxicated animals with histories of aggression in dyadic confrontations but not in animals with histories of submissive defensive responding (Blanchard, Hori, Blanchard, & Hall, 1987; Winslow & Miczek, 1985). Alcohol-induced aggression in high-status animals has also been demonstrated to be diminished markedly by benzodiazepine-GABA$_A$ receptor antagonists (Miczek *et al.,* 1993), which suggests that this site of neurotransmitter activity—also the site of action for many anxiolytic drugs—may be differentially responsive to the effects of alcohol in high- and low-aggressive animals.

In studies with human populations, converging lines of evidence suggest that predispositions to aggression, antisocial character traits, and alcohol abuse may moderate the aggression–alcohol link. Bailey and Taylor (1991) reported the only study that examined the moderating effects of aggressive disposition with experimental manipulations of alcohol in a competitive reaction-time paradigm. They hypothesized that alcohol might have the strongest aggression-inducing effect among persons disposed to interpret situations in a hostile manner and to respond aggressively to provocation. Intoxicated and sober subjects with high, moderate, and low self-rated aggressive dispositions administered electric shocks to opponents who increased provocations across blocks of trials. Under conditions of low provocation, intoxicated subjects at each level of aggressive disposition set higher shock levels than nonintoxicated subjects. The finding of alcohol-induced aggression under low provocation for low-aggressive subjects was somewhat unexpected. As provocation increased, however, low-aggressive subjects did not increase their aggression even after receiving alcohol; subjects with moderate and high levels of aggression disposition, on the other hand, escalated their own aggressive responding, and did so markedly when intoxicated as opposed to nonintoxicated. Thus, this study demonstrated that intoxicated persons with high and moderate levels of aggressive disposition are more likely to escalate aggressive responding than low-aggressive subjects, who seem as capable of inhibition of aggression in response to high provocation as do nonintoxicated persons.

Support for the moderating effect of an aggressive personality style has also been found in the marital violence area. Using a nationally representative sample of 320 men 23 years of age who were either married or living with partners, Leonard and Blane (1992) found that a pattern of risky drinking (a high score on the Alcohol Dependence scale) interacted with hostility and marital adjustment in predicting aggression toward the partner. Drinking patterns evidenced a strong association with husband-to-wife marital aggression among men with high hostility, regardless of marital adjustment level. However, among low-hostile men, alcohol use was associated with marital aggression only among those low in marital satisfaction. These findings are similar to the report by Kantor-Kaufman and Straus (1987) that alcohol consumption patterns were most strongly associated with marital violence in blue-collar men who approved of the use of aggression in the marriage.

Alcohol Expectancies

Expectancy effects have also been hypothesized to influence the alcohol–violence relationship, but very few studies have assessed this possibility directly. In a sample of college students, Dermen and George (1989) found modest support for the hypothesis that the expectancy for alcohol to cause aggression moderates the relationship between drinking patterns and aggressive behaviors. In regression analyses controlling for subjects' attitudes toward aggression, dispositional hostility, and age, the relationship between self-reported frequency of aggression and drinking habits increased significantly in proportion to the strength of beliefs that alcohol increases aggression. In contrast to this retrospective survey study, Chermack and Taylor (1995) administered alcohol or a placebo to men who either did or did not believe that alcohol caused aggressive behavior. Results indicated that alcohol administration led to increased shock setting in the competition paradigm, even among men who did not believe that alcohol caused aggression. These findings would suggest that supportive beliefs are not necessary for a relationship between alcohol and aggression to be observed.

Provocation, Threat, and Other Situational Variables

The settings within which interpersonally violent episodes emerge and transpire have been shown to be influential determinants in both naturalistic (Pernanen, 1991) and experimental (Lang, 1993; S. P. Taylor & Chermack, 1993) contexts. Situational manipulations of threat (S. P. Taylor, Gammon, & Capasso, 1976), provocation (Kelly, Cherek, Steinberg, & Robinson, 1988; S. P. Taylor, Schmutte, Leonard, & Cranston, 1979), and social pressure (S. P. Taylor & Sears, 1988) have been demonstrated to instigate increased levels of aggressive behaviors in intoxicated persons. Gustafson (1993) went so far as to argue that provoking conditions and the absence of nonaggressive response alternatives were essential to the production of observable experimental effects of alcohol on aggression. Although meta-analysis (Ito *et al.*, 1996) indicated that alcohol–aggression effect sizes were larger in studies where nonaggressive response options were unavailable, as noted previously, availability of nonaggressive response alternatives did not eliminate significant alcohol–aggression effects.

Comment

The literature reviewed here suggests that instances of alcohol-induced interpersonal aggression or violence are best conceptualized in frameworks wherein the main effects of and interactions between drinking (e.g., beverage type and dose, interaction with polypharmacy factors), persons (e.g., diverse biobehavioral dispositions and expectations), and situations (e.g., provoking and threatening circumstances, sociocultural background variables) are all seen as relevant to the multifactorial determination of a given violent episode (Lang, 1993; S. P. Taylor & Chermack, 1993). No simplistic direct-effect model suffices to account for what is known about the etiology of alcohol-related violence. Numerous factors, jointly and interactively considered, and spanning a broad range of scientific levels of analysis (biological, cultural, social-situational, cognitive-expectations, economic), are relevant to the causation of alcohol- related violent episodes (Goldstein, 1985; Lang, 1993; Miczek *et al.*, 1994; Pihl *et al.*, 1993; Reiss & Roth, 1993). Violent outcomes are seen, in this view, as the result of complex multifactorial inputs that are weighted in individual cases by relevant dispositional and situational variables which, in turn, affect the psychological processes of a behaving agent. In the case of a given violent episode enacted by a particular person, the multiple interacting factors combine with alcohol's cognitive, affective, and motivational psychopharmacological effects and ultimately devolve upon a final common pathway of influence—social-information processing and its relations to subsequent decision making and behavioral choice.

Clinical Implications: Risk Assessment and Treatment

Our review has focused on the covariation of alcohol and other substance use with various indices of violence, and on associated questions of causal influence and mechanisms of effect. Another approach to the use of information concerning substance use is to examine practical questions of risk assessment such as "How can knowledge of an individual's alcohol or substance use history inform clinical judgments of dangerousness of future violent offending?" In asking and attempting to address such questions one moves into the realm of clinical and actuarial risk assessment with specified populations. The risk assessment perspective conceives violence as a public health problem and emphasizes the possibilities of injury prevention that might accrue to society with the development of reliable and valid assessment protocols (Borum, 1996; Monahan and Steadman, 1994). Questions of risk assessment are of obvious relevance to the social agents responsible for supervising, managing, or otherwise treating individuals perceived to be at risk for violence or other forms of social deviance (e.g., courts, parole boards, probation and parole supervision officers, mental health and substance abuse personnel charged with monitoring outpatient commitments). Moreover, if risk can be assessed, it can be better managed through interventions that are tied to the risk variables. If a formalized decision process can demonstrate the predictive validity of alcohol and drug use assessment information when applied to specified at-risk groups, it can be argued that such information perhaps should be used by ethically informed social agents engaged in the violence-forecasting business (Grisso & Appelbaum, 1992).

Alcohol variables are included in several of the risk assessment protocols reviewed by Borum (1996) that appear promising for the assessment of risk of spousal violence and other domains of violent offending. The best validated of these schemes (Webster, Harris, Rice, Cormier, & Quinsey, 1994) is based on a study (Harris, Rice, & Quinsey, 1993) of Canadian violent criminal offenders, and includes assessment of the following alcohol variables: parental alcoholism, teenage alcohol problems, adult alcohol problems, alcohol involved in a prior offense, and alcohol involved in the index offense. Summary information about alcohol problems had a small but significant univariate correlation with the criterion "violent recidivism," and it contributed to the multiple discriminant function used to discriminate violent recidivists from nonrecidivists.

Alcohol variables certainly appear to hold promise in a risk assessment perspective (recall, e.g., that the data from the Epidemiological Catchment Area Study, reviewed earlier, showed that the risk of interpersonal violence is at least eight times higher in community populations with noted alcohol disorders compared with non-alcohol-disordered populations), but substantial research must be done to provide the validational underpinnings for their use as purely actuarial predictors. Specifically, more empirical research is needed that is directed at deriving the base rates for specific types of violence as stratified by relevant predictor variables, including the diversity of alcohol- and substance-use-related variables discussed in this review. Given our present state of knowledge, alcohol and substance use variables are most likely to be considered simply as clinical factors that are relevant to dispositional decision making and ongoing case management. Consider, for example, the decisional problem faced by a social agent attempting to design "conditions of release" for an incarcerated or hospitalized person who is known to have been interpersonally violent, known to have used alcohol as an explanation for his violence, known to have been intoxicated at the time of past crimes, known to have failed to progress in substance abuse treatment programs, and known to have an irritable, angry, hostile disposition in conjunction with an antisocial personality disorder of psychopathic proportions, and so on. Whether each "increment" in information in the fictitious case would contribute to increases in valid prediction is of course a question for future research. But one hardly needs a multiple regression equation to inform a risk management decision in such loaded circumstances.

We do, however, need to be able to evaluate the effectiveness of any intensive case management procedures designed around such persons and their conditions of living. Moreover, we need to know more precisely than we do currently how treatment for alcohol and other substance problems can successfully mitigate risk for future violence, and to what degree with what types of persons. At this point, there is very little known concerning the impact of alcohol or drug treatment on subsequent violent behaviors. There is some evidence that couples-based alcoholism treatment combined with behavioral marital therapy reduces the likelihood of marital violence, at least in the short term, and that those who are successful in the alcoholism treatment are more likely to be successful with respect to reductions in marital violence (O'Farrell & Murphy, 1995). However, it may be that the more seriously violent alcoholics simply had poorer outcomes both with respect to alcohol use and subsequent violence. There is also some evidence that treatment of drug-involved offenders can reduce both drug use and future arrests (e.g., Martin, Butzin, & Inciardi, 1995). Successful treatments tend to be fairly intensive interventions such as therapeutic communities which target more than drug and alcohol use. Consequently, the reductions in criminal recidivism (violent and nonviolent) may not be specifically tied to the successful reductions in drug use.

Summary

A simplistic model of the role of alcohol and drugs in the etiology of interpersonal violence can be rejected summarily: It is clear that alcohol and drugs are neither necessary nor sufficient to explain a violent act. Millions of Americans use alcohol, other drugs, or both, regularly without engaging in violent interpersonal acts. Heavy or irresponsible use of the substances does not alter the picture. Eleven percent of the U.S. population can be classified as heavy drinkers (U.S. Department of Health and Human Services, 1995) but only a small minority of drinking episodes eventuate in any type of violent outcome; despite a convincing association between marital aggression and drinking, more than two thirds of heavy drinking men do not aggress against their wives (Kantor & Straus, 1987). Violence also regularly occurs without any drug or alcohol involvement. Further, research suggests that a substantial proportion of violent substance abusers display premorbid aggressive and other antisocial characteristics such that, in many cases the violent tendencies of individual offenders predate the substance abuse itself. Nonetheless, it is clear that alcohol and drug use do have a significant influence on violent behavior.

It should not be surprising that the link between alcohol or drug use and a social behavior as variegated as human aggression would require a complex causal model to account for its determination. As the National Research Council has concluded in its recent volume on understanding and preventing violence, "The link among alcohol, other psychoactive drugs, and violence turns out to be not an example of straightforward causation, but rather, a network of interacting processes and feedback loops" (Reiss & Roth, 1993, p. 183). Among alcohol and drug researchers there appears to be a discernible and growing consensus that violent and aggressive outcomes associated with alcohol and drug consumption by humans are best conceptualized within such multifactorial frameworks (Lang, 1993; Leonard, 1993; Miczek *et al.*, 1994; Reiss & Roth, 1993; S. P. Taylor & Chermack, 1993). The available evidence suggests a pharmacologic role in violent events for alcohol and some benzodiazepines. Other drugs of abuse seem to be associated with violent events through nonpharmacologic, systemic, and economic processes (Goldstein, 1985). Alcohol and its combination with other drugs may contribute to phenotypically diverse violent outcomes through complex causal pathways involving activation of preexisting biobehavioral dispositions and cognitive expectancies in particular situational circumstances. Finally, alcohol and drug variables appear to have promise in risk assessment frameworks, and knowledge from research on effective alcohol and substance use treatment programs suggests their critical utility in the development of future violence risk management approaches.

ACKNOWLEDGMENTS

Preparation of this chapter was supported in part by grant K21-AA00149 awarded to Linda J. Roberts by the National Institute on Alcohol Abuse and Alcoholism and by grant RO1-AA07183 awarded to Kenneth E. Leonard by National Institute on Alcohol Abuse and Alcoholism.

References

Bailey, D., & Taylor, S. (1991). Effects of alcohol and aggressive disposition of human physical aggression. *Journal of Research in Personality, 25*, 334–342.

Beezley, D. A., Gantner, A. B., Bailey, D. S., & Taylor, S. P. (1987). Amphetamines and human physical aggression. *Journal of Research in Personality, 21*, 52–60.

Blanchard, R. J., Hori, K., Blanchard, D. C., & Hall, J. (1987). Ethanol effects on aggression of rats selected for different levels of aggressiveness. *Pharmacology, Biochemistry and Behavior, 26*, 61–64.

Borum, R. (1996). Improving the clinical practice of violence risk assessment: Technology, guidelines, and training. *American Psychologist, 51*, 945–956.

Bushman, B. J., & Cooper, H. M. (1990). Effects of alcohol on human aggression: An integrative research review. *Psychological Bulletin, 107*, 341–354.

Cervantes, R. C. (Ed.). (1992). *Substance abuse and gang violence.* New York: Sage.

Chaiken, J., & Chaiken, M. (1982). *Varieties of criminal behavior.* Santa Monica, CA: Rand.

Chermack, S. T., & Taylor, S. P. (1995) Alcohol and human physical aggression: Pharmacological versus expectancy effects. *Journal of Studies of Alcohol, 56*, 449–456.

Coleman, D. J., & Straus, M. A. (1979, August). *Alcohol abuse and family violence.* Paper presented at the annual meeting of the American Sociological Association, Boston.

Collins, J. J. (1989). Alcohol and interpersonal violence: Less than meets the eye. In N. A. Weiner & M. E. Wolfgang (Eds.), *Pathways to criminal violence* (pp. 49–67). New York: Sage.

Collins, J. J. (1993). Drinking and violence: An individual offender focus. In S. E. Martin (Ed.), *Alcohol and interpersonal violence: Fostering interdisciplinary research* (NIAAA Research Monograph No. 24, NIH Pub. No. 93-3496). Rockville, MD: National Institutes of Health (pp. 221–236).

Collins, J. J., & Messerschmidt, M. A. (1993). Epidemiology of alcohol-related violence. *Alcohol Health and Research World, 17*(2), 93–100.

Critchlow, B. (1986). The powers of John Barleycorn—Beliefs about the effects of alcohol on social behavior. *American Psychologist, 41*, 751–764.

DeLaRosa, M. R., & Soriano, F. I. (1992). Understanding criminal activity and use of alcohol and cocaine derivatives by multi-ethnic gang members. In R. C. Cervantes (Ed.), *Substance abuse and gang violence* (pp. 24–39). Newbury Park, CA: Sage.

Dermen, K. H., & George, W. H. (1989). Alcohol expectancy and the relationship between drinking and physical aggression. *The Journal of Psychology, 123*(2), 153–161.

Ellinwood, E. H. (1971). Assault and homicide associated with amphetamine abuse. *American Journal of Psychiatry, 127*, 90–95.

Fagan, J. (1990). Intoxication and aggression. In M. Tonry & J. Q. Wilson (Eds.), *Drugs and crime* (pp. 241–320). Chicago: University of Chicago Press.

Fagan, J. (1993). Set and setting revisited: Influences of alcohol and illicit drugs on the social context of violent events. In S. E. Martin (Ed.), *Alcohol and interpersonal violence: Fostering interdisciplinary research* (NIAAA Research Monograph No. 24, NIH Pub. No. 93-3496) (pp. 161–192). Rockville, MD: National Institutes of Health.

Gantner, A. B., & Taylor, S. P. (1988). Human physical aggression as a function of diazepam. *Personality and Social Psychology Bulletin, 14,* 479–484.

Goldstein, P. J. (1985). The drugs–violence nexus: A tripartite conceptual framework. *Journal of Drug Issues, 15,* 493–506.

Goldstein, P. J. (1989). Drugs and violent crime. In N. A. Weiner & M. E. Wolfgang (Eds.), *Pathways to criminal violence* (pp. 16–48). New York: Sage.

Graham, K. (1980). Theories of intoxicated aggression. *Canadian Journal of Behavioral Science, 12,* 141–158.

Greenberg, S. W. (1981). Alcohol and crime: A methodological critique of the literature. In J. J. Collins (Ed.), *Drinking and crime* (pp. 70–109). New York: Guilford.

Grisso, T., & Appelbaum, P. S. (1992). Is it unethical to offer predictions of future violence? *Law & Human Behavior, 16*(6), 621–633.

Gustafson, R. (1993). What do experimental paradigms tell us about alcohol-related aggressive responding? *Journal of Studies on Alcohol, 11,* 20–29.

Hamilton, C. J., & Collins, J. J. (1981). The role of alcohol in wife beating and child abuse: A review of the literature. In J. J. Collins (Ed.), *Drinking and crime* (pp. 253–287). New York: Guilford.

Harris, G. T., Rice, M. E., & Quinsey, V. L. (1993). Violent recidivism of mentally disordered offenders: The development of a statistical prediction instrument. *Criminal Justice and Behavior, 20,* 315–335.

Harrison, L., & Gfroerer, J. (1992). The intersection of drug use and criminal behavior: Results from the National Household Survey on Drug Abuse. *Crime and Delinquency, 38*(4), 422–443.

Hechtman, L., Weiss, G., & Perlman, T. (1984). Hyperactives as young adults: Past and current substance abuse and antisocial behavior. *American Journal of Orthopsychiatry, 54,* 415–425.

Heyman, R. E., O'Leary, K. D., & Jouriles, E. N. (1995). Alcohol and aggressive personality styles: Potentiators of serious physical aggression against wives? *Journal of Family Psychology, 9*(1), 44–57.

Ito, T. A., Miller, N., & Pollock, V. E. (1996). Alcohol and aggression: A meta-analysis on the moderating effects of inhibitory cues, triggering events, and self-focused attention. *Psychological Bulletin, 120*(1), 60–82.

Kantor, G. K., & Straus, M. A. (1987). The drunken bum theory of wife beating. *Social Problems, 34,* 213–230.

Kantor, G. K., & Straus, M. A. (1989). Substance abuse as a precipitant of wife abuse victimizations. *American Journal of Drug and Alcohol Abuse, 15,* 173–189.

Kaufman Kantor, G.K, & Straus, M. A. (1987). The "drunken bum" theory of wife beating. *Social Problems, 34,* 213–231.

Kelly, T., Cherek, D., Steinberg, J., & Robinson, D. (1988). The effects of provocation and alcohol on human aggressive behavior. *Drug and Alcohol Dependency, 21,* 105–112.

Kennedy, L.W., & Dutton, D. G. (1987). *The incidence of wife assault in Alberta* (Edmonton Area Series Report No. 53). Edmonton, Alberta, Canada: University of Alberta, Population Research Laboratory.

Koss, M. P., Gidycz, C. A., & Wisniewski, N. (1987). The scope of rape: Incidence and prevalence of sexual aggression and victimization in a national sample of higher education students. *Journal of Consulting and Clinical Psychology, 2,* 162–170.

Koss, M. P., Dinero, T. E., Seibel, C. A., & Cox, S. L. (1988). Stranger, acquaintance and date rape: Is there a difference in the victim's experience? *Psychology of Women Quarterly, 12,* 1–24.

Lang, A. R. (1993). Alcohol-related violence: Psychological perspectives. In S. E. Martin (Ed.), *Alcohol and interpersonal violence: Fostering multidisciplinary perspectives* (Research Monograph No. 24, pp. 121–147). Rockville, MD: U.S. Department of Health and Human Services.

Leonard, K. E. (1984). Alcohol consumption and escalatory aggression in intoxicated and sober dyads. *Journal of Studies on Alcohol, 45*(1), 75–80.

Leonard, K. E. (1993). Drinking patterns and intoxication in marital violence: Review, critique, and future directions for research. In S. E. Martin (Ed.), *Alcohol and interpersonal violence: Fostering multidisciplinary perspectives* (Research Monograph No. 24, pp. 253–280). Rockville, MD: U.S. Department of Health and Human Services.

Leonard, K. E., & Blane, H. T. (1992). Alcohol and marital aggression in a national sample of young men. *Journal of Interpersonal Violence, 7,* 19–30.

Leonard, K. E., & Jacob, T. (1988). Alcohol, alcoholism, and family violence. In V. B. Van Hasselt, R. L. Morrison, A. S. Bellack, & M. Hersen (Eds.), *Handbook of family violence* (pp. 383–406). New York: Plenum.

Leonard, K. E., & Senchak, M. (1993). Alcohol and premarital aggression among newlywed couples. *Journal of Studies on Alcohol, 11,* 96–108.

Leonard, K. E., & Senchak, M. (1996). The prospective prediction of husband marital aggression among newlywed couples. *Journal of Abnormal Psychology, 105,* 369–380.

Leonard, K. E., Bromet, E. J., Parkinson, D. K., Day, N. L., & Ryan, C. M. (1985). Patterns of alcohol use and physically aggressive behavior in men. *Journal of Studies on Alcohol, 46,* 279–282.

MacAndrew, C., & Edgerton, R. B. (1969). *Drunken comportment.* Chicago: Aldine.

Martin, S. S., Butzin, C. A., & Inciardi, J. A. (1995). Assessment of a multistage therapeutic community for drug-involved offenders. *Journal of Psychoactive Drugs, 27,* 109–116.

Martinez, F. B. (1992). The impact of gangs and drugs in the community. In R. C. Cervantes (Ed.), *Substance abuse and gang violence* (pp. 60–73). Newbury Park, CA: Sage.

McLaughlin, I. G., Leonard, K. E., & Senchak, M. (1992). Prevalence and distribution of premarital aggression among couples applying for a marriage license. *Journal of Family Violence, 7*(4), 61–71.

Meredith, W. H., Abbott, D. A., & Adams, S. L. (1986). Family violence: Its relations to marital and parental satisfaction and family strengths. *Journal of Family Violence, 1,* 299–305.

Miczek, K. A., Weerts, M. S., & DeBold, J. F. (1993). Alcohol, benzodiazepine-GABA$_A$ receptor complex and aggression: Ethological analysis of individual differences in rodents and primates. *Journal of Studies on Alcohol, 11,* 170–179.

Miczek, K. A., DeBold, J. F., Haney, M., Tidey, J., Vivian, J., & Weerts, E. M. (1994). Alcohol, drugs of abuse, aggression, and violence. In A. J. Reiss & J. A. Roth (Eds.), *Understanding and preventing violence: Vol.3, Social influences* (pp. 377–570). Washington, DC: National Academy Press.

Monahan, J., & Steadman, H. J. (1994). Toward a rejuvenation of risk assessment research. In J. Monahan and H. Steadman (Eds.), *Violence and mental disorder: Developments in risk assessment* (pp. 1–17). Chicago: University of Chicago Press.

Muntaner, D., Nagoshi, C., & Jaffe, J. H. (1989). Correlates of self-reported early childhood aggression in subjects volunteering for drug studies. *American Journal of Drug and Alcohol Abuse, 15,* 383–402.

Murdoch, D., Pihl, R.O., & Ross, D. (1990). Alcohol and crimes of violence: Present issues. *International Journal of Addictions, 25,* 1065–1081.

National Institute on Drug Abuse. (1993). *National Household Survey on Drug Abuse: Main findings.* (DHHS Publication No. (SMA)93-1980). Washington, DC: U.S. Government Printing Office.

O'Farrell, T. J., & Murphy, C. M. (1995). Marital violence before and after alcoholism treatment. *Journal of Consulting and Clinical Psychology, 63,* 256–262.

O'Leary, K. D., Barling, J., Arias, I., Rosenbaum, A., Malone, J., & Tyree, A. (1989). Prevalence and stability of physical aggression between spouses: A longitudinal analysis. *Journal of Consulting and Clinical Psychology, 57,* 263–268.

Osgood, D. W., Johnston, L. D., O'Malley, P. M., & Bachman J. G. (1988). The generality of deviance in late adolescence and early adulthood. *American Sociological Review, 53,* 81–93.

Pan, H. D., Neidig, P. H., & O'Leary, K. D. (1994). Predicting mild and severe husband-to-wife physical aggression. *Journal of Consulting and Clinical Psychology, 62,* 975–981.

Pernanen, K. (1976). Alcohol and crimes of violence. In B. Kissin & H. Begletier (Eds.), *The biology of alcoholism: Social aspects of alcoholism* (Vol. 4, pp. 351–444). New York: Plenum.

Pernanen, K. (1981). Theoretical aspects of the relationship between alcohol and crime. In J. J. Collins (Ed.), *Drinking and crime* (pp. 1–69). New York: Guilford.

Pernanen, K. (1991). *Alcohol in human violence.* New York: Guilford.

Peterson, J. T., & Pohorecky, L. (1989). Effect of chronic ethanol administration on intermale aggression in rats. *Aggressive Behavior, 15,* 201–215.

Pihl, R. O., Peterson, J. B., & Lau, M. A. (1993). A biosocial model of the alcohol–aggression relationship. *Journal of Studies on Alcohol, Supplement 11,* 128–139.

Pulkinnen, L. (1983). Youthful smoking and drinking in a longitudinal perspective. *Journal of Youth and Adolescence, 12,* 253–283.

Reiss, A. J., & Roth, J. A. (1993). *Understanding and preventing violence.* Washington, DC: National Academy Press.

Robbins, B. J., & Brotherton, P. L. Mood change with alcohol intoxication. *British Journal of Social & Clinical Psychology.* Vol 19(2), Jun 1980, 149–155.

Robins, L. (1966). *Deviant children grown up: A sociological and psychiatric study of sociopathic personality.* Baltimore: Williams & Wilkins.

Robins, L. N., & Regier, D. A. (Eds.). (1991). *Psychiatric disorders in America: The epidemiologic catchment area study.* New York: Free Press.

Roizen, J. (1982). Estimating alcohol involvement in serious events. In *Alcohol consumption and related problems* (Alcohol and Health Monograph No. 1, pp. 179–222). Washington, DC: U.S. Government Printing Office.

Roizen, J. (1983). Loosening up: General population views of the effects of alcohol. In R. Room & G. Collins (Eds), *Drinking and disinhibition: Nature and meaning of the link* (DHHS Publication No. (ADM) 83–1246; NIAAA Research Monograph No. 12, pp. 236–257).Washington, DC: U.S. Government Printing Office.

Roizen, J. (1993). *Alcohol, causalties and crime: The epidemiology of serious events.* Berkeley, CA: Alcohol Research Group.

Roizen, J., & Schneberk, D. (1977). Alcohol and crime. In M. Aarens, T. Cameron, J. Roizen, R. Roizen, R. Room, D. Schneberk, & D. Wingard (Eds.), *Alcohol, casualties and crime* (Alcohol, casualties and crime project final report, No. C-18, pp. 289–421). Berkeley: University of California, Social Research Group.

Salzman, C., Van Der Kolk, B. A., & Shader, R. I. (1976). Marijuana and hostility in a small-group setting. *American Journal of Psychiatry, 133,* 1029–1033.

Sayette, M., Wilson, G. T., & Elias, M. J. (1993). Alcohol and aggression: A social information processing analysis. *Journal of Studies on Alcohol, 54*(4), 399–407.

Shuntich, R. J., & Taylor, S. P. (1972). The effects of alcohol on human physical aggression. *Journal of Experimental Research in Personality, 6,* 34–38.

Stark, E., & Flitcraft, A. (1988). Violence among inmates: An epidemiological review. In V. B. Van Hasselt, R. L. Morrison, A. S. Bellack, & M. Hersen (Eds), *Handbook of Family Violence* (pp. 293–318). New York: Plenum.

Steele, C. M., & Josephs, R. A. (1990). Alcohol myopia: Its prized and dangerous effects. *American Psychologist, 45,* 921–933.

Straus, M. A., & Gelles, R. J. (1990). *Physical violence in American families. Risk factors and adaptions to violence in 8,145 families.* New Brunswick, NJ: Transaction.

Straus, M. A., Gelles, R. J., & Steinmetz, S. K. (1980). *Behind closed doors: Violence in the American family.* New York: Doubleday/Anchor.

Swanson, J. W. (1993). Alcohol abuse, mental disorder, and violent behavior: An epidemiologic inquiry. *Alcohol Health and Research World, 17*(2), 123–132.

Swanson, J. W. (1994). Mental disorder, substance abuse, and community violence. In J. Monahan. and H. Steadman (Eds.), *Violence and mental disorder: Developments in risk assessment* (pp. 101–136). Chicago: University of Chicago Press.

Taylor, S. (1993). Experimental investigation of alcohol-induced aggression in humans. *Alcohol Health and Research World, 17*(2), 108–112.

Taylor, S. P., & Chermack, S. T. (1993). Alcohol, drugs and human physical aggression. *Journal of Studies on Alcohol* (Suppl. 11), 78–88.

Taylor, S. P., & Gammon, C. B. (1975). Effects of type and dose of alcohol on human physical aggression. *Journal of Personality and Social Psychology, 32*(1), 169–175.

Taylor, S. P., & Leonard, K. E. (1983). Alcohol and human physical aggression. In R. G. Geen and E. I. Donnerstein (Eds.), *Aggression: Theoretical and empirical reviews: Vol. 2. Issues in research* (pp. 77–101). New York: Academic Press.

Taylor, S. P., & Sears, J. D. (1988). The effects of alcohol and persuasive social pressure on human physical aggression. *Aggressive Behavior, 14,* 237–243.

Taylor, S. P., Gammon, C. B., & Capasso, D. R. (1976). Aggression as a function of alcohol and threat. *Journal of Personality and Social Psychology, 34,* 938–941.

Taylor, S. P., Vardaris, R. M., Rawitch, A. B., Gammon, C. B., Cranston, J. W., & Lubetkin, A. I. (1976). The effects of alcohol and delta-9 tetrahydrocannabinol on human physical aggression. *Aggressive Behavior, 2,* 153–161.

Taylor, S. P., Schmuttte, G. T., Leonard, K. E., & Cranston, J. W. (1979). The effects of alcohol and extreme provocation on the use of a highly noxious electric shock. *Motivation and Emotion, 3,* 73–81.

Testa, M., & Parks, K. (1996). The role of woman's alcohol consumption in sexual victimization. *Aggression and Violent Behavior, 1,* 217–234.

U.S. Bureau of the Census (1992). *Statistical abstract of the United States: 1992* (112th ed.). Washington, DC: U.S. Government Printing Office.

U.S. Department of Health and Human Services. (1995). *National Household Survey on Drug Abuse: Main findings 1993* (DHSS Publication No. SMA 95-3020). Rockville, MD: Author.

U.S. Department of Justice. (1993). *Survey of state prison inmates, 1991* (Publication No. NCJ-136949). Washington, DC: U.S. Government Printing Office, Bureau of Justice Statistics.

U.S. Department of Justice. (1994). *Criminal victimization in the United States, 1992* (Publication No. NCJ-145125). Washington DC: U.S. Government Printing Office, Bureau of Justice Statistics.

U.S. Department of Justice. (1996). *1995 drug use forecasting annual report on adult and juvenile arrestees* (Publication No. NCJ-161721). Washington, DC: U.S. Government Printing Office, National Institute of Justice.

Webster, C. D., Harris, G. T., Rice, M. E., Cormier, C., & Quinsey, V. L. (1994). *The violence prediction scheme: Assessing dangerousness in high risk men.* Toronto, Ontario, Canada: University of Toronto, Centre of Criminology.

Welte, J. W. & Miller, B. A. (1987). Alcohol use by violent and property offenders. *Drug and Alcohol Dependence, 19,* 313–324.

Widiger, T. A., & Trull, T. J. (1994). Personality disorders and violence. In J. Monahan and H. Steadman (Eds.), *Violence and mental disorder: Developments in risk assessment* (pp. 203–226). Chicago: University of Chicago Press.

Wilkinson, C. J. (1985). Effects of diazepam (valium) and trait anxiety on human physical aggression and emotional state. *Journal of Behavioral Medicine, 8,* 101–114.

Winslow, J. T., & Miczek, K. A. (1985). Social status as determinant of alcohol effects on aggressive behavior in squirrel monkeys (Saimiri sciureus). *Psychopharmacology, 85,* 167–172.

Wish, E. D., & Johnson, B. D. (1986). The impact of substance abuse on criminal careers. In A. Blumstein, J. Cohen, J. A. Roth, & C. A. Visher (Eds.), *Criminal careers and career criminals* (Vol. 2, pp. 52–88). Washington, DC: National Academy Press.

Wright, K. N. (1993). Alcohol use by prisoners. *Alcohol Health and Research World, 17*(2), 157–161.

Index

ISBN 0-306-45845-4

90000